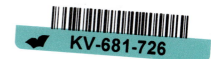
1995
YEAR BOOK OF
SPORTS MEDICINE®

Statement of Purpose

The YEAR BOOK Service

The YEAR BOOK series was devised in 1901 by practicing health professionals who observed that the literature of medicine and related disciplines had become so voluminous that no one individual could read and place in perspective every potential advance in a major specialty. In the final decade of the 20th century, this recognition is more acutely true than it was in 1901.

More than merely a series of books, YEAR BOOK volumes are the tangible results of a unique service designed to accomplish the following:

- to *survey* a wide range of journals of proven value
- to *select* from those journals papers representing significant advances and statements of important clinical principles
- to provide *abstracts* of those articles that are readable, convenient summaries of their key points
- to provide *commentary* about those articles to place them in perspective

These publications grow out of a unique process that calls on the talents of outstanding authorities in clinical and fundamental disciplines, trained literature specialists, and professional writers, all supported by the resources of Mosby, the world's preeminent publisher for the health professions.

The Literature Base

Mosby subscribes to nearly 1,000 journals published worldwide, covering the full range of the health professions. On an annual basis, the publisher examines usage patterns and polls its expert authorities to add new journals to the literature base and to delete journals that are no longer useful as potential YEAR BOOK sources.

The Literature Survey

The publisher's team of literature specialists, all of whom are trained and experienced health professionals, examines every original, peer-reviewed article in each journal issue. More than 250,000 articles per year are scanned systematically, including title, text, illustrations, tables, and references. Each scan is compared, article by article, to the search strategies that the publisher has developed in consultation with the 270 outside experts who form the pool of YEAR BOOK editors. A given article may be reviewed by any number of editors, from one to a dozen or more, regardless of the discipline for which the paper was originally published. In turn, each editor who receives the article reviews it to determine whether or not the article should be included in the YEAR BOOK. This decision is based on the article's inherent quality, its probable usefulness to readers of that YEAR BOOK, and the editor's goal to represent a balanced picture of a given field in each volume of the YEAR BOOK. In addition, the editor indicates when to include figures and tables from the article to help the YEAR BOOK reader better understand the information.

Of the quarter million articles scanned each year, only 5% are selected for detailed analysis within the YEAR BOOK series, thereby assuring readers of the high value of every selection.

The Abstract

The publisher's abstracting staff is headed by a physician-writer and includes individuals with training in the life sciences, medicine, and other areas, plus extensive experience in writing for the health professions and related industries. Each selected article is assigned to a specific writer on this abstracting staff. The abstracter, guided in many cases by notations supplied by the expert editor, writes a structured, condensed summary designed so that the reader can rapidly acquire the essential information contained in the article.

The Commentary

The YEAR BOOK editorial boards, sometimes assisted by guest commentators, write comments that place each article in perspective for the reader. This provides the reader with the equivalent of a personal consultation with a leading international authority—an opportunity to better understand the value of the article and to benefit from the authority's thought processes in assessing the article.

Additional Editorial Features

The editorial boards of each YEAR BOOK organize the abstracts and comments to provide a logical and satisfying sequence of information. To enhance the organization, editors also provide introductions to sections or individual chapters, comments linking a number of abstracts, citations to additional literature, and other features.

The published YEAR BOOK contains enhanced bibliographic citations for each selected article, including extended listings of multiple authors and identification of author affiliations. Each YEAR BOOK contains a Table of Contents specific to that year's volume. From year to year, the Table of Contents for a given YEAR BOOK will vary depending on developments within the field.

Every YEAR BOOK contains a list of the journals from which papers have been selected. This list represents a subset of the nearly 1,000 journals surveyed by the publisher and occasionally reflects a particularly pertinent article from a journal that is not surveyed on a routine basis.

Finally, each volume contains a comprehensive subject index and an index to authors of each selected paper.

The 1995 Year Book Series

Year Book of Allergy, Asthma, and Clinical Immunology: Drs. Rosenwasser, Borish, Gelfand, Leung, Nelson, and Szefler

Year Book of Anesthesiology and Pain Management: Drs. Tinker, Abram, Chestnut, Roizen, Rothenberg, and Wood

Year Book of Cardiology®: Drs. Schlant, Collins, Engle, Gersh, Kaplan, and Waldo

Year Book of Chiropractic®: Dr. Lawrence

Year Book of Critical Care Medicine®: Drs. Parrillo, Balk, Calvin, Franklin, and Shapiro

Year Book of Dentistry®: Drs. Meskin, Berry, Currier, Kennedy, Leinfelder, Roser, and Zakariasen

Year Book of Dermatologic Surgery®: Drs. Swanson, Glogau, and Salasche

Year Book of Dermatology®: Drs. Sober and Fitzpatrick

Year Book of Diagnostic Radiology®: Drs. Federle, Clark, Gross, Latchaw, Madewell, Maynard, and Young

Year Book of Digestive Diseases®: Drs. Greenberger and Moody

Year Book of Drug Therapy®: Drs. Lasagna and Weintraub

Year Book of Emergency Medicine®: Drs. Wagner, Dronen, Davidson, King, Niemann, and Roberts

Year Book of Endocrinology®: Drs. Bagdade, Braverman, Horton, Kannan, Landsberg, Molitch, Morley, Nathan, Odell, Poehlman, Rogol, and Ryan

Year Book of Family Practice®: Drs. Berg, Bowman, Davidson, Dexter, Dietrich, and Scherger

Year Book of Geriatrics and Gerontology®: Drs. Beck, Burton, Goldstein, Reuben, Small, and Whitehouse

Year Book of Hand Surgery®: Drs. Amadio and Hentz

Year Book of Hematology®: Drs. Spivak, Bell, Ness, Quesenberry, Wiernik, and Blume

Year Book of Infectious Diseases®: Drs. Keusch, Barza, Bennish, Gelfand, Klempner, Snydman, and Skolnik

Year Book of Infertility and Reproductive Endocrinology: Drs. Mishell, Lobo, and Sokol

Year Book of Medicine®: Drs. Bone, Cline, Epstein, Greenberger, Malawista, Mandell, O'Rourke, and Utiger

Year Book of Neonatal and Perinatal Medicine®: Drs. Fanaroff and Klaus

Year Book of Nephrology®: Drs. Coe, Favus, Henderson, Kashgarian, Luke, and Curtis

Year Book of Neurology and Neurosurgery®: Drs. Bradley and Wilkins

Year Book of Neuroradiology: Drs. Osborn, Eskridge, Grossman, Hudgins, and Ross

Year Book of Nuclear Medicine®: Drs. Gottschalk, Blaufox, McAfee, Wackers, and Zubal

Year Book of Obstetrics and Gynecology®: Drs. Mishell, Kirschbaum, and Morrow

Year Book of Occupational and Environmental Medicine: Drs. Emmett, Frank, Gochfeld, and Hessl

Year Book of Oncology®: Drs. Simone, Bosl, Glatstein, Ozols, and Steele

Year Book of Ophthalmology®: Drs. Cohen, Adams, Augsburger, Benson, Eagle, Flanagan, Grossman, Laibson, Nelson, Rapuano, Reinecke, Sergott, Tasman, Tipperman, and Wilson

Year Book of Orthopedics®: Drs. Sledge, Cofield, Dobyns, Griffin, Poss, Springfield, Swiontkowski, Wiesel, and Wilson

Year Book of Otolaryngology-Head and Neck Surgery®: Drs. Paparella and Holt

Year Book of Pain: Drs. Gebhart, Haddox, Jacox, Janjan, Marcus, Rudy, and Shapiro

Year Book of Pathology and Laboratory Medicine: Drs. Mills, Bruns, Gaffey, and Stoler

Year Book of Pediatrics®: Dr. Stockman

Year Book of Plastic, Reconstructive, and Aesthetic Surgery: Drs. Miller, Cohen, McKinney, Robson, Ruberg, and Whitaker

Year Book of Podiatric Medicine and Surgery®: Dr. Kominsky

Year Book of Psychiatry and Applied Mental Health®: Drs. Talbott, Breier, Frances, Meltzer, Schowalter, Tasman, and Yudofsky

Year Book of Pulmonary Disease®: Drs. Bone and Petty

Year Book of Rheumatology: Drs. Sergent, LeRoy, Meenan, Panush, and Reichlin

Year Book of Sports Medicine®: Drs. Shephard, Drinkwater, Eichner, Torg, Col. Anderson, and Mr. George

Year Book of Surgery®: Drs. Copeland, Bland, Deitch, Eberlein, Howard, Luce, Seeger, Souba, and Sugarbaker

Year Book of Thoracic and Cardiovascular Surgery®: Drs. Ginsberg, Lofland, and Wechsler

Year Book of Transplantation®: Drs. Sollinger, Eckhoff, Hullett, Knechtle, Longo, Mentzer, and Pirsch

Year Book of Ultrasound®: Drs. Merritt, Babcock, Carroll, Fagan, Finberg, and Fleischer

Year Book of Urology®: Drs. DeKernion and Howards

Year Book of Vascular Surgery®: Dr. Porter

1995

The Year Book of SPORTS MEDICINE®

Editor-in-Chief

Roy J. Shephard, M.D., Ph.D., D.P.E.
School of Physical and Health Education and Professor Emeritus of Applied Physiology, Department of Preventive Medicine and Biostatistics, University of Toronto; and CTAL Resident Scholar in Health Studies, Brock University, St. Catherine, Ontario

Editors

Col. James L. Anderson, PE.D.
Director of Physical Education, United States Military Academy, West Point

Barbara L. Drinkwater, Ph.D.
Research Physiologist, Department of Medicine, Pacific Medical Center, Seattle

Edward R. Eichner, M.D.
Professor of Medicine, University of Oklahoma Health Sciences Center, Oklahoma City

Francis J. George, A.T.C., P.T.
Head Athletic Trainer, Brown University, Providence

Joseph S. Torg, M.D.
Professor of Orthopaedic Surgery, and Director, Sports Medicine Center, Hahnemann University, Philadelphia

American College of Sports Medicine Liaison Representative

Kent B. Pandolf, Ph.D.
Director, Environmental Physiology and Medicine Directorate, U.S. Army Research Institute of Environmental Medicine, Natick, Massachusetts

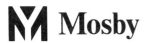 Mosby

St. Louis Baltimore Boston Carlsbad Chicago Naples New York Philadelphia Portland
London Madrid Mexico City Singapore Sydney Tokyo Toronto Wiesbaden

Vice President and Publisher, Continuity Publishing: Kenneth H. Killion
Director, Editorial Development: Gretchen C. Murphy
Acquisitions Editor: Linda Steiner
Illustrations and Permissions Coordinator: Steven J. Ramay
Manager, Continuity–EDP: Maria Nevinger
Project Supervisor, Editing: Rebecca Nordbrock
Assistant Project Supervisor, Production: Laura Higgins
Freelance Staff Supervisor: Barbara M. Kelly
Director Editorial Services: Edith M. Podrazik, R.N.
Senior Information Specialist: Terri Santo, R.N.
Senior Medical Writer: David A. Cramer, M.D.
Vice President, Professional Sales and Marketing: George M. Parker
Senior Marketing Manager: Eileen M. Lynch
Marketing Specialist: Lynn D. Stevenson

1995 EDITION
Copyright © December 1995 by Mosby-Year Book, Inc.

Printed in the United States of America
Composition by Reed Technology and Information Services, Inc.
Printing/binding by Maple-Vail

Mosby-Year Book, Inc.
11830 Westline Industrial Drive
St. Louis, MO 63146

Editorial Office:
Mosby-Year Book, Inc.
200 North LaSalle Street
Chicago, IL 60601
International Standard Serial Number: 0162-0908
International Standard Book Number: 0-8151-7705-4

Table of Contents

Mosby Document Express

Copies of the full text of the original source documents of articles abstracted or referenced in this publication are available by calling Mosby Document Express, toll-free, at **1 (800) 55-MOSBY.**

With Mosby Document Express, you have convenient, 24-hour-a-day access to literally every article on which this publication is based. In fact, through Mosby Document Express, virtually any medical or scientific article can be located and delivered by FAX, overnight delivery service, international airmail, electronic transmission of bitmapped images (via Internet), or regular mail. The average cost of a complete, delivered copy of an article, including up to $4 in copyright clearance charges and first-class mail delivery, is $12.

For inquiries and pricing information, please call the toll-free number shown above. To expedite your order for material appearing in this publication, please be prepared with the code shown next to the bibliographic citation for each abstract.

Journals Represented

Mosby subscribes to and surveys nearly 1,000 U.S. and foreign medical and allied health journals. From these journals, the Editors select the articles to be abstracted. Journals represented in this YEAR BOOK are listed below.

Acta Orthopaedica Scandinavica
Acta Radiologica
Allergy
American Heart Journal
American Journal of Cardiology
American Journal of Clinical Nutrition
American Journal of Epidemiology
American Journal of Hypertension
American Journal of Knee Surgery
American Journal of Perinatology
American Journal of Physiology
American Journal of Preventive Medicine
American Journal of Respiratory and Critical Care Medicine
American Journal of Roentgenology
American Journal of Sports Medicine
Annals of Allergy
Annals of Epidemiology
Annals of Internal Medicine
Archives of Pediatrics and Adolescent Medicine
Archives of Physical Medicine and Rehabilitation
Arthroscopy
Australian Journal of Science and Medicine in Sport
British Heart Journal
British Journal of Ophthalmology
British Journal of Sports Medicine
British Journal of Urology
British Medical Journal
Calcified Tissue International
Canadian Journal of Applied Physiology
Canadian Medical Association Journal
Chest
Chiropractic Technique
Circulation
Clinical Biomechanics
Clinical Chemistry
Clinical Orthopaedics and Related Research
Clinical Science
Clinical Sports Medicine
Diabetes
Digestive Diseases and Sciences
Ergonomics
European Heart Journal
European Journal of Applied Physiology and Occupational Physiology
European Journal of Nuclear Medicine
European Respiratory Journal
Foot & Ankle International
Foot and Ankle
International Journal of Obesity
International Journal of Sport Nutrition
International Journal of Sports Medicine

Journal of Adolescent Health
Journal of Applied Physiology: Respiratory, Environmental and Exercise
Physiology
Journal of Arthroscopic and Related Surgery
Journal of Athletic Training
Journal of Biomechanics
Journal of Bone and Joint Surgery (American Volume)
Journal of Bone and Joint Surgery (British Volume)
Journal of Bone and Mineral Research
Journal of Cardiopulmonary Rehabilitation
Journal of Clinical Endocrinology and Metabolism
Journal of Computer Assisted Tomography
Journal of Emergency Medicine
Journal of Endocrinology
Journal of Gerontology
Journal of Hand Surgery (British)
Journal of Hypertension
Journal of Manipulative and Physiological Therapeutics
Journal of Orthopaedic Research
Journal of Orthopaedic Trauma
Journal of Orthopaedic and Sports Physical Therapy
Journal of Psychosocial Nursing and Mental Health Services
Journal of Sport & Exercise Psychology
Journal of Sports Medicine and Physical Fitness
Journal of Sports Sciences
Journal of Trauma
Journal of the American Academy of Orthopaedic Surgeons
Journal of the American Board of Family Practice
Journal of the American College of Cardiology
Journal of the American Medical Association
Journal of the National Cancer Institute
Mayo Clinic Proceedings
Medecine du Sport
Medical Journal of Australia
Medical Problems of Peforming Artists
Medicine and Science in Sports and Exercise
Metabolism
Movement Disorders
Neuropediatrics
Neuropsychologia
Neurosurgery
New England Journal of Medicine
Obstetrics and Gynecology
Orthopaedic Review
Orthopedics
Pediatrics
Physical Therapy
Physician and Sportsmedicine
Psychological Medicine
Radiology
Regional Anesthesia
Scandinavian Journal of Rheumatology
Science
Spine
Sports Medicine

Sports Medicine, Training, and Rehabilitation
Sports Training, Medicine, and Rehabilitation

Standard Abbreviations

The following terms are abbreviated in this edition: acquired immunodeficiency syndrome (AIDS), cardiopulmonary resuscitation (CPR), central nervous system (CNS), cerebrospinal fluid (CSF), computed tomography (CT), deoxyribonucleic acid (DNA), electrocardiography (ECG), health maintenance organization (HMO), human immunodeficiency virus (HIV), intensive care unit (ICU), intramuscular (IM), intravenous (IV), magnetic resonance (MR) imaging (MRI), and ribonucleic acid (RNA).

Note: The YEAR BOOK OF SPORTS MEDICINE is a literature survey service providing abstracts of articles published in the professional literature. Every effort is made to ensure the accuracy of the information presented in these pages. Neither the editors nor the publisher of the YEAR BOOK OF SPORTS MEDICINE can be responsible for errors in the original materials. The editors' comments are their own opinions. Mention of specific products within this publication does not constitute endorsement.

Introduction

As always, a major part of this volume is devoted to that staple diet of the sports physician—the prevention, diagnosis, and treatment of athletic injuries. The broad range of causation is highlighted by papers that range from a discussion of the contribution of poor diet to injuries to a group of papers on the optimal biomechanics of walking and running in both young adults and the elderly. Each year, injuries are discussed in relation to new adventure crazes. This year, 2 papers look at the intraocular complications of bungee jumping, and another examines the risks of asphyxia during snowboarding.

Some of the newer diagnostic techniques, e.g., radionuclide bone imaging, MRI, and stress radiography, continue to attract both attention and controversy. Interscalene brachial plexus block is again coming to the fore as anesthesia for shoulder surgery. Repetitive strain injury of the carpal tunnel, so common in video display terminal operators, is also attracting attention among wheelchair competitors. Displacement of the patella and methods of preventing it continue to preoccupy many authors. The 6 degrees of movement around the knee still perplex those who wish to examine the mechanics of this joint.

There remains a need for more long-term follow-up of surgical treatments, but studies that have followed patients prospectively over a number of years are showing that anterior cruciate ligament reconstruction does not necessarily give perfect results; risk factors for a poor operative outcome and optimization of insurance coverage are now being reviewed. Artificial substitute ligaments for the anterior cruciate ligament are becoming ever more popular, and electrical stimulation is now being recommended as therapy not only for weak muscles but also for long bones that fail to unite after fractures.

It is difficult to assign whole populations on a random basis between a lifetime of vigorous physical activity and a lifetime of inactivity, but increasingly sophisticated epidemiologic studies are uncovering the effects of such a lifestyle choice, as exemplified by 2 papers from Paffenbarger and his associates. Another elegant epidemiologic study suggests for the first time that vigorous exercise can have a protective effect against testicular cancer, probably by reducing the levels of testosterone.

In the promotion of physical activity, the emphasis seems to be moving away from complicated and regimented fitness programs; instead, people are being encouraged to incorporate physical activity into daily activities such as commuting. However, there are still some benefits from more structured programs; for example, there is a 20–25 mm Hg reduction of systolic and diastolic blood pressures during exercise that can be realized through a well-designed weight training program.

Methods of regulating the intensity of prescribed exercise continue to attract concern; papers in this volume compare walking and jogging and note that heart rate is more useful than the rating of perceived exertion. One intriguing study shows that the aerobic condition of an athlete can be maintained over a year of very light activity by the simple expedient of providing extra fluids and salt.

The optimal walking distance for testing the capacity of the elderly patient also continues to be debated. One paper discussed in this volume suggests that although a 6-minute test is well correlated with peak aerobic performance, gains in condition are better correlated with the distance covered in 12 minutes. Overtraining of the high-performance athlete continues to be a concern, and a number of new papers suggest that some form of the Profile of Mood States test is a useful way to detect athletes in whom a stress response is developing.

Distance runners will follow with interest both the report on at least a temporary impairment of semen quality in those running 104 km/wk and Dr. Eichner's advice on how to avoid the "trots." Physicians should also be careful to distinguish between this physiologic response and amebiasis. A paper on necrotizing fasciitis reminds us that this dangerous disease seems to be increasing in prevalence; moreover, it can affect athletes as well as the leader of Canada's Bloc Québecois! A training regimen for pregnant women is presented, and it is shown that responses (sometimes quite substantial) can be monitored in terms of changes in blood lactate accumulation.

Among interesting papers regarding the female athlete, questions are raised about the accuracy of standard prediction equations developed using data from male subjects and about injuries associated with the gender-specific differences of anatomy. New information is also offered on eating disorders, menstrual disturbances, and osteoporosis. Aging athletes will be encouraged by a report suggesting that their β-receptors can still enhance cardiac filling during exercise, thus enabling an increase of stroke volume that can compensate for a declining maximal heart rate. Training can also enhance the production of insulin-like growth factor-1; a decreased output of this peptide may be to blame for the decrease of lean tissue mass commonly observed in old age, although another paper challenges the view that administration of recombinant growth hormone can increase muscle mass over that which can be developed by resistance exercises. Finally, regular exercise seems to reduce the risks of gastrointestinal hemorrhage in the older patient.

Cardiac patients will be encouraged to learn that regular activity enhances the thrombolytic effect of an acute exercise bout. A controversial report from Finland recommends that patients with inflammatory arthritis should be encouraged to exercise, even in the early stages of the disease.

As our cities expand, and reliance on the automobile increases, anxiety about ozone levels also increases. A paper examines possible interactions between exercise-induced asthma and ozone exposure. Many athletes will continue to compete under hot conditions (including the athletes participating in the Olympics in Atlanta), and thus the report showing that the tendency to renal failure is exacerbated by indomethacin is particularly important. A proportion of divers will experience dangerous (and potentially fatal) incidents of decompression illness. Wilmshurst and associates suggest that in some of these individuals, small airway disease may play a role. For astronauts and athletes with paraplegia, it is encouraging to note that postural pooling can be minimized by arm exercise, with a single bout upregulating autonomic reflexes for as long as 24 hours.

Myocardial infarction, prostatic enlargement, obstruction of the urinary tract, severe liver damage, and acute renal failure can now seemingly be added to the complications of steroid injection. Doping experts still struggle to stay one move ahead of the athletes. A ketoconazole test seems to be a nice way to distinguish between individuals with a high testosterone/episterone ratio who are doping and those with a naturally high ratio. There are also efforts under way to lower the permissible standard of human gonadotropic hormone, now that methods of detection have become more precise.

Exercise immunology continues to make rapid strides. Increases in monocyte adhesion molecules for rhinoviruses may explain some of the protection that has been observed with moderate training programs. The neutrophil response to eccentric exercise seems less well-developed in older subjects. Concern about HIV infection is focusing attention on the more common problem of hepatitis B virus infection among athletic trainers; appropriate precautions include immunization and modification of CPR recommendations.

There are many more outstanding abstracts in this year's edition of the YEAR BOOK OF SPORTS MEDICINE, but these examples are enough to illustrate the rapid progress that the discipline is making. I am delighted that the timely efforts of the Year Book publishers and my colleagues on the editorial board continue to make available to us this important resource that allows us to keep abreast of the latest developments in sports medicine and the sports sciences.

Roy J. Shephard, M.D., Ph.D., D.P.E.

Metabolic Issues in Winter Sport

ROY J. SHEPHARD, M.D., PH.D., D.P.E.

School of Physical and Health Education and Professor Emeritus of Applied Physiology, Department of Preventive Medicine and Biostatistics, University of Toronto; and CTAL Resident Scholar in Health Studies, Brock University, St. Catherine, Ontario

Introduction

The influence of a cold environment on body metabolism is of interest to the sports physician for several reasons. Perhaps most importantly, an increase of metabolic rate helps to bring the body back into thermal equilibrium when the protection offered by clothing is insufficient to sustain the body temperature of an individual who is exercising under winter conditions. An understanding of the extent of such metabolic adjustments should help the physician to advise the winter athlete how to avoid the hazard of hypothermia and to recommend the amount of food that is needed when planning a prolonged winter expedition. Cold-induced depletion of body food reserves may also have practical significance in terms of the treatment of obesity and the planning of diets for those seeking high levels of performance in winter sports.

Metabolism and Thermal Equilibrium

The body often responds to cold by redistributing blood flow away from the skin, thus limiting body heat loss (1). However, here we will focus on compensatory increases of body heat production induced by a combination of exercising, shivering, and increases in resting metabolism.

EXERCISE

Exercise is performed with a low mechanical efficiency in any environment, and a large percentage (75% or more) of the energy content of the food that is consumed during physical exertion appears as heat (2). If the insulation provided by available clothing is insufficient to maintain body temperature at rest, it might thus seem a simple matter to warm the body by exercising.

Sometimes, the tactic is effective—indeed, when vigorous exercise is performed in the cold, it may be necessary to reduce the number of clothing layers so that the body does not become overheated and saturate the garments with sweat. However, if exercise is continued for several hours, it becomes difficult for the average person to sustain more than about 40% of peak aerobic effort. If the cold exposure is prolonged, the ability to exercise hard enough to maintain body temperature thus depends in part on the physical fitness of the individual. Reviewing incidents of clinical hypothermia during hill-walking contests in northern England, Pugh (3) noted that victims were the least fit contestants. Not only were such individuals less able to increase their heat production by hard exercise, they also covered the journey more slowly, thus being exposed to cold for a longer time.

Furthermore, if an individual attempts to generate the necessary additional heat by exercising harder, the rate of body cooling is controlled much less efficiently than might be expected. Vigorous movement of the limbs displaces the thin, insulating film of still air that normally surrounds the body. Unless the outer garments are closed very effectively at the wrists and ankles, body movement also pumps cold air underneath the clothing. Moreover, if the exercise is vigorous enough to cause sweating, clothing may become saturated with fluid to the point that it loses 50% to 60% of its initial insulation (3). If environmental conditions are such that a person is losing heat at a rate of 10 kJ/min while resting, it may be necessary to exercise at a rate of 70 kJ/min (7 METS) in order to compensate for this heat loss (4).

SHIVERING

Shivering is an involuntary tremor produced by the simultaneous contraction of the muscles initiating a body movement and by their antagonists. Paroxysms of shivering interfere with any skilled movement, degrading the skilled performance of an athlete and adding to the danger of many winter pursuits. However, if an individual cannot sustain a high enough intensity of deliberate exercise to compensate for environmental conditions (because of an injury, inadequate clothing, or a soaking of garments by sweat or rain), then voluntary activity must be supplemented by shivering to slow body cooling (3, 5).

When a person is resting, a 3–4°C decrease of mean body temperature typically induces a 2.5-fold increase of metabolism related to an increase of muscle tone and/or overt shivering (6, 7). Under very severe environmental conditions, the increase of metabolism may be as much as fivefold (8). For any given decrease of skin temperature, the increase of metabolic rate is greatest in thin individuals, the response showing an inverse relationship to the square root of body fat content (8). The neck, chest, and abdominal muscles show increased activity within a few minutes of cold exposure, and shivering later spreads to the limbs (9). During vigorous exercise, many of the limb muscles are already active, and the potential metabolic impact of shivering is thus smaller than when a person is sitting at rest. Nevertheless, the cumulative metabolic cost of a day of exercise in the cold can be much higher than that of performing an equivalent activity in a temperate climate. For instance, Hong et al. (10) set the energy expenditure of Korean pearl divers (who work in very cold water) at 4 MJ per shift. If the metabolic demands of shivering are augmented by vigorous exercise, then the ability to maintain body temperature is commonly limited by the delivery of food energy to the muscles rather than by circulatory or cellular factors (11).

INCREASES OF RESTING METABOLISM

If an individual has been repeatedly exposed to cold conditions, a given exposure can increase his resting metabolism in the absence of shivering. This response reflects the development of a cold-sensitive type of adipose tissue ("brown fat"), a stimulation of resting metabolism in other tissues (e.g., by the initiation of "futile" cyclic metabolic reactions), and changes in the mechanical efficiency of simple body movements.

Brown Fat

Brown adipose tissue (BAT) is a special type of adipose tissue that is able to generate large quantities of heat by uncoupling the normal linkage between the oxidation of food substrates and the synthesis of the local adenosine triphosphate (ATP) energy stores used in muscle contraction. Free fatty acids, liberated by the neurohormone, norepinephrine, activate an "uncoupling protein" in the mitochondrial membrane; this allows a rapid leakage of protons across the membrane, and energy is expended in countering the resulting proton flux.

Triiodothyronine, the active metabolite of thyroid gland secretions, seems to be needed for the fat cells to express the messenger RNA that stimulates synthesis of the uncoupling protein (12). It is thus important that prolonged cold exposure tends to increase the secretion of thyroid hormone (13) and leads to a several hundred-fold increase in activity of the enzyme thyroxine-5-deiodinase, which converts the thyroid hormone into its active metabolite, triiodothyronine.

Substantial amounts of BAT are found in small mammals, and in young children, about one quarter of total fat (some 50–100 g) is BAT. However, the continued existence of BAT in adults has been hotly debated (14–22). Because of its high rate of metabolism—up to 70 J/g/min, compared with 3 J/g/min in active muscle (22–24)—a small quantity of BAT (not readily detected microscopically in a larger mass of white fat) could have a large impact on an individual's overall metabolic rate. Thermography has demonstrated certain body regions (e.g., the subcutaneous tissue between the scapulae) where cold exposure leads to a local increase of blood flow, and Rothwell and Stock (17) have suggested that these regions contain activated BAT.

Norepinephrine is known to induce large increases in the blood flow to BAT (25); some authors have reported values as high as 360 mL/min per 100 g of tissue (26). Needle biopsies of "hot" subcutaneous fat have not identified any BAT (27), but recent studies using specific antisera and metabolic inhibitors such as guanosine diphosphate have categorically demonstrated the presence of uncoupling protein in adult human beings (24, 28). What is still uncertain is the quantity of such tissue and its importance to thermoregulation.

Brown adipose tissue uses fat preferentially, both for its own growth and for subsequent heat production (29). In the short term, fatty acids are obtained (22) from triglyceride stores within the BAT itself. In the longer term, energy is obtained from 3 dietary sources: plasma fat droplets (chylomicrons) and lipoproteins (norepinephrine increases the lipoprotein lipase content of BAT, allowing metabolism of the neutral fat); plasma free fatty acids; and plasma glucose (the BAT synthesizes fat from the glucose, a mechanism that is suppressed by a high-fat diet).

The BAT cells are directly innervated by sympathetic nerves, which release the neurohormone norepinephrine. Cold exposure induces growth of BAT, apparently via an action of norepinephrine on specific (β-3) receptors (30). The same sympathetic nerve system signal increases the metabolic activity of BAT (22). However, the administration of thyroxine reduces the cold response of BAT, probably because this hormone increases the resting metabolic rate before cold exposure (31). Cold exposure leads to a rapid increase in the expression of genes regulating the synthesis of uncoupling protein, lipoprotein lipase, and thyroxine-5-deiodinase, and membrane glucose transporters are either translocated or synthesized. Conditions are thus optimized for both growth and vigorous heat production in BAT. In contrast, exposure to a warm or temperate climate leads to an atrophy of BAT, with reversal of the various enzyme changes that favor heat production.

Brown adipose tissue seems to be involved not only in thermoregulation but also in matching metabolism to food intake (17, 32). There is a small increase of resting metabolic rate immediately after eating (the "obligatory" component of diet-induced thermogenesis, which is greater with a high-fat meal) and a longer-lasting "adaptive" component of diet-induced thermogenesis. The latter apparently allows a 10% to 15% compensation of daily energy expenditure for overeating by increasing the uncoupling of metabolism in BAT. Conversely, metabolic uncoupling is reduced to meet energy needs during dietary restriction, possibly through the regulatory action of the pituitary hormone, prolactin (33).

Futile Cycles

The energy stored in food reserves can be converted into heat in tissues other than BAT, possibly including muscle, liver, and white fat (26, 34, 35). The suggested mechanisms for the release of heat include "futile" metabolic cycles and metabolism in structures other than the mitochondria, such as the peroxisomes (26, 36).

Cold exposure induces a catecholamine-linked increase in the activity of the enzyme, adenylate cyclase (37), and this in turn leads to an energy-wasting (i.e., heat-liberating) breakdown and resynthesis of various substances, including neutral fat (38, 39), glycogen, and protein (40, 41). Other possible "futile" cycles involve hexose phosphates and cholesterol esters (42). For instance, cold induces a catecholamine-mediated conversion of glucose-6-phosphate to free glucose (43), and energy is subsequently spent in its rephosphorylation. Likewise, ATP is converted to cyclic adenosine monophosphate (AMP), with a later energy-consuming regeneration of ATP (44). Heat is also generated by an increased activity of the "pump" transferring sodium ions across cell membranes (45).

The secretion of thyroid hormone is increased slightly by some months of cold exposure (13). This impacts on nonshivering thermogenesis, as discussed above, and probably also leads to a more general increase of metabolism, either by a direct stimulation of "futile" cycling or by increasing the sensitivity of such cycling to norepinephrine (42). The overall hormonal effects of cold can augment the metabolic cost of sleeping by up to 10% (46), and the total 24-hour energy expenditure is increased by at least 6% (47), so that the cumulative added energy cost of life in a cold environment is often about 3.0 MJ/wk.

Studies of Korean diving women (ama) with and without protection against cold water have given an interesting confirmation that repeated cold exposure induces some or all of these various tactics for heat generation. Since the divers have taken to wearing insulated wet suits, there has been a dramatic drop in the energy demands of their work, and they no longer show an increase of resting metabolism during the winter months (10).

Mechanical Efficiency of Effort

Cold exposure (48) and cold-induced dehydration (49) both reduce the mechanical efficiency of muscular contraction, thus increasing the total energy cost of many simple physical tasks and causing a larger fraction of this energy to appear as heat. Vascular dilatation may occur more slowly if the limbs are cold, and the resulting early accumulation of lactate further increases the steady oxygen cost of exercise (50).

Nevertheless, the overall energy cost of physical activity in the cold often shows only a small increase relative to temperate conditions (51). More energy is required to walk over ice or snow than to move on dry ground. Heavy boots and the hobbling effect of clothing further increase metabolic demand during outdoor winter activities, but these effects are at least partially offset by a decrease of local temperature and thus of metabolic rate in the inactive regions of the body. According to the "Law" of Arrhenius, resting metabolism is approximately halved for every 10°C decrease in local tissue temperature (although because of countervailing sympathetic stimulation, BAT is an important exception to this rule).

Fuel Needs During Acute Cold Exposure

If the energy needed to maintain body temperature were derived entirely from carbohydrate, as assumed by Wissler (52), then acute cold exposure would quickly deplete body glycogen stores. Certainly, carbohydrates provide the main fuel when exercising in the cold. A single bout of cold exposure thus improves glucose tolerance (53), but it has little effect on tolerance to a test dose of fat (7). On average, a 3–4°C decrease of mean body temperature causes a 588% increase of carbohydrate oxidation and a 63% increase of fat oxidation, but it causes no change in the rate of protein metabolism (6). The increased oxidation of fat persists if subjects are given nicotinic acid, which prevents the liberation of free fatty acids from white fat depots. This suggests that both the shivering muscles and BAT metabolize alternative sources of fat, including droplets of neutral triglycerides stored in muscle and triglycerides in the plasma (7, 54).

When an individual is exercising, cold exposure that is sufficient to induce some shivering speeds the rate of muscle glycogen depletion relative to the performance of an equivalent amount of exercise in a temperate environment (55, 56). Faster glycogen depletion is particularly marked in thin subjects (57). Cold stress also increases the turnover of free fatty acids (58), and the breakdown of neutral fat is shown by increments of plasma glycerol (7, 56, 57). If a second cold exposure occurs within 24 hours of the first, the rate of fat utilization is further increased (7), probably because the previously depleted muscle glycogen reserves have not yet been fully replenished.

The catecholamines secreted in response to both cold exposure (59) and vigorous exercise (epinephrine and norepinephrine) stimulate the breakdown of glycogen to glucose (60) and of depot fat to free fatty acids and glycerol. If tissue reserves are initially well stocked, both glucose and fatty acids contribute to the maintenance of core temperature (56, 57). However, an increased metabolism of fatty acids apparently can compensate for any shortage of glucose or vice-versa (61, 62). Thus, the acute response to body cooling is unchanged over a wide range of initial intramuscular glycogen reserves, from 144 to 543 mmol/kg (57). In individuals with poor peripheral circulation, insulin is less readily available to the muscles, limiting their rate of glucose uptake and encouraging the metabolism of fat. Very low levels of plasma glucose (less than 2.5 mmol/L) increase the rate of body cooling (63, 64), but this seems to be a result of an impairment of the brain mechanisms that regulate shivering rather than of a lack of fuel for the muscles or BAT.

Glucose is essential for both cerebral metabolism and anaerobic muscle contractions. The relative proportions of carbohydrate and fat that are metabolized can have important implications for both physical performance and survival in the cold (52, 61, 62, 65, 66). At low levels of blood glucose, thinking becomes impaired, creating major problems for the cold weather athlete.

Prolonged Cold Exposure and Depletion of Body Fat

Animal experiments (67, 68) and human observations (69, 70) both suggest that prolonged exposure to a cold environment enhances the breakdown of depot fat that would normally be induced by exercise. However, with the exception of one laboratory experiment discussed below, the human studies have been uncontrolled, causing uncertainty regarding the relative contributions of exercise and cold exposure to the observed fat loss.

O'Hara et al. (71) noted a progressive loss of subcutaneous fat when male recruits undertook strenuous 2- to 3-week military field expeditions in the Arctic. Others have reported similar findings during circumpolar expeditions (49, 72–74). Likewise, the body mass of the traditional Korean pearl diver decreases by some 5 kg during the diving season (75), mainly as a result of a depletion of subcutaneous fat stores (76). In a recent 3-month transpolar ski trek (77), the thinner participants actually gained both body mass and fat, but a progressive fat loss was seen in the more obese team members.

Canadian Experiments on Moderate Activity in the Cold

Each of the soldiers studied by O'Hara et al. (71) traversed 70 km of Arctic tundra, carrying a 30-kg pack, and shared with 4 others the responsibility of dragging a heavy (180-kg) sledge. The cumulative energy consumption of 13–16 MJ per person per day was more than satisfied by survival rations. Nevertheless, project participants experienced a cumulative fat loss of about 4.2 kg. This was partly masked by the synthesis of a similar mass of lean tissue. The fat loss was more marked in obese than in lean personnel. Similar changes in skinfold readings and hydrostatic estimates of body fat (2.6 and 4.8 kg) were observed when young men (78) and obese middle-aged adults (79) were exposed to comparable combinations of exercise and cold in a controlled climatic chamber.

As in earlier studies of prolonged cold exposure and vigorous exercise (69, 80–84), all project participants showed a marked urinary excretion of ketones. An increased proportion of total energy requirements was met from the metabolism of fat (85). Blood levels of free fatty acids were also increased, despite the fact that cold exposure increased the muscle uptake of fat for a given plasma concentration of free fatty acids. In some of the cold exposures, as much as 70% of daily energy requirements were met from the metabolism of ingested and depot fat (86). A controlled crossover experiment in the climatic chamber confirmed the specificity of the cold response, with an equivalent amount of exercise producing a much smaller fat loss when it was performed under temperate conditions (86). A similar picture of an increased overall rate of metabolism, increased plasma levels of free fatty acids, and the urinary excretion of ketones has been reported in traditional (thermally unprotected) Korean pearl divers. The mediator of these responses seems to be the cold-induced release of norepinephrine (13, 87).

In the experiments of O'Hara and associates, there was little cooling of the body as a whole. However, the mean skin temperature decreased by some 10°C. The fat loss was correlated ($r = 0.88$) with skin temperatures; those subjects who were better able to sustain their skin temperatures showed a larger cold-induced fat loss. Himms-Hagen (88) has also demonstrated that cutaneous thermoreceptors can stimulate fat mobilization.

O'Hara found that the inspiration of cold air was sometimes in itself a sufficient stimulus to precipitate the fat loss. Hartung et al. (89) found no metabolic reaction when air was inhaled at a temperature of $-35°C$, but their subjects did not develop a large enough respired volume to bypass the normal air-conditioning mechanisms of the nose. More recently, Stroud (90) found that facial cooling decreased the gas exchange ratio in exercising subjects, implying that such conditions increased fat utilization. Plainly, there is a need for further study of the fat breakdown caused by an intense local cold exposure of the face and/or respiratory tract, relative to the fat loss induced by more general body cooling (91).

Explanations of Fat Loss

In the uncontrolled experiments of O'Hara et al. (71, 78, 79), the combination of exercise and prolonged cold exposure apparently caused a negative energy balance of 3–15 MJ/wk, and a similar deficit was observed in a controlled laboratory study. Several factors could have contributed to the negative energy balance, particularly under field conditions. Although the field rations had an adequate energy content, they were not very palatable. Because a high proportion of daily energy needs were met by fat, the heat yield was some 10% less per liter of oxygen consumption than would have occurred had the subjects been metabolizing carbohydrate (42). Synthesis of up to 4 kg of lean tissue also increased energy use during the 2 weeks of observation. Heavy boots and hobbling of movement by heavy clothing augmented the energy cost of moving by about 16% relative to performance of the same tasks under temperate conditions (51, 92). Other possible effects included ketonuria, an increase of resting metabolism of the type noted by Dauncey (47), and a decreased mechanical efficiency of muscle contraction.

KETONURIA

Incomplete metabolism of fat to ketone bodies wastes energy. Observations of patients with diabetes (93) have set a likely ceiling of ketone excretion in urine, sweat, and expired air at 200 g/day. The corresponding loss of energy could be as large as 4 MJ/day. O'Hara et al. (71, 78, 79) found a much more modest urinary excretion of 1–2 g of ketone per day, but the available measuring technique did not detect the usually dominant species of ketone (β-hydroxybutyrate). Moreover, there may have been a short-term accumulation of ketones in blood, tissue water, and fat, plus substantial losses of ketones in expired air. Certainly, the severity of urinary ketosis was related to the extent of the cold-induced fat loss (71, 78).

CHANGES OF RESTING METABOLISM

The resting metabolism of O'Hara's subjects was probably augmented relative to assumed normal values because of long-term effects of exercise on metabolic rate (94, 95), interactions of exercise with a dietary-induced stimulation of metabolism (61, 96, 97), undetected shivering, effects of catecholamines on resting muscle tone (44), and other forms of nonshivering thermogenesis (47).

SEX DIFFERENCES IN RESPONSE

The fat loss was much smaller and less readily demonstrated in women than in men (98). In the studies of O'Hara et al. (86), the men had access to caffeine, which would have helped to maintain body temperatures by mobilizing fat from their adipose tissue depots (99–101). However, others have found that the overall metabolic response to cold is more vigorous in men than in women (102–105). Perhaps for this reason, male subjects maintain a higher skin temperature even though they generally have less subcutaneous fat than women do (104, 106).

It is currently speculated that fat is less readily mobilized in women than in men (107) because of the potential energy needs of pregnancy and lactation. Potential mechanisms include sex differences in the number or sensitivity of catecholamine receptors (108) or prolactin secretion (33). The thermoregulatory areas of the hypothalamus also show sex-related structural differences (109).

Cold as a Potential Treatment of Obesity

Could prolonged cold exposure be used in the treatment of obesity? Some have argued that unless a person shivers, the energy cost of exercise is similar in cold and warm environments (3, 57, 110). Nevertheless, as discussed above, there are many other reasons prolonged cold exposure could increase energy usage. Moreover, the mere fact of feeling cold may provide the motivation for vigorous exercise, which the obese individual frequently lacks in a temperate climate.

Repeated cold exposure diminishes some components of the human sympathetic nerve response to cold, such as cutaneous vasoconstriction (16). However, there is also an increase in the sensitivity of catecholamine receptors in the fat depots, and thus there is an enhanced breakdown of neutral fat in response to the catecholamines that are secreted during a combination of exercise and cold exposure (111).

Obese subjects show a number of peculiarities of metabolism. Feeding stimulates metabolism in an obese individual less than it does in a thinner person, and cold exposure or exercise causes less sympathetic nerve activation (112–115). However, animal experiments suggest that obesity also reduces the stimulation of appetite by cold exposure (116), perhaps in part because the obese individual is better insulated and thus experiences a lesser decrease of body temperature in a given cold environment.

In essence, exposure to a combination of cold and exercise induces the local sympathetic secretion of a therapeutically useful dose of fat-mobilizing catecholamines in the fat depots without imposing an excessive physical stress on a person who is relatively unfit. The physical training resulting from a winter exercise program may further augment the sensitivity of the β-adrenergic system in an obese individual (117).

During acute cold exposure, the obese exerciser might be expected to use a higher proportion of carbohydrates than would a fitter individual. A lesser reactivity of their sympathetic nerves would reduce their fat mobilization, and the activity of fat metabolizing enzymes in their skeletal muscles would also be low (118, 119). However, experimental studies have shown that fat individuals have low rates of carbohydrate use for a given cold exposure; cold-induced muscle glycogen use is inversely correlated with body fat content (58, 59). The probable reasons are that better-insulated fat subjects shiver less, and their low sensitivity to catecholamines reduces the uncoupling of carbohydrate metabolism from ATP synthesis as discussed above.

O'Hara's subjects were exposed to quite severe arctic conditions. However, they were also wearing heavy arctic protective clothing, so that the personal microclimate was comparable to that which would be encountered by a more lightly clothed person who undertook winter sports such as cross-country skiing. Moreover, the total amount of exercise (an energy expenditure of 3–5 MJ/day) was comparable to what would be undertaken during a vigorous winter holiday. O'Hara placed no formal restrictions on food intake, but his subjects did have a limited menu. Vigorous exercise can lead to an immediate suppression of appetite (120). Nevertheless, success in reducing body fat stores would be less likely if a ski resort's gourmet menu were to replace the survival rations that were available to O'Hara's subjects. It is also disquieting that the response was less marked in women, because many of those who wish to lose body fat are women.

If cold exposure is to receive serious consideration as a treatment for obesity, it will finally be necessary to consider possible adverse effects of cold, including the risks of provoking systemic hypertension, angina, bronchospasm, and pulmonary hypertension.

Implications for the Winter Athlete

Both the acute metabolic reactions to cold and long-term adaptive reactions have some potential significance for the performance of the winter athlete. Prolonged cold exposure is likely to induce glycogen depletion in the slow-twitch muscle fibers of an endurance performer (58). Each gram of glycogen is linked to 3 g of water, so that a cold-induced glycogen depletion reduces not only the energy stores needed for anaerobic metabolism of the muscles (e.g., when climbing hills), but also body reserves of water. In some situations (e.g., mountain climbing), serious dehydration can develop.

A patient's blood glucose level may fall if a combination of exercise, shivering, and nonshivering thermogenesis imposes a large energy demand after intramuscular stores of glycogen have become depleted (58). The brain can only metabolize glucose, and if the blood glucose falls below a critical level, the judgment and skilled performance of the competitor will deteriorate. Frank hypoglycemia is unlikely in short- and medium-term athletic events, but it can occur during long-distance hill walks (3).

Carbohydrate metabolism and thus the physical performance of the muscles are adversely affected when muscle glycogen reserves drop below 175 mmol/L (121). Depending on the intensity of exercise and the athlete's psychological reactions, the output of catecholamines is increased during competition; this induces a mobilization of free fatty acids, compensating in part for the diminishing intramuscular stores of glycogen. More importantly, vigorous exercise causes a reduction of blood insulin (122), which facilitates the mobilization of fat (58).

Acclimation occurs with repeated exposure to cold conditions. Deliberate cold acclimation programs for the winter endurance competitor have commonly been considered in terms of their potential impact on aerobic fitness. However, there are also metabolic implications. As cold exposure is repeated, the normal adaptive mechanism is to reduce peripheral blood flow (an "insulative" type of reaction). This allows limb temperatures to fall (1, 10) but conserves the body's core temperature. Because of the insulative reaction, there is less need for shivering, and a well-acclimated individual uses less of the available glycogen stores in response to a given cold exposure. The slower depletion of glycogen reserves has a correspondingly favorable effect on endurance performance (123).

Endurance training further reduces the rate of glycogen depletion by increasing the activity of enzymes that metabolize fat in the working muscles (124). In such activities as hill walking, the larger maximal oxygen intake also allows the participant to exercise below the anaerobic threshold, at an intensity at which fat rather than carbohydrate can be metabolized. The metabolic response to sustained cold exposure can be further redirected toward fat metabolism by the provision of a fat-rich diet (125), and if the environment is very cold, such a diet carries the added bonus of an increase in obligatory dietary thermogenesis. Although glycogen loading of the muscles by a high-carbohydrate diet has a favorable impact on prolonged aerobic performance during a single cold exposure, repeated feeding of a high-carbohydrate diet is likely to increase the reliance on glycogen when exercising in the cold, with an adverse impact on both cold tolerance and endurance performance.

Summary

The cold encountered during outdoor winter activity has many effects on metabolism. Physical activity is often deliberately increased, and shivering and various other forms of nonshivering heat production all increase the rate of metabolism. During a single, short cold exposure, the main metabolic fuel is glycogen. However, repeated bouts of exercise in the cold lead to an increased metabolism of depot fat, with a reduction of obesity. Potential factors contributing to fat loss in the cold include the metabolic cost of synthesizing lean tissue; a wasting of energy through a cold-induced excretion of ketones; a stimulation of resting metabolism (probably as much through nonspecific mechanisms as through a hypertrophy of brown fat); increases in the energy cost of movement (walking over snow, the weight of heavy boots, hobbling by winter clothing, and a decreased mechanical efficiency of dehydrated muscles); and a lower yield of energy per liter of oxygen consumed (resulting from reliance on fat as the energy source).

Biochemical explanations of the cold-induced fat mobilization include an increased secretion of catecholamines, an increased sensitivity of peripheral catecholamine receptors, and decreased circulating insulin. The fat loss induced by combinations of cold and exercise may be helpful in the treatment of moderate obesity, although the response seems less well developed in women than in men. The glycogen depletion induced by shivering has a negative effect on the performance of the endurance competitor. However, there are several important techniques of preparation. Repeated exposure leads to cold acclimation; the body then shows an insulative response, conserving core temperature by a restriction of peripheral blood flow; in consequence, the rate of depletion of glycogen stores is reduced. Endurance training can further protect glycogen reserves by enhancing the activity of fat-metabolizing enzymes in the skeletal muscles, not only those involved in the exercise itself, but also those contributing to shivering.

Acknowledgment

Dr. Shephard's research is supported in part by a research grant from Canadian Tire Acceptance Limited.

References

1. Shephard RJ: Adaptation to exercise in the cold. *Sports Med* 2:59–71, 1985.
2. Shepard RJ: *Physiology and Biochemistry of Exercise.* New York, Praeger Publications, 1982.
3. Pugh LGCE: Accidental hypothermia among hillwalkers and climbers in Britain, in Cumming GR, Snidal D, Taylor AW (eds): *Environmental Effects on Work Performance.* Ottawa, Canadian Assoc Spt Sci, 1972, pp 41–56.
4. Burton A, Edholm OG: *Man in a Cold Environment.* New York, Hafner Press, 1969.
5. Nadel ER, Holmér I, Bergh U, et al: Energy exchanges of swimming man. *J Appl Physiol* 36:465–471, 1974.
6. Vallerand AL, Jacobs I: Rates of energy substrates utilization during cold exposure. *Eur J Appl Physiol* 58:873–878, 1989.
7. Vallerand AL, Jacobs I: Influence of cold exposure on plasma triglyceride clearance in humans. *Metabolism* 39:1211–1218, 1990.
8. Tikusis P, Bell DG, Jacobs I: Shivering onset, metabolic response, and convective heat transfer during cold air exposure. *J Appl Physiol* 70:1996–2002, 1991.
9. Spurr GB, Hutt BK, Horvath SM: Shivering, oxygen consumption and body temperatures in acute exposure of men to two different cold environments. *J Appl Physiol* 11:58–64, 1957.
10. Hong SK, Rennie DW, Park YS: Cold acclimatization and deacclimatization of Korean women divers. *Exerc Sports Sci Rev* 14:231–268, 1986.
11. Wang LCH, Man SFP, Belcastro AN: Metabolic and hormonal responses in theophylline-increased cold resistance in males. *J Appl Physiol* 63:589–596, 1987.
12. Silva JE, Bianco AC: Role of local thyroxine-5-deiodinase on the response of brown adipose tissue (BAT) to adrenergic stimulation, in Bray GA, Ricquier D, Spiegelman BM (eds): *Obesity; Towards a Molecular Approach.* In press, cited by Himms-Hagen (1990).
13. Itoh S: *Physiology of Cold Adapted Man.* Sapporo, Hokkaido University School of Medicine, 1974.
14. Keatinge WR: *Survival in Cold Water.* Oxford, Blackwell, 1969, pp 1–140.
15. Kang BS, Han DS, Paik KS, et al: Calorigenic action of norepinephrine in the Korean women divers. *J Appl Physiol* 29:6–9, 1970.
16. LeBlanc J: *Man in the Cold.* Springfield, Ill, CC Thomas, 1975.
17. Rothwell NJ, Stock MJ: A role for brown adipose tissue in diet-induced thermogenesis. *Nature* 281:31–35, 1979.

18. Budd GM, Brotherhood JR, Thomas DW, et al: Infusion of noradrenaline, in Fortuine R (ed). *Proceedings of the Sixth International Symposium on Circumpolar Health*. Seattle, University of Washington Press, 1985.
19. Huttunen P, Hirvonen J, Kinnula V: The occurrence of brown adipose tissue in outdoor workers. *Eur J Appl Physiol* 46:339–345, 1981.
20. Hervey GR, Tobin G: Luxuskonsumption, diet-induced thermogenesis and brown fat: A critical review. *Clin Sci* 64:7–18, 1983.
21. Nicholls DG, Locke RM: Thermogenic mechanisms in brown fat. *Physiol Rev* 64:1–64, 1984.
22. Himms-Hagen J: Brown adipose tissue thermogenesis: Interdisciplinary studies. *FASEB J* 4:2890–2898, 1990.
23. Bukowiecki L, Follea N, Vallières J, et al: Beta adrenergic receptors in brown adipose tissue: Characteristics and alterations during acclimation of rats to cold. *Eur J Biochem* 92:189–196, 1978.
24. Lean M: Brown adipose tissue in humans. *Proc Nutr Soc* 48:243–256, 1989.
25. Foster DO: Quantitative role of brown adipose tissue in thermogenesis, in Trayhurn P, Nicholls DG (eds): *Brown Adipose Tissue*. London, Arnold, 1986, pp 31–51.
26. Alexander G: Cold thermogenesis, in Robertshaw D (ed): *International Review of Physiology Volume 20. Environmental Physiology III*. Baltimore, University Park Press, 1979, pp 43-155.
27. Åstrup A, Bülow J, Madsea J, et al: Ephedrine-induced thermogenesis in man: No role for interscapular brown adipose tissue. *Clin Sci* 66:179–186, 1984.
28. Lean M, James PT: Brown adipose tissue in man, in Trayhurn P, Nicholls DG (eds): *Brown Adipose Tissue*. London, Arnold, 1986, pp 339–365.
29. Johnson TS, Murray S, Young JB, et al: Restricted food intake limits brown adipose tissue hypertrophy in cold exposure. *Life Sci* 30:17, 1982.
30. Arch JRC: The brown adipocyte beta adrenoceptor. *Proc Nutr Soc* 48:215–223, 1989.
31. Sundin U: The influence of thyroxine on brown fat thermogenesis, in Szelenyi Z, Szekely M (eds): *Advances in Physiological Sciences 32*. Oxford, Pergamon Press, 1980, pp 499–502.
32. Rothwell NJ, Stock MJ: Brown adipose tissue and diet-induced thermogenesis, in Trayhurn P, Nicholls DG (eds): *Brown Adipose Tissue*. London, Arnold, 1986, pp 269–298.
33. Prentice AM: Adaptations to long term low energy intake, in Pollitt E, Amante P (eds): *Energy Intake and Activity*. New York, Alan Liss, 1984, pp 3–31.
34. Newsholme EA, Crabtree B: Substrate cycles in metabolic regulation and in heat generation. *Biochem Soc Symp* 41:61–109, 1976.
35. Åstrup A, Bülow J, Madsen J, et al: Contribution of BAT and skeletal muscle to thermogenesis by ephedrine in man. *Am J Physiol* 248:E507–E514, 1985.
36. Alexson S, Nedergard J, Osmundsen H, et al: *Advances in Physiological Sciences 32*. Szelenyi Z, Szekely M (eds). Oxford, Pergamon Press, 1980, pp 483–485.
37. Masironi R, Depocas F: Effect of cold exposure on respiratory $c^{14}O_2$ production during infusion of albumin bound palmitate $1-C^{14}$ in white rats. *Can J Biochem Physiol* 39:219–224, 1961.
38. Theriault DG, Mellin DB: Cellularity of adipose tissue in cold-exposed rats and the calorigenic effect of norepinephrine. *Lipids* 6:486–491, 1971.
39. Itoh S, Kuroshima K: Lipid metabolism of cold adapted man, in Itoh S, Ogata K, Yoshimura H (eds): *Advances in Climatic Physiology*. Tokyo, Igaku Shoin, 1972, pp 260–277.
40. Yousef MK, Chaffee RRJ: Studies on protein turnover rates in cold-acclimated rats. *Proc Soc Exp Med* 133:801–804, 1970.
41. Goodenough RD, Royle GT, Nadel ER, et al: Leucine and urea metabolism in acute human cold exposure. *J Appl Physiol* 53:367–372, 1982.
42. Newsholme EA, Leech AR: *Biochemistry for the Medical Sciences*. London, Wiley, 1983.

43. Bray GA: The energetics of obesity. *Med Sci Sports Exerc* 15:32–40, 1983.
44. Webster AJF: Physiological effects of cold exposure, in Robertshaw D (ed). *Environmental Physiology*. Baltimore, University Park Press, 1974.
45. Guernsey DL, Stevens ED: The cell membrane sodium pump as a mechanism for increasing thermogenesis during cold acclimation in rats. *Science* 196:908–910, 1977.
46. Bray GA: The obese patient. *Major Probl Intern Med* 9:1–450, 1976.
47. Dauncey MF: Influence of mild cold on 24 hour energy expenditure, resting metabolism and diet-induced thermogenesis. *Br J Nutr* 45:257–267, 1981.
48. Blomstrand E, Essen-Gustavsson B: Influence of reduced muscle temperature on metabolism in type I and type II human muscle fibers during intensive exercise. *Acta Physiol Scand* 131:569–576, 1987.
49. Tappan DV, Jacey MJ, Heyder E: Blood volume responses in partially dehydrated subjects working in the cold. *Aviat Space Environ Med* 55:296–301, 1984.
50. Beelen A, Sargeant AJ: Effect of lowered muscle temperature on the physiological response to exercise in men. *Eur J Appl Physiol* 63:387–392, 1991.
51. Romet TT, Shephard RJ, Frim J: The metabolic cost of exercising in cold air. *Arctic Med Res* 44:29–36, 1986.
52. Wissler EH: Mathematical simulation of human thermal behavior using whole body models, in Shitzer A, Eberhart RC (eds): *Heat Transfer in Medicine and Biology*. New York, Plenum Press, 1985, pp 325–373.
53. Vallerand AL, Frim J, Kavanagh ML: Plasma glucose and insulin responses to oral and intravenous glucose in cold-exposed men. *J Appl Physiol* 65:2395–2399, 1988.
54. Theriault DG, Poe RH: The effect of acute and chronic cold exposure on tissue lipids in the rat. *Can J Biochem* 43:1427–1435, 1965.
55. Jacobs I, Romet T, Kerrigan-Brown D: Muscle glycogen depletion during exercise at 9°C and 21°C. *Eur J Appl Physiol* 46:47–53, 1985.
56. Martineau L, Jacobs I: Muscle glycogen utilization during shivering thermogenesis in humans. *J Appl Physiol* 65:2046–2050, 1988.
57. Young AJ, Sawka MN, Neufer PD, et al: Thermoregulation during cold water immersion is unimpaired by low muscle glycogen levels. *J Appl Physiol* 66:1809–1816, 1989.
58. Thompson GE: Physiological effects of cold exposure, in Robertshaw D (ed): *Environmental Physiology II*. Baltimore, Md, University Park Press, 1977, pp 29–69.
59. Young JB, Treadway JL, Balon TW, et al: Prior exercise potentiates the thermic effect of a carbohydrate load. *Metabolism* 35:1048–1053, 1986.
60. Himms-Hagen J: Sympathetic regulation of metabolism. *Pharmcol Rev* 19:367–461, 1967.
61. Martineau L, Jacobs I: Muscle glycogen availability and temperature regulation in humans. *J Appl Physiol* 66:72–78, 1989.
62. Martineau L, Jacobs I: Free fatty acid availability and temperature regulation in cold water. *J Appl Physiol* 67:2466–2472, 1989.
63. Haight JSL, Keatinge WR: Failure of thermoregulation induced by exercise and alcohol in man. *J Physiol* 229:87–97, 1973.
64. Gale EAM, Bennett T, Hilary Green J, et al: Hypoglycemia, hypothermia, and shivering in man. *Clin Sci* 61:463–469, 1981.
65. Parker GH, George JC: Glycogen utilization by the white fibres in the pigeon pectoralis as main energy process during shivering thermogenesis. *Comp Biochem Physiol A* 50:433–437, 1975.
66. LeBlanc J, LaBrie A: Glycogen and non-specific adaptations to cold. *J Appl Physiol* 51:1428–1432, 1981.
67. Grafnetter DJ, Grafnetterova J, Grossi E, et al: The effect of catecholamines and cold exposure on the lipolytic activity of rat heart. *Med Pharmacologica Experimentalia* 12:266–273, 1965.

68. Masoro EJ: Effect of cold on metabolic use of lipids. *Physiol Rev* 46:67–101, 1966.
69. Hanson PG, Johnson RE: Variations of plasma ketones and free fatty acids during acute cold exposure in man. *J Appl Physiol* 20:56–60, 1965.
70. Passmore R, Johnson RE: The modification of post-exercise ketosis (the Courtice-Douglas effect) by environmental temperature and water balance. *Q J Exp Physiol* 43:352–361, 1958.
71. O'Hara WJ, Allen C, Shephard RJ: Loss of body weight and fat during an arctic winter expedition. *Can J Physiol Pharmacol* 55:1235–1241, 1977.
72. Boyd JJ: Role of energy and fluid imbalance in weight changes found during field work in Antarctica. *Br J Nutr* 34:191–200, 1975.
73. Brotherhood JR, Budd GM, Reynard J, et al: Subjects, in Foruine R (ed): *Proceedings of the Sixth International Symposium on Circumpolar Health.* Seattle, University of Washington Press, 1985.
74. Campbell IT: Energy intakes on sledding expedition. *Br J Nutr* 45:89–94, 1981.
75. Yokoyama T, Iwasaki S: Ecology of the Japanese ama, in Yoshimura H, Kobayashi S (eds): *JIBS Synthesis. Human Adaptability, vol 3. Physiologica Adaptability and Nutritional Status of the Japanese. A. Thermal Adaptability of the Japanese and Physiology of the Ama.* Tokyo, Japan Committee for International Biological Programme, 1975, pp 199–209.
76. Yoshimura H: Lipid metabolism of the ama, in Shiraki K, Matsuoka S (eds): *Hyperbaric Medicine and Underwater Physiology.* Japan, Fukuoka Printing Co, 1983, pp 69–78.
77. Rode A, Shephard RJ: Observations on the Soviet/Canadian Transpolar Skitrek. Basel, S. Karger, 1991.
78. O'Hara WJ, Allen C, Shephard RJ: Loss of body weight and fat during exercise in a cold chamber. *Eur J Appl Physiol* 37:205–218, 1977.
79. O'Hara WJ, Allen C, Shephard RJ: Treatment of obesity by exercise in the cold. *Can Med Assoc J* 117:773–778, 1977.
80. Basu A, Passmore R, Strong JA: The effect of exercise on the level of non-esterified fatty acid in the blood. *Qu J Exp Physiol* 45:312–317, 1960.
81. Carlson LA, Pernow B: Studies on blood lipids during exercise: II. The arterial plasma free fatty acid concentration during and after exercise. *J Lab Clin Med* 58:673–681, 1961.
82. Lloyd RM: Ketonuria in the Antarctic: A detailed study. *Br Antarctic Surv Bull* 20:59–68, 1969.
83. Muir AL: Ketonuria in the Antarctic: A preliminary study. *Br Antarctic Surv Bull* 20:53–68, 1969.
84. St. Rose JEM, Allen CL, Myles WS, et al: *A Study of Energy Expenditure, Dehydration and Health in Canadian Troops During a Spring Exercise in the Sub-Arctic-Northern Ramble.* Toronto, Defence and Civil Institute of Environmental Medicine, 1972.
85. Murray SJ, Shephard RJ, Greaves S, et al: Effects of cold stress and exercise on fat loss in females. *Eur J Appl Physiol* 55:610–618, 1986.
86. O'Hara WJ, Allen C, Shephard RJ, et al: Fat loss in the cold: A controlled study. *J Appl Physiol* 46:872–877, 1979.
87. Hong SK: Pattern of cold adaptation in women divers of Korea (ama). *Fed Proc* 32:1614–1621, 1973.
88. Himms-Hagen J: Non-shivering thermogenesis. *Brain Res Bull* 12:151–160, 1984.
89. Hartung GH, Myhre LG, Nunneley SA: Physiological effects of cold air inhalation during exercise. *Aviat Space Environ Med* 51:591–594, 1980.
90. Stroud MA: Effects of energy expenditure on facial cooling. *Eur J Appl Physiol* 63:376–380, 1991.
91. Timmons BA, Araujo J, Thomas TR: Fat utilization enhanced by exercise in a cold environment. *Med Sci Sports Exerc* 17:673–678, 1985.

92. Smolander J, Louhevaara V, Hakola T, et al: Cardiorespiratory strain during walking in snow with boots of differing weights. *Ergonomics* 32:3–13, 1989.

93. Duncan GG: Diabetes mellitus, in Duncan GG (ed): *Diseases of Metabolism: Detailed Methods of Diagnosis and Treatment.* Philadelphia, WB Saunders Co, 1964, p 955.

94. Bielinski R, Schutz Y, Jequier E: Energy metabolism during the postexercise recovery in man. *Am J Clin Nutr* 42:69–82, 1985.

95. Lennon D, Nagel F, Stratman F, et al: Diet and exercise training effects on resting metabolic rate. *Int J Obes* 9:39–47, 1985.

96. Tremblay A, Fontaine E, Nadeau A: Contribution of post exercise increment in glucose storage to variations in glucose-induced thermogenesis in endurance athletes. *Can J Physiol Pharmacol* 63:1165–1169, 1985.

97. Thörne A, Wahren J: Diet-induced thermogenesis in well-trained subjects. *Clin Physiol* 9:295–305, 1989.

98. Murray SJ, Shephard RJ, Montelpare WJ, et al: Fat loss during moderate exercise in cold environments in relation to fitness level. *Arctic Med Res* 47:277S–279S, 1988.

99. Wilcox AR: The effects of caffeine and exercise on body weight, fat-pad weight and fat cell size. *Med Sci Sports Exerc* 14:317–321, 1982.

100. Tarnopolsky MA, Atkinson SA, MacDougall JD, et al: Physiological responses to caffeine during endurance running in habitual caffeine users. *Med Sci Sports Exerc* 21:418–424, 1989.

101. Doubt TJ, Hsieh SS: Additive effects of caffeine and cold water during submaximal leg exercise. *Med Sci Sports Exerc* 23:435–442, 1991.

102. McArdle WD, Magel JR, Spina RJ, et al: Thermal adjustment to cold water exposure in resting men and women. *J Appl Physiol* 56:1565–1571, 1984.

103. Stevens GHJ, Graham A, Van Dijk JP: Cardiovascular adjustments in a cold environment. *Med Sci Sports Exerc* 17:186, 1985.

104. Stevens GHJ, Graham TE, Wilson BA: Gender differences in cardiovascular and metabolic responses to cold and exercise. *Can J Physiol Pharmacol* 65:165–171, 1987.

105. Graham TE: Thermal, metabolic and cardiovascular changes in men and women during cold stress. *Med Sci Sports Exerc* 20:185S–192S, 1988.

106. Bernstein LM, Johnson LC, Ryan R, et al: Body composition as related to heat regulation in women. *J Appl Physiol* 9:241–256, 1956.

107. Desprès JP, Bouchard C, Savard R, et al: The effects of a 20-week endurance training program on adipose tissue morphology and lipolysis in men and women. *Metabolism* 33:235–238, 1984.

108. Altura BM: Sex and estrogens and responsiveness of terminal arterioles to neurohypophyseal hormones and catecholamines. *J Pharmacol Exp Ther* 193:403–412, 1975.

109. Swaab DF, Fliers E: A sexually dimorphic nucleus in the human brain. *Science* 228:1112–1115, 1985.

110. Hart JS: Commentary. *Can Med Assoc J* 96:803, 1967.

111. James WPT, Trayhurn P, Davies H, et al: Interaction of food intake and energy expenditure: An overview, in Cioffi LA, James WPT, Van Itallie TB (eds): *The Body Weight Regulatory System: Normal and Disturbed Mechanisms.* New York, Raven Press, 1981.

112. Keatinge WR: The effects of subcutaneous fat and previous exposure to cold on the body temperature peripheral blood flow, and metabolic rate of men in cold water. *J Physiol* 153:166–178, 1960.

113. James WPT, Trayhurn P: Thermogenesis and obesity. *Br Med Bull* 37:43–48, 1981.

114. Contaldo F: The development of obesity in genetically obese rodents, in Cioffi LA, James WPT, Van Itallie TB (eds): *The body weight regulatory system: Normal and disturbed mechanisms.* New York, Raven Press, 1981.

115. Bittel JHM, Nonotte-Varly C, Livecchi-Gonnot H, et al: Physical fitness and

thermoregulatory reactions in a cold environment in men. *J Appl Physiol* 65:1984–1989, 1988.

116. Hamilton CL: Food and temperature, in Code CF (ed): *Handbook of Physiology, Section 6. Alimentary Canal I.* Washington, DC, American Physiology Society, 1967, pp 302–317.

117. Krotkiewski M, Maudroukas K, Morgan L, et al: Effects of physical training on adrenergic sensitivity in obesity. *J Appl Physiol* 55:1811–1817, 1983.

118. Holloszy JO, Rennie MJ, Hickson RC, et al: Physiological consequences of the biochemical adaptations to endurance exercise. *Ann NY Acad Sci* 301:440–450, 1977.

119. Molé PA: Exercise metabolism, in Bove AA, Lowenthal DT (eds): *Exercise Medicine.* New York, Academic Press, 1983, pp 43–88.

120. Stevenson JAF: Exercise, food intake and health in experimental animals. *Can Med Assoc J* 96:862–866, 1967.

121. Shephard RJ: Meeting carbohydrate and fluid needs in soccer. *Can J Sport Sci* 15:165–171, 1990.

122. Smith OLK, Huszar G, Davidson SB, et al: Effects of acute cold exposure on muscle amino acid and protein in rats. *J Appl Physiol* 52:1250–1256, 1982.

123. Saltin B: Unpublished experiment, cited by: Astrand PO, Rodahl K. *Textbook of Work Physiology.* New York, McGraw Hill, 1970, p 466.

124. Holloszy JO: Biochemical adaptations to exercise: Aerobic metabolism. *Exerc Sport Sci Rev* 1:45–71, 1973.

125. Kuroshima A, Doi M, Kurahashi M, et al: Effects of diets on cold tolerance and metabolic responses in fasted rats. *Jpn J Physiol* 26:177–187, 1976.

Suggested Reading

The following articles are recommended to the reader:

Young AJ, Muza SR, Sawka MN, et al: Human thermoregulatory responses to cold air are altered by repeated cold water immersion. *J Appl Physiol* 60:1542–1548, 1986.

Hanson PG, Johnson RE, Engel G: Plasma free fatty acid changes in man during acute cold exposure and nicotinic acid ingestion. *Aerospace Med* 36:1054–1058, 1965.

McNaughton KW, Sathasivam P, Vallerand AL, et al: Influence of caffeine on metabolic responses of men at rest in 28 and 5°C. *J Appl Physiol* 68:1889–1895, 1990.

Trayhurn P, James WPT: Thermogenesis, dietary and non-shivering aspects, in Cioffi LA, James WPT, Van Itallie TB (eds): *The Body Weight Regulatory System: Normal and Distributed Mechanisms.* New York, Raven Press, 1981.

1 Epidemiology and Prevention

Athletic Medical Insurance Practices at NCAA Division I Institutions
Street SA, Yates CS, Lavery ES, Lavery KM (Wake Forest Univ, Winston-Salem, NC)
J Athletic Train 29:9–13, 1994   139-95-1–1

Background.—As the price of athletic medical insurance continues to increase, athletic departments are searching for ways to provide quality coverage while containing costs. The types of athletic medical insurance coverage used by universities and their policies regarding staff and medical coverage were assessed in members of the National Collegiate Athletic Association (NCAA).

Method.—An 18-item questionnaire was mailed to the head athletic trainers of the 295 active Division I member schools of the NCAA. The questionnaire was completed by the individual primarily responsible for the athletic department's athletic medical insurance. The data were compiled into summary tables, and simple percentages were calculated.

Results.—Of the 295 questionnaires sent, 207 were returned. The athletic training staff were primarily responsible for gathering information and filing insurance claims in 85% of the responding programs. The percentage of the workday required to manage athletic medical insurance was as follows: head athletic trainer (15%, range 1-60), assistant athletic trainer (25%, range 1-60), and secretary/clerical (50%, range 10–100). Most respondents had received no formal training in dealing with medical insurance policies. They reported using 16 different insurance companies. A total of 85% were enrolled in a secondary insurance plan, with 69% using a deductible ranging from $50 to $5,000. The respondents reported that in 91% of their programs, scholarship and nonscholarship athletes were treated the same with regard to medical insurance coverage; however, 9% reported that they require the nonscholarship athlete to provide his or her own insurance. There was a wide range of premiums used (table). Schools with more sports and larger teams generally paid higher premiums, but some smaller programs reported paying premiums as large as those paid by schools participating in Division I football. Many discrepancies were found in premiums paid and coverage received by individual schools.

Conclusion.—As the cost of medical insurance continues to rise, it is vital for athletic trainers and administrators to understand and take an

Athletic Insurance Premiums

Premium	NCAA Football Division					
	I	IAA	II*	III*	No Football	Total
0–$10,000	4 (2%)	2 (1%)	4 (2%)	4 (2%)	14 (7%)	29 (14%)
$10–$20,000	4 (2%)	10 (5%)	0	4 (2%)	23 (11%)	41 (20%)
$20–$30,000	8 (4%)	8 (4%)	0	2 (1%)	10 (5%)	29 (14%)
$30–$40,000	17 (8%)	8 (4%)	2 (1%)	2 (1%)	2 (1%)	31 (15%)
$40–$50,000	10 (5%)	8 (4%)	0 (0%)	0 (0%)	4 (2%)	23 (11%)
$50–$60,000	6 (3%)	4 (2%)	0	0	0	10 (5%)
$60–$70,000	10 (5%)	4 (2%)	0	0	0	15 (7%)
over $70,000	25 (12%)	4 (2%)	0	0	0	29 (14%)
Total	85 (41%)	50 (24%)	6 (3%)	12 (6%)	54 (26%)	207 (100%)

* Institutions that are classified as Division I but play football at a different level.
(Courtesy of Street SA, Yates CS, Lavery ES, et al: J Athletic Train 29:9–13, 1994.)

interest in the different options available to athletes to obtain the best coverage for the right price.

▶ We often speak of how the role of the athletic trainer has changed significantly over the years. This area of athletic medical insurance is a prime example of how our world has expanded. I find myself on the "University Student Health Insurance Committee." A good portion of almost every day is spent on insurance matters or essentially finding payment for medical bills. Now that more and more of our students belong to HMOs or other types of managed care programs, these problems are increasing rapidly.

All students at Brown University are billed through the bursar's office for the student medical insurance, which also covers athletes. They must buy this policy or show proof that they have equivalent coverage; however, it can be difficult to define equivalent coverage. With higher deductibles and managed care and HMOs in our future, this problem is going to become more severe. Athletic trainers must have a working knowledge of the athletic medical insurance policy at their schools.—F.J. George, A.T.C., P.T.

Exercise, Training and Injuries
Jones BH, Cowan DN, Knapik JJ (Army Research Inst of Environmental Medicine, Natick, Mass; Walter Reed Army Inst of Research, Washington, DC; Army War College, Carlisle Barracks, Pa)
Sports Med 18:202–214, 1994   139-95-1–2

Purpose.—The benefits of exercise include improved physical fitness, better health, and greater life expectancy; one risk is the increased chance of sustaining musculoskeletal injuries. Because identifying the various risk factors for exercise-related injuries is integral to reducing this risk, the aspects of exercise and training that most influence the risk of injuries were identified through review of the literature.

Findings and Conclusions.—The rates of injury associated with vigorous weight-bearing exercise, such as running and training of military recruits are high. A strong and consistent correlation exists between greater total amount of exercise and higher injury risk; the total amount of exercise is a function of intensity, duration, and frequency. Greater duration and greater frequency of exercise contribute significantly to the total and are therefore associated with higher injury rates, but speed (intensity) contributes less to the total and thereby has a smaller effect on injury risks. Military research shows that higher rates of injury are associated with a greater amount of running (miles) per week, which in some instances does not impart any additional increase in fitness. However, greater physical activity in the past (especially previous running) decreases the risk of training-related injuries. Studies using multivariate analysis to simultaneously control for the influence of multiple risk factors have consistently shown that an increased amount of running and previous injuries are associated with an increased risk of injury. When military trainees were the subjects of multivariate analysis, older age, cigarette smoking, sedentary job and lifestyle, high and low flexibility, high foot arches, and low previous running mileage and unit training were identified as risk factors for training-related injuries.

Conclusion.—To best achieve the benefits of exercise while minimizing the risk of injury, better knowledge of the effects of the various aspects of training or other factors on this risk is necessary. The risks associated with common physical fitness activities other than running, such as walking, aerobics, bicycling, and tennis, should be quantified. In addition, individuals and fitness health professionals need better information on the effect of personal (individual) host characteristics and environmental factors on injury risk to better determine which exercise type and plan is most likely to yield optimal health benefits.

▶ Although this study indicates that greater amounts of training result in greater risks of exercise-related injury, data on military recruits undergoing basic training indicate that prior physical activity, exercise, and in particular running, protect new recruits from training-related injuries. Clearly, what is needed are critical exercise levels to maintain fitness but avoid destruction. Such information was not forthcoming from this article.—J.S. Torg, M.D.

Relationship of Fatigued Run and Rapid Stop to Ground Reaction Forces, Lower Extremity Kinematics, and Muscle Activation
Nyland JA, Shapiro R, Stine RL, Horn TS, Ireland ML (Univ of Kentucky, Lexington)
J Orthop Sports Phys Ther 20:132–137, 1994   139-95-1–3

Introduction.—Knee and ankle injuries have recently been occurring more frequently among female athletes than among male athletes. Injuries related to overuse, such as patellar tendinitis and patellofemoral stress syndrome, are seen more often among female athletes. Lower extremity injury may be related to fatigue.

Methods.—The manner in which lower extremity fatigue influences ground reaction force production, lower extremity kinematics, and muscle activation during the landing phase of a run and rapid stop was investigated. Nineteen female volleyball or basketball players participated in the study (average age, 20.8 years). The women did 3 trials of a run and rapid stop. Lower extremity fatigue was induced when the women walked on an uphill treadmill that started at a 10% grade and was raised 2% every minute thereafter, until the women stated they could not continue. At 2,000 Hz, dominant leg ground reaction and muscle activation were sampled. At 200 Hz, lower extremity kinematic data were sampled, and 3-dimensional analysis was done.

Results.—During fatigue, knee extensor–flexor muscle activation tended to be delayed. Maximum knee flexion occurred earlier. According to stepwise multiple regression, the knee may be the primary site of force attenuation after fatigue. Differences in knee kinematics and muscle activation times show that during fatigue, biodynamic compensations in the mechanical properties of the knee extensor may enhance knee stability. After fatigue, run and rapid stop performance showed trends toward later onset of muscle activations of the rectus femoris, vastus lateralis, biceps femoris, and medial hamstrings and earlier occurrence of maximal knee flexion.

Conclusion.—The run and rapid stop maneuver depends on the shock absorption or damping muscle properties. The study results may be explained by the delayed onset of muscle activation found during fatigue for the rectus femoris, biceps femoris, vastus lateralis, and medial hamstring muscles and by the earlier achievement of maximum knee flexion, which could serve as compensation to enhance shock absorption. Futher studies should include training periods for test maneuvers and a fatigue method that more closely mimics specific sports performance.

▶ Why do athletes become injured? Do female athletes sustain more lower extremity injuries than their male counterparts? Studies such as this will help us determine what causes these injuries. Once that is determined, hopefully we can develop training programs that will reduce the number and severity of these injuries. These studies will also assist us in developing rehabilitation programs to prevent the recurrence of these injuries.—F.J. George, A.T.C., P.T.

Seizures Induced by Physical Exercise: Report of Two Cases
Schmitt B, Thun-Hohenstein L, Vontobel H, Boltshauser E (Univ Children's Hosp, Zürich, Switzerland)
Neuropediatrics 25:51–53, 1994   139-95-1-4

Introduction.—Two types of movement-induced seizures have been described: those induced by sudden, unexpected movements and those induced by passive or active movements. On the basis of the scarcity of reports in the literature, seizures provoked by physical exercise seem to be uncommon. Two patients with seizures induced by physical exercise were described.

Case 1.—An 18-month-old boy had a history of generalized tonic-clonic and absence-like seizures. Generalized tonic-clonic and complex partial seizures were first noted during febrile episodes at age 4 and 6 months. Electroencephalogram (EEG), cranial MRI, and metabolic evaluations were found to be normal. Seizure activity continued during subsequent months despite anticonvulsant therapy. Absence-like seizures, lasting as long as 1 minute, were also observed. Electroencephalograms, including ambulatory 24-hour cassette, were normal; moderate slowing of background activity was only detected once after a grand-mal seizure. At age 18 months, generalized tonic-clonic seizures were noted when the child walked a short distance; this occurred daily. Seizures were also noted occasionally when the child was resting, sometimes as a series of myoclonic jerks. Although not provoked by walking, generalized tonic-clonic seizures were later noted when the patient played football. Generalized spike waves and postictal slowing of background activity were seen on cassette EEG with a normal ECG. Short-lasting left hemispheric discharges were recorded with EEG before the onset of seizures. The seizures could not be controlled.

Case 2.—A 3½-year-old boy was found to have seizure activity provoked by vigorous physical activity. Seizure activity was first noted at age 5 months with a complex partial seizure during a febrile episode. Seizure activity—generalized, partial, and complex partial—continued over several months. Cranial CT, EEG, and CSF examinations were normal. Anticonvulsant therapy and ketogenic diet were not effective. Developmental retardation, hyperactivity, and an abnormal gait were apparent at 2 years of age. At age 3½ years, seizure activity associated with physical exercise—climbing stairs and playing football—was observed. When these activities were avoided, seizure activity was reduced. Just before seizure activity, EEG and ECG were normal. The latter was normal during seizure activity, whereas generalized spike wave discharges and postictal generalized high-voltage delta activity were noted on EEG. Anticonvulsant agents were ineffective in controlling seizures; only strict avoidance of physical exercise reduced seizure frequency.

Discussion.—The cause of exercise-induced seizures is unknown. Cardiac arrhythmias resulting in cerebral anoxia have been associated with seizure activity in some patients. However, in these 2 patients, ECG recordings were normal. Hyperventilation was also considered as a cause of the exercise-induced seizures in these patients. However, voluntary hyperventilation, a known technique for provoking seizures, produces pathophysiologic effects that differ from those the ventilation produced with exercise. In addition, characteristics associated with stress convulsions—abnormal interictal EEG, absence of unprovoked seizures, and good prognosis—were not found in these 2 patients. The exercise-induced seizures described in these 2 patients probably represent a form of reflex epilepsy. The consistent association with exercise and specific seizure activity in these patients justifies this classification.

▶ More than 4 million Americans have epilepsy. It is believed, although not on the basis of a rigorous controlled trial, that physical training and sports participation either decrease or at least do not increase the rate of seizures for most patients with epilepsy (1). Certainly, most people with epilepsy can participate safely in most sports. However, this report and others (2) note that in some epileptics, vigorous exercise—climbing stairs or playing football—can trigger seizures in the absence of cardiac arrhythmias. Exactly how exercise does this is unknown; imaging studies of the brain generally are normal. On the other hand, in 3 healthy adults who had generalized seizures shortly after jogging, CT scans revealed small frontal cortical lesions: an arteriovenous malformation, an astrocytoma, and a cyst (3).—E.R. Eichner, M.D.

References

1. 1992 Year Book of Sports Medicine, pp 257–258.
2. Ogunyemi AO, et al: *Neurology* 38:633, 1988.
3. 1993 Year Book of Sports Medicine, pp 236–237.

Childhood Lightning Injuries on the Playing Field
Cherington M, Martorano FJ, Siebuhr LV, Stieg RL, Yarnell PR (St Anthony Hosp, Denver)
J Emerg Med 12:39–41, 1994   139-95-1-5

Background.—A literature review has shown that the most frequently reported locations of childhood lightning injuries are on the playing field, at the swimming pool, or in tents (table). Cases of 2 children struck by lightning during outdoor activities were reviewed.

Case 1.—Boy, 11 years, was struck by lightning while playing football. The entrance wound was under the metal snap of his football helmet. Cardiopulmonary resuscitation was immediately administered. Paramedics arrived within 4 minutes, and the patient was intubated and countershocked for ventricular fibrillation. On the patient's arrival at the emergency department, blood pressure was only palpable at 70 mm Hg. Plasmanate, dopamine, steroids, mannitol, and bicarbonate were given. Electrocardiogram results were consistent with an antero-inferior wall myocardial infarction, and a CT scan performed 10 days later showed hydrocephalus and cerebral atrophy. Low-density areas also were seen in the regions of the basal ganglia. The patient remained in a coma and died 5 months after the lightning strike.

Case 2.—Boy, 10 years, was struck by lightning while sitting in a tent at an altitude of approximately 11,000 feet. The patient experienced momentary loss of consciousness and transient paralysis of his arms and legs, which subsided within a few minutes. Superficial burns of the abdomen, legs, and left arm were noted. Complaints of tiredness, clumsiness, and flashbacks at night were also reported. Ten days after the accident, neurologic examination failed to show any abnormalities, and the patient's complaints had resolved. The patient's mother indicated that cognitive abilities and sports skills had returned to normal and believed that further medical follow-up was unnecessary.

Conclusion.—Knowledge of measures to lower the risk of lightning strikes should help decrease the numbers of childhood lightning injuries. New lightning detection technology also may serve to minimize these tragic events in the future.

▶ Cherington and colleagues present a tragic lightning death of a boy playing football. In the United States, about 100 people die because of lightning strikes each year. About 30% of lightning strikes prove fatal to human beings. The sports and activities associated with the most lightning injuries and

Childhood Injuries on the Playing Field (Literature Review)

No.	Age	Sex	Location/activity	Outcome	Reference
1.	9	F	Playground slide	Coma—recovered	Apfelberg (1974)
2.	14	M	Swimming pool	Coma—recovered	Apfelberg (1974)
3.	15	M	Mountain/Hiking	Stroke—recovered	Cherington (1992)
4.	9	M	Tent	Died	Hanson (1973)
5.	15	M	Tent	Died	Hanson (1973)
6.	9	M	Baseball field	Cataracts	Hubbell (1992)
7.	11	M	Soccer field	Depression—recovered	Kotagal (1982)
8.	11	M	Soccer field	Depression—recovered	Kotagal (1982)
9.	9	M	Soccer field	Died	Kotagal (1982)
10.	11	M	Soccer field	Forgetful—recovered	Kotagal (1982)
11.	17	M	Football field	Died	Maggied (1973)
12.	16	M	Football field	Died	Maggied (1973)
13.	14	M	Football field	Died	Maggied (1973)
14.	14	M	Football field	Died	Maggied (1973)
15.	14	M	Football field	Coma—improved	Maggied (1973)
16.	14	F	Swimming pool	Died	Myers (1977)
17.	7	F	Swimming pool	Cerebral hypoxia	Myers (1977)
18.	15	F	Swimming pool	Spinal atrophy	Myers (1977)
19.	10	M	Swimming pool	Burns	Myers (1977)
20.	10	M	Bicycling	Coma—recovered	Ravitch (1961)
21.	15	M	Lacrosse field	Died	Shannon (1992)
22.	11	M	Soccer field	Intracerebral hematoma—improved	Stanley (1985)

(Courtesy of Cherington M, Martorano FJ, Siebuhr LV, et al: *J Emerg Med* 12:39-41, 1994.)

deaths are water sports, golf, camping, hiking, baseball, and football. This article includes practical tips on prevention and information on new devices that may foretell lightning. Other practical, clinical articles on lightning injuries are recommended (1–3).—E.R. Eichner, M.D.

References

1. Ghezzi KT: *Postgrad Med* 85:197, 1989.
2. Blount BW: *Am Fam Physician* 42:405, 1990.
3. Cherington M, Vervalin C: *Physician Sportsmed* 18:59, 1990.

Minimizing Liability Risks of Head and Neck Injuries in Football

Heck JF, Weis MP, Gartland JM, Weis CR (Richard Stockton College, Pomona, NJ; Professional Sports Care Meadowlands, East Rutherford, NJ; Homestead Insurance Company, Secaucus, NJ; et al)

J Athletic Train 29:128–139, 1994   139-95-1–6

Background.—Head and neck injuries in football are among the most devastating in all sports and almost always result in litigation. The athletic trainer's responsibilities center around the prevention and treatment

Athlete's Name: _____

I understand that the game and sport of football is an inherently dangerous activity and that there are genuine and real serious risks to anyone who engages in this activity.

I also understand that football is the highest risk sport for injury on the high school level. Due to the nature of the physical violence and collisions that are a part of the game and sport of football, I understand that the risk of serious physical injury, including catastrophic injury resulting in permanent paralysis, brain injury or death does exist.

I also understand that other participants, the coaching staff, athletic trainer, team physician and/or spectators may engage in conduct, including negligent conduct, that may increase the risk of injury to me.

I knowingly assume responsibility for any and all such risks and any and all resulting injuries, including death. I promise to accept and assume responsibility and risk for injury, death, illness, or disease, or damage to property arising from my traveling to, participation in, or returning from this activity. And I do hereby voluntarily choose to participate in this event in spite of the risks.

Furthermore I attest that I am physically fit and have sufficiently trained for this event. I do not have any medical record or history that could be aggravated by my participation in this activity.

My signature below indicates I have read this entire document, understood it completely, and agree to be bound by its terms.

Printed Name _____

Address _____

Phone _____

_____ _____ Parent/Guardian SignatureDate

Parent/ Guardian must execute form if the athlete is under the age of eighteen (18) years.

_____ _____ Athletes Signature Date

Signature of Witness _____

Fig 1–1.—Example of an acknowledgement of assumption of risk form for a high school athlete. (Courtesy of Heck JF, Weis MP, Gartland JM, et al: *J Athletic Train* 29:128-139, 1994.)

of these injuries and are part of a comprehensive risk management program of the athletic department.

Legal Terms.—The foundation of a risk management program is an understanding of pertinent legal terms. Litigation related to sports injuries is based on the common law concept of tort, a civil wrong resulting in damages that are caused by the acts or omissions of others. Negligence, conduct that falls below the standard of what a reasonable individual would do under similar circumstances, is the most common tort related to injury. Gross negligence and willful, wanton, or reckless negligence are more extreme forms of negligence.

Claims Against Athletic Staffs.—The most common claims by injured athletes allege breaches of duty by athletic department staff in 1 or more of 5 areas: failure to give adequate instruction; failure to supply proper equipment; failure to reasonably select or match participants; failure to provide adequate supervision, and failure to use proper postinjury procedures.

Risk Reduction.—Defenses to claims of negligence must demonstrate proactive efforts to reduce risk and to inform participants of potential risk and document individual assumption of risk and informed consent. Athletic departments should have standard acknowledgement of assumption of risk (Fig 1-1) and release of liability forms signed by the players and, if they are minors, by the players' parents. Additionally, complete medical histories and physical examination records should be on file, along with consent for treatment if injured. Only helmets approved by the National Operating Committee on Standards for Athletic Equipment should be purchased and used. The fitting of helmets must be rigorous and supervised. Comprehensive instruction of the athletes regarding techniques and safety must be given regularly and be documented. Rules must be rigorously enforced. Standardized procedures for handling injuries should be established, and all athletes and staff should be knowledgeable regarding the procedures.

Conclusion.—A risk management program provides a general framework that can both reduce legal liabilities and, perhaps more importantly, prevent injuries.

▶ In his comments on this article, K.L. Knight states, the authors "present recommendations aimed at minimizing the risk of head and neck injuries" and this article is "an excellent primer for students and a review for the practicing professional" (1).

Athletic trainers are responsible for instructing the football team as a group and players as individuals concerning the dangers of spearing. This should be done at a team meeting before the first practice and on an individual basis when unsafe techniques are observed. The subject should be discussed with the coaching staff, and all coaches must see the videotape "Prevent Paralysis: Don't Hit With Your Head," with Joe Torg, M.D. and coach Dick Verneal. This tape is provided by the Riddell All-American Company [1 (800)

275-5338]. It is a must. After coaches see this video, they should ensure that their athletes use proper blocking and tackling techniques.—F.J. George, A.T.C., P.T.

Reference

1.   Knight KL: *Athletic Train: Sports Health Care Perspectives* Vol. 1, No. 1, p 98.

Clinical Implications of Secondary Impingement of the Shoulder in Freestyle Swimmers

Allegrucci M, Whitney SL, Irrgang JJ (Univ of Pittsburgh, Pa)
J Orthop Sports Phys Ther 20:307–318, 1994   139-95-1-7

Introduction.—Swimming places physical demands on the shoulder that can increase shoulder laxity through a cumulative mechanism of injury. Anterior and superior translation of the humeral head may, through prolonged fatigue, develop in the rotator cuff and scapula stabilizers, leading to secondary impingement and rotator cuff tears. The pathology of primary and secondary impingement experienced by freestyle swimmers and the requirements for rehabilitation were studied.

Pathology.—Primary shoulder impingement is characterized by the mechanical obstruction of rotator cuff tendons located under the acromion, the coracoacromial ligament, or the acromioclavicular joint. Secondary shoulder impingement is characterized by a reduction of subacromial space caused by glenohumeral instability, which can be caused by

---

TABLE 1.—Typical Signs and Symptoms and Possible Causes of Swimmer's Shoulder

Signs and Symptoms	Possible Cause
Postural deformities of rounded shoulders and thoracic kyphosis	Tightness of the pectoralis minor
Weakness of the posterior cuff muscles and scapular stabilizers	Weakness can be due to strength imbalances between the anterior and posterior muscles secondary to the demands of the sport and to stretch weakness
Limited internal rotation and excessive external rotation range of motion	Tightness of the posterior capsule or posterior cuff muscles which causes a shift in the available range of motion
Decay of normal scapulothoracic rhythm	Tightness of the anterior chest musculature and weakness of the scapular stabilizers

(Courtesy of Allegrucci M, Whitney SL, Irrgang JJ: *J Orthop Sports Phys Ther* 20:307–318, 1994.)

TABLE 2.—Basic Guidelines for Progression of Treatment for Swimmer's Shoulder With Secondary Impingement

Phase I
- *Modalities for pain control*
- *Address range of motion losses*
- *Rotator cuff strengthening at 0°*
  Side lying ER
  Theraband ER/IR at 0°
- *Scapulothoracic muscle in neutral*
  Shrugs
  Prone arm raise at 0°
  Scapular retraction (row)
- *Aerobic conditioning*
  Bike
- *Kicking in water*

Phase II (0–90°)
- *Rotator cuff*
  Prone ER
  Theraband ER
  Prone arm raise with ER at 90°, progress to
      120°
  Elevation in scapular plane with IR (empty can)
- *Scapulothoracic exercises*
  Scapular protraction
  Stabilization exercises
      Bilateral → unilateral
      Add dynamic resistance
      Progress to stabilizing on a ball
  Push-up "plus" progression
      Wall → table → modified (on knees) →
          regular
- *Axial humeral muscles*
  Flexion
  Abduction in the plane of the scapula
  Lat pull-down
  Chest press
  Bench press
- *Proprioception*
  Active and passive matching
- *Aerobic conditioning*
  Upper body ergometer
  Rower
  Kicking in water

Phase III—Functional Training
- *Full range flexion and abduction*
- *Combined movement patterns*
      Proprioceptive neuromuscular facilitation D1
          and D2 (Theraband or manual)
- *Stroke-specific exercise*
  Stimulation of recovery
  Pull-through and reverse pull-through with
          Theraband
- *Plyometric exercises*
- *Swim bench*

Phase IV—Return to Sport

Abbreviations: ER, external rotation; IR, internal rotation; D1, flexion, adduction, IR; D2, flexion, abduction, ER.

(Courtesy of Allegrucci M, Whitney SL, Irrgang JJ: *J Orthop Sports Phys Ther* 20:307–318, 1994.)

either rotator cuff dysfunction, resulting from fatigue or injury, or instability resulting from laxity of the dynamic stabilizers. Range of motion tends to be reduced in patients who have primary impingement and excessive in patients who have secondary impingement. Swimmers, like throwing athletes, may exhibit injuries that overlap impingement and instability during the different biomechanical phases of swimming. The positioning of the joint in adduction and internal rotation during mid-pull-through presents a risk of mechanical impingement. Shoulder adduction during late pull-through can twist and stretch the supraspinatus tendon. During recovery, positioning may cause primary impingement or anterior laxity, and rotator cuff fatigue may cause secondary impingement. Swimmers may exhibit a range of signs and symptoms (Table 1).

Rehabilitation.—Upper extremity plyometric exercises, which reflect the open kinetic chain activity nature of swimming, can promote elasticity in the muscle tendon unit and enhance synchrony of movement. In addition, closed chain activities can mimic pulling the body over the arms.

Conclusion.—Freestyle swimmers may have any combination of signs and symptoms of shoulder instability and impingement. Because stability at the glenohumeral joint is dependent primarily on the rotator cuff muscles, rehabilitation efforts must focus on correcting the structural context for these muscles by establishing proper stability and relationships of the scapula and all the muscles in the shoulder complex (Table 2). Because the biomechanics of the freestyle stroke can cause either impingement or instability, training should emphasize maintaining equilibrium of the shoulder complex.

▶ The authors stress the importance of maintaining equilibrium of the shoulder complex. This particular concept must be foremost in conditioning, training, and, of course, all rehabilitation programs of the shoulder. The scapula stabilizers play a very important role in this equilibrium and must not be overlooked. Too often, our treatment programs center on the rotator cuff and neglect the scapula stabilizers.

The coach plays an important role in the evaluation of the swimming stroke. The authors recommend that the coach "watch for a dropped elbow during late recovery, which is the universal sign of fatigue. Observe the position of hand entry into the water. During hand entry, the shoulder should be in internal rotation with the palm facing out. . . . Modification of stroke mechanics must be done cautiously so that productivity is not altered, particularly with elite swimmers."—F.J. George, A.T.C., P.T.

Carbohydrate Strategies for Injury Prevention

Schlabach G (Northern Illinois Univ, DeKalb)
J Athletic Train 29:244–246, 249–254, 1994   139-95-1-8

Background.—The specific mechanism of skeletal muscle fatigue depends on the patient's level of fitness. In unfit individuals, the mechanism of fatigue is usually lactic acid accumulation. Conversely, fit individuals exercising at intensities of 75% to 90% maximal oxygen output for long durations may experience fatigue caused by muscle glycogen depletion. Muscle glycogen is derived primarily from carbohydrates. Nutritional strategies that can maximize glycogen stores and delay the onset of fatigue were studied.

Nutritional Strategies.—In general, carbohydrate consumption should account for approximately 60% to 70% of the total caloric intake in all adults. Carbohydrate loading, pre-event meals, and carbohydrate intake before, during, and after exercise are also recommended for active individuals participating in events lasting longer than 60 minutes and requiring repeated bouts of high-intensity exercise. Carbohydrate loading should commence 7 days before a scheduled event. A modified loading method, which avoids the side effects associated with the standard version, begins with gradual tapering of activity and normal carbohydrate intake on days 7, 6, 5, and 4. Carbohydrate intake is then increased to 500 to 600 g/day and maintained until the day of the event. A pre-event meal is also advised. Generally, carbohydrate intake per kilogram of body weight should coincide with the number of hours before the event. For example, 4 g of carbohydrate per kilogram of body weight should be consumed 4 hours before the event, 3 g should be consumed 3 hours before the event, and so forth. Liquid carbohydrate meals or drinks are recommended before exercise, and dry glucose polymers mixed in water are recommended during exercise. Immediately after exercise, approximately 50 g of a high-to-moderate glycemic carbohydrate should be consumed to enhance muscle glycogen resynthesis. Recommended foods and beverages include glucose and sucrose (4.2 tbsp), bagels (1.6), bread (3.5 slices), baked potatoes, rice (1 cup), macaroni (1.5 cups), oranges, corn (1.2 cups), 6% sucrose solution (3.5 cups), 10% corn syrup (2.1 cups of a carbonated drink), and 20% maltodextrin solution (1.1 cups). Fructose, found in fruits and honey, has a low glycemic index and is thus associated with a slow rate of muscle glycogen resynthesis.

Conclusion.—Muscle glycogen depletion is a risk factor for fatigue and injury. Because muscle glycogen is the predominant fuel in exercise of moderate-to-heavy intensities, the nutritional emphasis should be on carbohydrate intake.

▶ Hopefully, by now everyone associated with an athlete's nutrition realizes the importance carbohydrates play in optimizing performance and recovery. Unfortunately, many athletes continue to consume large amounts of protein and expensive protein supplements. All too often, these are recommended to athletes by people who are making a profit on the sale of these substances. Athletes should be educated in sound dietary practices not only for pregame meals and carbohydrate loading but for a lifetime of healthy eating.—F.J. George, A.T.C., P.T.

Identification of Risk Components in Exercises for the Low Back
Tornatora B, Karagiannis J, Polus BI, Walsh MJ (RMIT, Bundoora, Australia)
Chiroprac Tech 6:79–83, 1994   139-95-1–9

Introduction.—Up to 80% of the population has low back pain; lack of fitness is considered to be a risk factor. Exercises are often prescribed for the low back to decrease pain, strengthen weak muscles, improve fitness level to prevent injury, improve posture, and improve mobility. However, some exercises are dangerous, and safe principles should be applied.

Injurious Exercises.—A literature search found several exercises associated with possible low back insult: straight-leg sit-ups; double straight-leg raises; hydrant position with hands and knees on floor; push-ups; cobra position/back arching; star jumps; repetitive foot strike; and rotation/twisting on a fixed base.

Risk Factors.—Four major risk factors or movements associated with exercises involved in aggravating low back injury are rotation, hyperextension, axial loading, and increased intradiskal pressure. The lumbar spine is extended by posterior movement of the trunk. An average maximum extension of 3.2 ± 2 degrees occurs in the lumbar spine during normal movement; however, severe, repeated, or sudden extension may cause minor damage that could lead to more severe damage. Microdamage to the diskal structures occurs with rotation beyond the normal average range of 2.6 degrees, along with impaction of the zygapophyseal joints. Jumping can create considerable axial loading, and although 1 jump may not cause injury, multiple, repetitive jumping movements are of concern.

Protocol for Exercises.—Prolonged extension movements should be avoided, as should sustained extension of the lumbar spine. If extension is done, movements should be as slow as possible. Repetitions of movement and extreme movements should be avoided, and all exercise postures for inadvertent extension should be examined. Reaching full end-range limits for all rotational movements of the spine and repetitive foot-strike patterns should be avoided. Rotation should be done over a mobile rather than a fixed base. Lower axial loading movements should be used instead of higher loading movements, (e.g., jogging rather than jumping). Sit-ups should not be greater than 20 degrees of lumbar flexion.

▶ The authors have identified a number of risk factors that may cause back problems. Some of these exercises are used in exercise conditioning programs, and some continue to be used in back rehabilitation programs. In general, the authors propose a good protocol for performing exercises of the lumbar spine. Each component of their protocol should be evaluated and modified to meet patients' needs.—F.J. George, A.T.C., P.T.

Outcome in the Treatment of Chronic Overuse Sports Injuries: A Retrospective Study

Almekinders LC, Almekinders SV (Univ of North Carolina, Chapel Hill; North Carolina State Univ, Raleigh)
J Orthop Sports Phys Ther 19:157–161, 1994   139-95-1–10

Objective.—Chronic overuse injuries are common among recreational and elite athletes, who frequently do not seek immediate medical help. Little information is available about the long-term outcome of treating such injuries. The outcome of and compliance with treatment of chronic overuse injuries were studied.

Methods.—Sports medicine records between 1987 and 1989 were reviewed for 102 patients aged 14–73 years. The patients had symptoms of pain for more than 3 weeks in an extremity resulting from soft tissue injury where no cause could be identified, and they had normal radiographs and no history of joint disease or instability or previous treatment. Patients' activities were modified. Patients were given daily home exercises and reported to a physical therapist 2–3 times weekly for at least 6 weeks. Patients were followed up by telephone and questionnaire for an average of 27 months.

Results.—The most common injuries were to the foot, shoulder, or knee. Thirty-seven percent of patients said they were completely better, 28% were improved, and 35% were no better or worse. Patients with knee injuries had a significantly poorer outcome than did patients with other types of injuries. Excluding patients with knee injuries, 71.4% were improved or completely better. Noncompliance rates were 9% for nonsteroidal anti-inflammatory drugs (NSAIDs) and 13% for exercise. The length of time between onset of pain and onset of treatment had no significant effect on outcome.

Conclusion.—The long-term effects of chronic overuse injuries are not affected by activity modification, exercise, or NSAID treatment, either alone or in combination. Additional analyses need to be done to determine the effectiveness of such treatments.

▶ The authors state, "Until the efficacy of potentially dangerous medication as well as several weeks of therapist-supervised exercises is firmly established, correction of training errors and activity modifications should remain the mainstay of our treatment of overuse sports injuries." I have never seen this type of injury improve completely unless there is a change in the causative factor. Big words that mean the source of the problem must be identified and modified. The fact that there may be a combination of causative factors confounds the solutions. Many areas must be closely evaluated, including the level of conditioning, flexibility, strength, biomechanical probems, diet, and training errors. I'm sure that, depending on the injury, there are other areas that must be considered.

An example is "tennis elbow." This injury will not be cured unless all the areas of flexibility, strengthening stroke modification, and overuse are addressed. Unfortunately, you have to learn to hit the ball correctly. There isn't a magic pill, exercise, or treatment modality that will cure these overuse injuries. The anterior knee appears to be the biggest problem area for long-term resolution of these injuries.—F.J. George, A.T.C., P.T.

Persistent Visuospatial Attention Deficits Following Mild Head Injury in Australian Rules Football Players

Cremona-Meteyard SL, Geffen GM (Univ of Queensland, Brisbane, Australia)
Neuropsychologia 32:649–662, 1994   139-95-1-11

Introduction.—Controversy exists over whether fundamental deficits in cognition persist for several months after a mild head injury (MHI). Two groups of Australian Rules football players who sustained an MHI during competition were evaluated to determine the extent and duration of visuospatial attention deficits.

Methods.—In the first experiment, 9 players from the South Australian National Football League (SANFL) who sustained an MHI with a change in consciousness from 2 to 20 minutes, were tested within 2 weeks and again at 1 year after injury. Seven of 9 players had sustained previous MHIs. In experiment 2, 8 SANFL players who had sustained an MHI at least 1 year previously were tested. Six had sustained multiple previous MHIs. The control group consisted of 12 non-MHI athletes from varying sporting events. There were not enough non-MHI SANFL players to comprise a control group. Visuospatial attention was tested

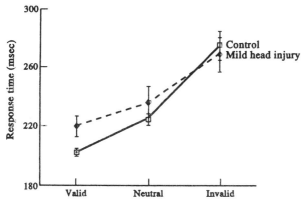

Fig 1–2.—Mean of median reaction times (ms) to onset of target following valid, neutral, and invalid cues in the control ($n = 12$) and previous head injury ($n = 8$) groups from the retrospective study. Reaction times have been averaged over left and right target presentations. *Vertical bars* represent the standard error of the mean. (Courtesy of Cremona-Meteyard SL, Geffen GM: *Neuropsychologia* 32:649–662, 1994.)

using a cued reaction time (RT) task to measure the RT benefit of valid directional cueing and the RT cost of miscueing.

Results.—Athletes in experiment 1 showed an average cost of the same magnitude as controls. However, the benefit in speed of response to cues was significantly reduced compared with controls. At 1 year after injury, these athletes, as well as those in experiment 2 who sustained an MHI at least 1 year previously, also displayed normal costs but reduced benefits. This trend was observed in RTs for each of the cue conditions for each group (Fig 1–2). A patient's history of MHIs was not significant.

Conclusion.—A persistent impairment was seen in visuospatial attention at least 1 year after MHI in Australian Rules football players. Because visuospatial skills are important for optimal performance on the football field, the inability to respond quickly to spatial events may put these players at risk for further injury.

▶ Visuospatial deficits are important not only in terms of the cerebral injury that has already been sustained, but also because the individual who is slow to react is at increased risk of a further head injury. The performance deficit relative to control athletes is not very convincing evidence of long-lasting effects (the athletes concerned may have been injured the first time because they were slow to react), but the difference in performance between 2 and 52 weeks after injury shows that there was a real impact on brain function. Clearly, it is necessary to be vigilant with a head injury, even if it does not seem to be very severe.—R.J. Shephard, M.D., Ph.D.

Trends in Head Injuries Among Child Bicyclists
Pitt WR, Thomas S, Nixon J, Clark R, Battistutta D, Acton C (Master Children's Hosp, South Brisbane, Queensland, Australia; Inst of Med Research, Herston, Queensland, Australia; Univ of Queensland Herston, Australia; et al)
BMJ 308:177–178, 1994   139-95-1–12

Purpose.—The wearing of approved helmets by bicyclists is mandatory in some areas of the United States and Australia. Proponents of this legislation cite evidence of a decrease in the number of head injuries and a reduced risk of bicycle-related head injury among helmet wearers. Trends in the incidence of head injuries and bicycle-related injuries in children in Brisbane, Australia, were evaluated retrospectively with injury surveillance data.

Methods and Results.—The records of all children admitted to a hospital and 75% of children attending emergency departments in Brisbane (population 600,000) during a 6-year period were studied. The most common injury category was bicycle injury. The rate of head injury resulting from bicycle accidents decreased from 47.34/100,000 in 1985 to 18.32/100,000 in 1991. Hospital admissions for bicycle-related injuries other than head injuries did not change. Helmet use became compulsory in Brisbane in June 1991; the proportion of primary school–children wearing helmets increased from 2.5% to 59% between 1986 and June 1991.

Conclusion.—Some critics of mandatory helmet laws charge that helmets are not effective in collisions with motor vehicles. However, the helmets are designed to protect the head in accidents that do not involve vehicles; only 8% of bicycle-related injuries and 25% of bicycle-related head injuries were caused by collision with a motor vehicle. The noted decrease in bicycle-related injuries started before helmets were widely used and occurred concomitant with a steady rate of hospital admissions for other bicycle-related injuries and a decreased rate of head injuries from other causes. The protective effect of helmets is supported, as evidenced by the large decrease in head injuries occurring in the year before the legislation (when public debate significantly increased awareness and helmet wearing), but the reason for the decrease in bicycle-related head injury is more complex than just an increase in the wearing of helmets.

▶ Granted, the reason for the decrease in bicycle-related head injuries is more complex than just wearing helmets, but the sharp decrease in head injuries in the year leading up to the compulsory law suggests that public awareness of the need for helmets leads to greater use and greater safety for kids. In fact, a recent case-control study of bicycle-related injuries in the emergency departments of the 2 main children's hospitals in Brisbane, Australia, finds that the risk reduction for helmet wearers was 63% for head injury and 86% for loss of consciousness (1). See the 1994 YEAR BOOK OF SPORTS MEDICINE for the risks of "drunk cycling" (2).—E.R. Eichner, M.D.

References

1. Thomas S, et al: *BMJ* 308:173, 1994.
2. 1994 YEAR BOOK OF SPORTS MEDICINE, pp 8–9.

Injury Patterns in Cyclists Attending an Accident and Emergency Department: A Comparison of Helmet Wearers and Non-Wearers
Maimaris C, Summers CL, Browning C, Palmer CR (Addenbrooke's Hosp, Cambridge, England; Univ of Cambridge, England)
BMJ 308:1537–1540, 1994   139-95-1–13

Background.—Bicycle-related injury and its resultant morbidity and mortality have serious economic costs in terms of both direct health care expenditures and lost working time. Compared were the nature and extent of injuries sustained by cyclists with and without helmets. Patients seen with bicycle-related injuries at the study hospital in 1992 were prospectively studied.

Results.—During 1992, 1,107 patients were seen in the emergency department because of cycle injuries. Complete data were available for

1,040, and 114 were wearing a safety helmet. With respect to the type or nature of accidents or the nature and distribution of injuries other than injuries to the head, there were no significant differences between the 2 groups. The incidence rate of head injuries was significantly higher in the group of cyclists not wearing helmets (100/928 or 11%) compared with the helmet-wearing group (4/114 or 4%). Using multiple logistic regression analysis, only 2 variables were significant predictors of head injury: involvement of a motor vehicle and helmet use. Involvement of a motor vehicle increased the odds of head injury by 2.95 times, whereas wearing a helmet provided a protective factor, decreasing the odds of head injury by 3.25 times.

Conclusion.— The significant protective effect of wearing a helmet in decreasing the risk of head injury in any bicycle accident was confirmed. Legislative mandates requiring protective helmets worn during cycling have proven effective in increasing compliance.

▶ This article substantiates that which is obvious, i.e., bicyclists who wore safety helmets were just as likely to be involved in an accident as those who didn't, but they were 3 times less likely to have received a head injury, and the head injuries sustained were much less severe.—J.S. Torg, M.D.

Helmets and Horseback Riders
Nelson DE, Rivara FP, Condie C (Ctrs for Disease Control and Prevention, Atlanta, Ga; Univ of Washington, Seattle; Univ of Canberra Faculty of Management, Belconnen, Australia)
Am J Prev Med 10:15–19, 1994   139-95-1–14

Objective.—Almost 20% of all horseback riding injuries occur to the neck and head and, according to some studies, are responsible for 70% of horse-related deaths. Although no studies have examined the effectiveness of hard helmets in preventing injury, preliminary information indicates that helmets are effective. Data from a national survey were studied to determine riders' attitudes about wearing helmets.

Methods.—Two questionnaires, 1 for adults and 1 for children, were mailed to 4,000 riding households.

Results.—A total of 1,834 individuals responded. More than half were aged 25–44 years, most were women, most had been riding for more than 10 years, and most rode at least 15 hours per month. A total of 58% of English-style riders wore helmets compared with 12% of Western-style riders. Nonowners of helmets believed helmets were not necessary (44%), were uncomfortable (30%), were expensive, or looked silly. Riders younger than 25 years of age or older than 55 years of age, Western-style riders, and men were most likely to believe that helmets were unnecessary or looked silly. Almost two thirds of helmet owners had at least 1 complaint about helmets, most commonly that helmets were too hot or too heavy. However, 41% believed that helmets had prevented at least 1 head injury. Less than half of helmet owners had American Society for Testing Materials (ASTM)-approved helmets.

Conclusion.—To increase the use of helmets, manufacturers will have to improve ventilation or lower heat build-up, improve the fit for adults and children, and make lighter-weight and more attractive helmets.

▶ Helmets can reduce the risk of injuries in horseback riding accidents. As with bicycle helmets, riders must wear helmets for them to be effective. To achieve this, the design and fit of the helmets must be improved.—F.J. George, A.T.C., P.T.

An Evaluation of Cervical Orthoses in Limiting Hyperextension and Lateral Flexion in Football
Hovis WD, Limbird TJ (Vanderbilt Univ, Nashville, Tenn)
Med Sci Sports Exerc 26:872–876, 1994   139-95-1-15

Background.—The cervical nerve pinch syndrome has not been thoroughly researched. Players with such injuries often are placed in a protective orthosis during games and practice to limit hyperextension and lateral flexion, thus protecting them against reinjury. The efficacy of 3 cervical orthoses in restricting hyperextension and lateral flexion in football players was investigated.

Methods and Findings.—Five collegiate football players who routinely wore cervical orthoses while playing participated in the study. The average percent decrease of angular displacement in hyperextension was

A 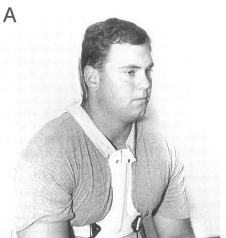 B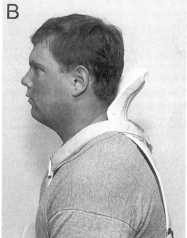

Fig 1–3.—**A**, anteroposterior view of custom orthosis. **B**, tangential view. (Courtesy of Hovis WD, Limbird TJ: *Med Sci Sports Exerc* 26:872–876, 1994.)

3.5% with shoulder pads alone, 33.2% with a neck roll, 32.4% with the Cowboy Collar, and 48.4% with a customized orthosis. The custom brace was most effective in restricting motion, measured as an angular range, compared with the other braces (Fig 1–3). No significant reduction in lateral range of motion was observed.

Conclusion.—All of the braces assessed in this study provided some degree of limitation of hyperextension. However, the braces inconsistently limit lateral bending.

▶ Once an athete has sustained an injury that causes a neurapraxia of a branch of the brachial plexus, it is almost impossible to prevent this injury from recurring. The athletes call them "burners" or "stingers," and they are often worn as a badge of courage. Prevention of this injury must be paramount when coaches teach blocking and tackling techniques. Off-season conditioning programs designed to improve neck, upper back, and shoulder strength are a necessity. Protective equipment should be worn by any athlete who has had a previous injury or may be susceptible to this injury because of the position played, body composition, or poor blocking and tackling technique. However, as G.D. Delforge stated in his comments on this abstract, "As the authors of this article correctly point out. . .the efficacy of cervical collars in restriction of cervical motions that cause 'burners' suffers from a lack of objective substantiation" (1). If the injury occurs, it must be allowed to heal before the athlete returns to participation. The severity of the injury will determine the amount of time an athlete must stay away from competition, which may range from a few minutes to a number of months.—F.J. George, A.T.C., P.T.

Reference

1. Delforge GD: *Athletic Train: Sports Health Care Perspectives* Vol. 1, No. 1, p 87.

Use of the Hollywood Impact Base and Standard Stationary Base to Reduce Sliding and Base-Running Injuries in Baseball and Softball
Sendre RA, Keating TM, Hornak JE, Newitt PA (Central Michigan Univ, Mount Pleasant)
Am J Sports Med 22:450–453, 1994   139-95-1–16

Background.—Baseball and softball are attracting growing numbers of participants. Most significant injuries occurring in baseball and softball players result from sliding and base running. The efficacy of the Hollywood Impact Base in reducing the frequency of sliding and base-running injuries was investigated.

Methods.—Injury data were recorded for several teams that used these bases in addition to standard stationary bases. Injured participants were

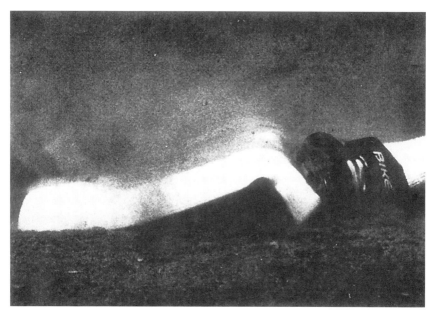

Fig 1–4.—The Hollywood Impact Base compresses as the player slides into it. (Courtesy of Sendre RA, Keating TM, Hornak JE, et al: *Am J Sports Med* 22:450–453, 1994.)

later contacted. Study participants included interscholastic, intercollegiate, recreational, and intramural softball and baseball players.

Findings.—In 1990 and 1991, 33,153 athlete exposures occurred with the impact base, and 3,999 occurred with the standard stationary base. Four injuries could be directly attributed to the standard base compared with 1 attributed to the impact base. The Hollywood Impact Base significantly decreased the frequency of sliding and base-running injuries (Fig 1-4). The injury rate with the impact base was 0.08% per game, which compares favorably with the rate reported with use of a breakaway base.

Conclusion.—Compared with the standard stationary base, the Hollywood Impact Base significantly reduces the possibility of injury in baseball and softball games. These findings are consistent with previous results showing that more injuries in sliding players occur with a stationary base than with a breakaway base.

▶ This study corroborates the findings of Janda et al. (1), who demonstrated that injuries were reduced from 45 per 627 games when the stationary base was used to 2 per 633 games when the breakaway base was used. The implications of the results of these 2 studies are obvious: modifying baseball games can alter the frequency pattern of sliding injuries. The standard stationary base should go the way of spear tackling.

The ball, so to speak, is now in the hands of those responsible for administering the game.—J.S. Torg, M.D.

Reference

1. Janda DH, et al: *JAMA* 259:1848–1850, 1988.

Incidence and Mechanisms of Acute Ankle Inversion Injuries in Volleyball: A Retrospective Cohort Study

Bahr R, Karlsen R, Lian Ø, Øvrebø RV (Norwegian Volleyball Federation, Rud, Norway; Norwegian Univ of Sport and Physical Education, Oslo, Norway)
Am J Sports Med 22:595–600, 1994   139-95-1–17

Introduction.—Ankle sprains account for 25% to 50% of all acute injuries sustained by volleyball players. To develop preventive strategies, the incidence and mechanisms of ankle inversion injuries were retrospectively studied in a group of volleyball players.

Methods.—Data on ankle inversion injuries were obtained by questionnaires returned by 13 men's and 14 women's volleyball teams. General information gathered included the number of training hours per week, the training participation rate, the number of matches played, and players' demographic data. Information gathered on each injury included the use of ankle protection devices, the mechanism of injury, court position, the skill performed at the time of injury, treatment, and absence from training or competition.

Results.—The men averaged 8.6 hours per week of training and played 1.1 matches per week; they sustained 10 injuries during matches and 15 during training. The women averaged 7.7 hours of training and 1 match per week; they sustained 12 injuries during matches and 26 during training. Overall, the relative risk of injury during match play compared with training was 3.9. The mean injury rate among women was 0.8 during training and 2.9 during match play. The mean injury rate among men was 0.5 during training and 2.3 during match play. None of the injured players used prophylactic taping, and 10% wore ankle braces at the time of injury. Injury occurred most frequently in the net zone and were most often caused by landing on another player's foot. Almost all injuries were treated with immediate icing; only 27% received further physician attention. Most injuries were mild to moderate. None required surgical treatment.

Discussion.—Volleyball players sustain approximately 1 ankle inversion injury per 1,000 playing hours. The risk of injury increases considerably during competition, and most injuries are caused by landing on another player's foot after blocking or attacking within the net zone. Therefore, the incidence and severity of these injuries could be reduced by making a rule change (to create a safety zone under the net where no player can step, reducing the incidence of landing on an opponent's foot), increasing technical training (particularly of takeoff and landing techniques), and using prophylactic taping or bracing.

▶ It is noteworthy that 78% of the players injured in this series had experienced previous ankle injuries. The authors raise the question whether inadequate rehabilitation was the reason for the frequency of reinjury. It would appear that, rather than changing rules, a more reasonable approach would be to ensure adequate rehabilitation and prophylactic taping of patients with previous injuries.—J.S. Torg, M.D.

Sledding Trauma in a Northeastern Ontario Community
Wynne AD, Bota GW, Rowe BH (Northeastern Ontario Family Medicine Residency Program, Sudbury, Ont, Canada; Northeastern Ontario Lead Trauma Program, Sudbury Gen Hosp, Sudbury, Ont, Canada; Sudbury Gen Hosp Lead Trauma Programs, Sudbury, Ont, Canada)
J Trauma 37:820–825, 1994   139-95-1–18

Background.—Sledding-related trauma is common, with an estimated 33,000 injuries occurring per year in the United States. Furthermore, such injuries can result in death. According to unpublished data from the Chief Coroner's Office in Ontario, Canada, sledding-related injuries are responsible for 1 death per year. The incidence of sledding injuries was prospectively investigated in a Northeastern Ontario community, as were factors and behaviors associated with these events.

Patients and Methods.—One hundred one patients with sledding-related injuries were included. Data forms for each patient were completed by physicians at 1 of 2 emergency departments in Sudbury, Ontario. Information was verified by examining the emergency room records. Follow-up telephone interviews were then conducted 1–2 weeks after the initial emergency room visit to determine residual disability and requirements for further physician follow-up.

Results.—The mean age of the injured patients was 16 years, with a range of 4–46 years. A higher incidence of injuries was noted among males (59%). The GT-racer, used by 44% of the patients, was the sled type most frequently associated with injury. Most injuries were sustained during periods of suboptimal lighting and on weekends. In addition, most of these events occurred on nondesignated sledding hills. Extremity and spinal trauma was noted in 49% and 17% of the patients, respectively. The mean Injury Severity Score was 2.5, although 7% of the patients were admitted to the hospital and 58% required follow-up by a family physician or specialist. Patients missed an average of 3.7 days of school or work as a result of their injuries.

Conclusion.—Despite their low incidence compared with all traumatic events, sledding accidents can lead to serious injury requiring hospitalization and may result in disability and time lost from work or school. Operator, sled type, and environmental factors play a role in these types of injuries.

▶ Despite the fact that not all the injury forms were completed and exposure data were not available, this is an excellent paper. The authors present a comprehensive analysis of circumstances surrounding sledding injuries as they relate to operator, vehicle, and environment. Also of note was the variety of devices i.e., toboggans, GT-racers, crazy carpets, flying saucers, and inner tubes, as well as classic sleds involved in this activity.—J.S. Torg, M.D.

Comparison of In-Line Skating Injuries With Rollerskating and Skateboarding Injuries
Schieber RA, Branche-Dorsey CM, Ryan GW (Natl Ctr for Injury Prevention and Control, Atlanta, Ga; US Dept of Health and Human Services, Atlanta, Ga)
JAMA 271:1856–1858, 1994   139-95-1–19

Background.—In-line skating is a fast-growing recreational sport in the United States. The risk of injury from in-line skating is unknown. Experienced skaters reach speeds of 10–17 mph. Outdoor skaters share the roadway with motor vehicles, pedestrians, and pets, and they sustain falls on relatively hard surfaces. Estimates of injuries of in-line skaters were compared with estimates of injuries associated with roller skating and skateboarding in a nationwide study.

Methods.—Data were obtained from the National Electronic Injury Surveillance System, which is a random sample of all hospitals in the United States with a 24-hour emergency department. Its probability sample of hospitals offers a reliable estimate of the incidence of injuries related to a given product for the entire nation.

Results.—During the 1-year study, more than 30,800 individuals were treated for injuries related to in-line skating. For every in-line skating injury, there were approximately 3.3 injuries related to roller skating and 1.2 injuries related to skateboarding. The median age of the participants was 15 years for in-line skating, 12 years for roller skating, and 13 years for skateboarding. Of those injured while in-line skating, 63% had a musculoskeletal injury, including 37% with a wrist injury, of which two thirds were fractures, dislocations, or both. Five percent of all the injured in-line skaters had a head injury; and 3.5% of the injured in-line skaters were hospitalized.

Conclusion.—The incidence of injuries related to in-line skating and skateboarding is similar, but it is lower than that of injuries related to roller skating. Wrist protection is needed for participants of all 3 sports. The effectiveness of wrist guards in protecting against sudden, forceful wrist extension should be evaluated. The wearing of helmets is recommended.

▶ This paper represents the first report dealing with in-line skating injuries. The data reported were obtained from the National Electronic Injury Surveillance System (NEISS), which is maintained by the U.S. Consumer Product Safety Commission. There are several problems with data obtained in this manner. First, injury incidence is not discernible. The NEISS data also lack detailed information concerning both the mechanisms of injury and subsequent disability incidence. Also, the database does not include a validated Injury Severity Score or full medical report. Regardless, it would appear that on the basis of 30,000 injuries documented by this report, in-line skating is a significant at-risk activity.—J.S. Torg, M.D.

Incidence of Injury in Indoor Soccer
Lindenfeld TN, Schmitt DJ, Hendy MP, Mangine RE, Noyes FR (Cincinnati Sportsmedicine and Orthopaedic Ctr, Ohio; Deaconess Hosp, Cincinnati, Ohio)
Am J Sports Med 22:364–371, 1994   139-95-1–20

Background.—Until recently, soccer has been considered a minor sport in the United States. The United States Soccer Federation is sponsoring more and more leagues at the youth, high school, and college levels, making soccer the fastest growing team sport in the country. One possible reason for this is the perception that it is a safe sport. Soccer is relatively safe, but injuries do occur. Studies have reported that in Europe, 50% to 60% of all sports injuries and 3.5% of all injuries treated in hospital are related to soccer. The incidence and type of injuries in indoor soccer were explored.

Methods.—An on-field examiner attended all soccer games at an indoor soccer arena and documented all injuries occurring in 7 weeks. The examiner was either a certified medical doctor, a physical therapist, or an athletic trainer. A study representative examined each injury after the game and assisted the injured player in completing a questionnaire.

Results.—A total of 300 games and 2,700 player-hours were monitored. The overall injury rates were similar for male and female players. Male players aged 19–24 years had fewer injuries than expected. Male players aged 25 years or older had the highest injury rate. The most common activity at the time of injury was collision with another player, which accounted for 31% of all injuries; 16% of all injuries occurred when a player was kicked by an opponent. There was no significant difference in the rate of ligament injuries for male and female players. However, male players had a significantly higher rate of overall ankle injuries. Female players had a significantly higher rate of knee ligament injuries than did male players. The injury rates were similar for goalkeepers and non-goalkeepers. Goalkeepers more often injured fingers, heads, elbows or hands, and non-goalkeepers more often injured ankles or thighs.

Discussion.—A large percentage of athletes who play indoor soccer also play outdoor soccer, and the similarity of the 2 populations allows comparisons. Two previous studies have reported both a higher and a lower rate of injury for indoor vs. outdoor soccer. Because of the methods used for data collection, some injuries may have been missed.

▶ It is pointed out that soccer has rapidly increased in popularity because of the perception that it is a safe sport. As stated, "Compared with American football, soccer appears to be a relatively safe sport for younger players, who sustain 2 to 5 times fewer injuries than their counterparts playing football." Similar to football, however, the incidence of injury was observed to increase as the average age of the participants rose. Thus, 14- to 16-year-old players sustained 5 times more injuries than did players under the age of 12 years.—J.S. Torg, M.D.

Save the Trees: A Comparative Review of Skier–Tree Collisions
Friermood TG, Messner DG, Brugman JL, Brennan R (Lakewood Orthopaedic Clinic, Colo; St Anthony's Hosp, Denver)
J Orthop Trauma 8:116–118, 1994   139-95-1–21

Background.—With the growing popularity of alpine skiing, collision injuries have become more frequent. Skier–tree collision injuries were compared with ski injuries not involving collision with a tree.

Methods.—A retrospective review was undertaken of all hospital records of patients admitted to the study hospital from 1981 to 1989 secondary to skiing injuries. Patients were divided into 2 groups: those with injuries related to skier–tree collisions and those who did not collide with a tree.

Results.—One hundred seven of the total 323 (33%) patients admitted for skiing-related injuries were injured as a result of skier–tree injuries. Both groups had similar numbers of beginner, intermediate, and advanced skiers. Those injured in tree collisions were significantly younger and had a significantly greater proportion of male skiers. Skiers injured in tree collisions were, on initial examination, significantly more physiologically unstable as measured by their revised trauma scores and Injury Severity Scores. Skull fractures, head injuries, pulmonary contusions, rib fractures, pneumothoraces, and pelvic fractures were more common in the tree collision group. Mortality was higher among those in tree collisions than other injuries (6.5% vs. 2.3%), but this difference was not significant.

Conclusion.—Skier–tree injuries are increasing because of the increasing speed of skiers and more crowded slopes. There is a need for further data collection on these injuries. Skiers should be made aware that injuries sustained from a skier–tree collision are severe and cause significant mortality.

► This study clearly demonstrates that skiers who hit a tree had a significantly higher Injury Severity Score—a retrospective indicator of the magnitude of the injury—than did skier who did not. Also, 9 skier deaths were reported in Colorado in 1990, 6 of which were caused by skier–tree collisions. Interestingly, the authors state that "one piece of information that is still unclear is why skiers hit trees. Trees are large, highly visible, immovable objects. Luckily, in our series no trees were injured."—J.S. Torg, M.D.

Bungee Jumping and Intraocular Haemorrhage
Jain BK, Talbot EM (Royal Preston Hosp, Fulwood, England)
Br J Ophthalmol 78:236–237, 1994   139-95-1–22

Background.—Bungee jumping involves wearing a full-body or ankle harness attached to a bungee cord. The jumper dives off a 200- to 400-foot-high platform, and approaches but does not touch the ground, rebounds a significant distance, and bounces several times again until stopping. When the participant jumps head first, the load is distributed through the padded shoulder straps or through both legs and hips, depending on the type of harness worn.

Case Report.—Man, 22, bungee-jumped from 200 feet. When released from the harness, he noticed that vision in his right eye was blurred. He was in good general health. On examination, his best corrected vision was 6/9 in the right eye and 6/6 in the left eye. No relative afferent pupillary defect was observed. Anterior segments were normal. Binocular indirect ophthalmoscopy showed subhyaloid hemorrhages nasal to the disc and in the inferior temporal quadrant below the inferior arcade. The latter had ruptured through the internal limiting membrane into the vitreous gel inferiorly. Intraocular pressure was 12 mm Hg. One month later, the patient's blurred vision had cleared, and visual acuity was 6/6, N6 in each eye. The subhyaloid and vitreous gel hemorrhages were resolving.

Discussion.—Rupture of small capillaries and subhyaloid hemorrhage can result from a sudden increase in venous pressure. This patient's hemorrhage resulted from a dive, which increased venous return to the heart; tensed abdominal muscles against a closed glottis, increased venous pressure, and reduced venous return to the head. During acute deceleration, the kinetic energy of the liver might act as a headward plunger on the diaphragm and compress the thoracic contents, thereby additionally increasing thoracic venous pressure, which would be transmitted to the head and neck veins. Other reported complications of bungee jumping include hormonal changes, quadriplegia, and gluteal hematoma.

Ocular Complications Associated With Bungee Jumping

David DB, Mears T, Quinlan MP (Victoria Eye Hosp, Hereford, England)
Br J Ophthalmol 78:234–235, 1994   139-95-1–23

Background.—Bungee jumping originated in the South Pacific islands as a means of initiating boys into manhood. Originally, a length of vine was attached to their legs, but today this is replaced with a bungee rope. Bungee jumping is becoming more and more popular, in spite of lethal accidents caused by miscalculations of the extent to which the rope will stretch and, in 1 case, a jumper who forgot to attach his rope. Other reported complications include a nonfatal hanging injury and quadriplegia secondary to a locked facet joint. One jumper had acute diminution of vision after a bunjee jump.

Case Report.—Man, 31, bungee jumped from 185 feet and remained bobbing up and down in the air for 1 minute. When released from the harness, he noticed his vision was blurred. When he was examined 2 hours later, his unaided vision was right 6/60, not improving with pinhole, and left 6/18, with pinhole 6/9. The anterior segments were normal with clear media, but the fundi had scattered superficial retinal and preretinal hemorrhages and various cotton wool spots in the macular area of each eye. The results of the general and neurologic examinations were normal. The next day, the patient had a subconjunctival hemorrhage in the right eye. One week later, his vision improved to right 6/18 and left 6/6. One month later, the patient's unaided vision was 6/6 in both eyes. There was almost complete resolution of the retinal changes and there were only minimal residual hemorrhages in the right eye.

Discussion.—This retinopathy is typical of Purtscher's traumatic retinal angiopathy believed to be caused by a sudden rise of intravascular pressure in the upper portion of the body, often after sudden compression of the chest. The rise in intravascular pressure is probably a result of the sudden deceleration when the downward momentum of the bungee jumper is overcome by the tensile strength of the cord. Caution is advised in bungee jumping because of these ocular complications in an otherwise healthy person.

▶ The authors' conclusion that "We would advise caution in the sport of bungee jumping in light of the reported ocular complications" is certainly an understatement.—J.S. Torg, M.D.

Deep Snow Immersion Deaths: A Snowboarding Danger

Kizer KW, MacQuarrie MB, Kuhn BJ, Scannell PD (Univ of California, Davis; Tahoe Forest Hosp, Truckee, Calif)
Physician Sportsmed 22:49–50, 55–56, 61, 1994   139-95-1–24

Objective.—Snowboarding is becoming increasingly popular, and the injury rate is rising. More than 95% of snowboarding injuries occur to males between 21 and 30 years of age. After a heavy snowstorm in the Lake Tahoe area, 3 snowboarders died in separate accidents when they became vertically buried head down in the snow. The 3 cases were reported, and suggestions regarding improved education and equipment were made.

Cases.—Three males, aged 15, 22, and 19 years, were found on separate occasions between 2½ and 4½ hours after last seen head down at the base of a tree. All 3 patients were pulseless, cold and stiff, and apneic. Resuscitation efforts failed in all 3 cases.

Surviving Snow Immersion.—Avalanche studies have shown that survival is rare when a person is buried in snow for more than 30 minutes.

Prevention Considerations.—Boarders are advised to find out snow conditions, to know the equipment and be sure it fits, to dress for the weather, not to exceed skills or physical limits, not to go alone in deep powder, to keep edges sharp, not to ski or board when visibility is poor, to stay on groomed trails, to avoid tree wells, to obey signs, to be on the alert for avalanches and know what to do if caught in one, to know the dangers of hypothermia, and not to drink and ski or board.

Equipment Modifications.—The use of contrasting color on the bottom of boards might make it easier to locate victims. Releasable bindings cannot be recommended until more studies are done.

Conclusion.—Snowboarders need to be educated to develop a safety-conscious attitude.

▶ This practical article has useful tips and suggested equipment changes to prevent a new danger of snowboarding: ending up head down and dead at the base of a tree. These 3 deaths show the need for education about the hazards of deep powder, tree wells, and snowboarding outside groomed areas. See also a recent report of a 29-year-old expert male skier who had been drinking alcohol and fell on a difficult slope. He died of bleeding from traumatic transection of the subclavian vein (1).—E.R. Eichner, M.D.

Reference

1. Fiore DC: *Physician Sportsmed* 22:46, 1994.

Biomechanical Factors Associated With Shoe/Pedal Interfaces: Implications for Injury
Gregor RJ, Wheeler JB (Univ of California, Los Angeles)
Sports Med 17:117–131, 1994   139-95-1–25

Background.—Cycling puts considerable strain on the lower extremities, often adversely affecting joint tissues, which typically results in knee injuries. Historically, biomechanical analyses of lower extremity injury in cycling have considered either the rider or the bike and paid little attention to the link between the two. In fact, the mechanics of knee load during the pedaling cycle are affected by the interaction between the rider and the bicycle, primarily at the shoe/pedal interface. The shoe/pedal interface allows for power transmission from the cyclist to the bicycle, but it also results in reactive forces that, in the constrained environment of the pedaling cycle, transmit load to the lower limbs, often contributing to overuse injuries.

Changes in Pedal Designs.—Significant changes in pedal design have been seen during the past decade from traditional toe-clip and strap systems to step-in clipless devices. In response to complaints of knee pain, the cycling component industry developed shoe/pedal interfaces that permit varying degrees of float about the axis perpendicular to the pedal surface, resulting in a toe-in/heel-out and toe-out/heel-in movement. For many years, instrumented force pedal systems have been in use to conduct biomechanical analyses of lower extremity function, including applied pedal forces, intersegmental dynamics, and, more recently, applied pedal torsion. Laboratory studies have shown that torsion at the shoe/pedal interface is a primary factor in load transmission through the lower leg and the resulting moment. Past investigations of the effect of force pedal system incorporating the clipless designs on lower extremity dynamics showed that permitting float at the shoe/pedal interface attenuates the twisting moment M_z at the pedal surface and subsequently reduces predicted knee loads. Cyclists with knee pain tend to have exaggerated M_z patterns compared with those without knee pain, which support the hypothesis that M_z at the pedal surface and M_z at the knee are principal contributors to cycling-related knee pain.

Conclusion.—Cyclists can significantly reduce undesirable knee loads, especially the twisting moment, by using shoe/pedal systems with float features. Although the industry's philosophy that float is good evolved from purely anecdotal evidence, recent scientific studies support recommendations to use float systems as a means of alleviating existing cycling-related knee pain or as a preventive measure. Contrary to concerns circulated in the cycling community regarding the loss of power associated with float systems, these devices have not been found to compromise effective force transmission at the shoe/pedal interface.

▶ This paper represents a comprehensive review of the subject and, as well, includes an extensive list of references.—J.S. Torg, M.D.

Morphological and Clinical Aspects of Heterotopic Ossification in Sports: A Case Study
Bosse A, Wanner KF, Müller K-M (Univ of Bochum, Germany; Martin Luther

Hosp, Bochum, Germany)
Int J Sports Med 15:325–329, 1994   139-95-1–26

Background.—Heterotopic ossification—new bone formation—may originate in muscle tissue, tendons, fascies, and periosteal and subcutaneous fatty tissue. In sports, it is generally the result of injuries, but often no adequate trauma can be identified. A case of heterotopic ossification in sports was presented.

Case Report.—Man, 34, active in cycling and volleyball, was seen with an increasingly painful swelling of the soft tissue of the right proximal femoral adductor. It had been apparent for the past 2 weeks and no evidence of traumatic injury could be established. A firm-to-hard mass was felt in the adductor femoris that was tense, nonpulsatile, noncollapsible, and not warm. Internal rotation and adduction were each terminally restricted by 10 degrees. Radiographs revealed no pathologic findings, whereas ultrasound examination of the femur showed a tumor with clear demarcation from the surrounding soft tissue. The patient refused further radiographic studies, so a surgical procedure was performed. A solid, oval-shaped tumor with clear demarcation from the surrounding muscle tissue was found in the medium part of the musculus adductor longus. No vessels or nerves were compressed, and the tumor was easy to mobilize and showed no connection to the femur. It was excised completely. Pathomorphologic characteristics of the $5 \times 4 \times 2$ cm tumor led to the diagnosis of atraumatic heterotopic ossification. The patient's postoperative course was uneventful, and after 22 weeks, the patient was actively playing volleyball again. There was no recurrence after 16 months of follow-up.

Conclusions.— The nontraumatic variant of heterotopic ossification in sports presents many diagnostic problems. A correct diagnosis will result from a combination of clinical and radiologic findings together with pathomorphologic features.

▶ As pointed out by the authors, "Only exact knowledge of the morphological different stages in the development of heterotopic ossification in combination with the clinical picture, especially radiological findings, will lead to the correct evaluation of heterotopic nontraumatic ossification."—J.S. Torg, M.D.

Corticosteroid Injections: Their Use and Abuse

Fadale PD, Wiggins ME (Brown Univ School of Medicine, Providence, RI)
J Am Acad Orthop Surg 2:133–140, 1994   139-95-1–27

Background.—On the assumption that they will diminish the pain of inflammation and accelerate healing, local injections of corticosteroids are commonly used in orthopedic practice. A literature review was undertaken to identify the indications, mechanism of action, recommendations for use, and methods to avoid complications in corticosteroid therapy in orthopedic disease.

Mechanism of Action.—Produced in the adrenal glands, corticosteroids are naturally occurring 21-carbon steroid hormones that are synthesized from cholesterol. The metabolism of most tissues of the body is affected by them directly or indirectly. Corticosteroids exert their anti-inflammatory effects by inhibiting the synthesis of leukotrienes, prostaglandins, and thromboxanes, thus inhibiting both the cyclooxygenase and lipoxygenase pathways. Because inflammation is an important part of the healing process, corticosteroids can be detrimental.

Selection.—There are a variety of corticosteroid preparations, each with a different plasma half-life and solubility. The decision about which preparation to use should be based on general guidelines. For acute inflammatory conditions, a more water-soluble preparation or a mixture of short- and long-acting preparations is advised. More water-insoluble preparations should be selected for chronic inflammatory conditions. Dosage is not standardized, and the commonly accepted practice is to select the dose on the basis of the size of the area that will receive the injection.

Effects on Types of Tissue.—Intra-articular injections, common in the treatment of osteoarthritis and rheumatoid arthritis, have varying results, apparently depending on the joint treated. For example, little benefit is reported for injections into the hip or the knee, whereas smaller joints, like the carpometacarpal, seem to have a better response. Chronic back pain has not been effectively treated with intra-articular facet injections, with the exception of pain caused by facet-joint degenerative cysts. Steroid injection into the periligamentous tissue is a common and controversial treatment for ligamentous injury. Only extremely judicious use of corticosteroids in and around an injured ligament is warranted. Some forms of tendinitis and tenosynovitis respond well to steroid injection, but here, too, a conservative approach is warranted. A number of peripheral nerve compression syndromes are treated with corticosteroid injection, most commonly carpal tunnel syndrome. Steroid injection into unicameral bone cysts is an accepted treatment, often requiring 2 or 3 injections to succeed.

Injection Technique.—Sterile gloves are worn for all injections of corticosteroids. The injection is made after antiseptic cleansing, palpation of landmarks, and cutaneous anesthesia. For small joints, a 0.5-inch, 30-gauge needle is used; a 1.5-inch, 25-gauge needle is used in larger or deeper joints.

Contraindications.—An absolute contraindication for corticosteroid injection is infection of the proposed area. Injections should not be made directly into a ligament or tendon. Multiple injections should be avoided, with the exception of unicameral bone cysts, rheumatoid arthritis, and selected cases of osteoarthritis.

▌ The authors present a comprehensive review of the place of corticosteroid injections in clinical practice. Appropriately, they point out that "there is a paucity of well-controlled studies that provide definitive recommendations for nonrheumatologic use of corticosteroids." However, they do believe that the use of corticosteroids is appropriate in those conditions that have been proven to be positively influenced by them. In my own experience, such conditions include traumatic hemarthrosis, traumatic myositis, and nonligamentous soft tissue trauma.—J.S. Torg, M.D.

The Goalkeeper's Fear of the Nets

Scerri GV, Ratcliffe RJ (Canniesburn Hosp, Bearsden, Glasgow, Scotland)
J Hand Surg (Br) 19-B:4:459–460, 1994   139-95-1–28

Introduction.—The soccer goalkeeper is highly respected for a willingness to be exposed to physical injury. Considerable psychological morbidity may also attend this activity. Injuries may occur even before the game begins.

Series.—Three goalkeepers incurred ring avulsion injuries when the goal nets were being set up before kickoff. All were amateur players and were less than 1.68 meters tall, requiring them to jump to reach the hooks with which the net is attached to the crossbar. The patients failed to wear gloves. Injuries occurred when a finger ring caught on 1 of the hooks. One player had an amputation at the proximal interphalangeal joint level and another distal to this joint (Fig 1–5). The third patient had

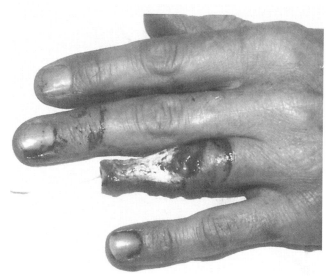

Fig 1–5.—An injury sustained in which there was a complete amputation and therefore an Urbaniak grade 3 injury. (Courtesy of Scerri GV, Ratcliffe RJ: *J Hand Surg (Br)* 19-B:4:459–460, 1994.)

a degloving injury and a middle phalangeal shaft fracture; the avulsion was incomplete.

Suggestions.—A safer device for attaching the goal net might prevent these injuries. Amateur goalkeepers should use a ladder if necessary.

▶ It would appear that wearing no rings and wearing gloves would be the solution to this problem.—J.S. Torg, M.D.

Discrepancies in Perceptions Held by Injured Athletes and Athletic Trainers During the Initial Injury Evaluation
Kahanov L, Fairchild PC (San Francisco State Univ, Calif; Univ of Arizona, Tucson)
J Athletic Train 29:70–75, 1994   139-95-1–29

Background.—The importance of effective communication between athletic trainers and athletes has recently been highlighted. The nature of this communication was investigated during the initial injury evaluation, and attempts were made to identify whether the resulting perceptions held by the athlete and the trainer were similar.

Method.—Fifty collegiate athletes who were injured during the 1992–1993 athletic season and 6 athletic trainers who did their initial injury evaluation completed a questionnaire. The questions examined the effectiveness of the trainer's communication in relation to the athlete's understanding of the injury and rehabilitation program, objective elements of the interchange, the athlete's frame of reference, short-term and long-term goals, and the development of a rehabilitation strategy and a written rehabilitation protocol. The yes–no answers to the questionnaire were put into an agreement matrix on the basis of agreement-disagreement between the athletic trainer and the athlete for each item.

Results.—Significant disagreement was seen between the trainer and the athlete regarding the athlete's understanding of the rehabilitation program, the athlete's frame of reference related to the comfort and motivation level, 2 items related to type of communication, whether objectives and goals were discussed, and whether the athlete was given a written protocol. There was agreement between the two parties only on 1 item: whether the trainer asked questions.

Discussion.—There is a significant lack of communication between athletic trainers and athletes regarding the nature of the injury and the rehabilitation program. It is well known that the athlete's perceptions of the injury and the program greatly affect his or her compliance with rehabilitation. It is therefore the trainer's responsibility to influence these perceptions so that maximum motivation and adherence to the program are achieved. An essential feature of good communication is the maintenance of eye contact. This indicates attentiveness on the part of the trainer and evokes trust in the athlete. Distractions that interrupt the evaluation lead to a breakdown of communication and trust. Therefore, an important skill for the trainer to develop is active listening, which involves rephrasing back to the athlete not only the athlete's verbal messages but also his or her nonverbal messages.

Conclusion.—A significant number of athletes failed to understand rehabilitation strategies because of poor communication during the initial evaluation with athletic trainers. It is thus important for trainers to develop stronger communication skills. Undergraduate and graduate training programs should incorporate communication skills instruction into their curriculum.

▶ This study was an eye-opener for me. Too often, we believe that because we have said something, patients understand what we have said. Communication is a skill that all athletic trainers must develop if they are to be effective. After an evaluation or the development of a rehabilitation program, the athlete should be asked a very simple question: "Do you understand . . . ?" They should know what their injury involves and the what and why of the treatment and rehabilitation program. Goals should be set that involve a time frame for their accomplishment. The more serious the injury, the more involved this communication process becomes.—F.J. George, A.T.C., P.T.

2 Shoulder and Upper Extremity

Anatomy and Actions of the Trapezius Muscle
Johnson G, Bogduk N, Nowitzke A, House D (Univ of Newcastle upon Tyne, England; The Univ of Newcastle, New South Wales, Australia)
Clin Biomech 9:44–50, 1994

139-95-2–1

Objective.—There are notable inconsistencies between and within published descriptions of the trapezius muscle and its actions. None of the descriptions provide sufficiently detailed data on the point-to-point attachments of the trapezius for use in biomechanical modeling. The anatomy of the trapezius and its functions were formally reappraised.

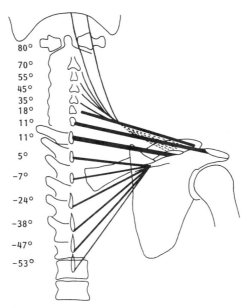

Fig 2–1.—Tracing of a radiograph of a normal individual standing upright at rest, on which the disposition of the fibers of trapezius has been depicted. The lines depicting the various fascicles have been drawn semiquantitatively to depict their relative size in terms of cross-sectional area. The orientations of the fascicles are indicated in degrees from the horizontal. (Courtesy of Johnson G, Bogduk N, Nowitzke A, et al: *Clin Biomech* 9:44–50, 1994.)

Methods and Findings.—The cervical trapezius was dissected bilaterally in 2 elderly adult cadavers, including the thoracic trapezius in 3 cadavers and the entire trapezius in 2 cadavers. The occipital and nuchal fibers of the muscle passed transversely, with only a slight downward inclination, to insert into the clavicle (Fig 2–1). The acromion and spine of the scapula received transversely oriented fibers from C7 and T1, and the thoracic fibers of the trapezius converged to the deltoid tubercle of the scapula. On volumetric studies, the fibers from C7, T1, and the lower half of the ligamentum nuchae were found to be the largest.

Conclusion.—Because the upper and middle fibers of the trapezius muscle are essentially oriented transversely, their commonly described action as being elevators of the scapula is impossible. Instead, these fibers act to draw the scapula and clavicle backward or to raise the scapula by rotating the clavicle about the sternoclavicular joint. The cervical spine is relieved of compression loads through balancing moments of the trapezius.

▶ This article may come as a surprise to those who learned in their human anatomy class that the function of the trapezius was to elevate the scapula. The authors also emphasized the role of the sternoclavicular joint in sustaining downward loads that are applied to the upper limbs.—Col. J.L. Anderson, PE.D.

Subjective and Objective Evaluation of Shoulder Muscle Fatigue
Öberg T, Sandsjö L, Kadefors R (Univ College of Health Sciences, Jönköping, Sweden; Chalmers Univ of Technology, Göteborg, Sweden; Lindholmen Development Ctr, Göteborg, Sweden)
Ergonomics 37:1323–1333, 1994 139-95-2–2

Background.—Although the colloquial definition of "fatigue" is well known, as a scientific concept the term is poorly defined. Fatigue can be quantified by both psychological and physiologic methods; characterization of this interrelationship is an important question of validity. The respective objective and subjective signs of fatigue, as represented by mean power frequency (MPF) and the Borg's category rating (CR) scale, were compared in the trapezius muscle at different load levels to determine whether these methods of fatigue measurement provided essentially equivalent information.

Results.—Twenty healthy volunteers exposed their right trapezius muscle by raising their arm to 90 degrees of abduction and performed 2 contractions: a 0-kg hand load over a 5-minute period and a 2-kg hand load over a 2.5-minute period. A significant correlation occurred between MPF and CR scores at the high but not at the low load level. A linear decrease of MPF with increasing load dose occurred at the high load level; however, despite significant reported research subject fatigue, the MPF did not change at the low load level. Category rating scores showed a linear rise with increased load dose that was more pronounced at the high load level.

Conclusion.—Essentially the same information was not provided by the MPF and CR scores, at least not at the lower load levels, which are common to many static load situations in working life. Therefore, MPF may be unsatisfactory as an estimator of localized muscle fatigue in the trapezius muscle. The MPF changes in muscle fatigue may be the result of the opposing actions of the fatigue of currently active motor units and the recruitment of new motor units. The fatiguing effects dominate at high load levels, but they are counterbalanced by recruitment of new motor units at low load levels. The differences in subjective fatigue observed at high and low load levels may be explained by the nonlinear relationship between load dose and endurance time. If load and running time are treated as separate variables, the results may be better explained, because the subjective sensation of fatigue seems to be more closely connected to the load itself than to the load dose.

▶ These questions have been studied for years. What is fatigue? Is it better measured using physiologic or psychological variables? Some people appear to withstand fatigue better than others. I think we will all agree that this is a mental phenomenon that is probably learned through practice.—Col. J.L. Anderson, PE.D.

The Normal and the Painful Shoulders During the Breaststroke: Electromyographic and Cinematographic Analysis of Twelve Muscles
Ruwe PA, Pink M, Jobe FW, Perry J, Scovazzo ML (Centinela Hosp Med Ctr, Inglewood, Calif)
Am J Sports Med 22:789–796, 1994   139-95-2–3

Introduction.—The electrical muscle activity patterns in 12 shoulder muscles used during the breaststroke were described and compared (Fig 2-2) in competitive swimmers with normal and painful shoulders.

Methods.—A total of 25 normal and 14 painful shoulders were evaluated in 34 collegiate and master's level competitive swimmers. Respectively, swimmers with normal and painful shoulders had a mean of 9 and 11 years of competitive swimming, trained 2,500–4,000 and 2,500–3,700 meters daily, 3–5 times weekly, and had a mean age of 39 and 31 years. Testing was done in pools equipped with underwater windows. High-speed cameras recorded pull-through and recovery phases of the stroke cycle. Electromyograms and maximal isometric manual muscle tests (MMTs) for 12 shoulder muscles were recorded with swimmers resting and swimming.

Results.—During pull-through, activity was increased in the subscapularis muscle and decreased in swimmers with painful shoulders. This resulted in a relative internal rotation of the shoulder, with subsequent

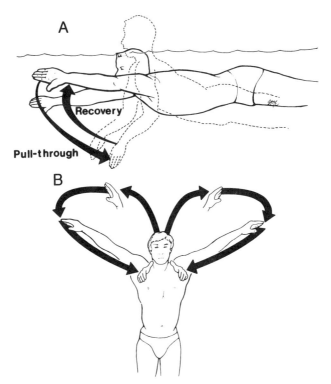

Fig 2–2.—Phases of the breaststroke. (Courtesy of Ruwe PA, Pink M, Jobe FW, et al: *Am J Sports Med* 22:789–796, 1994.)

predisposition to impingement in the forward flexed position. During recovery, significantly decreased activity in the middle deltoid, upper trapezius, and supraspinatus was observed in swimmers with painful shoulders. Impingement was exacerbated by decreased supraspinatus activity, allowing proximal migration during middle-to-late recovery, and by decreased scapular elevation resulting from decreased upper trapezius muscle function. The serratus anterior and teres minor muscles fired at or above 15% of MMT consistently throughout the breaststroke cycle and were therefore subject to fatigue.

Conclusion.—Rehabilitation efforts for swimmers with painful shoulders should focus on building endurance of the serratus anterior and teres minor muscles and reestablishing the balance between the internal and external rotators and the deltoid and supraspinatus muscles.

▶ Rehabilitation of the shoulder muscle is very difficult because of the complicated muscular patterns that comprise it. It is not a job for an amateur personal trainer, as these authors point out.—Col. J.L. Anderson, PE.D.

EMG Mean Power Frequency: Obtaining a Reference Value

Öberg T, Sandsjö L, Kadefors R (Univ College of Health Sciences, Jönköping, Sweden; Univ of Linköping, Sweden; Univ of Technology and Lindholmen Development Ctr, Göteborg, Sweden)
Clin Biomech 9:253–257, 1994

139-95-2-4

Background.—The mean power frequency (MPF) and the median frequency are the 2 single parameters most often used to estimate muscle fatigue as measured with electromyographic (EMG) techniques. Factors such as skin impedance and electrode position have a negative effect on the standardization of EMG data. Procedures for establishing a reference value for normalization of MPF that can counteract these negative effects were compared, and the best method for establishing a reference value was identified.

Method.—Twenty healthy adults with no shoulder pathology were included. Five procedures were studied with the research subjects in a seated position: calibration contractions with a 0-kg hand load (twice) and a 2-kg hand load, and regression routines with a 0-kg and a 2-kg hand load (Fig 2–3). Data on EMG were recorded by electrodes placed over the right trapezius muscle. The reference value was designated as being the mean of 20 segments. A random design analysis of variance and regression analysis were used to analyze data.

Results.—Only the between-subject variation was statistically significant. The variance caused by routine, load, and time could be included in the error variance. No significant interaction effects were found with routine, load, and time.

Conclusion.—To determine a reference value, the following method is recommended: Elevate the straight arm with the hand loaded with a 2-kg weight to 90 degrees of abduction in the scapular plane. Record the

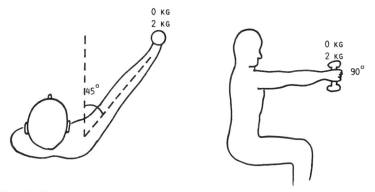

Fig 2–3.—Test position and hand loads for testing different routines to establish an initial reference value. (Courtesy of Öberg T, Sandsjö L, Kadefors R: *Clin Biomech* 9:253–257, 1994.)

EMG for 10 seconds. Repeat this procedure several times, with rest periods of 20 seconds between contractions.

▶ The authors provide a recommended method for determining an EMG MPF reference value using the trapezius muscle. They suggest that this procedure, using short, repeated 10-second calibration contractions, is a more practical way of establishing the reference value than is the more complicated regression routine. They believe that this procedure could also be applied to other muscles.—Col. J.L. Anderson, PE.D.

Magnetic Resonance Imaging of the Glenoid Labrum in Anterior Shoulder Instability

Green MR, Christensen KP (Tripler Army Med Ctr, Honolulu, Hawaii)
Am J Sports Med 22:493–498, 1994   139-95-2-5

Objective.—Because an accurate assessment of the glenoid labrum is a key aspect of treating shoulder problems, the results of MRI were compared with the surgical findings in a prospective double-blind series of 33 patients with possible anterior shoulder instability.

Method.—Both T1 and T2 images were recorded at 3-mm multiplane cuts using a 1.5-T unit and a shoulder coil. All studies were interpreted by the same radiologist before operative assessment.

Findings.—Of 28 patients who were found to have a detached glenoid labrum and inferior glenohumeral ligament complex, 21 (75%) were correctly diagnosed by preoperative MRI. The examination was 100% specific and had an overall accuracy of 79%. Its respective positive and negative predictive values were 10% and 41%. Only 21% of labra were correctly classified by MRI, and it was seldom possible to precisely determine the site and size of the tear or detachment.

Conclusion.—Current MR techniques cannot reliably distinguish between glenoid labral lesions that are reparable arthroscopically and those that are not.

▶ This is an extremely limited investigation in which 28 patients were reviewed by a single radiologist. The conclusions of the authors, with reference to the MRI evaluation of the glenoid labrum for anterior shoulder instability (e.g., "We recommend careful discretion and very restrictive use . . .") are not warranted. Their comparison of a noninvasive technique (MRI) with an invasive and costly diagnostic procedure (arthroscopy) is not appropriate for the investigation of subtle instability, especially in those instances in which repair may not be indicated.

Magnetic resonance imaging is an evolving tool for which imaging sequences and interpreter expertise are improving exponentially. The accuracy of the MR examination for the interpretation of the glenoid labrum can be directly correlated with the time, effort, and experience of the interpreter and the MR protocol and units used. When surgical intervention is based on an MR interpretation, it is prudent for the surgeon to be fully aware of the experience of the radiologist.—J.S. Torg, M.D.

Labral-Ligamentous Complex of the Shoulder: Evaluation With MR Arthrography

Palmer WE, Brown JH, Rosenthal DI (Massachusetts Gen Hosp, Boston)
Radiology 190:645–651, 1994   139-95-2–6

Background.—Instability of the shoulder can be caused by a number of different pathologic processes. The articular surfaces, the glenoid labrum, the glenohumeral ligaments (GHLs), and the rotator cuff are the structures most often involved. Of the GHLs stabilizing the joint, the inferior may have the most critical function. The use of MRI has met with only limited success in diagnosing shoulder problems. Arthrography, in combination with MRI, was examined after injecting the joint with the contrast medium gadopentetate dimeglumine. This technique was examined in diagnosing the labral-ligamentous complex and the significance of inferior GHL strength in shoulder instability.

Materials and Methods.—Magnetic resonance images of the shoulder were obtained from 121 consecutive patients with clinically suspected rotator cuff or labral injury. Of them, 48 later received an examination of the labrum by arthroscopy or open surgery; these patients were enrolled in this study. Nine of the patients had previous surgery on the shoulder. Gadopentetate dimeglumine was injected into the joint 30 minutes before the MRIs were obtained with a 1.5-T scanner. Radiologists reading the scans were blinded to information about the patients; they based their judgment of whether the labra were normal, torn, or deficient on the MRI evidence. The results indicated that MRI was capable of imaging displaced and partially attached labral tears (Fig 2-4). The GHLs were identified by MRI, and they were fully examined and assessed. During surgery, the exact location of labral abnormalities were noted relative to the position of the GHL.

Results.—Surgical examination revealed 14 normal, 29 torn, and 6 deficient labra. Using these observations as a gold standard, MRI was 91% sensitive, 93% specific, and 92% accurate. Excluding those with previous shoulder surgery, only 3 of the 45 patients did not have a superior GHL, and 2 of the 3 reported recurrent dislocations. Considerable variability was seen in the exact configuration of the GHL. Ninety-two percent of the torn labra occurred at the origin of 1 of the GHLs. Anterior instability was diagnosed in 23 of these shoulders; in 22 MRI identified a labral tear or a defective inferior GHL attachment. Tears were not seen at the position of the inferior GHL in patients without instability.

Discussion.—Magnetic resonance imaging is a good method for diagnosing labral injury; tears can be visualized with a high degree of sensitivity and specificity. This is particularly important in cases of anterior joint

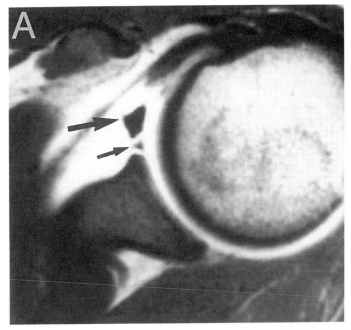

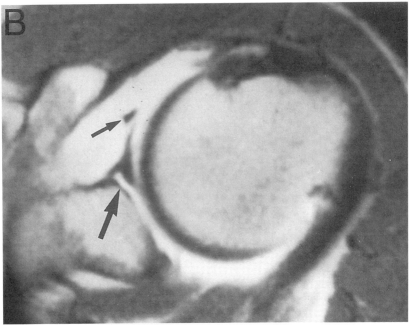

(continued)

instability, where MRI can be used to determine the stability of labral injury associated with the inferior GHL attachment site.

▶ Although MR arthrography is an interesting adjunct to conventional MRI, it adds time, pain, possible infection, and additional cost to an otherwise noninvasive, painless, and already expensive study. Although the sensitivity and specificity are impressive, this study is limited, with only 32 patients having surgical confirmation. Additional investigations that use newer sequences and image acquisition on conventional MR should be explored before invasive MR arthrography is advocated for the routine evaluation of the labral ligamentous complex.—J.S. Torg, M.D.

Prevalence of Latent and Manifest Suprascapular Neuropathy in High-Performance Volleyball Players
Holzgraefe M, Kukowski B, Eggert S (Univ Hosp, Göttingen, Germany)
Br J Sports Med 28:177–179, 1994   139-95-2-7

Introduction.—Whereas direct trauma is the most common cause of acute isolated lesions of the suprascapular nerve, chronic nerve damage usually results from an entrapment neuropathy. The nerve is usually compressed as it traverses the suprascapular notch, possibly as a result of repetitive microtrauma caused by forceful movements around the shoulder joint. This mechanism has been reported in tennis and volleyball players, weight lifters, and boxers. The features of suprascapular neuropathy include weakness of abduction and external rotation of the arm as a result of supraspinatus and infraspinatus muscle denervation, often with vague shoulder pain. Clinical and electrophysiologic assessments were used to screen high-level volleyball players for latent and manifest suprascapular neuropathy.

Methods.—The study included 30 players from the top German men's volleyball team. In addition to history and clinical examination, all had concentric needle electromyographic recordings from 5 different regions of the supraspinatus and infraspinatus muscles on both sides. Clinical examinations were also completed in another 36 international-level men's volleyball players.

Fig 2–4   (cont).

Fig 2–4.—Displaced and partially attached labral tears in (**A**) a male patient 24 years of age and (**B**) a male patient 32 years of age. **A**, after intra-articular injection of gadopentetate dimeglumine, T1-weighted (repetition time ms/echo time ms = 450/18) axial MR arthrogram at the level of the subscapularis tendon shows a thick middle glenohumeral ligament (MGHL) (*large arrow*) and detached labral fragment (*small arrow*) that has been displaced from the glenoid rim. **B**, T1-weighted (450/18) axial MR image from another patient. The MGHL (*small arrow*) is smaller than that in (**A**), but it is clearly distinguished from the glenoid labrum. A linear region of contrast material (*large arrow*) extends under the anterior labrum, which remains partially attached to the glenoid rim. (Courtesy of Palmer WE, Brown JH, Rosenthal DI: *Radiology* 190:645-651, 1994.)

Findings.—Four of the 30 German athletes had severe atrophy of the infraspinatus muscle, with dull pain in the lateral shoulder. All had marked paresis of external arm rotation; they denied any impairment in playing their sport but had some difficulty with daily activities. These athletes all had EMG evidence of complete denervation of the infraspinatus muscle—with more than 3 fibrillations and a loss of recruitable motor unit potentials—and chronic nerve damage in the supraspinatus muscle. Another 8 players had electromyographic evidence of partial denervation of both the supraspinatus and infraspinatus muscles, despite having normal clinical findings. All cases of suprascapular neuropathy were on the same side as the player's smashing arm. Severe infraspinatus muscle atrophy was also found on clinical examination in 10 of the 36 international players.

Conclusion.—As many as one third of top-level volleyball players may show evidence of suprascapular neuropathy. Early diagnosis of this condition is key to preventing more severe damage. Careful monitoring of suprascapular nerve function may be beneficial in high-performance volleyball players.

▶ Once again, a severe penalty is being incurred by playing a sport at the international level. The suprascapular nerve is fixed at 3 points: its origin, the suprascapular notch, and the lateral edge of the scapula. Because both the supraspinatus and infraspinatus muscles are affected, the suprascapular notch seems to be the likely site of injury. The problem, as in other sports, is excessive training—a top player makes more than 1,000 maximum-force serves per week. The lesion is particularly insidious because most of the affected players do not note any deterioration in their competitive performance. This suggests the importance of regular examinations of volleyball competitors for this type of nerve injury.—R.J. Shephard, M.D., Ph.D., D.P.E.

Use of the Suture Anchor in Open Bankart Reconstruction: A Follow-Up Report
Levine WN, Richmond JC, Donaldson WR (Tufts Univ, Boston)
Am J Sports Med 22:723–726, 1994   139-95-2–8

Background.—Bankart's reconstructive method for shoulder dislocation has high success and minimal recurrence rates, but it is technically difficult. A technical modification—the use of a suture anchor—was introduced to facilitate the Bankart repair. Long-term follow-up data on patients undergoing this procedure were analyzed.

Methods and Findings.—Fifty-three patients with recurrent anterior glenohumeral instability underwent a modified Bankart reconstruction with the use of a suture anchor between April 1988 and August 1991. Thirty-two met the inclusion criteria of an identifiable Bankart lesion, an open repair with suture anchors, and a minimum 2-year follow-up. Four patients were lost to follow-up. No complications resulted from this technique. Ninety-three percent of the patients had objectively excellent or good results. Two failures occurred with recurrent anterior dislocation.

Conclusion.—The suture anchor used in this series enables the surgeon to reattach the capsulolabral complex to the glenoid rim. The use of curved drill holes, large metallic implants, special awls, or osteotomes can be avoided. However, to avoid technical failure careful attention to anchor placement at the junction of articular cartilage and the glenoid neck is needed.

Soft Tissue Reconstruction in the Shoulder: Comparison of Suture Anchors, Absorbable Staples, and Absorbable Tacks
Shall LM, Cawley PW (Orthopaedic Associates of Virginia, Ltd, Norfolk; Smith & Nephew DonJoy, Carlsbad, Calif)
Am J Sports Med 22:715–718, 1994   139-95-2–9

Introduction.—Anterior instability of the shoulder, which is common in throwing athletes, was traditionally treated with open repair. Increasingly, however, open techniques, including stapling and Bankart technique modifications, are being adapted to arthroscopic procedures. There have been a number of complications related to stapling techniques, prompting the development of new soft tissue–to–bone anchoring devices especially for use in arthroscopic procedures. The failure strengths and modes of failure were studied in 3 of these devices.

Methods.—The glenoid, scapular neck, and a 5-cm blade of the scapular body along with a segment of the subscapularis tendon for each specimen were removed from 20 cadaveric shoulders and prepared for soft tissue repair. The repairs were performed at a randomly selected site on the anterior glenoid (superior, middle, or inferior) with a randomly selected anchor device (the Mitek SuperAnchor, Acufex 8-mm Suretac, or Instrument Makar Staple). The glenoid specimen was fixed in a cylinder in a 3-axis vise with a humeral head surrogate. Force and displacement data were obtained with a computerized system.

Results.—The SuperAnchor demonstrated a significantly higher ultimate failure load than the Instrument Makar Staple or the Suretac, which were comparable. Suture breakage at the knot was the predominant mode of failure for the SuperAnchor, whereas 93.75% of the Suretac failures resulted from the staples pulling out of bone. Staple breakage and pullout from bone were both common modes of failure with the Instrument Makar Staple.

Discussion.—The SuperAnchor device withstood forces to failure that were nearly twice those withstood by the 2 bioabsorbable devices, and it rarely pulled out from the bone. These data may be useful in determining the degree of aggressiveness of the postoperative rehabilitation protocol. However, these data do not consider other important factors that have an impact on the success of ligament repair, including biocompatibility and host effects.

▶ The suture anchor is a first-generation device manufactured by Mitek Surgical Products of Norwood, Massachusetts. It has been my experience that use of this device renders the open Bankart procedure user-friendly. Notably, the authors point out that it is rare for the anchor to pull out of bone and that the majority of failures were suture knot failures.—J.S. Torg, M.D.

Arthroscopic Repair of Combined Bankart and Superior Labral Detachment Anterior and Posterior Lesions: Technique and Preliminary Results

Warner JJP, Kann S, Marks P (Univ of Pittsburgh, Pa)
Arthroscopy 10:383–391, 1994   139-95-2–10

Background.—The superior labral detachment anterior and posterior (SLAP) lesion is now a recognized cause of shoulder pain. However, its incidence and treatment remain controversial.

Methods.—From 1991 to 1993, 585 arthroscopic and open procedures were performed for shoulder pain. Nine of the patients were found to have a SLAP lesion. Seven patients also had a Bankart lesion and had arthroscopic repair of the entire anterior-inferior-superior-posterior labral detachment using the Suretac fixation device. The technique required an accessory anterolateral portal access to the superior-posterior labral detachment and an accessory anteroinferior portal to access the Bankart lesion. Three to 4 Suretacs were needed in these patients.

Outcomes.—At a mean follow-up of 19 months, 5 of 7 patients had no pain, full range of motion, and a full premorbid activity level. One patient had a redislocation at 4 months after surgery and was managed successfully with arthroscopic release and manipulation.

Conclusion.—The technique used was helpful for managing extensive labral detachment in selected patients. In 2 of the 3 patients undergoing second-look arthroscopy, the labral repair had healed. Five of the 7 patients resumed sports participation that required overhead reaching. No complications occurred.

▶ The small size of this series and the short long-term follow-up do not support the conclusion of the authors that "this arthroscopic technique is a useful method to manage extension labral detachment in selected patients." However, considering the alternatives, this approach is certainly not unreasonable.—J.S. Torg, M.D.

Functional Outcomes in Athletes After Modified Anterior Capsulolabral Reconstruction

Montgomery WH III, Jobe FW (Kerlan-Jobe Orthopaedic Clinic, Inglewood, Calif)

Am J Sports Med 22:352–358, 1994   139-95-2–11

Introduction.—The anterior capsulolabral reconstruction was developed for athletes with anterior glenohumeral instability who participate in overhead activities. The results with a modification of the anterior capsulolabral reconstruction were reviewed. The modification involved the use of a horizontal capsulotomy rather than a T capsulotomy and Mitek suture anchors rather than drill holes.

Technique.—After the drill holes are made near the glenoid rim at approximately the 3-, 4-, and 5:30-o'clock positions, the Mitek anchors with No. 2 braided nonabsorbable suture are placed in each hole, with the single barb facing away from the articular surface. (Fig 2–5). Tension is placed on each suture to set the anchors. The superior flap is shifted inferiorly, thereby overlapping and reinforcing the inferior flap (Fig 2–6). The remaining gap in the capsule is loosely closed. The reconstruction has 2 layers of reinforced capsule outside the joint (Fig 2–7).

Patients.—During a 7-month period, 32 athletes with recurrent anterior subluxation or dislocation who had failed to respond to conservative treatment underwent the modified procedure. All but 1 were involved in overhead athletics. Thirty-one patients were available for follow-up study, which included physical examination, radiography, and an interview.

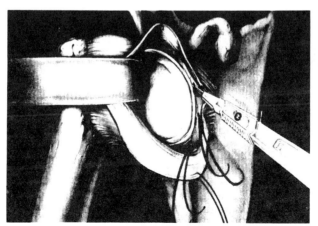

Fig 2–5.—Placement of the Mitek anchors. (Courtesy of Montgomery WH III, Jobe FW: *Am J Sports Med* 22:352–358, 1994.)

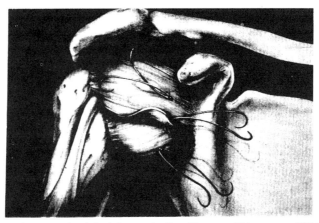

Fig 2–6.—Inferior capsular shift of the superior flap. (Courtesy of Montgomery WH III, Jobe FW: *Am J Sports Med* 22:352–358, 1994.)

Results.—After a follow-up of 24–31 months, the objective results were excellent in 24 patients (77%) and good in 6 (20%). The operation was considered a failure in 1 patient (3%) who had an episode of recurrent instability secondary to a new traumatic event. Rehabilitation therapy enabled him to return to competitive swimming at the previous level. All patients were satisfied with the outcome. Twenty-five patients (81%) were able to return to their sports at the same level of competition after an average of 12 months; 4 (13%) returned to the same sport but at a lower level of competition; and 2 (6%) did not return to competitive sports. At follow-up, none of the patients had positive impingement signs or a positive relocation test, and only 2 patients had lost 5–15 de-

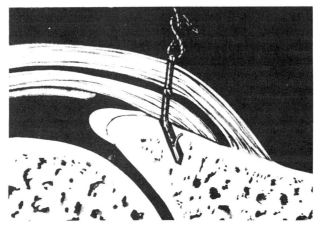

Fig 2–7.—Cross-section of the reconstruction. (Courtesy of Montgomery WH III, Jobe FW: *Am J Sports Med* 22:352–358, 1994.)

grees of shoulder motion. Three baseball pitchers with posterior shoulder pain underwent arthroscopic débridement of the posterior labrum.

Conclusion.—The modified anterior capsulolabral reconstruction using Mitek suture anchors and horizontal capsulotomy simplified the original procedure and allowed more aggressive early rehabilitation.

Inferior Capsular Shift Procedure for Anterior-Inferior Shoulder Instability in Athletes
Bigliani LU, Kurzweil PR, Schwartzbach CC, Wolfe IN, Flatow EL (New York Orthopaedic Hosp; Columbia-Presbyterian Med Ctr, New York)
Am J Sports Med 22:578–584, 1994   139-95-2–12

Introduction.—Recurrent anterior glenohumeral instability can disable athletes. Many of those in overhead sports are unable to return, despite operative repair. The tendency today is to perform a more anatomical repair by correcting the actual lesion, which generally consists of both capsular laxity and avulsion of the glenohumeral ligament from the glenoid.

Series.—Sixty-three athletic patients had 68 shoulders repaired by an anteroinferior capsular shift operation. They included 42 men and 21 women whose average age was 23 years. Patients with a glenoid fracture, mainly posterior instability, or only anterior instability were not included. Forty-two patients, including all 31 overhead-throwing athletes, had their dominant arm operated on. Forty-six shoulders had recurrent anterior dislocations and 22 had recurrent subluxation.

Management.—The extent of capsular shift was geared to the degree of laxity found at exploration. The inferior capsule was mobilized and shifted in 56 of the 68 operated shoulders. Twenty-one patients had repair of the capsular detachment to the glenoid rim before undergoing a capsular shift. At first, the arm was kept in a sling for 6 weeks, but exercises out of the sling were allowed after 10 days.

Results.—The average follow-up was 4 years. The outcome was rated as excellent in 67% of patients, good in 27%, and fair in 3%. Two patients had a poor result. Ninety-two percent of patients returned to their previous sports activity, the majority of them at the same competitive level. However, 5 of the 10 elite throwing athletes could not compete as well as before. Loss of external rotation averaged 7 degrees, and the average forward elevation was 175 degrees. Two patients had a recurrent dislocation after a violent fall.

Conclusion.—More than 90% of the athletic patients had excellent or good results and were able to return to sports activity, although not always at the same competitive level.

Arthroscopic Bankart Repair Versus Nonoperative Treatment for Acute, Initial Anterior Shoulder Dislocations

Arciero RA, Wheeler JH, Ryan JB, McBride JT (United States Military Academy, West Point, NY)
Am J Sports Med 22:589–594, 1994   139-95-2-13

Background.—Traditionally, traumatic anterior shoulder dislocations are managed nonoperatively when they first occur, but recurrences continue to be frequent in young patients. Recurrent shoulder instability impeded the academic progress and athletic activities of cadets.

Objective.—The outcome of acute first-time traumatic anterior shoulder dislocation that was managed nonoperatively was compared with the result of arthroscopic Bankart repair.

Patient Population.—Only patients who lacked a history of impingement or occult subluxation were included in the study. All required manual reduction of the dislocation. The 36 athletes in the study had an average age of 20 years. Fifteen patients had their extremity immobilized for 1 month and were then rehabilitated. Full activity was allowed at 4 months. Twenty-one other patients had arthroscopic repair.

Results.—Twelve of the 15 conservatively treated patients (80%) had recurrent instability during an average follow-up of 23 months. Collision sports were responsible in most instances. Seven patients had an open Bankart repair. Two of the patients without recurrent instability were rated as having an excellent and 1 a good outcome. During an average follow-up of 32 months, 86% of the arthroscopically treated patients were free of recurrent instability and had returned to their preinjury levels of participation. There were 3 recurrences, all of which occurred during collision sports. Three patients had postoperative complications.

Recommendation.—Young, active patients with an initial traumatic anterior shoulder dislocation are currently offered an arthroscopic repair. However, should instability recur, an open repair can be carried out.

▶ Abstracts 139-95-2–11, 139-95-2–12, and 139-95-2–13 describe 2 open and 1 arthroscopic technique for addressing the pathoanatomy responsible for glenohumeral instability. Montgomery and Jobe report 77% excellent results, with an average follow-up of 27 months. Bigliani and associates report 67% excellent results, with an average of 4 years of follow-up. Arciero and co-workers report an 86% success rate, with an average follow-up of 32 months.

Because no surgical procedure for glenohumeral instability has truly withstood the test of time (that is, a minimum follow-up of 10 years), these investigators are encouraged to reevaluate these groups after adequate long-term follow-up. It is hoped that these procedures will not go the way of all other operations for glenohumeral instability.—J.S. Torg, M.D.

Electromyographic Biofeedback Use in the Treatment of Voluntary Posterior Dislocation of the Shoulder: A Case Study
Young MS (Orthopedic and Sports Physical Therapy, Mission Viejo, Calif)
J Orthop Sports Phys Ther 20:171–175, 1994   139-95-2–14

Introduction.—In 3 previous case studies, electromyographic biofeedback has been used successfully as a nonsurgical treatment measure for voluntary posterior dislocation of the shoulder. This condition is the result of voluntary muscle action in which habitual or voluntary instability can begin with minor or no trauma in the adolescent years. A case report of the successful use of electromyographic biofeedback was described.

Case Report.—Girl, 15 years, could voluntarily dislocate both shoulders, and her right shoulder dislocated easily with gymnastics. She had participated in a weight training program to strengthen her shoulder; however, she could not reduce her shoulder herself and required medical intervention. She had pain at the tuberosity with resistance to external rotation. She initially began treatment that emphasized strengthening the rotator cuff. An electromyographic study showed that the posterior deltoid muscle was not active during forward flexion, descent from forward flexion, and dislocation. During the electromyographic biofeedback program, the patient reeducated the posterior deltoid muscle and was discharged after 5 weeks of treatment with a home biofeedback unit. She resumed therapy 6 months later when she dislocated her shoulder, and she indicated that she had stopped her home exercises. After 8 weeks of biofeedback therapy, she was discharged and returned to sports. One year later, her shoulder had not dislocated.

Protocol.—The protocol involved a clinical program and a home exercise program. A dual-channel biofeedback unit was used in which 1 electrode was placed on the posterior deltoid muscle and the other was placed on the anterior deltoid, allowing the patient to compare the output of the 2 muscles. The program included 30 minutes of exercises. She used isometric exercises to isolate the muscle with auditory and visual feedback from the monitor. She practiced humeral flexion and external rotation. If her shoulder was about to dislocate, she was told to stop what she was doing.

Discussion.—To ensure effective results, the exercise program should be continued over a long period. Using biofeedback, the patient could prevent dislocation of her shoulder by recruiting the posterior deltoid. A larger sample size is needed to confirm the effectiveness of this treatment; a long-term follow-up also would be beneficial.

▶ The use of biofeedback to train muscles has been shown to be effective in some studies. As the authors note, more studies with larger numbers of subjects that use controls and proper scientific protocol must be done to prove the effectiveness of this modality.—F.J. George, A.T.C., P.T.

Rehabilitation Following Total Shoulder Arthroplasty

Brems JJ (Cleveland Clinic Found, Ohio)
Clin Orthop 307:70–85, 1994   139-95-2-15

Background.—A successful total shoulder arthroplasty depends on a well-designed and well-executed physical therapy program. Proper post-arthroplasty rehabilitation should follow a logical sequence that allows for tissue healing, joint mobilization, and muscle strengthening. More-over, the patient must participate actively and not be a passive receiver of care. Preoperative and postoperative steps for such rehabilitation were presented.

Preoperative Rehabilitation.—The therapist should meet with the patient before surgery, examine the involved shoulder for range of motion (ROM) and muscle tone, and discuss these findings with the patient and surgeon. The therapist will discuss pain and stiffness and the ROM program that follows joint replacement. Effective communication between the therapist and the patient and between the therapist and the surgeon is essential to the success of the rehabilitation program. Examination of the joint should include assessment of external rotation, which is best carried out with the patient supine and the elbow held off the table by towels to maintain the long axis of the humerus parallel to the long axis of the spine and body of the scapula (Fig 2–8). The elbow should be brought away from the side to establish perpendicularity between the long axis of the humerus and the central axis of the glenoid, allowing for maximal capsule relaxation, which enables improved external rotation (Fig 2–9).

Rehabilitation Program.—Four principles should be followed in establishing a program: (1) initiate rehabilitation as early as possible; (2) allow

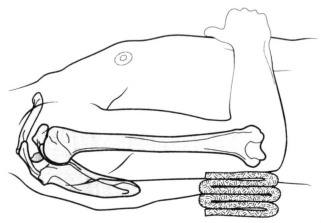

Fig 2–8.—Supine external rotation. Patient lies supine with the elbow held off the table by towels to maintain the long axis of the humerus parallel to the long axis of the spine and body of the scapula. (Courtesy of Brems JJ: *Clin Orthop* 307:70–85, 1994.)

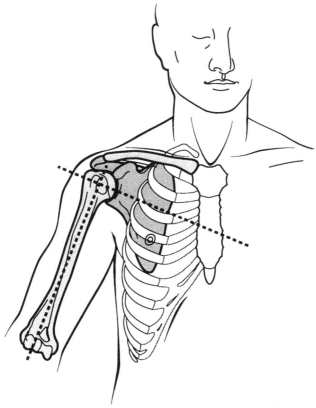

Fig 2–9.—Supine passive external rotation. The elbow should be brought away from the side to establish perpendicularity between the long axis of the humerus and the central axis of the glenoid. This ensures maximal capsule relaxation allowing improved external rotation. (Courtesy of Brems JJ: *Clin Orthop* 307:70-85, 1994.)

early active motion; (3) eliminate or limit the use of supportive devices such as slings and immobilizers; and (4) maximize passive joint motion in the cardinal planes before starting a strengthening program. Frequent short periods of stretching exercises are more helpful than fewer prolonged sessions. It is preferable to spend no more than 5 minutes 3 or 4 times daily in therapy to avoid prolonged periods of pain. The program should start with phase 1 stretching 24–48 hours after surgery. Phase 2 stretching should begin after suture removal. Phase 3 should begin anywhere from 3 to 6 weeks later. As the patient progresses through the stretching programs, strengthening programs can begin.

Conclusion.—Proper rehabilitation after total shoulder replacement is critical to a successful outcome. The role of the surgeon is to direct, modify, and evaluate the progress of the program. Rehabilitation normally begins 48 hours after surgery, starting with joint mobilization to maximize ROM in the cardinal planes. Strengthening follows and proceeds in a stepwise fashion until maximum strength has been attained.

▶ This is an excellent teaching article on techniques to use in the evaluation process and the rehabilitation program. The author has outlined a sound philosophical approach to rehabilitation, stressing early active motion with short (5 minutes) and frequent (3–4 times daily) bouts of exercise.

A number of different rehabilitation exercises with adequate explanations are described and illustrated in this article. These illustrations could easily be reproduced for the patient to use in a home exercise program. This article stresses the importance of the surgeon's ongoing involvement in the rehabilitation process as well as the responsibility of the patient as an active participant.—F.J. George, A.T.C., P.T.

The Effect of Medical Exercise Therapy on a Patient With Chronic Supraspinatus Tendinitis. Diagnostic Ultrasound—Tissue Regeneration: A Case Study

Torstensen TA, Meen HD, Stiris M (Centre for Physiotherapy Research and Development, Oslo, Norway; Norwegian Univ of Sports and Physical Education, Oslo Norway; Univ of Oslo, Norway)
J Orthop Sports Phys Ther 20:319–327, 1994   139-95-2-16

Objective.—Supraspinatus or impinging syndrome can cause tendinitis and degeneration of the rotator cuff; this syndrome can have many causes. A recent study showed that supervised exercise was just as effective and much less expensive than arthroscopic surgery in treating it. The amount, type, and effect of exercise in regenerating low metabolic tissue was examined in a patient with chronic supraspinatus syndrome.

Case Report.—Man, 73, was physically active until he experienced a sharp pain in his right shoulder. Chronic supraspinatus syndrome was diagnosed. After almost 1 year and 12 ultrasound sessions, physiotherapy, analgesics, and steroid injections, he did not improve. At this time he received a diagnosis of rotator cuff dysfunction caused by chronic supraspinatus tendinitis. He had pain that limited his range of motion, and an ultrasound scan showed a widening of the tendon from inflammation with no rupture.

Treatment.—The patient received a personal medical exercise program with 4 or 5 other patients. In phase 1, the patient was rendered symptom free using graded exercises and performing the required movements at least 1,000 times at each 1-hour session. When free of pain, the patient progressed to phase 2, which provided increased weight resistance to improve tolerance for loading. Nine exercises were repeated 3 times with 30–40 repetitions per set. The patient received fifty-six 1-hour treatments during a period of about 5 months. The width of the tendon decreased by 1.4 mm, and 4 years later the patient was as physically active as before the injury, with no symptoms.

Conclusion.—Chronic supraspinatus syndrome can be treated successfully with graded exercises alone. Ultrasound is a valuable diagnostic tool.

▶ The authors note that their findings are encouraging and support the possibility of tendon repair using biomechanical stresses from exercise. They go on to observe that most treatment regimens for chronic supraspinatus syndrome fail because they are directed at relieving the pain by only applying passive treatment modalities instead of giving the tendon biomechanical stresses that stimulate regeneration through graded exercises. Another factor is that most treatment methods aim to treat "the painful spot" and forget that the supraspinatus has to be treated in its functional setting together with the other rotator cuff, shoulder girdle, and arm muscles."

The exercises in this program were performed within the pain-free range-of-motion areas. They were performed using specifically designed apparatus. Treatment sessions lasted at least 1 hour. Exercises were done in a group of 4–5 patients. Very high numbers of repetitions with light resistance were used in the first phase. As the symptoms improved, lower repetitions with increased resistance were used.

This is an interesting concept of exercise that was developed in Norway. It produced good results in this case study. More studies with larger numbers of subjects should be done to repeat the results reported by these authors.—F.J. George, A.T.C., P.T.

Isolated Paralysis of the Infraspinatus Muscle

Takagishi K, Saitoh A, Tonegawa M, Ikeda T, Itoman M (Kitasato Univ, Japan)
J Bone Joint Surg (Br) 76-B:584–587, 1994   139-95-2–17

Introduction.—Isolated paralysis of the infraspinatus muscle is thought to be rare and therefore is seldom considered in the differential diagnosis of patients with shoulder pain and muscle weakness. Six patients with isolated paralysis of the infraspinatus were studied.

Patients.—Six men aged 17–42 years had consultations for shoulder pain and weakness. Five patients had been active in sports for at least 5 years. Physical examination showed atrophy of the infraspinatus muscle but not the supraspinatus and weakness of external rotation and abduction. Electromyography confirmed isolated paralysis of the infraspinatus muscle. Radiographs were normal. Ultrasonography showed space-occupying lesions in 4 patients and infraspinatus atrophy in 2. Fast-scan MRI was normal in 2 and not performed in 1. These 3 patients were managed conservatively. The MRI scans of the other 3 patients showed space-occupying lesions at the spinoglenoid notch (Fig 2–10). These 3 patients were operated on after conservative treatment had failed. A ganglion

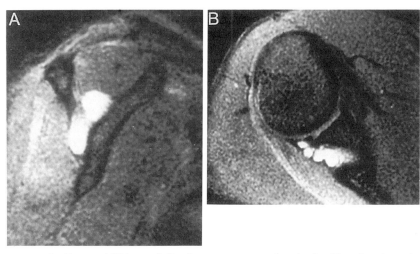

Fig 2–10.—Fast-scan MRI in case 2. Ganglion cysts are seen at the spinoglenoid notch on images in the sagittal oblique plane **(A)** and the horizontal plane **(B)**. (Courtesy of Takagishi K, Saitoh A, Tonegawa M, et al: *J Bone Joint Surg (Br)* 76-B:584–587, 1994.)

arising from the posterior capsule of the shoulder that compressed the inferior branch of the suprascapular nerve was found and removed in all 3 patients. The fourth patient, who had a space-occupying lesion, was managed conservatively with good results.

Outcome.—After a mean follow-up of 33 months, all patients were free of pain and had returned to full activity. Reinnervation was confirmed by electromyography in 5 patients; 1 patient did not undergo electromyography.

Conclusion.—Isolated paralysis of the infraspinatus muscle caused by ganglia is not as uncommon as was previously thought.

▶ Fritz and associates pointed out that ganglion cysts in the spinoglenoid notch can result in both supraspinatus and infraspinatus muscle involvement if there is proximal suprascapular nerve entrapment, whereas isolated atrophy of the infraspinatus muscle is associated with posteriorally located masses and distal nerve entrapment (1). Involvement of 1 or both of these muscles is an indication for MRI.—J.S. Torg, M.D.

Reference

1. Fritz RC, Helms CA, Steinbach LS, et al: Suprascapular nerve entrapment: Evaluation with MR imaging. *Radiology* 182:437–444, 1992.

Posterior Ossification of the Shoulder: The Bennett Lesion

Ferrari JD, Ferrari DA, Coumas J, Pappas AM (Univ of Massachusetts,

Worcester)
Am J Sports Med 22:171–176, 1994   139-95-2–18

Background.—The Bennett lesion is an extra-articular ossification of the posterior inferior glenoid that can occur in throwing athletes. The records of all athletes treated for a Bennett lesion during a 6-year period were evaluated.

Patients.—Between 1985 and 1991, 7 elite baseball players with shoulder pain underwent arthroscopic examination, plain radiography, and CT or MRI. In addition to generalized nonspecific shoulder complaints, all players had pain on palpation of the posterior glenoid.

Findings.—Arthroscopic examination identified posterior labral lesions in all cases. Four players also had posterior rotator cuff fibrillation and 2 had posterior undersurface rotator cuff tears. None of the players had an anterior capsular injury or posteroinferior glenoid ossification. The lesions were débrided arthroscopically; none required operative re-

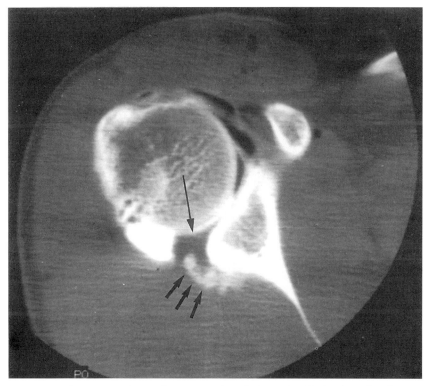

Fig 2–11.—A repeat examination shows progressive soft tissue mineralization (*arrow*) and a new posterior labral tear (*thin arrow*), which was confirmed at arthroscopy. Computed tomography-arthrogram shows posterior subluxation of the humeral head with reference to the bony glenoid. (Courtesy of Ferrari JD, Ferrari DA, Coumas J, et al: *Am J Sports Med* 22:171-176, 1994.)

moval. Rehabilitation therapy was usually started 1–2 months after arthroscopic surgery. After an average postoperative follow-up of 41 months, 6 of the 7 players had returned to preinjury performance levels, and 1 had stopped playing competitive baseball. This player had the most tissue damage, including a posterior labral and capsular tear, because he had continued to throw after the lesion had been diagnosed (Fig 2–11).

Conclusion.—A Bennett lesion should be suspected in throwing athletes who complain of posterior shoulder pain and have posterior tenderness on palpation. The mechanism responsible for the production of this lesion is still unknown.

▶ It is important to note that the authors think that "operative removal of the lesion is not necessary, but that arthroscopic treatment of the associated intra-articular pathologic tissue is warranted. Furthermore, arthroscopic removal of the extra-articular Bennett lesion with the synovial resector may jeopardize the integrity of the posterior capsule."—J.S. Torg, M.D.

Interscalene Brachial Plexus Block for Shoulder Surgery

Tetzlaff JE, Yoon HJ, Brems J (Cleveland Clinic Found, Ohio)
Reg Anesth 19:339–343, 1994   139-95-2–19

Objective.—The efficacy of interscalene brachial plexus block was evaluated as the primary anesthesia for shoulder surgery.

Procedures.—Between 1984 and 1990, 676 reconstructive surgical procedures of the shoulder were performed. Of these, 563 were performed under interscalene brachial plexus block alone and 117 under general anesthesia. The majority of the interscalene blocks involved intentional elicitation of paresthesia, and only 32 involved nerve stimulation. The most frequently used agent was 1.4% mepivacaine with 1:200,000 epinephrine followed by 0.625% bupivacaine and 0.5% bupivacaine.

Outcome.—Of the 563 interscalene blocks attempted, 39 required general anesthesia either to initiate or complete the surgery, for an overall success rate of 94.1%. Twenty failures occurred in the 0.5% bupivacaine group, 10 in the mepivacaine group, and 9 in the 0.625% bupivacaine group. Operative blood loss was significantly less with interscalene anesthesia compared with general anesthesia, particularly with rotator cuff repairs. Mean blood loss was also less, although not significantly, for total shoulder replacement and capsular advancements under interscalene block. Other complications included 2 seizures and 2 subdural injections.

Conclusion.—Interscalene brachial plexus block is a satisfactory anesthesia for elective reconstructive surgery of the shoulder; it has a high success rate and good safety.

▶ We initially reported the use of interscalene brachial plexus block anesthesia for shoulder surgery in 1982 (1). It is refreshing to see that others have finally come around to accepting our view that it is an effective and practical anesthetic for both major and minor orthopedic procedures involving the shoulder.—J.S. Torg, M.D.

Reference

1. Mitchell EI, Murphy FL, Wyche MQ, et al: Interscalene brachial plexus block anesthesia for the modified Bristow procedure. *Am J Sports Med* 10:79–81, 1982.

Atraumatic Osteolysis of the Distal Clavicle
Slawski DP, Cahill BR (Great Plains Sports Medicine and Rehabilitation Ctr, Peoria, Ill)
Am J Sports Med 22:267–271, 1994   139-95-2–20

Introduction.—Athletes and those doing manual work are at risk of osteolysis of the distal clavicle developing without incurring acute shoulder trauma. Repeated loading of the acromioclavicular joint appears to be responsible. Excision of the distal clavicle is warranted if conservative measures are ineffective.

Patients.—Fourteen patients with atraumatic osteolysis of the distal clavicle who had failed to respond adequately to conservative management had 17 open operations to excise the distal clavicle. Twelve patients engaged in weight training and 2 repeatedly lifted heavy objects overhead in their work. Conservative measures had been tried for at least 6 months. The average patient age at the time of operation was 28 years.

Surgery.—The distal clavicle was directly exposed, subperiosteal dissection was carried out, and the distal 1–2 cm of the bone was removed. Patients began motion immediately after surgery and returned to activities as tolerated. A sling was used to provide comfort for no longer than 48 hours.

Results.—All patients returned to sports and employment an average of 9 weeks after surgery with no sacrifice of competitiveness or productivity. Eight patients had an excellent outcome, and 9 had a good outcome, as judged by the University of California at Los Angeles Shoulder Rating scores. Eight patients had some residual pain, and 3 were slightly restricted in their activities. During an average follow-up of 25 months, 7 of the 10 patients who had unilateral clavicular excisions had symptoms develop on the other side.

Discussion.—Distal clavicular excision is an effective approach to atraumatic osteolysis that does not respond to conservative treatment.

Patients should be aware of the high risk that symptoms may ultimately develop on the unaffected side.

▶ Reporting on what they describe as nontraumatic clavicular osteolysis, Scavenius and Iversen (1) noted a 28% prevalence of this problem in weight lifters. Patients were treated surgically with open arthrotomy of the acromio-clavicular joint. Recently, others (2, 3) have reported and I have experienced results using arthroscopic resection of the distal clavicle comparable to those used in conventional open surgery.—J.S. Torg, M.D.

References

1. Scavenius M, Iversen BF: Nontraumatic clavicular osteolysis in weight lifters. *Am J Sports Med* 20:463–467, 1992.
2. Jartsman GM: Arthroscopic resection of the acromioclavicular joint. *Am J Sports Med* 21:71–77, 1993.
3. Flatow EL, et al: Arthroscopic resection of the outer end of the clavicle from a superior approach: A critical, quantitative radiographic assessment of bone removal. *Arthroscopy* 8:55–64, 1992.

Rupture of the Distal Biceps Tendon: Evaluation With MR Imaging
Falchook FS, Zlatkin MB, Erbacher GE, Moulton JS, Bisset GS, Murphy BJ
(Univ of Miami, Fla; Mem Hosp, Hollywood, Fla; Univ of Cincinnati, Ohio)
Radiology 190:659–663, 1994   139-95-2-21

Background.—A distal biceps tendon tear is diagnosed in 3% of all biceps tendon injuries, and it occurs most often in males older than 40 years. The dominant arm is usually involved, and the injury is usually palpable as a defect at the distal tendon and a lump in the region of the retracted muscle. Rupture of the distal biceps tendon is a relatively rare event as is the use of MRI in diagnosing elbow complaints. Descriptions of MRI use in cases of distal biceps rupture are even less common. Possibly because clinical findings alone are often enough to make diagnoses of the elbow, little is known about the MRI of pathologic lesions. Images of ruptures were obtained to determine the usefulness of MRI in this condition.

Materials and Methods.—A retrospective evaluation of all elbow imagings during a 3-year period at 3 institutions was undertaken, and 20 images with suspected injury to the distal tendon were found. Eight healthy volunteers submitted to MRI assessment of the elbow as controls. Imaging of the volunteers and 14 of the patients took place with a 1.5-T unit. One patient was imaged with a 0.5-T unit and 5 with a 1.0-T unit. Standard MRI protocols were used. All images were evaluated by blinded radiologists who were experienced in musculoskeletal imaging. The biceps tendon was assessed for tendinosis, which was present if there was an intratendinous signal intensity on long repetition time (TR)/short echo time (TE) images that attenuated with long TR/TE images. Tenosynovitis was diagnosed when fluid was present, whether these conditions prevailed or not. Partial tendon tears were indicated by the presence of fluid on long TR/TE images at the distal tendon but without evidence of tendon retraction. Complete rupture was indicated when the distal tendon was not seen at the insertion site, the sheath was full of fluid, the retracted distal tendon could be seen proximally, and edema or hemorrhage was present in tissues surrounding the tendon.

Results.—The biceps tendon follows a complicated course and is best imaged by axial and sagittal sections. Of the 20 patients, 10 had a diagnosis of complete tendon rupture. Two patients had tendinosis or tenosynovitis. Two others had abnormalities of the muscle. Seven of 10 ruptures diagnosed with MRI were confirmed surgically.

Discussion.—Although imaging may not be needed in most cases of distal biceps tendon rupture, it can be a helpful adjunct in difficult-to-diagnose cases of elbow injury or in distinguishing complete from partial tears.

▶ Rupture of the distal biceps tendon is an uncommon clinical entity that is seen with typical signs and symptoms for which further imaging may not be indicated. However, in patients with an atypical presentation, e.g., a palpable mass unrelated to trauma, MRI is an excellent method of diagnosis. The MR examination sensitivity in differentiating a complete from a partial tendon tear can be beneficial in determining the appropriateness of aggressive management and surgical intervention.—J.S. Torg, M.D.

Brachial Artery Compression by the Lacertus Fibrosus

Bassett FH III, Spinner RJ, Schroeter TA (Duke Univ, Durham, NC)
Clin Orthop 307:110–116, 1994   139-95-2-22

Introduction.—Five patients had classic findings of compression of the brachial artery at the level of the elbow by the lacertus fibrosis, or bicipital aponeurosis. All study patients were men aged 17–36 years.

Clinical Findings.—All patients had findings of intermittent claudication, including pallor of the hand, paresthesias in the fingertips, cramping pain in the forearm and anteromedial aspect of the elbow, and easy fatigability. The symptoms were worsened by raising the hand overhead or pronating the forearm. No patient had a history of trauma. The forearm muscles appeared hypertrophic. Resisted elbow flexion or pronation of the forearm obliterated the radial pulse and also reproduced the symptoms. The pulse deficit was confirmed by Doppler study. Two patients also had findings of ulnar neuropathy at the elbow.

Management.—Surgery was done after conservative measures had failed. Four patients had surgery under local anesthesia. An incision in the antecubital fossa revealed a tight lacertus fibrosis indenting the brachial artery (Fig 2–12). The structure was fully released and partially ex-

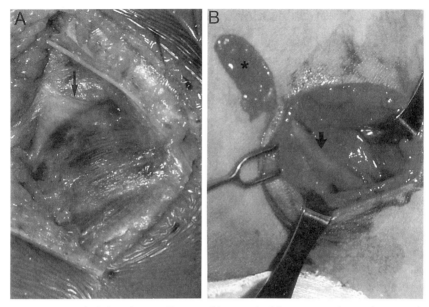

Fig 2–12.—A, the bulging lacertus fibrosus and hypertrophied forearm musculature. The proximal edge of the lacertus fibrosus can be seen (*arrow*). **B,** indentation of the brachial artery (*arrow*) and excised lacertus fibrosis (*asterisk*). (Courtesy of Bassett FH III, Spinner RJ, Schroeter TA: *Clin Orthop* 307:110–116, 1994.)

cised. In 1 of the patients with coexisting ulnar neuropathy, the nerve was transposed subcutaneously.

Results.—Four of the patients had dramatic relief and could resume their normal work and athletic activities within 3 weeks. One patient subsequently had ulnar nerve decompression but continued to have symptoms of brachial artery compression. Symptoms of musculocutaneous nerve entrapment developed in 1 patient, who did well after decompression.

Conclusion.—Hypertrophy of the elbow muscles and lacertus fibrosis from excessive use can produce vascular, neural, or combined neurovascular lesions.

▶ Although I cannot recall having recognized intermittent claudication resulting from brachial artery compression by the lacertus fibrosus, the authors certainly present a well-documented experience with this problem. What is somewhat ambiguous is the most precise and preferred method of establishing the diagnosis. Differential blood pressure cuff measurements, Doppler findings, CT scans, MRI and MR or dynamic angiography, electromyography, and nerve conduction studies are mentioned. However, no precise diagnostic criteria have been established.—J.S. Torg, M.D.

Preoperative Evaluation of the Ulnar Collateral Ligament by Magnetic Resonance Imaging and Computed Tomography Arthrography: Evaluation in 25 Baseball Players With Surgical Confirmation

Timmerman LA, Schwartz ML, Andrews JR (American Sports Medicine Inst, Birmingham, Ala)

Am J Sports Med 22:26–32, 1994   139-95-2–23

Background.—Elbow pain is a frequent complaint of baseball pitchers, which is not surprising, as pitching imposes huge valgus forces across the medial side of the elbow, consequently stretching the soft tissues at this site. The chief stabilizer to valgus stress at the elbow is the anterior bundle of the ulnar collateral ligament (UCL). The cause of medial elbow pain in a thrower may be difficult to identify noninvasively.

Objective and Methods.—Twenty-five consecutive baseball players seen in a 6-month period with persistent pain in the medial side of the elbow prospectively underwent CT arthrography and MRI, followed by arthroscopic assessment. If an abnormal UCL was present, the ligament was examined at open operation.

Arthroscopic and Operative Findings.—Valgus laxity was evident in 15 patients at arthroscopy. Four patients had osteophytes of the posteromedial olecranon, and 3 had loose bodies. Only 5 patients had normal arthroscopic findings. Valgus instability was not very evident clinically in most cases. It was consistently associated with an abnormal anterior bundle of the UCL. Open surgery revealed an abnormal UCL in 16 of the 19 patients who underwent exploration. There were 7 full-thickness and 7 partial tears as well as 2 degenerated, lax ligaments. In 14 patients, the anterior bundle was reconstructed using autogenous palmaris longus tendon or toe extensor tendon. Two ligaments were directly repaired.

Imaging Results.—Computed tomographic arthrography was 86% sensitive in detecting tears of the UCL and it was positive in all 7 patients having full-thickness injuries. The study was 91% specific. Five of the 7 patients with partial tears had contrast leakage about the detachment of the ligament from its bony insertion. Magnetic resonance imaging was 57% sensitive, and all complete ligament tears were also detected. The MR study was totally specific.

Clinical Correlations.—A tender UCL was a very nonspecific finding, but it was 94% sensitive in detecting an abnormal ligament. Valgus instability testing correlated only moderately with the operative findings. The valgus extension overload test was negative in several patients with osteophytes or an abnormal UCL.

Conclusions.—Both CT arthrography and MRI accurately detect complete tears of the UCL. Computed tomographic arthrography is preferred at present, although contrast MRI might provide comparable diagnostic results.

▶ The authors document similar accuracies between MRI and the CT arthrogram for diagnosing a complete tear of the UCL; however, the CT arthrogram is more sensitive for evaluating partial undersurface tears. This article is severely compromised by the inadequate description of the MRI method used (e.g., multiplanar, using a 5-inch general-purpose surface coil).

The sensitivity of an MRI examination is dependent not only on the observer's acumen˙ and familiarity with various injury patterns but also on the manner in which the MRI examination is performed. Various sequences, imaging planes, slice thicknesses, and 3-dimensional acquisitions are required to demonstrate subtle findings. The newer fast spin-echo sequences with fat suppression are especially sensitive to subtle muscle and tendon injuries. For the authors to promote an invasive, time-consuming CT arthrographic modality vs. a noninvasive MRI modality on the basis of this study is not justified.—J.S. Torg, M.D.

Stress Radiography of the Medial Elbow Ligaments
Rijke AM, Goitz HT, McCue FC, Andrews JR, Berr SS (Univ of Virginia Health Sciences Ctr, Charlottesville; Alabama Sports Medicine Inst, Birmingham; Henry Ford Hosp, Detroit)
Radiology 191:213–216, 1994   139-95-2–24

Background.—In baseball players and other athletes, injury to the ligaments of the elbow joint is relatively common. The usefulness of stress radiography in assessing injury to the medial collateral ligament (MCL) was investigated.

Methods.—Forty-two injured and 4 asymptomatic athletes were examined with a stress device. The increase in joint space width between the medial epicondyle and coronoid process was measured on anteroposterior radiographs obtained after 0- and 15-daN force was applied to the lateral elbow joint. That measurement was then used to assess the extent of ligament tear. The validity of this method was tested on selectively severed cadaveric MCLs.

Findings.—When the increase in the width of joint space was greater by 0.5 mm in the affected elbow compared with the opposite normal elbow, all complete and large partial tears were diagnosed correctly with stress radiography. In research subjects in whom the measurements were less than 0.5 mm, the MCLs were normal or showed a small tear that could be managed with conservative treatment.

Conclusion.—Stress radiography performed with commercially available equipment with force monitoring ability can be used to accurately diagnose the extent of injury to the medial elbow ligaments. Large or complete tears and small or normal ligaments can be distinguished with

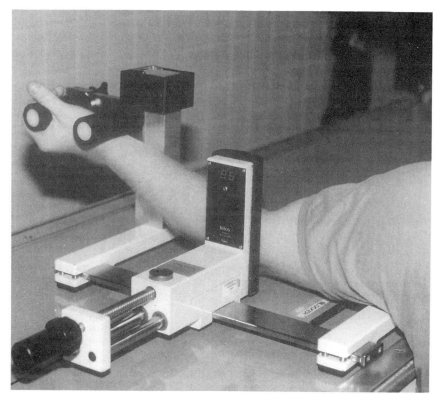

Fig 2–13.—Illustration of stress examination of the left elbow joint. (Courtesy of Rijke AM, Goitz HT, McCue FC, et al: *Radiology* 191:213–216, 1994.)

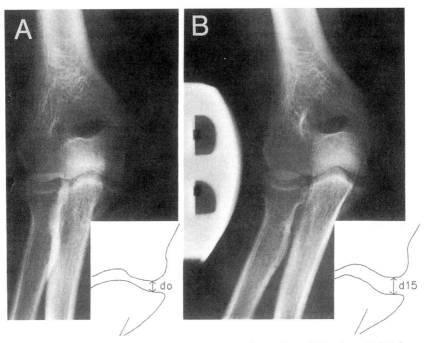

Fig 2–14.—Anteroposterior radiograph of left elbow with **(A)** 0 force (*d0*) and **(B)** 15 daN force (*d15*) applied to the radiohumeral joint shows increase in medial joint spacing. (Courtesy of Rijke AM, Goitz HT, McCue FC, et al: *Radiology* 191:213-216, 1994.)

great accuracy. The technique is cost-effective and can be done in less than 10 minutes (Figs 2–13 and 2–14).

Histology and Arthroscopic Anatomy of the Ulnar Collateral Ligament of the Elbow

Timmerman LA, Andrews JR (American Sports Medicine Inst, Birmingham, Ala)
Am J Sports Med 22:667–673, 1994   139-95-2–25

Introduction.—Injuries to the ulnar collateral ligament can result in symptomatic medial instability of the elbow, particularly in throwing athletes. Arthroscopy can be a useful adjuvant in the evaluation of elbow pain; however, the intra-articular arthroscopic appearance of the ulnar collateral ligament and its anatomical relationship to the medial capsule have not been clearly defined. A series of cadaveric studies were performed to evaluate the histology and arthroscopic anatomy of the ulnar collateral ligament.

Methods and Findings.—Ten fresh-frozen paired cadaveric elbows—one joint was used for arthroscopy and the other for histologic examination—were examined. The medial capsule comprised 2 layers of collagen fibers. There were 2 distinct ligamentous bundles corresponding to the anterior and posterior parts of the ulnar collateral ligament. Distinct collagen bundles within the capsule layers made up the posterior bundle. A similar thickening within the capsule layers comprised the anterior bundle, along with another ligament complex superficial to the capsular layers. Using arthroscopy, only the anterior 20% to 30% of the anterior bundle of the ulnar collateral ligament could be visualized through the anterior portal. Similarly, only the posterior 30% to 50% of the posterior bundle was seen through the posterior arthroscopic portals. Sectioning of the anterior bundle led to joint instability. Arthroscopically, this appeared as increased opening of the ulnohumeral joint in response to valgus stress.

Conclusion.—It was suggested that arthroscopy may not permit complete visualization of tears of the ulnar collateral ligament. Although medial capsular defects and tears of the ulnar collateral ligament can be partially visualized, complete tears may be missed. The diagnosis of ligamentous laxity or tearing abnormalities may be enhanced by the finding of an increased opening of the ulnohumeral joint in response to valgus stress.

▶ It would appear that the bottom line for these 2 articles (Abstracts 139-95-2-24 and 139-95-2-25) is that stress radiography performed using commercially available equipment with a force-monitoring capability is both more accurate and cost-effective than MRI or elbow arthroscopy in determining both partial and complete tears of the various components of the ulnar collateral ligament.—J.S. Torg, M.D.

Arthroscopic Treatment of Posttraumatic Elbow Pain and Stiffness
Timmerman LA, Andrews JR (American Sports Med Inst, Birmingham, Ala)
Am J Sports Med 22:230–235, 1994   139-95-2-26

Patients.—Nineteen consecutive patients with arthrofibrosis of the elbow secondary to a fracture or fracture-dislocation had arthroscopic débridement after a trial of conservative management. The 12 men and 7 women were 12–62 years of age when they had surgery. Six patients had an elbow dislocation, and 15 were injured in a fall. All patients had a flexion contracture of at least 15 degrees. Ten patients had previously had surgery, 3 of them more than once. Pain was consistently present, and 15 of the 19 patients had locking or catching in the elbow. All patients were limited in their activities.

Management.—Surgery was done at an average of 53 months after injury. The anterolateral portal usually served as the initial viewing point. All patients had extensive scarring in the anterior compartment. An overgrown coronoid was osteotomized or débrided before the anterior capsule was débrided. The capsule was released from its humeral attachment but not excised. Lateral scar tissue was then removed followed by débridement in the posterior compartment as needed.

Results.—Overall ratings indicated an excellent outcome in 6 patients and good results in 9 others. Three patients had fair results, and 1 had treatment failure. Symptoms lessened after surgery in all patients. The average flexion contracture improved from 29 degrees to 11 degrees. The average arc of motion increased from 94 degrees to 123 degrees. One patient required a repeat arthroscopic procedure, and the 1 patient in whom treatment had failed underwent open arthrotomy.

Summary.—Good-to-excellent overall results were achieved with arthroscopy in 84% of patients with post-traumatic arthrofibrosis of the elbow. The procedure caused minimal morbidity.

▶ The authors report encouraging results in the management of what in my experience has been a most difficult problem—post-traumatic elbow arthrofibrosis. It was noted that although complete return of preinjury motion was not obtained, each patient showed a significant improvement in motion and subjective symptoms. Notably, this procedure is of limited value in patients who have radiographic evidence of severe degenerative or post-traumatic arthritis.—J.S. Torg, M.D.

Treating—and Preventing—Little League Elbow

Congeni J, Tanner S (Children's Hosp Med Ctr, Akron, Ohio; Univ of Colorado, Denver)
Physician Sportsmed 22:54–55, 59–64, 1994   139-95-2–27

Introduction.—Little League elbow is a common overuse injury that is seen mainly in pitchers 8–16 years of age. It results from repetitive valgus stress placed on the elbow by throwing, creating tension on the medial supporting structures, including the medial epicondyle, medial epicondylar apophysis, and medial collateral ligaments, and compressing the lateral structures (radial head and capitellum). Progression results in inflammation, fragmentation, and avulsion of the apophysis, loose bodies, osteochondritis dissecans, and eventually even osteoarthritis of the affected elbow.

Causes and Complaints.—Contributing factors include training error or excessive repeated overhand throwing; lack of flexibility and muscle imbalance in the forearm muscles; biomechanical factors such as specific errors that add to the excessive valgus stress on the elbow; anatomical variances; specific pitching motions such as throwing breaking pitches or pitching sidearm; and the "too much, too soon" mentality at the start of the season. Early complaints include pulling, popping, giving out, or mild tenderness around the medial joint line with throwing. Swelling and limitation of elbow motion are signs of more advanced involvement.

Treatment.—Treatment always involves complete rest from throwing, typically from 2 to 6 weeks, until elbow tenderness disappears. Pitching is not a "no pain, no gain" activity, and the player must fully recover strength, range of motion, and pain-free throwing before returning to competition. Stretching and strengthening exercises for the flexor and extensor muscles of the forearm should be delayed until the patient can perform them without pain. The return to throwing should be accomplished through a carefully planned, functional progression program that gradually increases the number, distance, and intensity of the throws. The progression varies with the patient's age, degree of involvement in baseball, and amount of rest after injury. Physicians should convince parents and coaches that excessive throwing is the major cause of this condition, particularly during practice. Pitch count limitation may have to be considered in young pitchers who throw 30 pitches per inning. For players without elbow or shoulder injuries, limits in the range of 90–110 pitches per game or practice are reasonable. Preventive measures include proper warmup and stretching and strengthening exercises for the forearm, upper arm, shoulder, and trunk during the off-season or at a minimum of 6 weeks before the "live" pitch; rehabilitation of previous injuries; and correction of improper mechanics.

▶ This is a comprehensive, practical article on the probable causes, clinical features, treatment, and prevention of Little League elbow. A key cause is not so much throwing *breaking* pitches as throwing *too many* pitches, that is, 30 per inning in games and who knows how many in practice. When it comes to kids and pitching, more is not always better. The authors argue that pitching is not a "no pain, no gain" activity, and they warn about the "too much, too soon" mentality.—E.R. Eichner, M.D.

Upper Extremity Peripheral Nerve Entrapments Among Wheelchair Athletes: Prevalence, Location, and Risk Factors
Burnham RS, Steadward RD (Univ of Alberta, Edmonton)
Arch Phys Med Rehabil 75:519–524, 1994   139-95-2–28

Background.—Soft tissue injuries of the arms and hands are some of the most common among athletes with disabilities. Peripheral nerve entrapments make up a portion of these injuries. Some injuries may be caused by repetitive extrinsic hand pressure from using devices for mobility and frequent high intracarpal pressures from wrist extension posturing. There is a need to protect these nerves, but until the specific location of maximal nerve injury can be identified, the placement of protective devices will be imprecise. The prevalence of peripheral nerve entrapments of the upper extremities of wheelchair athletes was determined using clinical and electrophysiologic criteria, and sites of nerve entrapment were localized. In addition, the demographic factors and training associated with electrodiagnostic evidence of nerve entrapment were identified.

Methods.—The clinical and electrodiagnostic assessments were performed on 52 upper extremities of 28 wheelchair athletes and 30 able-bodied controls. Short-segment stimulation techniques of the median nerve across the carpal tunnel and the ulnar nerve across the elbow were used.

Results.—When clinical criteria were used, the incidence of nerve entrapment was 23% among wheelchair athletes, but the rate was 64% when electrodiagnostic methods were used. The most common dysfunction detected electrodiagnostically was that of the median nerve at the carpal tunnel in 46% of research subjects. The portion of the nerve within the proximal carpal tunnel was most often affected. The second most common entrapment detected electrodiagnostically was ulnar neuropathy at the wrist and forearm segments. The duration of the research subject's disability was significantly correlated with the electrophysiologic median nerve dysfunction.

Discussion.—The variation between the clinical and electrodiagnostic findings presents a treatment dilemma. It would be tragic to let hand impairment continue in an individual who relies on the upper extremities to compensate for other disabilities. However, unnecessary surgery, postoperative immobilization, and possible complications would cause exceptional further disability. Strategies to minimize the cumulative stress and pressure of the peripheral nerves of the upper extremities must be identified so preventive and conservative methods of treatment can be found.

▶ This article is recommended reading for those who care for disabled athletes. It should be noted that because the research subject selection for this study was not randomized, the potential for selection bias exists.—J.S. Torg, M.D.

Carpal Tunnel Syndrome

Zimmerman GR (Nova Univ, Fort Lauderdale, Fla)
J Athletic Train 29:22–30, 1994   139-95-2–29

Objective.—Carpal tunnel syndrome has a variety of causes, but it usually results from repetitive daily activities that place the wrists in repeated flexion or abnormal positions, causing compression of the median nerve. The evaluation and management of the disorder were examined.

Mechanisms.—Compression of the median nerve can result from systemic diseases, congenital defects, wrist shape, acute trauma, or ergonomic factors. Pregnancy, oral contraceptive use, menopause, and gyne-

Rehabilitation Exercises

Stretch	Strength
Finger stretch	Wrist extensors
Wrist circles	Wrist flexors
Wrist flexor stretch	Forearm pronators
Wrist extensor stretch	Forearm supinators
Forearm pronator stretch	Radial deviation
Forearm supinator stretch	Ulnar deviation
	Grip squeeze

(Courtesy of Zimmerman GR: *J Athletic Train* 29:22–30, 1994.)

cologic surgery are other causes, and this may explain why 3 times as many women as men have the syndrome.

Signs and Symptoms.—Symptoms include paresthesia of the hand with or without pain that can radiate up the arm and worsen at night as the syndrome progresses. Those who have carpal tunnel syndrome drop things and have difficulty performing daily activities involving twisting motions.

Differential Diagnosis.—The differential diagnosis includes cervical radiculopathy, cervical syndrome, cervical osteoarthritis to thoracic outlet compression, anterior interosseous nerve entrapment, double crush, and polymyalgia rheumatica.

Treatment.—Nonoperative treatment involves splinting to immobilize the wrist, rehabilitation to cause release of the nerve by decreasing edema, nonsteroidal anti-inflammatory drugs, and stretching and strengthening exercises (table). Pyridoxine treatment has not been shown to improve localized nerve lesions, but it may provide some benefit for systemic neuropathy. Surgical intervention may be necessary if nonoperative measures fail.

Special Considerations.—Occupational factors that can help to prevent the condition include early diagnosis, job reassignment, job modification, job rotation, and tool redesign.

Conclusion.—Although the condition is not common in athletes, trainers should be knowledgeable about the consequences of cumulative trauma injuries.

▶ The author cautions us about mismanagement of this problem, because it may be considered to be simply tendinitis. We must be aware of the signs and symptoms of this disorder and refer the patient to the proper physician.—F.J. George, A.T.C., P.T.

Scaphoid Fracture as a "Puncher's Fracture"

Horii E, Nakamura R, Watanabe K, Tsunoda K (Nagoya Univ, Japan)
J Orthop Trauma 8:107–110, 1994   139-95-2–30

Purpose.—Most scaphoid fractures are produced by falling on an out-stretched hand, but they can also be caused by punching. The features of

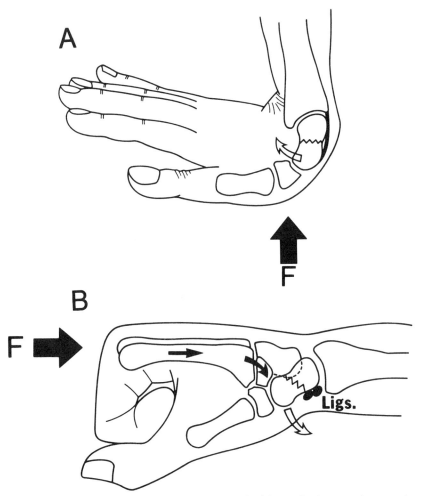

Fig 2–15.—Mechanism of scaphoid fracture. **A,** the scaphoid fracture has been stated to occur in extension. The bending force at the distal pole of the scaphoid (*white arrow*) is the main factor producing fracture. **B,** in neutral or slight palmar flexed position, the external force (F) transmitted through the second metacarpal disperses to the trapezoid and trapezium (shown by *black arrows*), resulting in flexion moment on the distal pole of the scaphoid (*white arrow*). The palmar ligaments (*Ligs.*), which hold the proximal pole of the scaphoid, are the fulcrum. Because of the obliquity of the scaphoid, the external force creates shear stress at the waist of the navicular. (Courtesy of Horii E, Nakamura R, Watanabe K, et al: *J Orthop Trauma* 8:107–110, 1994.)

scaphoid fractures produced by falling were compared with those produced by punching.

Patients.—Of 125 patients who were treated for scaphoid fractures, 18 (14%) acquired their fracture by punching and 107 (86%) acquired it by other mechanisms. All punching fractures were transverse fractures. Seventeen fractures were located at the waist, and 1 was located proximally. Of the 10 patients with acute fractures, 8 were treated by cast immobilization and 2 were treated by Herbert screw fixation without bone grafting. The other 8 patients had delayed or nonunion of a chronic fracture and required screw fixation with bone grafting. Seven of these fractures (38%) had not been diagnosed on the original radiographs. The average interval between injury and diagnosis for these patients was 14 weeks.

Discussion.—Most wrist injuries occur in extension, but the wrist position while punching usually is neutral to slight palmar flexion. When a punching scaphoid fracture occurs in extension, the bending force at the distal pole of the scaphoid is the main cause of the fracture (Fig 2-15, A). When a scaphoid fracture occurs with the wrist in a neutral or slight palmar flexion, the external force is transmitted through the second metacarpal and dispersed to the trapezium and trapezoid, producing shear stress at the waist of the navicular (Fig 2-15, B).

▶ This interesting observation has significant clinical implications. The author observes that "because the fracture lines were often oriented more vertically in the coronal plane, shear stress easily displaced the fragments, consequently causing delayed union." This phenomenon, coupled with the failure to recognize these injuries, initially resulted in high nonunion rates.—J.S. Torg, M.D.

Lunate and Perilunate Dislocations in Professional Football Players: A Five-Year Retrospective Analysis
Raab DJ, Fischer DA, Quick DC (Minneapolis Sports Medicine Ctr)
Am J Sports Med 22:841–845, 1994   139-95-2-31

Background.—The final stage of dorsal perilunate dislocations is considered to be volar dislocation of the lunate. There is disagreement about the appropriate method of stabilization after reduction. The treatment and prognosis of lunate and perilunate carpal dislocations in professional football players over a 5-year period were reviewed.

Methods.—Survey forms were sent to National Football League team physicians to elicit data on carpal dislocation injuries sustained by players between 1986 and 1990; all 28 physicians responded. Additional information was then obtained on the 10 players who sustained volar lunate and dorsal perilunate carpal dislocations.

Findings.—Seven lunate and 3 perilunate dislocations occurred in the 10 players (Figs 2-16 and 2-17). In 9 players, the mechanism of injury

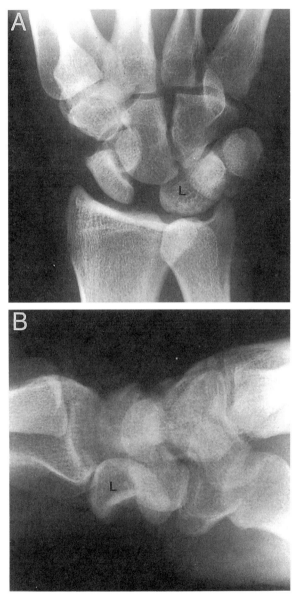

Fig 2–16.—Anteroposterior (**A**) and lateral (**B**) radiographs taken at the time of injury showed volar dislocation of the lunate (L). (Courtesy of Raab DJ, Fischer DA, Quick DC: *Am J Sports Med* 22:841–845, 1994.)

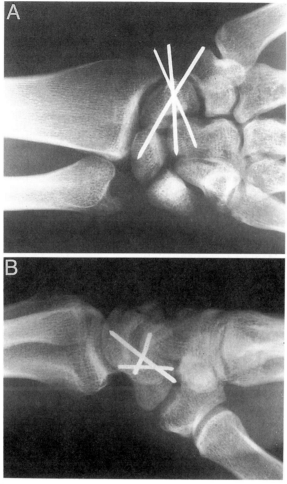

Fig 2–17.—Anteroposterior **(A)** and lateral **(B)** radiographs showing percutaneous pinning of the scaphocapitate and scapholunate joints. (Courtesy of Raab DJ, Fischer DA, Quick DC: *Am J Sports Med* 22:841–845, 1994.)

was hyperextension. Five players were subsequently treated by closed reduction and percutaneous pinning, and 5 underwent open reduction and K-wire fixation. No player was treated by cast immobilization alone. Although at least 4 weeks of playing time were lost, these injuries did not end the professional careers of these players.

Conclusion.—Treatment for these players differed in terms of the use of open or closed reductions, placement of pins, casts, and time of immobilization. None of the variations was clearly superior or detrimental.

However, 4 of the 5 players who returned to play in the same season were treated by closed reduction with percutaneous pinning.

▶ Follow-up evaluation of this group was performed between 4 months and 3 years. "Various players" experienced persistent pain; 2 had crepitus, 4 had persistent widening of the scapholunate joint, 1 had degenerative changes, and all players lost range of motion. Four players also experienced complications that included neurapraxia of the superficial branch of the radial nerve, deep wound infection, reflex sympathetic dystrophy, and early pin removal because of pin migration.—J.S. Torg, M.D.

Alternative Management of Midthird Scaphoid Fractures in the Athlete
Rettig AC, Weidenbener EJ, Gloyeske R (Methodist Sports Medicine Ctr, Indianapolis, Ind)
Am J Sports Med 22:711–714, 1994   139-95-2–32

Background.—Treatment of scaphoid fractures is designed to achieve clinical and radiographic union, thereby preventing post-traumatic arthrosis of the wrist; however, the best means of achieving union remains uncertain. Traditionally, the wrist is immobilized for as long as 24 weeks if the fracture is unstable. An alternative approach would be helpful for in-season athletes who wish to return to play.

Objective.—The efficacy of internal fixation using a Herbert screw was compared with the use of a playing cast in 30 athletes who incurred a stable fracture of the middle third of the scaphoid during the preseason or early in the season or who wanted to play a different sport in the ensuing season.

Management.—Eighteen athletes who were unable to participate with a playing cast underwent immediate open reduction and internal fixation (group 1). Bone grafts from the distal radius or ilium were used in 10 of these patients. Twelve other patients (group 2) were managed nonoperatively in a playing cast.

Outcome.—Patients in group 1 returned to sports activity after an average of 8 weeks, whereas those in group 2 returned in 4.3 weeks. Six of the latter athletes were able to resume activity immediately. The time to clinical healing averaged 11 weeks in group 1 patients and 14 weeks in group 2 patients. One subacute fracture in a group 2 patient failed to heal and was later treated operatively. No complications occurred in either group.

Conclusion.—Athletes who incur a mid–third scaphoid fracture can be effectively managed by either a playing cast or immediate screw fixation. The choice can be guided by the athlete's preference.

▶ This is a good retrospective article that provides concise and definitive management plans for mid–third scaphoid fractures based on the credible experience of the senior author. That the radiographic determinations were made by the senior author represents something of a bias. No mention was made of the preoperative stability of the lesions.—J.S. Torg, M.D.

Gamekeeper's Thumb: Early Diagnosis and Treatment
Kozin SH, Bishop AT (Temple Univ, Philadelphia; Mayo Clinic and Found, Rochester, Minn)
Orthop Rev 23:797–804, 1994   139-95-2-33

Background.—The term "gamekeeper's thumb" refers to chronic laxity of the ulnar collateral ligament (UCL) of the thumb that may result in an unstable metacarpophalangeal (MCP) joint. When killing a wounded hare, the English gamekeeper holds the head in 1 hand while strongly pulling on the rear legs and at the same time sharply extends the animal's neck with the thumb and index cleft. The so-called "skier's thumb" is an acute tear of the thumb UCL.

Diagnosis.—Rupture of the UCL results from either forceful abduction or valgus stress. Typically, there is a painful, swollen, ecchymotic MCP joint, sometimes with direct tenderness over the insertion of the ligament. The integrity of the UCL is examined by stressing the ligament in 20–30 degrees of flexion after obtaining radiographs. Volar subluxation of the proximal phalanx on the lateral radiograph indicates a complete UCL rupture.

Management.—An acute partial tear or sprain can be effectively treated nonoperatively using a thumb spica cast for 4-6 weeks with the MCP joint slightly flexed. Operative repair is recommended for all complete UCL injuries. Primary repair yields better results than late attempts at repair or reconstruction. Cast immobilization is indicated if radiographs show a nondisplaced fracture fragment at the site of insertion of the UCL. If a chronic UCL injury is complicated by significant arthritis, arthrodesis of the MCP joint is indicated. Chronic instability without arthritis can be managed by advancing the adductor tendon or reconstructing the ligament.

▶ This article presents a credible review of the anatomy and biomechanics as well as the diagnosis and treatment guidelines for what might be more appropriately called "skier's thumb." The Stener lesion is well defined in a situation in which the ruptured end of the UCL becomes trapped outside the abductor aponeurosis. This abnormal placement prevents anatomical healing and is an indication for surgical intervention.—J.S. Torg, M.D.

Casting in Sport

DeCarlo M, Malone K, Darmelio J, Rettig A (Methodist Sports Medicine Ctr/ Thomas A. Brady Clinic, Indianapolis, Ind)

J Athletic Train 29:37–38, 41–43, 1994   139-95-2–34

Background.—Much confusion and debate surround sports medicine clinicians' attempts to quickly return to competition high school athletes who have hand and wrist injuries. Authorities disagree on the appropriateness of the use of playing casts in high school football and on the best material for playing cast construction. Materials used for playing casts must be hard enough to provide adequate stabilization and include enough padding to absorb blunt impact forces.

Methods and Findings.—A biomechanical study was done to determine the most appropriate materials for use in constructing playing casts for the hand and wrist. Different materials were assessed for hardness, using a Shore durometer, and for their ability to absorb impact, using a force platform. The RTV11 and Scotchcast were the least hard of the underlying casting materials. Temper Stick foam greatly increased the ability of RTV11 to absorb impact.

Conclusion.—Playing casts should have the internal hardness to ensure immobilization of the injured part and the external impact absorption to act as a cushion during contact. Safe participation is the main goal of such casts. Sports physicians and trainers must consider the specific needs of the athlete as well as the nature and severity of the injury.

▶ Should high school athletes be allowed to participate in football wearing a cast to protect an injury? Why not? If the team physician or orthopedist believes that the injury can be adequately protected from further damage, then the athlete should be allowed to participate. The only negative I've heard is that the injured athlete may use the cast as a "weapon" and cause an injury to an opponent. Proper padding and close officiating can certainly prevent this from occurring.—F.J. George, A.T.C., P.T.

3   Knee

Relationships Between Alignment, Kinematic and Kinetic Measures of the Knee of Normal Elderly Subjects in Level Walking
Wang H, Olney SJ (Queen's Univ, Kingston, Ontario)
Clin Biomech 9:245–252, 1994   139-95-3–1

Background.—Correction of lower limb angular deformities and re-distribution of joint forces have been considered important components of osteotomy, arthroplasty, and other knee surgeries. However, few studies have examined the relationship between lower limb alignment and in vivo biomechanical measurements of the knee. Relationships between static and dynamic alignment and kinetic performance of the knee were assessed in normal elderly subjects during level walking.

Methods.—The study sample comprised 12 men and women (mean age, 68 years) who had no history of lower limb problems. In each individual, static lower limb alignment was measured using a standard precision radiograph (Fig 3–1). The biomechanical performance of the knee during level walking was measured using a 3-dimensional optoelectric system. These data were used to calculate the relationships between static and dynamic knee angular measures, dynamic knee forces, and dynamic knee moments during gait in corresponding motion planes and between dynamic knee angular measures, forces, and moments during gait and in corresponding motion planes.

Results.—Static lower limb alignment measurements did not closely correlate with kinetic measures of the knee in gait. However, about half the static angular alignment measures were significantly related to some of the dynamic knee angular measures. Of 9 dynamic angular measures of the knee, 6 were significantly related to the dynamic forces and force moments in the corresponding motion planes.

Conclusion.—Static alignment measures do not closely correlate with dynamic force and moment measures during gait in asymptomatic elderly individuals. Therefore, static measures alone are not sufficient to predict dynamic forces in intact knees in which some compensation mechanism may exist. Significant correlations are noted between many dynamic knee angle variables and dynamic kinetic measures, which may be useful in evaluating biomechanical forces. Further studies of the po-

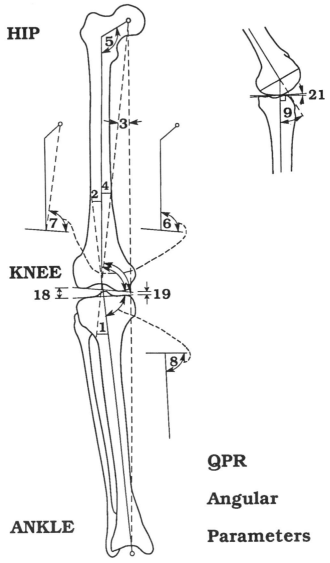

Fig 3–1.—Questor Precision Radiograph (*QPR*) angular parameters. *Coronal plane:* Q1, capito mid-condylar-tibial shaft angle (*CMTS*), Q2, femoral shaft-tibial shaft angle (*FSTS*); Q3, capito-mid-condylar–capito mid-malleolar angle (*CMCM*); Q4, capito-mid-condylar-femoral shaft angle (*CMFS*); Q5, femoral neck–femoral shaft angle (*FNFS*); Q6, femoral shaft–transcondylar angle (*FSXC*), difference from 90 degrees; Q7, capito-mid-condylar–transcondylar angle (*CMXC*), difference from 90 degrees; Q8, tibial plateau–tibial shaft angle (*TPTS*), difference from 90 degrees; Q18, lateral joint space (*LJS*); Q19, medial joint space (*MJS*). *Sagittal plane:* Q9, standing femoral shaft–tibial shaft flexion angle (*SFSTSF*); Q21, anterior-posterior tilt (*APT*). *Transverse plane:* Q10, foot rotation angle (not known). (Courtesy of Wang H, Olney SJ: *Clin Biomech* 9:245–252, 1994.)

tential complex interrelationships between static and dynamic knee measures are indicated.

▶ Although this study did not show that the static alignment measures correlated with the dynamic force and moment measures in gait, the authors believe their results support the use of dynamic gait analysis in surgical decision-making. They also recognize that there is still much work to be done in this area before the roles of important parameters are understood. That the authors used only 12 research subjects would require higher correlations to identify significant relationships.

Was there inadvertent error introduced, because half the research subjects were women and half were men? I was surprised that there was no relationship between the static foot placement, or foot rotation angle, and the dynamic force and moment measurements in gait. I often notice that in gait the knee follows the direction the toes are pointing. Is it possible that some compensation mechanism is more likely to be present when people are research subjects in studies than when they are walking normally?—Col. J.L. Anderson, PE.D.

The Effect of the Squat Exercise on Anterior-Posterior Knee Translation in Professional Football Players
Panariello RA, Backus SI, Parker JW (Sports Medicine, Performance, and Research Ctr, New York; Hosp for Special Surgery, New York)
Am J Sports Med 22:768–773, 1994   139-95-3–2

Introduction.—Weight training techniques are widely used in athletic training regimens. Although the squat exercise is generally considered to be essential for optimal training, the safety of this exercise and its effect on the stability of knee ligaments are controversial. The effect of the squat exercise on knee ligament stability was studied in professional football players.

Methods.—Thirty-two professional football players with no evidence or history of knee injury participated in an off-season 21-week strengthening and conditioning program. The squat exercise was performed lifting an average of 130% to 200% of the participant's body weight during at least 2 sessions each week. Ligament stability was assessed passively and actively with a knee ligament arthrometer at flexion angles of 30 degrees and 90 degrees at the beginning of the program and at 12 and 21 weeks (Fig 3-2).

Results.—There were no significant changes in anteroposterior knee translation in either active or passive tests during the training period. Only 8 tests—5 active and 3 passive—showed excursions that were increased by more than 2 mm. Ten tests—2 passive, 8 active; 9 in 1 participant—revealed excursions that decreased by more than 4 mm.

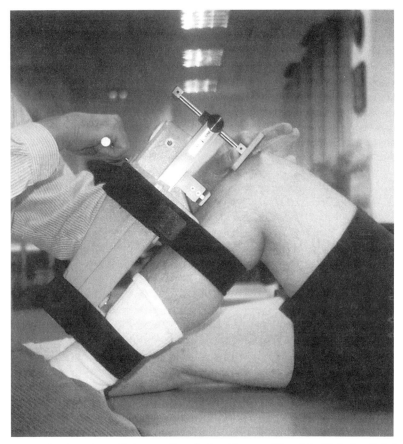

Fig 3–2.—Passive testing at 90 degrees of knee flexion. (Courtesy of Panariello RA, Backus SI, Parker JW: *Am J Sports Med* 22:768–773, 1994.)

Discussion.—The squat exercise does not have deleterious effects on anteroposterior knee translation. Therefore, it can be safely included in athletic training and conditioning programs with healthy individuals. However, more study is needed to determine the effects of the squat exercise on individuals who have increased passive anteroposterior knee translation.

▶ The authors have performed an excellent service with this study. There has been considerable confusion within athletic training circles concerning the use of the full squat, because of the threat of damage to the ligaments of the knees. We should remember that when the original work was done that called into question the use of the full squat exercise, the instrument used for testing the medial and lateral collateral ligament stability was in its first generation of development. That was more than 30 years ago.

This may be a good lesson for us. Maybe we should revisit our research from time to time as our measuring instrumentation improves. Of course, we should also remember that the research subjects in this test were all mature men, with an average age older than 25 years. Can we be certain that the same results will be obtained if the research subjects are of high school age?—Col. J.L. Anderson, PE.D.

Role of the Medial Structures in the Intact and Anterior Cruciate Ligament-Deficient Knee: Limits of Motion in the Human Knee
Haimes JL, Wroble RR, Grood ES, Noyes FR (Univ of Cincinnati, Ohio; Sportsmedicine and Orthopaedic Ctr, Cincinnati, Ohio; Deaconess Hosp, Cincinnati, Ohio)
Am J Sports Med 22:402–409, 1994   139-95-3–3

Objective.—Injuries to knee ligaments result in changes in motion limits that are characteristic of the particular ligament injured. The anterior cruciate ligament (ACL) primarily controls the anterior translation limit, whereas the superficial portion of the medial collateral ligament (MCL) mainly restrains the abduction rotation limit. There is less information regarding the control of internal-external rotation. The changes in knee motion limits with and without ACL injury were examined.

Methods.—The ACL, MCL, posterior oblique ligament, and the posterior medial capsule were sequentially cut in 19 unembalmed normal lower limbs from 12 donors aged 28–71 years. Motion limits of the tibia were measured before and after the ligaments and capsular structures were cut.

Results.—The anterior translation limit of the ACL-deficient knee was significantly greater at 30 degrees of flexion than at 90 degrees of flexion. With the intact ACL that had the medial structures severed, there was no increase in the anterior limit. The external rotation limit grew with an increasing angle of flexion for both the ACL-sectioned and ACL-intact knee. Severing the posterior oblique ligament–posterior medial capsule in ACL knees, MCL-deficient knees, or both increased the external limit significantly at all angles of flexion. The abduction limit increased at zero degrees of flexion when the ACL alone was cut and at all flexion angles except zero degrees when the MCL alone was cut; cutting both produced an additional increase. Severing the posterior oblique ligament–posterior medial capsule increased the limit significantly only when the ACL, MCL, or both were also cut. Severing the MCL alone reversed the direction of coupled external rotation compared with the intact knee.

Conclusion.—In addition to determining the extent of external tibial rotation, it is necessary to ascertain the final anteroposterior position of each plateau to decide which ligaments have been injured. Additional research needs to be done to clinically facilitate this diagnosis.

▶ This study should be helpful to all clinicians in diagnosing knee injuries. In an earlier study, these authors found that experienced clinicians frequently assumed increased external rotation was caused by posterolateral ligamentous injury, whereas the actual injury was to the medial structures. They reported that clinical testing of only the magnitude of increased external tibial rotation was not sufficient to indicate whether medial structures, lateral structures, or both are injured.

To determine which ligaments have been injured, the final anteroposterior position of each plateau must also be known. The authors note that it is often clinically difficult to accurately determine the position of both tibial plateaus with respect to the femoral condyle.—Col. J.L. Anderson, PE.D.

Proprioception in the Knee and Reflex Hamstring Contraction Latency
Jennings AG, Seedhom BB (Univ of Leeds, England)
J Bone Joint Surg (Br) 76-B:491–494, 1994   139-95-3–4

Objective.—Because the anterior cruciate ligament (ACL) plays an important role in proprioception of the knee, injury to it affects the position and movement of the joint. One method of determining proprioception involves measuring the delay in the reflex hamstring contraction in ACL-deficient knees, as reported by some investigators. An attempt was made to reproduce and compare those results in injured and noninjured legs.

Methods.—Six tests were performed on each knee of 11 patients aged 23–33 years who had ACL injuries. In 3 tests, hamstring reaction times were determined when a 140-N force was applied to the posterior proximal tibia of the weight-bearing leg. The non–weight-bearing leg was similarly tested in each patient.

Results.—In 7 patients, there was no difference between legs in the reflex hamstring contraction latency (RHCL). Two patients showed a significant delay in the injured leg and 1 patient in the noninjured leg. Another patient had conflicting results.

Conclusion.—The investigators were not able to reproduce the results of the earlier study. Instead, no significant differences were found between injured and uninjured legs with regard to the RHCL.

▶ In our search for facts it is important that we call into question research that we have been unable to replicate. These authors question whether the RHCL is actually a valid method of measuring proprioception. They believe that there are too many unknown factors in the experiment.—Col. J.L. Anderson, PE.D.

Load and Length Changes in an Artificial Ligament Substitute: 10 Cases of Anterior Cruciate Ligament Reconstruction

Gillquist J, Good L (Univ Hosp, Linköping, Sweden)
Acta Orthop Scand 64:575–579, 1993   139-95-3–5

Background.—Reconstructive surgery for an unstable anterior cruciate ligament entails replacement of the natural ligament with an artificial substitute ligament. Accurate placement of the substitute is important, because length changes will affect the load level in the substitute. Length changes were analyzed to determine whether they can predict the load level in an artificial substitute during passive knee motion.

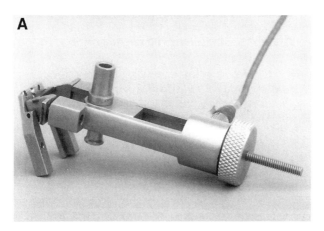

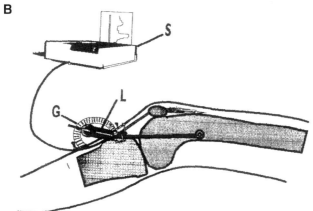

Fig 3–3.—The load cell assembly. **A,** details of the load cell assembly. **B,** the load cell (L) was connected to the ligament, which was fixed to the femur by a bicortical screw. The flexion angles were measured by a liquid goniometer (G). The signals from the load cell were recorded on a strip chart recorder (S). (Courtesy of Gillquist J, Good L: *Acta Orthop Scand* 64:575-579, 1993.)

Method.—Ten patients undergoing anterior cruciate ligament reconstruction received a ligament prosthesis. The flexion angle was measured in increments of 10 degrees, and the ligament was preloaded with 40 N. The change in load was measured from 90 degrees of flexion to full extension. A Kistler piezoelectric load cell was fixed to the anterior tibia (Fig 3–3). During surgery, the anteroposterior displacement of the tibia was measured at 20 degrees of knee flexion before and after the ligament was placed. Data were analyzed with the Student's *t*-test.

Results.—The respective mean ligament positions on the femur and the tibia were 0.67 (0.02) and 0.41 (0.05). The mean change in length was 2.5 (0.9) mm. Ligament preload was always lost during the first extension and flexion cycle, but it was maintained during the last cycle. There was a good correlation between the isometer curves and load curves, but individual length changes could not predict the magnitude of load change. The more anterior the ligament position on the tibia, the greater the change in length.

Conclusion.—High loads in knee joint extension can occur in artificial ligament reconstructions. To avoid overextending the substitute, the final preload should be applied midway between full extension and the flexion angle with the shortest intra-articular length.

▶ The use of artificial substitute ligaments in reconstructive surgery of the unstable anterior cruciate ligament is becoming increasingly popular. The authors analyzed whether length changes recorded by a spring-loaded isometer can be used to predict load levels in artificial substitute ligaments during passive knee motion. The load levels reached during clinical implantation of the artificial ligament were also related to ligament placement. Of the 10 patients used in this study, 6 showed acceptable values with a preload of 40 N; in 3 cases a preload of 20 N was used, and in 1 case the preload was 60 N. The authors found that in the mean they achieved a slight overtightening of the knees, but considering the measurement error, they thought it was safer on the tight side.—Col. J.L. Anderson, PE.D.

Axial Rotation of the Prosthetically Replaced Knee
Minns RJ, Sibly TF (Dryburn Hosp, Durham, England; Hereford Gen Hosp, England)
Clin Biomech 9:199–202, 1994   139-95-3–6

Objective.—In contrast to total condylar replacements, the Minns meniscal total knee replacement permits axial rotation of the femoral component on the tibia. The result is reduced torque forces on the tibial component that may help prevent aseptic loosening. Axial rotation was assessed several months after placement of the Minns meniscal knee replacement.

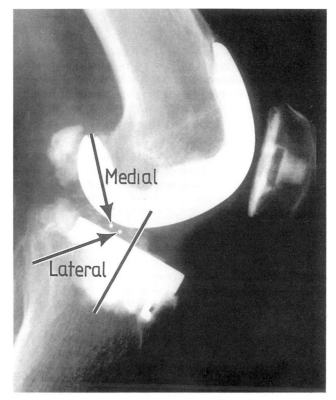

Fig 3–4.—Lateral radiograph showing the markers in the meniscus (*arrow*) and the center line of the tibial component (*line*). (Courtesy of Minns RJ, Sibly TF: *Clin Biomech* 9:199-202, 1994.)

Methods.—Forty-three meniscal knee replacements were investigated in 40 women a mean of 16 months after surgery. Radiographic measurements were made to compute the axial rotation from straight translation of both meniscal bearings and to assess the individual movement of each bearing in the anteroposterior direction (Fig 3-4).

Findings.—The average range of axial rotation was 6 degrees. The average movement of both polyethylene "menisci" was 3 mm. The meniscal range of movement and the position of the center of rotation during passive flexion were only slightly affected by the absence of 1 or both cruciate ligaments.

Conclusion.—In patients with meniscal total knee replacement, in vivo radiographic studies for detecting meniscal bearing movement can be used to compute the axial rotation of the tibial component relative to the femoral component. The polyethylene bearings still move several months after prosthesis implantation, which must lead to a large reduction in torsional forces transmitted to the tibial component, thereby reducing horizontal shear stresses at all interfaces beneath the tibial component, resulting in a reduced incidence of interface failure.

▶ This is an excellent study of the Minns meniscal total knee replacement 16 months after the operation. Although I am not familiar with the Minns technique, I know patients who have had knee replacement surgery and who are still very active in playing racquetball, tennis, and golf. It will be interesting to see how long the knee replacement will last and whether the patients will continue to be as physically active as they are now.—Col. J.L. Anderson, PE.D.

Modified Lachman Test for Anterior Cruciate Ligament Stability
Whitehill WR, Wright KE, Nelson K (Middle Tennessee State Univ, Murfreesboro; Univ of Alabama, Tuscaloosa)
J Athletic Train 29:256–257, 1994   139-95-3–7

Background.—The Lachman test is one of several stress tests commonly used to determine the integrity of the anterior cruciate ligament (ACL). However, the mechanics of this test make it hard to perform. A modification of the Lachman test for ACL stability that avoids some of the problems of the original test was described.

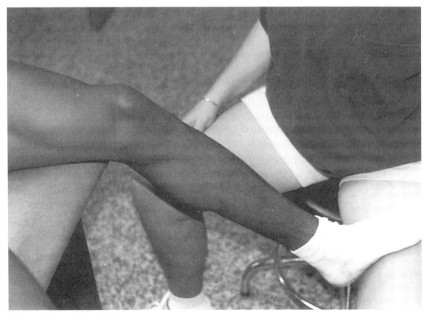

Fig 3–5.—Position of athlete for modified Lachman test. (Courtesy of Whitehill WR, Wright KE, Nelson K: *J Athletic Train* 29:256–257, 1994.)

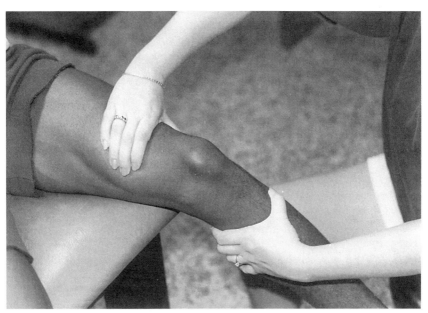

Fig 3–6.—Hand placement for modified Lachman test. (Courtesy of Whitehill WR, Wright KE, Nelson K: *J Athletic Train* 29:256–257, 1994.)

Technique.—In the athletic training facility, the modified test is performed with the athlete supine on an examination table, the knee at the edge of the table, the lower leg hanging off, and the foot on the examiner's thigh (Fig 3–5). When the left knee is stressed, the examiner's right hand is placed on the distal part of the thigh for stabilization. The left hand is cupped around the proximal part of the lower leg, pulling in the anterior plane (Fig 3-6). The examiner's thigh supports the lower leg and relieves ACL tension, and the anterior pull provides about 6 to 10 mm of displacement if the ACL is injured. As a result, the size and strength of the examiner's hands are less important than in the original Lachman test. When an ACL must be assessed in a setting where there is no examination table, the knee is supported by a rolled up towel or similar support, and the foot is stabilized by the playing surface rather than the examiner's thigh. The test is then performed in the same fashion, with the examiner's hand on the lower leg providing the anterior pull needed to displace the lower leg if the ACL is affected.

Conclusion.—The modified Lachman test differs from the original test in several ways. Two examiners are not needed to perform the modified test. In addition, the modified test permits full assessment in a training facility or at a competition. With the modification, the size and strength of the examiner's hands are not important factors.

▶ The traditional Lachman test is difficult for many of us to perform, for many of the reasons cited by the author. For the past several years, I have found a modified Lachman test with the patient in a prone position to be the easiest and most reliable method of testing for ACL laxity.

Since reading this article, I have tried the method described and will continue to use it in conjunction with the method I have been using. As with any new testing procedure, practice and repetition are needed to produce reliable results that can be reproduced. This method is a fairly easy way to evaluate ACL joint laxity.—F.J. George, A.T.C., P.T.

Assessment of Functional Tests After Anterior Cruciate Ligament Surgery

Risberg MA, Ekeland A (Ullevaal Hosp, Oslo, Norway; Univ of Oslo, Norway)
J Orthop Sports Phys Ther 19:212–217, 1994   139-95-3–8

Objective.—Functional testing after anterior cruciate ligament (ACL) surgery is important in assessing the stability of the knee joint. There are few studies evaluating these tests and their results after rehabilitation. Six functional tests were compared, and their ability to assess knee function was evaluated.

Methods.—Using the Lysholm score, the Tegner activity score, thigh atrophy, laxity test, and 6 functional tests, 35 patients aged 18–34 years rated their knee problems about 18 months after ACL reconstruction. The 6 functional tests included the vertical jump test; figure-of-eight test; stairs-running test; triple jump test; stairs hopple test, where the patients jumped up and down 22 steps on each leg; and the side jump test, where the patients jumped 1 leg at a time back and forth between 2 parallel lines 30 cm apart.

Results.—Functional tests fell into 2 areas: daily life function (factor 1) and strength/stability function (factor 2). Tests in these 2 areas helped assess functional progress during early and late postoperative phases. Daily life function can be assessed at 3 months using the figure-of-eight and stairs-running tests, whereas assessment of the degree of reestablishment of preinjury function can be made using the triple jump and stairs hopple tests.

Conclusion.—Two-leg tests evaluate daily living functions, whereas 1-leg tests assess knee stability. The Lysholm test did not accurately identify functional problems during testing.

▶ As I noted after the previous article, developing appropriate rehabilitation programs is a prime concern of athletic trainers and therapists. With studies such as this and the previous one, we can judge the efficacy of the programs we have designed. We must continually assess them to determine whether they are safe. They must certainly cause no damage or further injury and they must be effective. To determine their effectiveness, studies such as this must be done. Some of these tests may actually become a part of the final stages of the rehabilitation program.—F.J. George, A.T.C., P.T.

Instrumented Arthrometry for Diagnosing Partial Versus Complete Anterior Cruciate Ligament Tears
Rijke AM, Perrin DH, Goitz HT, McCue FC III (Univ of Virginia, Charlottesville)
Am J Sports Med 22:294–298, 1994   139-95-3-9

Introduction.—Because partial and complete tears of the anterior cruciate ligament (ACL) have significantly different prognoses with conservative management, the development of a ligament testing technique that could evaluate the extent of an ACL tear would be useful in planning treatment. Graded stress radiography, a procedure in which radiographs are taken of the lateral aspects of the knee while applying varying pressures to the calf, has resulted in 88% sensitivity and 75% specificity for diagnosing complete tears and 20% sensitivity and 90% specificity for diagnosing partial tears. The diagnostic usefulness of instrumented arthrometry with the graded stress technique was assessed.

Methods.—Nineteen patients with a clinical diagnosis of ACL injury underwent a modified KT-1000 arthrometric examination of both knees, with application of between zero and 30 pounds of stress the day before arthroscopy. The force required to induce more than 1 mm of anterior displacement was recorded. There were 5 patients with acute (less than 6 weeks), 4 with subacute (6 weeks to 3 months), and 10 with chronic (greater than 3 months) injuries.

Results.—Three patterns of force-anterior displacement relationships were identified. In the normal, contralateral knees, there was a linear force-anterior displacement relationship until the 6-mm displacement associated with a 12-lb force, after which the slope increased sharply. The second pattern was similar to the first but with a less sharply increasing slope. The third pattern was linear until the 10-mm displacement associated with a 15-pound force, after which the slope increased sharply. The first pattern was relatively consistent; there was more variability in the other 2 patterns. Arthroscopy revealed partial tears in all 4 knees with the second pattern and complete tears in 14 of 15 knees with the third pattern.

Discussion.—Instrumented arthrometry with the graded stress technique identified distinct force-anterior displacement relationships for both normal ACL and ACL with partial and complete tears. The resultant patterns could identify partial tears with a sensitivity of 80% and a specificity of 100% and complete tears with a sensitivity of 100% and a specificity of 80%. However, because there is great variability in these patterns between patients, a diagnostic distinction requires a comparison of both knees. There were no significant differences found among acute, subacute, and chronic injuries.

▶ This study is an interesting and well-designed approach to the problem of differentiating between partial and complete ACL tears. However, the study groups were small, and the data were not subjected to statistical analysis. Correlating the determination of ligament status with long-term follow-up would be worthwhile.

Clearly, the authors are onto something worthwhile, and I would agree with their statement that "the technique described . . . based on viscoelastic stress-strain behavior of the ACL, appears to allow successful diagnosis of partial vs. complete tears and to further extend the capabilities of the KT-1000 arthrometer in the evaluation of knee joint instability."—J.S. Torg, M.D.

Three-Phase Radionuclide Bone Imaging and Magnetic Resonance Imaging Detection of Occult Knee Fractures in Athletes

Giammarile F, Masciocchi C, Barile A, di Pietro M, Carducci A, Baschieri I (Cattedra di Medicina Nucleare, L'Aquila, Italy; Università L'Aquila, Italy; Ospedale San Salvatore, L'Aquila, Italy)
Eur J Nucl Med 21:493–496, 1994   139-95-3–10

Background.—Occult fractures in athletes are very important. In the acute phase, they may simulate soft tissue abnormalities. Acute knee pain after recent trauma that was associated with sports activity was studied by combining 3-phase radionuclide bone imaging (TPBI) with MRI to improve diagnosis and arrive at a correct therapeutic approach.

Methods and Findings.—Twelve athletes with acute knee injury with normal radiologic findings underwent TPBI and MRI. The combination of these very sensitive diagnostic procedures enabled detection of occult fractures in all patients. The areas of signal intensity changes on MRI corresponded to those of increased radionuclide uptake in blood pool images (Fig 3-7). These regions appeared to be more extended on delayed TPBI. Early diagnostic data about lesion sites and functional activities were obtained by TPBI. Magnetic resonance imaging provided better anatomical definition and specific information on associated soft tissue lesions, establishing the correct treatment approach and follow-up.

Conclusion.—In patients with clinically suspected occult fractures, TPBI correlated with a total body bone scintigraphy should be done first. The presence of osseous traumatic lesions can be excluded when osseous uptake is normal. Occult fractures, which are often multiple, are easily localized. Magnetic resonance imaging, which is indicated when soft tissue end endoarticular abnormalities are suspected clinically, will exclude unnecessary diagnostic arthrography. The information provided

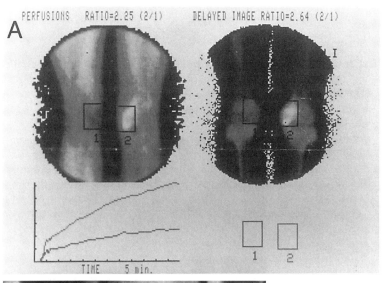

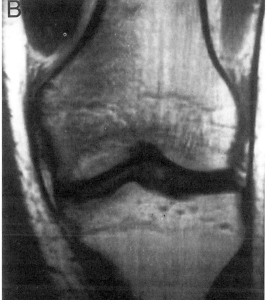

Fig 3–7.—Occult fracture of the medial femoral condyle in a 26-year-old soccer player. **A,** three-phase radionuclide bone images showed increased radionuclide uptake, already evident on the perfusion phase (*left image and curves*), corresponding to the area of low signal intensity on the T1-weighted coronal MR image **(B).** (Courtesy of Giammarile F, Masciocchi C, Barile A, et al: *Eur J Nucl Med* 21:493–496, 1994.)

by MRI in such cases is subsequently useful for assessing treatment response.

▶ The authors concluded that MRI provided more detailed and specific anatomical information compared with TPBI but that neither TPBI nor MRI characterized the microfracture itself.

The authors used low field strength (0.5 T and 0.2 T) magnets, which may account for the limited visualization. It was performed in Italy, so the authors' suggestion that in instances of clinically suspected occult fractures TPBI should be performed first and then an MRI investigation should be performed to evaluate soft tissue and endoarticular pathologies is not in keeping with the current United States health care environment and the need to be cost-conscious in ordering various imaging techniques. A 1.0-T or 1.5-T MRI examination that uses appropriate protocols should be more than sufficient to identify clinically suspected occult fractures.—J.S. Torg, M.D.

The Prevalence of Abnormal Magnetic Resonance Imaging Findings in Asymptomatic Knees: With Correlation of Magnetic Resonance Imaging to Arthroscopic Findings in Symptomatic Knees

LaPrade RF, Burnett QM II, Veenstra MA, Hodgman CG (Michigan State Univ, Kalamazoo)
Am J Sports Med 22:739–745, 1994   139-95-3–11

Background.—Although MRI has replaced arthrography as the diagnostic method of choice for intra-articular knee lesions, the proportion of asymptomatic patients with positive MRI findings of intra-articular pathologic changes is unknown. The prevalence of abnormal MRI scans of the knees of asymptomatic subjects was prospectively evaluated.

Methods.—Fifty-four patients (25 men, 29 women; average age, 28 years) with asymptomatic knees, no history of knee injury, and a negative physical examination of the knee underwent MRI scans. Analysis of MRI and arthroscopic findings in symptomatic knees in 72 patients was done concurrently and prospectively.

Results.—The prevalence of meniscal tears in asymptomatic knees was 5.6% (lateral meniscus, 3.7%; medial meniscus, 1.9%). Degenerative changes of the medial femoral condyle were present in 1.9% of patients; ganglion cysts and patellofemoral joint articular cartilage degenerative changes were each present in 3.7% of patients. No anterior cruciate ligament tears were found in the asymptomatic research subjects. The prevalence of grade II signal changes of the posterior horn of the medial meniscus was 24.1%. The findings of this study were compared statistically with previous studies. The results showed that the MRI scan readings on the asymptomatic knees in this study were accurate and lesions were correctly identified. When previous studies that reported intrasubstance grade II meniscal signal changes correlated with arthroscopy were compiled, an overall tear rate of 14.3% was found.

Conclusion.—Because of the 5.6% prevalence of meniscal tears in asymptomatic subjects, clinical signs and symptoms should be matched with the MRI scan findings before initiating surgical treatment. The significance of grade II MRI signal changes of the medial meniscus in asymptomatic knees is unknown.

▶ Although this is an important study that documents the possibility that there can be false positive MR findings, it is unfortunate that these studies are necessary, because the authors' conclusions should be apparent to all competent physicians: "A positive MR result should not be an indication for surgery unless the history and physical examination were found to be consistent with the MRI results," and "MRI should not be used as a screening device to replace the history and physical examination and should only be used when a patient has symptoms and the diagnosis is in doubt."—J.S. Torg, M.D.

Improvement of Full-Thickness Chondral Defect Healing in the Human Knee After Debridement and Microfracture Using Continuous Passive Motion

Rodrigo JJ, Steadman JR, Silliman JF, Fulstone HA (Univ of California, Davis-Sacramento; Univ of Texas, Dallas)
Am J Knee Surg 7:109–116, 1994   139-95-3–12

Background.—Biological resurfacing of joint surface defects has long been a goal of orthopedic surgeons. Resurfacing attempts have included various methods involving continuous passive motion (CPM). The appearance of the healing tissue in full-thickness chondral defects of the knee in patients with and without CPM after operation was investigated.

Methods.—Since 1985, 298 patients have been studied after treatment of full-thickness articular surface defects of the knee. Seventy-seven patients had second-look arthroscopy. Although CPM was recommended for 8 weeks after surgery for all patients, only 46 of the 77 could comply, mostly because of insurance restrictions.

Findings.—The mean improvement in grade for patients in the CPM group was 2.7 compared with 1.7 for those in the non-CPM group. Only 15% of the CPM group showed no grade improvement compared with 45% of the non-CPM group. The improvements in the CPM group were the same whether the lesion was patellofemoral or tibiofemoral, large or small, or in a young or older patient.

Conclusion.—Continuous passive motion for 6 hours daily for 8 weeks after débridement and microfracture for full-thickness cartilage defects in the knee apparently results in better gross healing of the lesion when assessed by arthroscopic visualization compared with the same treatment without CPM. Because this was not a functional outcome study, extrapolation to the functional outcome status of the patients cannot be made.

▶ The authors presented an innovative approach to dealing with a very difficult problem. Their observations substantiate those of Salter et al., which are based on animal investigations and show that CPM results in better healing than intermediate active motion (1). However, because of a lack of a real unoperated control group, the recommendation that full-thickness chondral lesions should be treated with débridement, microfracture, and a CPM regimen is not supported by the data presented.—J.S. Torg, M.D.

Reference

1. Salter RB, Simmonds DF, Malcolm BW, et al: The biological effect of continuous passive motion on the healing of full-thickness defects in articular cartilage: An experimental investigation in the rabbit. *J Bone Joint Surg* 62A:1232–1251, 1980.

Meniscal Lesions Treated With Suture: A Follow-up Study Using Survival Analysis

Valen B, Mølster A (Univ of Bergen, Norway)
Arthroscopy 10:654–658, 1994   139-95-3–13

Background.—Total meniscectomy increases the risk for long-term degenerative joint changes. As a result, meniscal suture repair may be the method of choice in select patients, such as younger persons with vertical, longitudinal, and preferably fresh lesions in the peripheral third of the meniscus and those with stable knees. Patients undergoing suture repair were evaluated to determine the meniscal healing rate and to identify the factors that influenced healing.

Patients and Methods.—Fifty-seven patients aged 8–56 years underwent meniscal refixation by suture between 1986 and 1991. An arthroscopic outside-in technique with PDS sutures was performed through injection cannulas. Thirty-six knees were stable and 21 had anterior insufficiency. Respectively, 5 and 2 of the latter knees underwent simultaneous and subsequent patellar tendon reconstruction. The mean follow-up was 2 years (range, 2 months to 5.5 years). The outcome was evaluated using the BMDP statistical package and the Kaplan–Meier survival analysis.

Results.—Fifty-one of the 57 patients were available for follow-up evaluation. No neurologic or vascular complications occurred. Twenty patients required reoperation for meniscal reloosening after an average of 1.5 years. Rerupture occurred during ordinary activities in 15 patients and during sports activities in 5. The cumulative 5-year survival rate was 50%. Smaller posterior lesions healed better than more extensive ones.

Factors such as medial or lateral localization, age of the patient or lesion, present displacement of the meniscus, instability of the knee, or experience of the surgeon did not appear to affect survival.

Conclusion.—The disadvantages of meniscal suture repair include a greater need for rehabilitation as a result of postoperative immobilization and potential meniscal rerupturing. The patient's age and level of activity must be considered when evaluating potential candidates for this type of repair. Patients also should be informed about other treatment options and actively participate in the decision-making process.

▶ To look at the data another way: The cumulative 5-year failure rate is really 50%. Certainly, this is most disconcerting. Of equal concern was the failure of the authors to identify the reasons for their poor results.—J.S. Torg, M.D.

Acute Torn Meniscus Combined With Acute Cruciate Ligament Injury: Second Look Arthroscopy After 3-Month Conservative Treatment

Ihara H, Miwa M, Takayanagi K, Nakayama A (Kyushu Rosai Hosp, Kitakyushu, Japan; Kyushu Rehabilitation College, Kitakyushu, Japan)
Clin Orthop 307:146–154, 1994   139-95-3–14

Background.—Surgical removal or repair is the most common approach to treatment of a meniscal injury that is associated with anterior or posterior cruciate ligament injury. Nonoperative treatment and natural healing of an acute torn meniscus combined with an acute cruciate ligament injury was evaluated.

Methods.—Consecutive patients seen with acute tears of the meniscus along with acute tears of the cruciate ligament had their knees arthroscopically examined under general anesthesia. After examination and confirmation of the tears, all were fitted with a Kyuro knee brace with a traction system. The braced knee was mobilized as early as possible using an open kinetic chain and no extension block. Dynamic joint control and muscle strengthening exercises were begun immediately. Partial weight-bearing began on day 10 for meniscal/posterior cruciate ligament injuries and on day 28 for meniscal/anterior cruciate ligament injuries. Full weight-bearing was achieved gradually within 2–3 weeks. All patients underwent arthroscopic examination of the injured knee 3 months after injury.

Results.—Twenty men and 12 women had acute tears of 30 lateral and 10 medial menisci. Most were injured during sports; their average age was 23 years (range, 11–64 years). Of the 39 tear regions in the lateral menisci, 27 healed completely, 7 healed partially, and 5 did not heal. Seven of the 12 tear regions in the medial menisci healed completely, whereas 5 did not heal. Overall, 67% of all the injuries healed completely and 19% did not heal at all. Twenty-nine of the 32 patients' knees achieved full range of motion.

Conclusion.—When early protected mobilization is provided by an appropriate knee brace, an acute torn meniscus can heal spontaneously. Whether the healed meniscus can withstand a return to strenuous activities will be known only with long-term follow-up.

▶ The authors' findings that acute meniscal tears will heal spontaneously with protracted immobilization is interesting. However, because of the propensity of the menisci to be reinjured in the anterior cruciate ligament–deficient knee, these findings are of limited practical value clinically.—J.S. Torg, M.D.

Meniscal Tears Missed on MR Imaging: Relationship to Meniscal Tear Patterns and Anterior Cruciate Ligament Tears

De Smet AA, Graf BK (Univ of Wisconsin, Madison)
AJR 162:905–911, 1994   139-95-3–15

Background.—Magnetic resonance imaging is considered to be a generally accurate means of detecting torn menisci, but occasionally subsequent arthroscopy reveals an injury of a meniscus that appeared intact on MR images.

Objective.—The findings were evaluated in 400 patients who had both MRI and arthroscopy of the knee to learn whether the chance of missing a tear depends on the site or pattern of injury or on the presence of a torn anterior cruciate ligament (ACL). The average interval between MRI and arthroscopy was 79 days.

Findings.—There were 211 medial meniscal tears and 122 lateral meniscal injuries. Thirteen partial and 132 complete ACL tears were found at arthroscopy. Magnetic resonance imaging was 88% sensitive in detecting medial meniscal tears if an ACL tear also was seen and 97% sensitive without an ACL tear. The respective figures for lateral meniscal tears were 69% and 94%. The sensitivity of MRI did not depend on whether surgery was done within 6 weeks of imaging or later. Tears in the posterior third of the lateral meniscus were especially likely to be missed. Peripheral tears of the lateral meniscus were missed more often than complex tears. Both peripheral tears and posterior injuries of the lateral meniscus were much more frequent in knees that also had a torn ACL.

Conclusion.—If an ACL tear is found on MRI, the posterior horn of the lateral meniscus should be carefully evaluated so as not to miss a subtle peripheral tear.

▶ This excellent study calls attention to the well-recognized association of disruption of the posterolateral corner (including meniscal tears) with ACL tears. The authors' recommendation that "when an ACL tear is detected on the MR study, specific attention should be paid to the posterior horn of the lateral meniscus, where a subtle peripheral tear may be present" is wholeheartedly supported.—J.S. Torg, M.D.

Biomechanical and Histological Concepts in the Rehabilitation of Patients With Anterior Cruciate Ligament Reconstructions

Parker MG (Parker Physical Therapy, Inc, Brooklyn Park, Minn)
J Orthop Sports Phys Ther 20:44–50, 1994   139-95-3–16

Objective.—Results of accelerated rehabilitation of patients who have anterior cruciate ligament (ACL) reconstruction surgery are impressive. Although the resumption of strenuous exercise when studies indicate that the graft is weakest does not conform to the standard medical practice regarding graft healing, knee joint stability does not seem to be affected. The mechanics of healing were studied to explain these discrepancies.

Biomechanics.—Activities of daily living place a variety of large anterior drawer forces on the graft and should be undertaken with caution during rehabilitation (table). Knee joint range-of-motion exercises with internal tibial rotation can produce ACL elongation. During eccentric and isometric quadriceps activity, terminal extension should be avoided because it also lengthens the ACL. Although the tissue length changes measured would not affect the integrity of the graft, incorrect graft placement can result in larger changes in tissue length and possible limi-

Anterior Drawer Forces on the Anterior Cruciate
Ligament During Selected Activities

Activity	Anterior Drawer Force	
	Newtons	(lbs)
Cycling	26.7	(6)
Single leg squat	71.2	(16)
Walking downstairs	90.0	(20)
Level walking	177.9	(40)
Active leg extension	355.9	(80)
Walking down ramp	444.8	(100)
Jogging	556.0	(125)
Active leg extension with weight*	622.7	(140)

* 31-N weight at ankle.
(From Parker MG: *J Orthop Sports Phys Ther* 20:44–50, 1994. Courtesy of Henning CE, Lynch MA, Glick KR: *Am J Sports Med* 13:22–26, 1985, and Paulos LE, Payne FC, Rosenberg TD: Rehabilitation after anterior cruciate ligament surgery. In: Jackson DW, Drez D (eds), *The Anterior Cruciate Deficient Knee*, p 296. St. Louis: CV Mosby Co, 1987.)

tations of motion or graft failure. At maximum load, an 80% "safety zone" exists for the graft, which may explain the good clinical outcomes for the accelerated exercise program, particularly because graft failure forces have been obtained from cadaver experiments.

Histology.—After grafting, revascularization takes place that produces collagen fibers and a histologically normal-looking ligament 12–18 months postoperatively. Exercise, by speeding the metabolic process, may aid in the synthesis of collagen.

Conclusion.—Accelerated rehabilitation of patients who have ACL reconstructive surgery is not harmful because it minimizes anterior drawer forces on the graft early on and gradually increases the strenuousness of exercises that do not compromise joint stability. Additional research into the consequences of strenuous activities should be done. Biomechanically, the greatest stress is placed on the graft during terminal extension of the knee joint and internal tibial rotation. Change in graft length depends on graft placement and on activities of daily living that generate anterior drawer forces.

▶ This is a very important study that should be read in conjunction with Abstracts 139-95-3–8, 139-95-3–19, and 139-95-4–13. A rehabilitation philosophy should be developed that involves concepts from these 4 studies.

First and foremost, the rehabilitation exercises must not damage, stretch, or compromise the graft. As a general concept, any exercise we teach should not cause injury or harm to any bodily structure. The exercises should be effective and efficient and provide good functional results. If we want to strengthen the hamstring muscle, we must be certain that the exercise we use will safely strengthen the muscle. We must test periodically during the rehabilitation program to determine whether the exercises are appropriate. We must include exercises that will restore function to the level at which the athlete wishes to participate.—F.J. George, A.T.C., P.T.

Rehabilitation After Meniscus Repair

McLaughlin J, DeMaio M, Noyes FR, Mangine RE (Kennedy Orthopedic Ctr, Neenah, Wis; United States Navy, Oakland, Calif; Cincinnati Sports Medicine and Orthopedic Ctr, Ohio; et al)
Orthopedics 17:463–471, 1994   139-95-3–17

Background.—The rehabilitation program after meniscal repair must consider anatomical, surgical, and healing factors. Anatomical factors include the location of the tear—peripheral, middle, or central—and the relative vascularity at the site of the tear. Surgical factors include the stability of the repair and the surgeon's ability to achieve soft tissue fixation. Healing varies according to site, and the rate of healing and the stability of the repair determine the rehabilitation program. A protocol was pres-

Evaluation-Based Rehabilitation
Rehabilitation After Meniscus Repair*

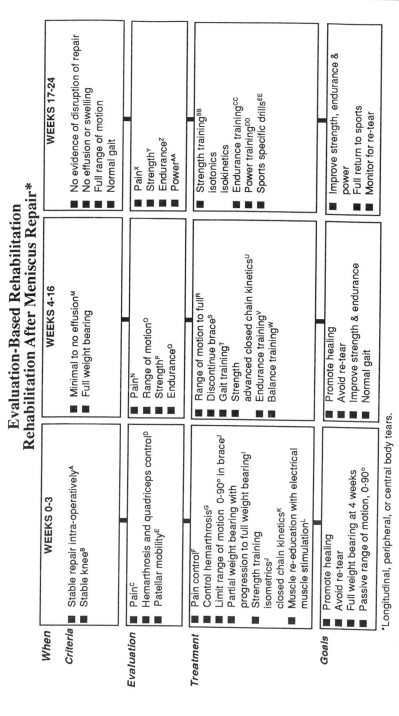

	WEEKS 0-3	**WEEKS 4-16**	**WEEKS 17-24**
When			
Criteria	■ Stable repair intra-operatively[A] ■ Stable knee[B]	■ Minimal to no effusion[M] ■ Full weight bearing	■ No evidence of disruption of repair ■ No effusion or swelling ■ Full range of motion ■ Normal gait
Evaluation	■ Pain[C] ■ Hemarthrosis and quadriceps control[D] ■ Patellar mobility[E]	■ Pain[N] ■ Range of motion[O] ■ Strength[P] ■ Endurance[Q]	■ Pain[X] ■ Strength[Y] ■ Endurance[Z] ■ Power[AA]

Treatment	■ Pain control[F]
	■ Control hemarthrosis[G]
	■ Limit range of motion 0-90° in brace[J]
	■ Partial weight bearing with progression to full weight bearing[I]
	■ Strength training isometrics[J]
	■ closed chain kinetics[K]
	■ Muscle re-education with electrical muscle stimulation[L]
		■ Range of motion to full[R]
		■ Discontinue brace[S]
		■ Gait training[T]
		■ Strength
		   advanced closed chain kinetics[U]
		■ Endurance training[V]
		■ Balance training[W]
			■ Strength training[BB]
			   isotonics
			   isokinetics
			■ Endurance training[CC]
			■ Power training[DD]
			■ Sports specific drills[EE]

Goals	■ Promote healing ■ Avoid re-tear ■ Full weight bearing at 4 weeks ■ Passive range of motion, 0-90°	■ Promote healing ■ Avoid re-tear ■ Improve strength & endurance ■ Normal gait	■ Improve strength, endurance & power ■ Full return to sports ■ Monitor for re-tear

*Longitudinal, peripheral, or central body tears.

Fig 3–8.—Flow sheet. (Courtesy of McLaughlin J, DeMaio M, Noyes FR, et al: *Orthopedics* 17:463–471, 1994.)

ented for longitudinal tears located in the central or peripheral portion (Fig 3–8).

Methods.—Repair of these longitudinal tears can be assisted by arthroscopy or by open techniques. Modifications may be required in cases with concomitant repair of radial tears or reconstruction of the anterior cruciate ligament (ACL). The protocol was followed in 66 patients having concurrent meniscal repair and ACL reconstruction; 80% of menisci completely healed, 14% partially healed, and 6% failed. Rim width was the only factor that significantly affected the rate of healing. The incidence of healing was higher for repairs in the outer third (98%) than for repairs in the central third (79%). No complications developed, and no adverse effects from immediate knee motion or early weight-bearing occurred. Goals of the initial phase of the program were full weight-bearing and full range of motion (ROM).

Discussion.—To withstand the forces of early weight-bearing and ROM, a stable repair and a stable knee are necessary. For the advancement of weight-bearing and muscle training, the ACL takes priority, whereas for the advancement of ROM the meniscus repair program takes precedence. Knee stability should be documented by clinical examination under anesthesia and monitored during the course of rehabilitation. Evaluation of the ability of the quadriceps to cause a superior patellar glide is valuable. Patellar mobility can be confirmed by passively gliding the patella in the superior-inferior and the medial-lateral positions. Continuous passive motion is used after surgery in patients who appear to be at risk for a postoperative motion problem. The goal is full weight-bearing at 3 weeks, at which time the patient is allowed unrestricted ROM with full weight-bearing out of the brace. Patients then receive isometric strength training, closed chain kinetic exercises, endurance evaluation, gait training, advanced closed-chain kinetic exercises, endurance training, balance training, and an evaluation of strength and power.

▶ Please read the previous 4 articles (Abstracts 139-95-3–13 through 139-95-3–16) and my comments after each. This article closely fits the philosophy I was attempting to describe. After a meniscal repair, we are very cautious about the types of exercises we prescribe. It is an area of rehabilitation in which a specific exercise could certainly undo the surgeon's repair. As we see more and more of these patients, our rehabilitation programs will change and evolve to a level where our goals will be achieved.

The program described by these authors certainly represents an advance from what we were doing 2 years ago, both in shortening the time restraints and increasing the demands on the knee joint.—F.J. George, A.T.C., P.T.

Comparison of the Effects of Exercise in Water and on Land on the Rehabilitation of Patients With Intra-Articular Anterior Cruciate Ligament Reconstructions

Tovin BJ, Wolf SL, Greenfield BH, Crouse J, Woodfin BA (Georgia Tech Athletic Assoc, Atlanta, Emory Univ, Atlanta, Ga; HealthSouth, Atlanta, Ga)
Phys Ther 74:710–719, 1994   139-95-3–18

Background.—Rehabilitation is considered the key to a beneficial outcome after anterior cruciate ligament reconstruction. The effects of exercises performed in water on joint effusion, thigh atrophy, range of motion, thigh musculature strength, and ability to perform the activities of daily living after anterior cruciate ligament reconstruction were compared with the effects of similar exercises performed on land.

Methods.—Fourteen male and 6 female research subjects aged 16–44 years who had first-time arthroscopically assisted intra-articular anterior cruciate ligament reconstruction were randomly assigned to either a traditional rehabilitation group or a pool rehabilitation group (Fig 3–9). After operation, both groups were given the same instructions and training for home-based exercises and the use of axillary crutches and a hinged knee brace. During the second through the eighth postoperative week each person performed a similar supervised rehabilitation program either in the pool or on land, according to his or her group assignment (table).

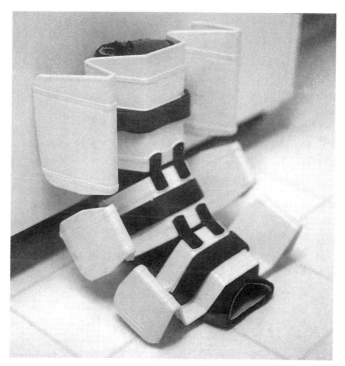

Fig 3–9.—Hydrotone resistance boot used by subjects in the water group. (Courtesy of Tovin BJ, Wolf SL, Greenfield BH, et al: *Phys Ther* 74:710-719, 1994.)

Rehabilitation Programs

Week 1 and Home Program Exercises (Both Groups)

1. Wall slides: 25 repetitions
2. Active-assistive range of motion: 25 repetitions
3. Passive knee extension: 10 minutes
4. Hamstring muscle and calf stretching: 10 minutes each
5. Quadriceps femoris muscle sets
6. Straight leg raises*: 3 sets × 10 repetitions for hip flexion, abduction, adduction, and extension
7. Active knee flexion*: 3 sets × 10 repetitions
8. Toe raises: 3 sets × 10 repetitions
9. Partial wall squats (usually added to the home program after first week): 3 sets × 10 repetitions

Week 2–8 Exercise Programs

Traditional Rehabilitation Group

1. Stationary cycling: 10 minutes
2. Gait training without brace, alternating forward and backward ambulation: 10 minutes
3. Side step-ups, front step-ups, step-downs: beginning with 3 sets of 10 repetitions, progressing to 3 sets of 15 repetitions
4. Hip flexion, extension, abduction, adduction in standing using a wall pulley with 4.54-kg (10-lb) plates: beginning with 3 sets of 10 repetitions, progressing to 3 sets of 15 repetitions
5. Knee flexion in sitting: 3 sets of 10 repetitions; boot: beginning with 3 sets of 10 repetitions, progressing to 3 sets of 15 repetitions

Pool Rehabilitation Group

1. Stationary cycling: 10 minutes†
2. Gait training without brace, alternating forward and backward ambulation: 10 minutes
3. Side step ups, front step-ups, step-downs: beginning with 3 sets of 10 repetitions, progressing to 3 sets of 15 repetitions‡
4. Hip flexion, extension, abduction, adduction in standing using the Hydrotone resistance boot: beginning with 3 sets of 10 repetitions and progressing to 3 sets of 15 repetitions
5. Knee flexion in standing using the Hydrotone resistance boot: beginning with 3 sets of 10 repetitions and progressing to 3 sets of 15 repetitions

*Cuff weights were added to straight leg raises and knee flexion in increments of 0.91 kg (2 lb).
†For stationary cycling in the pool rehabilitation group, a peddling device rather than a stationary bicycle was used.
‡Step-ups in the water were done with 20.32-cm (8-in.) and 40.64-cm (16-in.) steps.
(Courtesy of Tovin BJ, Wolf SL, Greenfield BH, et al: *Phys Ther* 74:710–719, 1994.)

Joint laxity was measured before operation and at 8 weeks after operation. Peak knee torques were measured at the end of 8 weeks after operation, and thigh girth and passive range of motion of the knee were measured at 2, 4, 6, and 8 weeks after operation. At the end of the eighth postoperative week, each person completed a questionnaire assessing the functional use of the repaired knee joint.

Results.—No significant differences were found between the groups for joint laxity, knee torque, passive range of motion, or thigh girth. The questionnaire scores were significantly higher in the pool group, indicating an increased self-assessed functional ability compared with the traditional group.

Conclusion.—A rehabilitation program performed in a pool by patients with intra-articular anterior cruciate ligament reconstruction resulted in better self-reports of functional improvement. Future studies should examine the effectiveness of programs that combine traditional and water-based exercises.

▶ With regard to the importance of eccentric muscle contractions for restoring muscle performance, the authors concluded that eccentric contractions "are more likely to occur on land than in water due to increased gravitational forces."

K.L. Knight, in his comments on this article, states that rehabilitation programs "should be goal-oriented rather than protocol- or cookbook-oriented." He goes on to note that squats or leg presses with the daily adjustable progressive resistive exercise technique "would have resulted in much greater muscle strength development." He observes that the "sooner strength is developed, the quicker other physical attributes develop" (1).

A combination of land- and water-based rehabilitation may prove to be the most effective method of rehabilitating these patients. Both methods have their advantages and disadvantages, and the best of both programs should be included in a total program.—F.J. George, A.T.C., P.T.

Reference

1. Knight KL: *Athletic Training: Sports Health Care Perspectives* Vol. 1, No. 1, pp 55–56.

Electromyographic Analysis of Knee Rehabilitation Exercises
Gryzlo SM, Patek RM, Pink M, Perry J (Northwestern Univ, Chicago; Centinela Hosp Med Ctr, Inglewood, Calif)
J Orthop Sports Phys Ther 20:36–43, 1994   139-95-3–19

Introduction.—Because knee injuries are so common, knee rehabilitation exercises are frequently necessary to restore function. Few studies have evaluated the safety and effectiveness of these exercises. Electromyographic activities of 5 leg muscles were compared during 5 rehabilitative exercises, and the EMG profile within a muscle during the full range of motion was determined.

Methods.—The EMG activities of 5 muscles were measured in 12 research subjects aged 25–32 years during the straight leg raise (SLR), short-arc knee extensions with (SAEXHS) and without (SAEX) hamstring co-contraction, squat, and isometric knee co-contraction (ICO).

Results.—Results obtained during SAEX showed that the vastus medialis oblique (VMO) and vastus lateralis (VL) demonstrated significantly more activity during the final 15 degrees of extension than in the other arcs. In SAEXHS, VMO, VL, and the rectus femoris (RF) were significantly more active than the biceps femoris (BF) and the semimembranosus (SM) during the last 15 degrees of extension. The VL, VMO, and RF also showed significantly more activity during all phases of squatting. The VMO and VL showed the most activity during the SAEX and the SAEXHS. The activity level of the RF remained relatively constant during all exercises. The BF showed highest activity during the ICO and the SAEXHS, whereas the SM showed most activity during the ICO. The SAEX and SAEXHS exercises would be most beneficial to patients who want to restore strength to VL, VMO, and RF muscles, as long as knee motion is not contraindicated. Anterior cruciate ligament (ACL) reconstruction patients can benefit from knee co-contraction exercises as long as EMG hamstring activity is high enough to provide a balanced co-contraction. Because of lack of evidence for co-contraction during the squat, this exercise should be used with caution in ACL reconstruction patients.

Conclusion.—In the SAEX and SAEXHS, the VMO and VL demonstrated the greatest activity during the last 15 degrees of arc. Balanced co-contractions occurred during the SAEXHS and ICO exercises, except during the last 15 degrees of extension. Squatting exercised the quadriceps but not the hamstring.

▶ Over the years we have continually changed our knee rehabilitation programs, attempting to protect the knee joint or surgical repair and to rebuild the necessary muscle strength. Many of our knee rehabilitation programs involve closed-chain exercises, including the squat exercise.

The results of this study indicate that the squat exercise is not the exercise of choice to increase hamstring strength. There are a number of studies now being done with EMG and fluoroscopy to measure the amount of tibial translation that occurs in ACL-deficient knees during exercise. Because more of these types of studies are being done, better rehabilitation programs will be developed.—F.J. George, A.T.C., P.T.

Effects of a Functional Knee Brace on Leg Muscle Function
Styf JR, Lundin O, Gershuni DH (Göteborg Univ, Sweden; Univ of California,

San Diego)
Am J Sports Med 22:830–834, 1994   139-95-3–20

Background.—When applied, a knee brace compresses the soft tissue of the thigh and leg. However, little is known about how a knee brace affects the soft tissues and neuromuscular function of the leg. External compression by a knee brace raises IM pressure at rest and muscle relaxation pressure during exercise to a degree that could hinder blood flow. The effect of a functional knee brace on IM pressure in the tibialis was investigated along with the time to elicit muscle fatigue in braced and unbraced legs during exercise.

Methods.—Six healthy volunteers were included in the study. The research subjects were 3 men and 3 women 22–36 years of age. A DonJoy Hinged Neoprene knee brace was used to compare right and left legs, braced and unbraced.

Findings.—The mean muscle relaxation pressures were significantly higher in braced legs at the beginning of exercise, increasing from 40 to 50 mm Hg at the start to 50-60 mm Hg afterward. The time to elicit muscle fatigue ranged from 81 and 86 seconds in the braced legs and from 123 and 131 seconds in the unbraced legs. Because of the increased muscle relaxation pressure, the calculated local blood perfusion pressure was reduced.

Conclusion.—Premature muscle fatigue in the braced leg resulted from the external compression of the brace, which leads to muscle relaxation pressure increases during exercise and local blood perfusion pressure reductions in the braced leg that can impede local muscle blood flow.

▶ The authors describe muscle relaxation pressure as being "the pressure in the relaxed muscle between contractions during dynamic exercise." They go on to note that "the application of a knee brace and the amount of tensile force used to tighten its straps are important." They recommend reducing the tensile force at each brace application.

We have all seen an athlete who wears a knee brace and complains that his leg feels tired; this article has given us a partial solution to that problem. We all have also had an athlete who complains that the brace continually slips down and is in the wrong place. A point must be found at which the least amount of tensile strength will hold the brace in the correct position. Proper fitting of the brace is necessary to find this position.—F.J. George, A.T.C., P.T.

Isolated Rupture of the Patellar Tendon in Athletes

Kuechle DK, Stuart MJ (Mayo Clinic and Found, Rochester, Minn)
Am J Sports Med 22:692–695, 1994   139-95-3–21

Objective.—The results of operative repair were examined in 5 athletic individuals who had 6 isolated patellar tendon ruptures and were followed for 6 years on average.

Patients.—The patients, all men, had a mean age of 36 years when they were injured. Four patients were competitive recreational athletes, and 1 was a high school basketball player. Four patients were injured while playing basketball, and 1 while playing softball. Three patients had preexisting symptoms of jumper's knee. Five tendons ruptured at the inferior patellar pole.

Management.—Repair was undertaken an average of $2\frac{1}{2}$ days after injury. The single midsubstance tear was reapproximated with heavy sutures. The other injuries were managed by débriding the tendon and reattaching it through vertical drill holes made in the patella. The repair was reinforced with permanent cerclage Dacron tape that was inserted through holes in the patella and tibial tubercle. Patients were placed in a cylinder cast for 6 weeks.

Results.—No patient was symptomatic when last evaluated, and all were able to resume their accustomed level of sports activity an average of 18 months after injury. All but 1 of the patients believed that his injured knee was at least as good as before injury; that patient rated his knee at 90%. Lateral patellar facet pressure syndrome developed in 1 patient, and he required arthroscopic release of the lateral retinaculum. None of the patients walked with a limp. Isokinetic testing of the quadriceps affirmed the excellent functional results.

Conclusion.—Prompt operative repair of an isolated patellar tendon rupture yields an excellent and lasting functional outcome in athletes who have no underlying systemic illness.

▶ I agree with the authors' conclusion that "after acute operative repair and aggressive rehabilitation, an excellent and enduring functional outcome can be expected" following isolated rupture of the patellar tendon.—J.S. Torg, M.D.

Operative Treatment of Partial Rupture of the Patellar Ligament
Raatikainen T, Karpakka J, Puranen J, Orava S (Deaconess Inst of Oulu, Finland; Univ Central Hosp, Oulu, Finland; Hosp Meditori, Turku, Finland)
Int J Sports Med 15:46–49, 1994   139-95-3-22

Introduction.—Although it is common in athletes whose sport involves jumping, partial rupture of the patellar ligament can be difficult to diagnose. Generally, partial ruptures of the patellar ligament are managed nonsurgically, with rest and physical therapy. Local corticosteroid or glycoaminoglycan polysulfate injections may also be given. However, refractory ruptures must be treated surgically. The results of surgical treatment of this overuse injury were evaluated.

Methods.—During a 14-year period, 124 patients underwent surgical treatment for partial rupture of the proximal patellar ligament in 138 knees after conservative management failed. Imaging studies included ultrasonographic examination in 45 knees and soft tissue radiographs of 22 tendons. Surgery involved removing devitalized tissue in the ligament. The tissue from 58 ligaments was examined histologically. The patients' satisfaction with the healing was assessed using a questionnaire at a mean of 19.8 months postoperatively.

Results.—Of the 45 patients who had ultrasonographic evaluation, 31 had ligaments with a hypoechogenic focus, 11 had a thickened ligament with a poorly defined focus, and 3 showed no abnormalities. Of the 22 ligaments that were examined with soft tissue radiography, 10 had a spindle-like swelling, and 4 showed an osteophyte of the patella. Surgery revealed a devitalized focus in all the ligaments that was usually located posteriorly inside the proximal end of the ligament. However, 17 knees had superficial diffuse degeneration. Macroscopic examination of the lesions revealed hyalinic-like tissue resembling scar tissue replacing normal longitudinal fibers. Microscopic examination revealed degenerated, fibrotic, neovascularized tissue with light-to-moderate inflammation. There were no major postoperative complications. Follow-up identified 111 knees in 97 patients with good or excellent results (i.e., return to preinjury sports activity level with no or minimal symptoms), 12 knees with fair results (i.e., some pain that limited activity), and 15 knees with poor results (i.e., excessive pain that precluded a return to sports). Thirteen of the 15 knees underwent repeat operation with further excision; 8 had good or excellent results and 5 had fair results.

Discussion.—Ultrasonography has significant diagnostic value; the identification of a hypogenic focus in the patellar ligament was highly predictive of finding devitalized tissue during surgery. By contrast, soft tissue radiographic findings were nonspecific and had little diagnostic value. Surgical excision of the devitalized tissue produced satisfactory results, enabling a return to sports in 86.2% of the patients.

▶ This is a well-documented and impressive series regarding what is referred to in the United States as "jumper's knee." Fifteen of the 124 operated patients were reported to have had poor results, with 13 requiring reoperation.

Although the authors do not describe the type of anesthesia used for the procedure, it has been my experience that when the procedure is done with local anesthesia, the painful site and therefore the pathology can be easily and accurately identified. The surgeon can then, so to speak, cut out the pain.—J.S. Torg, M.D.

Repair of Partial Quadriceps Tendon Rupture: Observations in 28 Cases

Raatikainen T, Karpakka J, Orava S (Deaconess Inst of Oulu, Finland; Univ Central Hosp of Oulu, Finland; Hosp Meditori, Turku, Finland)
Acta Orthop Scand 65:154–156, 1994   139-95-3-23

Background.—Tendinopathy of the knee extensor mechanism has been called "jumper's knee." Some cases progress, despite medical treatment, to a chronic condition with partial or complete rupture of the tendon. Such cases require surgical intervention. The results of such intervention in 28 cases of jumper's knee in the quadriceps tendon were reported.

Methods.—Six months to 5 years postoperatively, patients who had undergone excision of the scar tissue and closure of the quadriceps tendon were examined and interviewed regarding their sports activity and ability.

Results.—Seventeen of the 28 patients reported no pain and full resumption of their preinjury level of activity. Eight reported mild-to-moderate pain but a full return to preinjury activity. One of the 3 remaining patients reported severe pain and a significant decrease or no return to preinjury activity, whereas the remaining 2 reported a moderate level of pain and a minimal decrease in activity.

Conclusion.— For patients with jumper's knee who do not respond to medical treatment, a simple excision of the scar followed by suture of the healthy tendon provides excellent results overall in terms of pain and function.

▶ Although it is a small point, it is my understanding that what the authors are describing is disruption of the insertion of the rectus femoris in the superior pole of the patella. The reference to this as "jumper's knee" is a misnomer, because this condition entails involvement of the insertion of the infrapatellar tendon into the patella. The authors did not make a distinction between the insertion of the rectus femoris as opposed to the main bulk of the quadriceps tendon.—J.S. Torg, M.D.

Painful Bipartite Patella: A New Approach to Operative Treatment

Ogata K (Fukuoka Univ School of Medicine, Japan)
J Bone Joint Surg (Am) 76-A:573–578, 1994   139-95-3-24

Introduction.—Most patients with a painful bipartite patella will respond to conservative treatment. There have been few reports of those who required operative treatment, and the duration of follow-up has been limited. An operative approach was described that addressed the problems encountered in previously used techniques and enabled the patient to return to full sports activity free of pain.

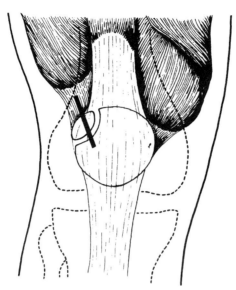

Fig 3–10.—First of 3 schematic drawings showing the operation. An oblique skin incision, extending just distal to the midportion of the separated area of the patella, is made over the distal portion of the vastus lateralis tendon. (Courtesy of Ogata K: *J Bone Joint Surg (Am)* 76-A:573–578, 1994.)

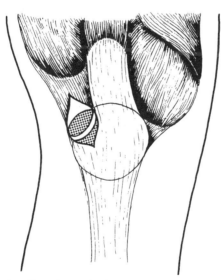

Fig 3–11.—The vastus lateralis tendon is split along its middle fibers, and its insertion to the painful patellar fragment is detached subperiosteally. The continuity of the tendon-periosteum complex to the main portion of the patella is preserved. (Courtesy of Ogata K: *J Bone Joint Surg (Am)* 76-A:573–578, 1994.)

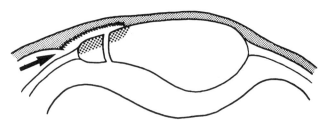

Fig 3–12.—The fragment is relieved from muscle traction without causing a medial-lateral imbalance that would affect patellofemoral tracking. Care is taken not to injure the synovial capsule to preserve some blood supply to the fragment. (Courtesy of Ogata K: *J Bone Joint Surg (Am)* 76-A:573–578, 1994.)

Patients.—Thirteen patients with 15 painful bipartite patellae that had failed to respond to conservative treatment were operated on between 1982 and 1990; the average age of those in the group was 21 years. Six patellae were type II, with the fragment at the lateral margin, and 9 were type III, with the fragment at the superolateral pole. All patients had pain during and after strenuous activities. Localized tenderness over the radiolucent area of the patella was a typical finding.

Technique.—The vastus lateralis tendon insertion to the painful patellar fragment is detatched subperiosteally, together with preservation of the continuity of the tendon-periosteum complex to the main portion of the patella (Figs 3-10, 3-11, and 3-12). A grossly mobile patellar fragment is removed from 3 of the type II and 2 of the type III patellae. Postoperative management consists of a splint applied with the knee in extension. Patients are allowed to walk immediately with full weight-bearing, and range-of-motion exercises are started in 4 or 5 days. The splint is removed at 1–2 weeks postoperatively.

Results.—The 5 patients who had removal of the painful fragment all had prompt relief of pain and could return to a full range of activities, with normal stability of the knee. One patient reported occasional pain at the latest follow-up, but the other 4 patients had results that were judged to be excellent. The 6 patients with type III patellae from which the fragment had not been removed remained asymptomatic and could participate in sports. All 3 type II fragments failed to unite, but results were excellent in 2 cases and good in 1.

Conclusion.—The simple operative technique of release of the vastus lateralis tendon yielded excellent results in 11 patients who had painful bipartite patellae and were followed for an average of 5 years postoperatively. The remaining results were good, and there were no major postoperative complications.

▶ This article offers a direct, simple approach to management of the painful bipartite patella. The original article is recommended reading for the interested surgeon.—J.S. Torg, M.D.

The Diagnosis and Treatment of Medial Subluxation of the Patella After Lateral Retinacular Release

Nonweiler DE, DeLee JC (Texas Orthopaedic and Sports Medicine Ctr, San Antonio)
Am J Sports Med 22:680–686, 1994   139-95-3–25

Patients.—Five patients were seen in a 4-year period with a medially subluxated patella after release of the lateral retinaculum. No other surgery had been done. The 4 women and 1 man were aged 19–28 years. The release procedure had been done for patellar instability or chondromalacia.

Diagnosis.—The patients had peripatellar pain with intermittent swelling and episodes of giving way during daily activities. They had noted clicking and popping sounds and had trouble climbing stairs. Minimal effusion was present, but there was a visible defect at the superior patellar border. Patients felt apprehensive when medial patellar displacement was attempted. This disorder can also be demonstrated by a gravity subluxation test in which the patient is in the lateral decubitus position and the leg is passively abducted with the knee extended so that the patella subluxates medially out of the patellofemoral groove.

Management.—After attempts to increase quadriceps strength had failed, the patients were operated on under sensory epidural anesthesia so that the effect of quadriceps contraction could be assessed. In all patients, the vastus lateralis muscle was found to be detached from the superior patellar pole. The remaining lateral retinacular tissue was isolated (Fig 3-13)—either divided or split in thickness—and imbricated (Fig

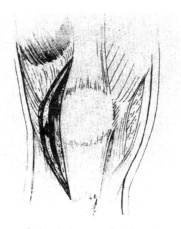

Fig 3–13.—The layer of scar residual in the location of the lateral retinaculum is split in its thickness, and medial and lateral leaves are developed. (Courtesy of Nonweiler DE, DeLee JC: *Am J Sports Med* 22:680-686, 1994.)

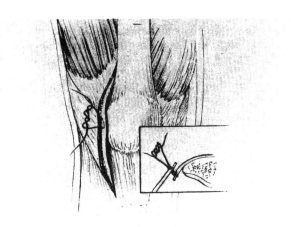

Fig 3–14.—The medial and lateral leaves are imbricated, thereby shortening and doubling the thickness of the tissue representing the lateral retinaculum. The patient is under selective sensory block anesthesia when each suture is tied. A quadriceps contraction is performed to test the tightness of the reconstruction. (Courtesy of Nonweiler DE, DeLee JC: *Am J Sports Med* 22:680–686, 1994.)

3–14). No patient required medial retinacular release. A knee immobilizer was used for 6 weeks postoperatively.

Results.—All patients were subjectively more stable when evaluated 1–7 years after surgery. One patient had a single episode of giving way. The patients were better able to climb stairs. Patellar stability approached that of the opposite knee. Three patients were considered to have had an excellent outcome, and 2 had a good outcome. All patients were satisfied with the functional and symptomatic results.

Conclusion.—In patients who have medial patellar instability after excessive release of the lateral retinaculum, reconstruction of this structure under sensory epidural anesthesia reliably relieves symptoms.

▶ It is essential that this procedure be performed under sensory epidural anesthesia. This allows the surgeon to evaluate the effect that each suture has on the imbricated retinaculum, i.e., the repair is evaluated after an active quadriceps contraction to prevent continued medial subluxation or inadvertent creation of lateral subluxation of the patella as a result of overzealous tightening of the retinaculum.—J.S. Torg, M.D.

Use of a Modified Elmslie-Trillat Procedure to Improve Abnormal Patellar Congruence Angle
Shelbourne KD, Porter DA, Rozzi W (Methodist Sports Medicine Ctr, Indianapolis, Ind)
Am J Sports Med 22:318–323, 1994   139-95-3–26

Background.—There is little information available concerning the effect of patellar realignment procedures on the postoperative patellar congruence angle. The relationship between postoperative angle correction and clinical outcome was evaluated in patients undergoing a modified Elmslie-Trillat procedure.

Patients and Findings.—Forty-five modified Elmslie-Trillat realignment procedures were performed in 40 patients. Surgical indications included refractory patellar instability in 34 and painful patellofemoral syndrome with malalignment in 11 knees. The mean follow-up was 2 years. The mean preoperative congruence angle was +21.5 degrees, which was significantly improved after surgery, with a mean angle of +3.4 degrees observed at 5 months. With "normal" congruence angles being defined as −20 to +4 degrees, this finding indicated appropriate surgical correction. No significant differences were observed at 24 months (mean angle, +6.3 degrees). None of the patients had postoperative patellar dislocations. Nine knees showed some postoperative subluxation. In 94% of the patients without subluxation, congruence angles of less than 15 degrees were observed, whereas 54% of those with subluxation had angles greater than 15 degrees. Early full activity after surgery did not affect the correction of the congruence angle over time.

Conclusion.—The modified Elmslie-Trillat procedure can predictably improve the patellar congruence angle. Sufficient correction may prevent patellar dislocation. Correction of the congruence angle to less than +15 degrees will also reduce the incidence of postoperative patellar instability. Further follow-up is needed to determine long-term effects.

▶ The authors indicated that the purpose of this study was to determine whether a modified Elmslie-Trillat procedure can correct the abnormal congruence angle, have it persist after a return to full activity, and enable patients to participate in an aggressive rehabilitation program. They appear to have accomplished these 3 goals.

However, they also propose to determine whether a correlation exists between postoperative patellar alignment and clinical outcome. Because of the short postoperative follow-up and because pain, chondral lesions, and degenerative changes were not evaluated, essentially this aspect was not addressed.—J.S. Torg, M.D.

Arthroscopic Suture Fixation of Displaced Tibial Eminence Fractures
Matthews DE, Geissler WB (Univ of Mississippi, Jackson)
Arthroscopy 10:418–423, 1994   139-95-3–27

Background.—The incidence of displaced tibial eminence fractures is increasing in adults with active lifestyles. Arthroscopic reduction and suture fixation were used to treat 6 avulsion fractures (5 type III and 1 type II) of the tibial eminence.

Patients and Findings.—The 5 men and 1 woman had an average age of 24 years. Arthroscopic evaluation was performed when closed reduction after aspiration failed to provide an anatomical reduction. The type II fracture was easily reduced after the interposed anterior horn of the lateral meniscus was manipulated. In the other 5 patients, the fragment was stabilized by arthroscopic placement of multiple 2-0 polydioxanone sutures on the base of the anterior cruciate ligament (ACL), which were pulled through a tibia drill hole and tied to a 4.5-mm screw post. All patients were placed on a standard postoperative ACL protocol, and radiographic healing was demonstrated by 8 weeks. No subjective complaints of instability were offered at 1 year. Full intraoperative extension was achieved in all patients, and only 1 patient had lost 2 degrees of terminal extension at the last follow-up.

Conclusion.—Arthroscopic reduction and suture fixation restore the length of the ACL; stabilize all the fragments; and promote early motion, minimal morbidity, and fracture union. Therefore, this technique is a useful adjunct in patients who sustain displaced tibial eminence fractures.

Arthroscopic Treatment of Fractures of the Tibial Spine

Medler RG, Jansson KA (Univ of Kansas, Wichita; St Francis Regional Med Ctr, Wichita, Kan)
Arthroscopy 10:292–295, 1994   139-95-3–28

Background.—Meyers and McKeever's classification of fractures of the tibial spine is generally accepted as a guide to treatment. Minimally displaced fractures (type I) and those with the anterior one third to one half elevated from the bony bed (type and II) can be treated in a long leg cast that is flexed about 20 degrees. Completely displaced fractures, or type III, are better managed with operative fixation, open or closed. An arthroscopic technique of internal fixation using the Accufex anterior cruciate ligament (ACL) tibial drill guide and absorbable sutures was performed in 2 patients with type III fractures.

Technique.—The leg is placed in the arthroscopic leg holder and the extremity is prepared and draped in the usual sterile fashion. The surgeon cleans the fracture site of all loose and unstable tissue so that it cannot become entrapped in the fracture site at the time of reduction. An anteromedial incision is made over the tibia, and the Accufex tibial aimer is used to place 2 drill-tipped guidewires through the tibia and tibial stump. Spade-tipped guide pins are inserted through the drill holes and bony fracture. The Accufex suture passer from the shoulder set is used to pass a no. 1 PDS through a 7-mm cannula in the anteromedial portal. The suture is threaded through the islet of the spade-tipped pin, and using a grabber it is brought back through the same portal. The surgeon then repeats this step for the other pin. Both pins are removed from the knee, and the double strands of suture are brought with it. The sutures protruding from the anteromedial portal are tied together and pulled snug into the joint (Fig 3–15),

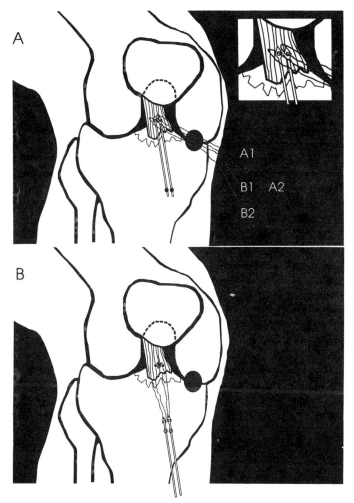

Fig 3–15.—Schematic drawing of the knee. **A,** order of suture tying—tie A1 to B1 and A2 to B2. **B,** pins are withdrawn pulling the knotted sutures over the anterior cruciate ligament insertion. (Courtesy of Medler RG, Jansson KA: *Arthroscopy* 10:292–295, 1994.)

forming a loop to snug down the avulsed fragment. The surgeon then ties the 2 suture loops together, exiting the anterior tibia over a small bony bridge.

Conclusion.—This arthroscopic technique has been used successfully to manage type III fractures. Its advantages include no morbidity from an arthrotomy, the ability to diagnose and treat concomitant injuries, anatomical reduction of the fragment, no retained hardware, and limited surgical time.

▶ The authors' experience in the arthroscopic management of displaced fractures of the tibial spine is similar to my own.—J.S. Torg, M.D.

Intraarticular Ganglion Between the Cruciate Ligaments of the Knee: A Case Report

Kaatee R, Kjartansson Ó , Brekkan Á (Univ Hosp, Reykjavik, Iceland)
Acta Radiol 35:434–436, 1994   139-95-3–29

Case Report.—Boy, 9 years, had pain in his right knee and progressive loss of full extension that started 4 years earlier. Examination showed a 15-degree extension deficit, muscle atrophy, and 1 cm of shortening of the right lower limb. The patient's x-ray films showed a 2-cm bony erosion with sclerotic borders in the intercondylar region of the proximal tibial epiphysis. Evaluation of radiographs obtained 2 years earlier revealed a small cavity. Computed tomography demonstrated a defined soft tissue mass in the intercondylar area and destruction of the cortical bone in both the tibial epiphysis and the medial femoral condyle. Magnetic resonance imaging showed a multilobulated cystic lesion resembling a ganglion. Coronal images demonstrated septations within the lesion (Fig 3–16, A). After arthroscopy failed, open exploration revealed a bluish cystic mass (Fig 3–16, B) that proved to be a ganglion cyst.

Discussion.—Cystic lesions are rarely found within the knee joint. Plain radiographic findings are often nonspecific, but MRI is a useful means of diagnosing meniscal and ganglion cysts. Multiplanar images can show how the lesion is related to intra-articular structures.

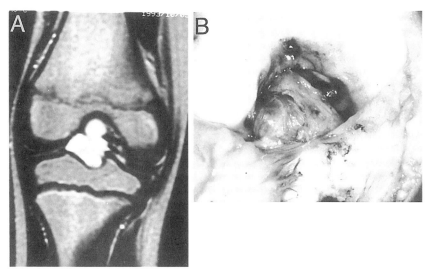

Fig 3–16.—**A,** coronal T2-weighted MR image: an intra-articular multilobulated cystic lesion arising from the tibial epiphysis is visualized with an increased signal intensity. **B,** intraoperative photograph demonstrates a large cystic mass adjacent to the posterior aspect of the anterior cruciate ligament. (Courtesy of Kaatee R, Kjartansson Ó, Brekkan Á: *Acta Radiol* 35:434–436, 1994.)

▶ This is an interesting case that is similar to one that we recently saw in our clinic. It appears that the diagnosis of this lesion is MRI specific.—J.S. Torg, M.D.

Biomechanical Function of the Human Anterior Cruciate Ligament
Takeda Y, Xerogeanes JW, Livesay GA, Fu FH, Woo SL-Y (Univ of Pittsburgh, Pa)
Arthroscopy 10:140–147, 1994   139-95-3-30

Introduction.—The management of the knee with anterior cruciate ligament (ACL) deficiency has improved substantially with recent advances in diagnosis, surgical technique, and rehabilitation. These advances are fueled by a greater understanding of ACL biomechanical function. An overview of current understanding of the biomechanical properties of the ACL was presented.

Normal Stabilizing Roles.—The ACL serves numerous stabilizing functions in the normal knee. It is the primary restraint to anterior tibial translation and to medial tibial displacement in both extension and flexion. It also provides a secondary restraint to tibial rotation, particularly internal tibial rotation in knee extension, and to varus-valgus angulation with the knee in full extension.

Properties of the ACL.—Tensile testing of the femur–ACL–tibia complex (FATC) in both the normal anatomical orientation and in the abnormal tibial orientation revealed distinct differences and values that could be used as guidelines for ACL replacement grafts. In the anatomical orientation, mean values were 242 N/mm for stiffness, 2,160 N for ultimate load, and 11.6 Nm for energy absorbed at failure. The structural values of the FATC were significantly reduced in the tibial orientation. Study of the mechanical properties of the ACL fibers revealed an average modulus of 278 megapascals and ultimate tensile strength of 35 megapascals, with the anteromedial and anterolateral bundles possessing greater modulus, ultimate tensile strength, and strain energy density than the posterior bundle. The bundles also lengthen and shorten differentially during knee motion and with different external loading conditions.

Effects of Muscle Stabilization.—Quadriceps muscle forces cause greater anterior tibial translation; graft tension is decreased between 100 degrees and 80 degrees of flexion, increased between 80 degrees and 5 degrees of flexion, and unaffected in full extension. Hamstring muscle forces diminish anterior tibial translation and internal tibial rotation during knee flexion, decreasing graft tension between 15 degrees and 45 degrees of flexion.

Discussion.—An understanding of the biomechanical function of the ACL is critical to the development of treatment strategies for the ACL-deficient knee. The techniques and mechanisms used to study the kinematics in normal and ACL-deficient knees can also be used to test the efficacy of ACL reconstructions.

Biologic and Synthetic Implants to Replace the Anterior Cruciate Ligament

Jackson DW, Heinrich JT, Simon TM (Long Beach Mem Med Ctr, Calif)
Arthroscopy 10:442–452, 1994   139-95-3–31

Introduction.—Current replacements for the anterior cruciate ligament (ACL) are intended to act as a "checkrein," limiting abnormal anterior translation of the tibia relative to the femur. The prospect of duplicating this dense connective tissue band, a microarchitecturally complex structure, is a considerable challenge. The ACL is heterogeneous at the level of fibers and also at the cellular level.

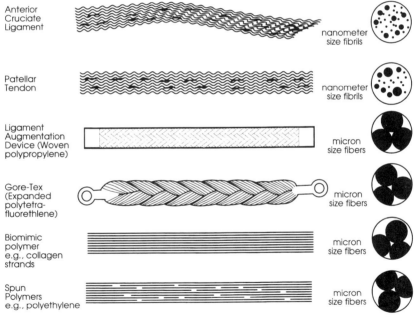

Fig 3–17.—Comparison of the anterior cruciate ligament (ACL) to biological substitutes and presently used synthetics. The ACL has nonparallel fibers and has small- and large-diameter collagen fibrils in the nanometer size range. The patellar tendon has parallel collagen fibers, a different crimp period than the ACL, and has small, large, and very large collagen fibrils in the nanometer size range. The ligament-augmentation device and Gore-Tex are synthetics and are either woven or braided into the final structure. Spun polymers have a linear molecular arrangement that imparts high strength and are made from synthetic fibers. Biomimic polymers such as reconstituted collagen can be formed into strands that can be assembled into a parallel fiber structure. None of the synthetic fibers or biomimic fibers have diameters in the size range of native collagen fibrils. (Courtesy of Jackson DW, Heinrich JT, Simon TM: *Arthroscopy* 10:442–452, 1994.)

Biopolymers.—The large molecules of the ACL are biologically synthesized polymers, predominantly type I collagen. About 10% of adult collagen is type II. Collagen is the major component of the autografts and allografts that are presently used to reconstruct the ACL. About 5% of the molecular framework of the ligament consists of elastin. Proteoglycans and glycoproteins also are present. The ACL normally is maintained through interaction between the constituent cells and the matrix.

Reconstructive Materials.—Currently, autogenous tendon is the standard material used to reconstruct the ACL. Autografts are more predictably incorporated than allografts, less costly, and do not carry a risk of transmitting disease. The ability to successfully transplant allograft fibroblasts, whether fresh or cryopreserved, remains uncertain. A number of materials are under study for use in reconstructing the ACL (Fig 3-17). Carbon fiber implants have performed better when covered by a coating of copolymer or collagen. Dacron implants have often failed, even when coated with silicone. The Gore-Tex II ligament is longer-lasting than its predecessor. Synthetic ligaments have been proposed for use as permanent ligaments, temporary stents, or scaffolds. Current research efforts are based on the use of embryonic cells, mesenchymal stem cells, or the recipient's cells to direct the final collagen pattern of the implant.

Anatomy of the Anterior Cruciate Ligament: A Blueprint for Repair and Reconstruction

Dodds JA, Arnoczky SP (Michigan State Univ, East Lansing)
Arthroscopy 10:132–139, 1994   139-95-3–32

Introduction.—The extraordinarily complex structure of the anterior cruciate ligament (ACL) reflects the complexity of its function as a constraint of joint motion. Its anatomical complexity also complicates the reconstruction of an injured or absent ACL. However, an understanding of the anatomy is required for orthopedic surgeons who are involved in knee repair.

Gross Anatomy.—The ACL connects the femur and tibia and is enveloped by the synovium. The proximal attachment of the ACL is at a fossa on the posterior aspect of the medial surface of the lateral femoral condyle, and it forms a segment of a circle with a convex posterior border. The distal attachment is at a fossa in front of and lateral to the anterior tibial spine, passing beneath and sometimes mingling minimally with the anterior and/or posterior attachment of the lateral meniscus. This attachment is flared, with a section that adopts the contour of the intercondylar roof. The ligaments cross each other between the femur and the tibia, and each demonstrates a slight outward twist. The fibers of the ligament perform in a continuum of tightness and looseness throughout the range of motion, depending on the anteromedial or posterolateral aspect of their tibial attachment.

Microanatomy.—Several collagen fiber bundles separated by columns of cells within fibrous capsules are grouped into fascicles of various sizes. Collagen fibers of the ligament are incorporated within the mineralized bone to form the attachments in a transition zone of fibrocartilage. The fiber bundles are composed of fibroblasts surrounded by a matrix that contains water and an arrangement of collagen, primarily with elastin, proteoglycans, and glycoproteins.

Blood and Nerve Supply.—Blood is supplied from the ligamentous branches of the middle genicular artery and some terminal branches of the medial and lateral inferior genicular arteries, primarily through the enveloping synovial membrane vessels and the infrapatellar fat pad. Both neurovascular bundles and specialized distinct nerve receptors and endings are located in the ligament.

Conclusion.—The structural complexity of the ACL has eluded exact replication. However, an understanding of the current anatomical research permits the best possibility of an optimally functional reconstruction.

▶ Takeda and associates (Abstract 139-95-3–30) predict that by using robotics in conjunction with a universal force-moments sensor, they will be able to control and measure both force and joint position with 6 degrees of freedom.

On the other hand, Jackson and colleagues (Abstract 139-95-3–31) note that "The next generation of biologic and synthetic implants for the ACL will be bioengineered in vitro or in vivo or synthesized by material engineers. The bioengineering of an implant to replace the damaged ACL will entail developing techniques using cells producing biopolymers and the selective use of bioactive molecules."

However, Dodds and Arnoczky (Abstract 139-95-3–32) conclude that the ACL is a complex structure at every level, ranging from its gross structure to its molecular organization, and exact replication of this structure has not been and may never be accomplished.

Only time will tell who is correct.—J.S. Torg, M.D.

Fate of the ACL-Injured Patient: A Prospective Outcome Study
Daniel DM, Stone ML, Dobson BE, Fithian DC, Rossman DJ, Kaufman KR
(San Diego Kaiser Med Ctr, Calif; San Diego Children's Hosp, Calif)
Am J Sports Med 22:632–644, 1994   139-95-3–33

Purpose.—Injuries to the anterior cruciate ligament (ACL) are common, particularly in sports involving deceleration, twisting, cutting, and jumping movements. The outcomes of these injuries vary significantly, with some patients being disabled for sports activity and others having only minimal impairment. This variability, along with the lack of proof that ACL surgery prevents degenerative arthritis, has led to debate over the indications for surgery. The outcome of ACL injury was studied prospectively, including an attempt to identify factors associated with an increased risk of functional impairment, secondary meniscal tears, and joint arthrosis.

Methods.—The study sample included 292 patients in 1 health plan who sustained an acute traumatic hemarthrosis of the knee. All were examined within 2 weeks of the injury and had lower limb injury only in the affected knee. The patients were 204 men and 88 women; 74% were injured during a sports activity, and 91% were between 15 and 44 years of age. The patients and their orthopedists made all management decisions. The patients were followed up—including clinical evaluation, radiographs, and in most cases, bone scans—for a mean of 64 months.

Results.—The KT-1000 arthrometer measurements performed within 90 days of the injury showed that the knee was unstable in 236 cases and stable in 56. Ninety-six percent of the patients with an arthroscopically documented ACL disruption had an injured minus normal knee displacement difference of 3 mm or more on the KT-1000 manual maximum test. Half of the patients with an acute ACL injury had a meniscal tear. An ACL reconstruction was performed within 90 days in 45 patients with unstable knees. Late ligament reconstruction, which was performed after 90 days, was done in 46 patients. Late surgery for a meniscal tear or ACL reconstruction was associated with hours of athletic participation before the injury, arthrometer measurements, and patient age.

Twenty-two patients were excluded from the follow-up analysis because of a subsequent injury to the other knee or reconstructive surgery of the injured ACL within 2 years of follow-up. The remaining 270 patients were grouped for follow-up analysis as follows: early stability with no reconstruction, 53 patients; early instability with no reconstruction, 139 patients; early reconstruction, 45 patients; and late reconstruction, 33 patients. In no instance did the knee injury require a patient to change occupation. All 4 groups had decreased hours per year and levels of sports participation. Patients with joint surface abnormalities who were seen at surgery and those undergoing meniscal surgery had more radiographic and bone scan abnormalities. Patients undergoing reconstructive surgery had a higher level of arthrosis, which was documented by radiography and bone scan. Only 13% of the patients whose knees were stable on instrumented examination experienced instability during follow-up.

Conclusion.—In patients with acute traumatic hemarthrosis of the knee, instrumented measurement of knee displacement is a sensitive test for complete ACL disruption. Knees that are stable on initial KT-1000 assessment are likely to remain stable. About half of the patients with acute ACL injury have a meniscal tear, but not all of these patients require meniscal surgery. Joint arthrosis is more common in patients who undergo meniscal surgery than in those who do not. Among patients who do not require meniscal surgery, ligament surgery is associated with a higher level of joint abnormalities on bone scan.

▶ This excellent article was the winner of the 1993 O'Donoghue Award of the American Orthopedic Society for Sports Medicine. The original article is recommended reading for those who care for patients with acute and chronic knee injuries.—J.S. Torg, M.D.

Bone Injuries Associated With Anterior Cruciate Ligament Disruption

Fowler PJ (Univ Hosp, London, Ont, Canada)
Arthroscopy 10:453–460, 1994   139-95-3–34

Background.—Magnetic resonance imaging has been an important aid in diagnosing soft tissue injury, especially in intra-articular knee ligament injuries. This imaging modality is highly accurate in confirming complete anterior cruciate ligament (ACL) ruptures.

Bone Injuries Associated With ACL Disruption.—Concomitant subchondral bone lesions occur in more than 80% of patients with complete ACL ruptures. Usually, these lesions are not visible on plain radiographs but are confirmed on bone scintigraphy as subchondral fractures. More than 80% of these lesions are found in the lateral compartment. Occult subchondral lesions occur in only 56% of acute knee hemarthrosis without an ACL tear on MRI. An MRI classification of infractions of the knee associated with ACL injury has been proposed. The category of occult subcortical infractions includes reticular, geographic I and II, and linear lesions. The osteochondral category includes chondral, displaced, and impaction lesions. In 1 study, reticular lesions comprised 70% of the occult fractures; linear occult lesions were rarely seen. Complete ACL tears were investigated in a subgroup of patients. Occult geographic I and II infractions were found in 25%. These lesions were characterized by increased density and immediate contiguity to adjacent cortical bone. Impaction fractures that had varying degrees of osteochondral surface depression were noted in 7%. In all patients, the occult geographic and impaction injuries were associated with reticular occult fractures of the posterior margin of the corresponding tibia. Eighty-four percent of the time, the lateral compartment was involved.

Conclusion.—More than 80% of knees with a complete ACL disruption have bone bruises that are detected by MRI. These bruises are an important component of the ACL injury and its outcome. Development of treatment methods to change the degenerative course of many of these lesions is one of the many challenges that face clinicians who treat patients with complete ACL disruption.

▶ This current concepts review points out that MRI-detected bone lesions may explain what have been generally accepted as "repetitive instability" lesions that lead to post-traumatic osteoarthritis in the ACL-deficient knee. As the author points out, "one of the many challenges facing those of us involved in the treatment of this injury is to develop treatment methods that will alter the degenerative course." An MRI classification of infractions of the knee associated with ACL injury is presented that has an excellent set of illustrations.—J.S. Torg, M.D.

Non-Operative Treatment of Ruptures of the Anterior Cruciate Ligament in Middle-Aged Patients
Ciccotti MG, Lombardo SJ, Nonweiler B, Pink M (Thomas Jefferson Univ Hosp, Philadelphia; Kerlan-Jobe Orthopaedic Clinic, Inglewood, Calif; Centinela Hosp, Inglewood, Calif)
J Bone Joint Surg (Am) 76-A:1315–1321, 1994   139-95-3-35

Objective.—Because relatively little is known of the outcome of a ruptured anterior cruciate ligament in middle-aged individuals, the results of nonoperative management were reviewed retrospectively in 52 patients aged 40–60 years. Thirty patients, whose mean age was 46 years, were evaluated after an average interval of 7 years.

Management.—Patients initially had the extremity immobilized and used crutches for 5–7 days; only 3 patients were casted. About three fourths of patients agreed to a formal program of physical therapy that lasted 8 weeks or longer. Rehabilitation focused on the thigh muscles, particularly the hamstrings. Many patients used a brace while doing manual labor that required climbing or pivoting or when engaging in sports activities.

Results.—The mean Lysholm and Gillquist score at follow-up was 82 points. Eight of 11 patients who were thought to have combined ligament injuries had a score less than 84. Although pain on strenuous exertion was frequent, only 3 patients had pain on moderate exertion. Eleven patients had 13 significant recurrent injuries during follow-up. All but 1 of the 30 patents had a grade 2 or 3 Lachman test, and 83% of patients had a positive pivot-shift test. The mean difference between the injured and normal knees in anteroposterior laxity was 5 mm with a 20-lb load. Magnetic resonance imaging showed a scarred ligament remnant in 6 of 9 patients examined.

Conclusion.—Most of the middle-aged patients had a satisfactory outcome without surgery. However, surgery may be considered for patients with combined injuries and those who are unwilling to modify their activities.

▶ Several important points bear reiterating. A substantial reinjury was noted in 37% of the patients in this series after they returned to activity. The use of braces did not affect the rate of reinjury. Ideally, a more meaningful evaluation of a nonoperative treatment of ACL ruptures in middle-aged patients would require comparison with a group that had undergone reconstruction.—J.S. Torg, M.D.

Measurements of the Intercondylar Notch by Plain Film Radiography and Magnetic Resonance Imaging

Herzog RJ, Silliman JF, Hutton K, Rodkey WG, Steadman JR (Steadman Sports Medicine Found, Vail, Colo)
Am J Sports Med 22:204–210, 1994   139-95-3–36

Introduction.—The incidence of anterior cruciate ligament (ACL) disruption has risen with more widespread sports participation. Several morphometric studies have implicated the presence of a femoral intercondylar notch as a predisposing factor for ACL disruption. However, the various morphometric methods make study comparison difficult. The relative accuracy of MRI imaging and plain film radiography was assessed in the morphometric assessment of the femoral intercondylar notch, and the predisposing factors for chronic ACL disruption were determined.

Methods.—Magnetic resonance imaging and plain film radiography were used to perform morphometric analysis of 10 cadaveric knees that were then dissected. The morphometric analyses were compared with direct osseus measurements. In the second part of the study, 1,200 skiing employees were examined clinically to evaluate knee stability. Any patients with asymmetry were further tested with a knee arthrometer. The 20 skiers with significant knee instability and 20 age-, sex-, and athletic activity–matched controls were evaluated with MRI and plain film radiography of both their normal and abnormal knees.

Results.—In part I, there were significant differences between the direct cadaveric measurements and the plain film radiographic morphometric measurements but not the MRI measurements for all parameters. Comparisons of the MRI and plain film measurements of control knees and ACL-deficient knees revealed no significant differences in the dimensions of the notch angle, lateral wall angle, notch widths, or notch ratio. Only 1 statistical difference was detected when comparing plain film measurements of the normal and ACL-deficient knees in each individual: The intercondylar notch at the level of the femoral articular margins in the ACL-deficient knees was narrower.

Discussion.—The accuracy of morphometric analysis of the knee with MRI was validated. Because there were no significant differences between the knees of participants with asymptomatic chronic ACL disruption and those with no documented ACL disruption, analysis failed to identify any predisposing factors, including intercondylar notch characteristics.

Detailed Analysis of Patients With Bilateral Anterior Cruciate Ligament Injuries

Harner CD, Paulos LE, Greenwald AE, Rosenberg TD, Cooley VC (Univ of Pittsburgh, Pa; Orthopedic Specialty Hosp, Salt Lake City, Utah)
Am J Sports Med 22:37–43, 1994   139-95-3–37

Introduction.—Many studies have attempted to define factors that predispose to injury of the anterior cruciate ligament (ACL). However, conclusions have been difficult to reach, partly because of differences in the methods used to measure intercondylar notch dimensions and in the results obtained. Anatomical and other predisposing causes of ACL rupture were sought in a thorough retrospective study of those with noncontact, bilateral ACL injuries.

Methods.—Thirty-one such patients were identified—22 men and 9 women with a mean age of 29 years. Twenty-three controls who had no history of knee injury and were matched for age, sex, height, weight, and activity level were also studied. All research subjects in both groups underwent a thorough evaluation, including a full clinical knee examination; joint hypermobility testing; hamstring tightness assessment; CT analysis, including measurement of specific notch and condyle dimensions; and plain view radiographic analysis. A complete history of knee injury in the immediate family was elicited as well. In the injured group, a KT-1000 arthrometer knee laxity examination was also performed. An injury profile was elicited from each patient, including information on the mechanisms of injury, the treatment received, and the interval between injuries.

Results.—Thirty-five percent of the injured patients had a family history of ACL injury compared with just 4% of the controls. There were few significant differences on physical examination. However, on CT analysis, those in the injured group had a significantly wider lateral femoral condyle than did the control group. The ratio of notch area to condylar area was significantly smaller in the injured group.

Conclusion.—This study, which used a repeatable CT technique of measuring condylar and intercondylar dimensions, suggests that patients with bilateral ACL injuries may have intercondylar notch stenosis secondary to increased lateral condylar width. The overall size of their distal femur is smaller than in normal controls, which perhaps reflects a smaller and weaker ACL. A congenital predisposition to ACL injury was suggested by the finding of an increased incidence of ACL injuries in the immediate families of patients with bilateral injuries.

Femoral Intercondylar Notch Stenosis and Correlation to Anterior Cruciate Ligament Injuries

LaPrade RF, Burnett QM II (Michigan State Univ, Kalamazoo)
Am J Sports Med 22:198–203, 1994   139-95-3–38

Introduction.—There is little understanding of the prevention of anterior cruciate ligament (ACL) tears. Some retrospective studies have reported an association between femoral intercondylar notch stenosis and ACL tears. This possible association was investigated in a prospective study of athletes who were involved in pivoting and cutting sports.

Methods.—A total of 213 college athletes with 415 ACL-intact knees who participated in football, ice hockey, basketball, soccer, gymnastics, or volleyball were studied for 2 years. Knees with ACL deficiency or that had undergone ACL reconstruction were excluded from the study. Bilateral notch-view radiographs were taken of all athletes on their hands and knees and with their knees flexed to 45 degrees. A notch width index, which was calculated as the ratio of the width of the anterior outlet of the femoral intercondylar notch divided by the total condylar width at the level of the popliteal groove, was measured for each knee.

Results.—There were 7 ACL tears in the cohort knees during the study. The average notch width index was 0.244 for men and 0.238 for women. The average notch width index in injured knees was 0.188 for men and 0.200 for women. The correlation between intercondylar notch stenosis and ACL tears was significant. There was stenosis in 6 of the 7 knees with ACL tears. Women had a slightly higher incidence of ACL tears.

Discussion.—These findings demonstrate a statistically significant relationship between anterior intercondylar notch stenosis and the incidence of ACL injuries among athletes who are involved in pivoting and cutting sports. Therefore, athletes with stenotic knees may be at higher risk for ACL injuries. It is recommended that a notchplasty of the medial aspect of the lateral femoral condyle be performed during ACL reconstruction to prevent notch impingement from compromising the success of the graft.

▶ Herzog and colleagues (Abstract 139-95-3–36) say there is no correlation between intercondylar notch stenosis and ACL tears, whereas Harner and associates (Abstract 139-95-3–37) argue that anatomical factors may predispose athletes to ACL injury, and LaPrade and Burnett (Abstract 139-95-3–38) conclude that there is a statistically significant relationship between intercondylar notch stenosis and ACL injuries; certainly, the evidence is inconclusive. However, the possibility of a congenital predisposition to ACL injury is important and deserves further investigation.—J.S. Torg, M.D.

The Measurement of Elongation of Anterior Cruciate-Ligament Grafts *In Vivo*

Beynnon BD, Johnson RJ, Fleming BC, Renström PA, Nichols CE, Pope MH, Haugh LD (Univ of Vermont, Burlington; Med Ctr Hosp of Vermont, Burlington; Univ Orthopaedics Sports Medicine Ctr, Colchester, Vt)

J Bone Joint Surg (Am) 76-A:520–531, 1994   139-95-3–39

Background.—Many researchers who study the mechanical behavior of anterior cruciate ligament grafts have attributed the increase in anterior translation of the tibia relative to the femur to the temporal changes in the strength and elastic properties of the graft that occur throughout the remodeling process. However, with the onset of joint motion, it is not clear whether the repeatable mechanical behavior of the graft remains unchanged just after fixation if the fixation slips or if the length of the graft changes and produces an increase in anterior translation of the tibia relative to the femur. Also, it is not known whether procedures done by different surgeons using similar graft material and similar operative methods can produce similar mechanical graft behavior or if graft behavior is similar to that of the normal anterior cruciate ligament.

Methods and Findings.—Two surgeons did a reconstruction of the anterior cruciate ligament on 10 patients; each used a bone–patellar ligament–bone graft. Immediately after graft fixation, a Hall-effect transducer was implanted to measure the changes in the length of the mid-

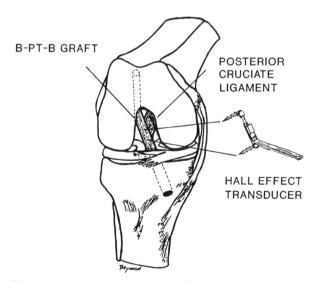

Fig 3–18.—Schematic drawing shows the orientation of the implanted Hall-effect transducer (Micro Strain) on the anteromedial aspect of the bone-patellar ligament-bone (*B-PT-B*) graft. Before it was used in vivo, the transducer was calibrated to measure the length (or relative displacement) between its attachment barbs. (Courtesy of Beynnon BD, Johnson RJ, Fleming BC, et al: *J Bone Joint Surg (Am)* 76-A:520–531, 1994.)

substance of the graft as the knee was moved through 20 cycles of passive flexion-extension. Unlike the length pattern of the normal anterior cruciate ligament, the length pattern of the graft changed cycles of passive motion of the knee. This phenomenon was defined as the cyclic response of the graft and was characterized by calculating the changes in the length of the graft at fixed positions of the knee across the multiple cycles of passive motion. The length of the graft increased through the initial passive-motion cycles in some patients and decreased in others. With the knee almost extended, the predicted increase in anterior translation of the tibia relative to the femur was at most 1 mm, indicating that increases in anterior translation of the tibia relative to the femur can occur immediately after reconstruction of the anterior cruciate ligament and that changes in the length of the graft occur after fixation at loads that are less than the ultimate failure load of the graft or the fixation. In a comparison of the local elongation behavior of the graft, there were no significant differences in the local elongation behavior between groups. Similar results were found when the local elongation data for the bone–patellar ligament–bone graft for the 20th cycle of passive motion were compared with data on the normal anterior cruciate ligament in vivo (Fig 3–18).

Conclusion.—The cyclic response of the graft, not just the structural properties of the graft or the ultimate failure load of the graft or fixation, should be considered during rehabilitation. Restoration of the local elongation behavior of the normal anterior cruciate ligament at the time of reconstruction may be possible.

An *In Vivo* Comparison Between Intraoperative Isometric Measurement and Local Elongation of the Graft After Reconstruction of the Anterior Cruciate Ligament
Fleming BC, Beynnon BD, Nichols CE, Renström PA, Johnson RJ, Pope MH (Univ of Vermont, Burlington; Med Ctr Hosp of Vermont, Burlington; Fanny Allen Hosp, Colchester, Vt)
J Bone Joint Surg (Am) 76-A:511–519, 1994   139-95-3–40

Background.—The intra-articular position of the graft during reconstruction of the anterior cruciate ligament is known to be important. Isometry was introduced in an attempt to determine the best position. Although there is controversy about the location of the near-isometric position, the use of isometers has been recommended for determining the optimal intra-articular graft placement. The utility of isometric measurement in predicting the pattern of elongation of a bone–patellar ligament–bone graft during passive flexion-extension of the knee at the time of anterior cruciate ligament reconstruction in vivo was investigated.

Methods.—Nine patients underwent a standard operative reconstruction procedure. Tunnel sites for the grafts were selected. The change in the distance between those sites was measured using a CA-5000 drill-

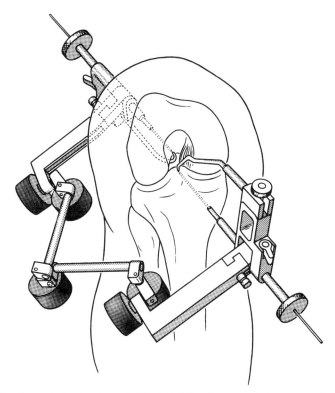

Fig 3–19.—Schematic drawing shows the CA-5000 drill-guide isometer linkage mounted to the knee joint. The femoral guide incorporates a rear-entry targeting hook, and the tibial targeting hook is placed through the medial arthroscopic portal, slightly anterior to the tibial spine. The guide-pins are inserted until their tips meet the targeting hooks of the drill-guide. (Courtesy of Fleming BC, Beynnon BD, Nichols CE, et al: *J Bone Joint Surg (Am)* 76-A:511–519, 1994.)

guide isometer as the knee was subjected to passive flexion-extension (Fig 3–19). After the reconstruction was finished, a Hall-effect transducer was implanted in the graft to measure the local displacement in the midsubstance of the graft produced by passive flexion-extension of the knee. For comparison, the isometric measurements and values for local displacement of the graft were normalized by calculating the percentage of change in length.

Findings.—With the knee in 10–30 degrees of flexion, the mean isometric measurements and the measurements of local displacement showed a reduction in length. However, the 2 techniques of measurement deviated at angles of flexion of 40 degrees and more. Generally, the isometric measurement of elongation between the trial insertion sites predicted that the graft would increase in length in flexion relative to extension, unlike the response of the graft after fixation. The isometric measurement and the local elongation of the graft were not significantly correlated.

Conclusion.—The CA-5000 drill-guide isometric measurements of elongation between the trial insertion sites did not correlate with the values for local elongation of the graft after fixation. Other commercially available isometric systems will probably provide comparable results, because they are based on similar principles of measurement.

▶ The authors developed a unique method for in vivo determination of anterior cruciate ligament (ACL) graft strain and displacement. Of concern is that reproducibility determinations were not performed for ACL grafts; instead, reliability of the method was assumed on the basis of determinations performed for a previous study with intact ligaments. I also question whether the size of the groups had sufficient power for real statistically significant conclusions to be drawn.—J.S. Torg, M.D.

Anterior Cruciate Ligament Reconstruction: Endoscopic Versus Two-Incision Technique
Harner CD, Marks PH, Fu FH, Irrgang JJ, Silby MB, Mengato R (Univ of Pittsburgh, Pa; Ctr for Sports Medicine and Rehabilitation, Pittsburgh, Pa)
Arthroscopy 10:502–512, 1994   139-95-3–41

Background.—Arthroscopically assisted anterior cruciate ligament reconstruction has been performed using a 2-incision technique. The single-incision endoscopic technique was developed relatively recently; before the technique was developed, the best tibial starting point for accurate graft placement was determined using cadavers. The most accurate graft placement was achieved by starting the tibial tunnel midway between the tibial tubercle and posterior border of the tibia. The single-incision endoscopic technique and the 2-incision rear-entry technique of anterior cruciate ligament reconstruction were compared.

Methods.—Of 60 patients, 30 underwent anterior cruciate ligament reconstruction using the 2-incision technique, and 30 underwent surgery with the single-incision technique. Rehabilitation protocol was standard for all patients. Follow-up evaluation included range-of-motion, thigh girth, vertical leap, hop test, and KT-1000 testing. Radiographs were assessed with a scoring system for tunnel location.

Results.—Of the 60 patients, 50 were available for follow-up. Patients were scored using the International Knee Documentation Committee protocol. Complications included 1 rerupture and loss of motion in 2 patients who underwent the 2-incision rear-entry technique and in 3 patients who underwent the single-incision endoscopic technique. Between the 2 groups, there were no significant differences on the International Knee Documentation Committee rating scale, in femoral and tibial tunnel placement shown by anteroposterior and lateral radiographs, or between the frequency and types of sports that patients were able to play before and after surgery.

Conclusion.—Radiographs revealed that consistent posterior placement of the femoral tunnel was achieved using the single-incision endoscopic technique. At a minimum follow-up of 2 years, there were no significant functional or radiographic differences between the 2 anterior cruciate ligament reconstruction techniques. The single-incision technique is less invasive and cosmetically superior.

▶ Although the authors found no significant functional or radiographic differences between these 2 methods, it is important to point out the observation that "fixation of the endoscopically placed femoral bone plug can be a challenge." Specifically, the authors noted that there was a potential risk of cutting the tendon off the bone plug with the screw. In addition, the screw may be divergent and thereby offer optimal fixation. The screw also may drop off the guidewire into the joint and require arthrotomy for retrieval. A posterior wall "blowout" may require the surgeon to make a second incision for completion of the procedure.—J.S. Torg, M.D.

Correlation of Remaining Patellar Tendon Width With Quadriceps Strength After Autogenous Bone-Patellar Tendon-Bone Anterior Cruciate Ligament Reconstruction
Shelbourne KD, Rubinstein RA Jr, VanMeter CD, McCarroll JR, Rettig AC
(Methodist Sports Medicine Ctr, Indianapolis, Ind)
Am J Sports Med 22:774–778, 1994   139-95-3–42

Introduction.—Although anterior cruciate ligament (ACL) knee reconstructions are usually performed using autogenous bone–patellar tendon–bone grafts, there are concerns about the morbidity associated with harvesting this graft, including the possibility of quadriceps muscle weakness. The effects of the size of the remaining patellar tendon on the rate and level of the recovery of quadriceps muscle strength after autogenous bone–patellar tendon–bone graft harvest were assessed in a prospective study.

Methods.—A total of 121 patients who underwent ACL reconstruction with an autogenous central bone–patellar tendon–bone graft were evaluated at 6 weeks, 3 months, 6 months, and 1 year postoperatively using isokinetic testing. The remaining patellar widths were measured intraoperatively at the level of the joint line. For analysis, the patients were assigned to groups that were defined by the remaining patellar tendon width: small (14–17 mm), medium (18–20 mm), and large (21–25 mm).

Results.—Patients in both the small-width and the medium-width group had significantly weaker mean isokinetic quadriceps scores than those in the large-width group at 6 weeks. At 3 months, there was significant comparative quadriceps weakness only in the small-width group. By the sixth postoperative month, there were no significant differences in quadriceps strength among the 3 groups. At 1 year, the mean quadriceps isokinetic score was 86% that of the uninjured leg.

Discussion.—Although there are differences in quadriceps strength that correspond to the width of the remaining patellar tendon after autogenous bone–patellar tendon–bone graft harvest for ACL reconstruction early in the recovery period, they diminish and become insignificant by 6 months after surgery. Therefore, the size of the remaining patellar tendon does not compromise the ultimate postoperative recovery of extensor strength.

▶ The authors have presented a relatively simple and well-documented 1-dimensional analysis of one factor that has been attributed to postoperative quadriceps weakness after ACL reconstruction. It is important because it will guide the surgeon in graft harvest. However, Shino and associates have previously observed that patients with allograft ACL reconstructions had a mean isokinetic extension score of 88% at an average follow-up of 57 months, indicating that other factors are involved (1). As the authors point out: "The explanation for quadriceps scores being less than 100% is multifactorial and likely includes the injury itself, the timing of surgery, the insult of intra-articular surgery, the rehabilitation, and the patient's motivation."—J.S. Torg, M.D.

Reference

1. Shino K, Inoue M, Horibe S, et al: Reconstruction of the anterior cruciate ligament using allogeneic tendon: Long-term followup. *Am J Sports Med* 18:457–465, 1990.

The Effects of Donor Age and Strain Rate on the Biomechanical Properties of Bone-Patellar Tendon-Bone Allografts
Blevins FT, Hecker AT, Bigler GT, Boland AL, Hayes WC (Charles A. Dana Research Inst, Boston; Beth Israel Hosp, Boston; Harvard Med School, Boston)
Am J Sports Med 22:328–333, 1994   139-95-3–43

Introduction.—Anterior cruciate ligament reconstruction using an isometrically placed bone–patellar tendon–bone autograft is currently the most effective method of knee stabilization. However, the use of patellar tendon autograft can result in significant morbidity. Consideration of the use of allografts has raised concerns such as the possibility of evoked immune response, decreased strength, and increased cartilage erosion. The relationship between donor age and biomechanical properties and the effects of strain rate on the biomechanical properties of bone–patellar tendon–bone allografts were investigated.

Methods.—Eighty-two medial and lateral bone–patellar tendon–bone allografts were obtained from 25 donors, aged 17–54 years. The medial and lateral allografts from each specimen were randomly assigned to be tested at strain rates of 10% or 100% elongation per second in a servohydraulic materials test system. The mode of failure was classified. Tensile strength and modulus were calculated using tendon length and cross-sectional area measurements obtained with an area micrometer.

Results.—Tendons tested at 10% elongation per second had a mean tensile strength of 35.9 megapascals and a mean modulus of 302 megapascals. Tendons tested at 100% elongation per second had a mean tensile strength of 37.1 megapascals and a mean modulus of 310 megapascals. There were no significant differences in tensile strength or modulus associated with the 2 strain rates, either overall or in the subgroup of specimens that failed because of ligamentous rupture. Age did not affect tensile strength at either strain rate. However, there was a weakly significant correlation between modulus and age only at a strain rate of 100% elongation per second. Modes of failure included midsubstance tears (46%), tendon failures at the tibial insertion (10%), tendon failures at the patellar insertion (11%), bony avulsions at the tibial bone plugs (12%), bony avulsions at the patellar bone plugs (2%), and tibial bone plug fractures (17%). The mode of failure was not associated with either age or strain rate.

Discussion.—Neither increased donor age nor increased strain rate diminishes the tensile strength of bone–patellar tendon–bone allografts or affects the mode of failure, although modulus is weakly negatively correlated with age at greater strain rates.

▶ The conclusions of this study are somewhat at variance with those of Noyes and Grood (1) and Paulos and colleagues (2), who reported a significant correlation between age and tensile strength of this graft material. However, the authors point out that although "the inclusion of specimens from donors over age 60 would likely increase the correlation between age and tensile strength, such specimens were excluded from the current study because 60 is the age limit for organ donors at most bone donor banks."—J.S. Torg, M.D.

References

1. Noyes FR, Grood ES: The strength of the anterior cruciate ligament in humans and rhesus monkeys: Age related and species related changes. *J Bone Joint Surg* 58:1074–1082, 1976.
2. Paulos LE, France EP, Rosenberg TD, et al: Comparative material properties of allograft tissues for ligament replacement: Effect of type, age, sterilization and preservation. *Trans Orthop Res Soc* 13:129, 1987.

Bone Tunnel Enlargement After Anterior Cruciate Ligament Replacement

Fahey M, Indelicato PA (Univ of Florida, Gainesville)
Am J Sports Med 22:410–414, 1994   139-95-3–44

Background.—Disruption of the anterior cruciate ligament is a common injury that often results in function instability. Intra-articular reconstruction of the anterior cruciate ligament is frequently recommended. Early studies of allograft anterior cruciate ligament replacement are encouraging, but there are concerns about transmission of viral disease, graft bacterial contamination, postoperative infection, immune response, and graft rejection. Increases in the tibial and femoral bone tunnels have been observed. Tunnel enlargements in allograft and autograft patellar tendon replacements were compared, and their clinical implications were assessed.

Methods.—At 1 year, 87 patients with allograft and 56 patients with autograft anterior cruciate ligament replacements had complete follow-up evaluations. Sclerotic margins of the tibial tunnel were measured 1 cm below the joint line. Exact tunnel dimension was calculated using a magnification factor determined by the interference screw of known diameter within the same tunnel.

Results.—The average allograft tunnel enlargement was 1.2 mm, and the average autograft tunnel enlargement was 0.26 mm, a significant difference. There was no significant difference in KT-1000 arthrometer measurements between the allograft and autograft groups and no correlation between increased tunnel size and clinical outcome, as determined by the modified Hughston knee evaluation system. Independent repeated measurements confirmed the reproducibility of the tunnel measurement.

Conclusions.—The cause of bone-tunnel enlargement is unknown. Possible explanations include immune response with resorption; stress-shielding proximal to the interference screw and bone plug, which results in resorption; or an inflammatory response by synovium in the tunnel. Tunnel enlargement does not seem to adversely affect clinical outcome.

▶ This study agrees with the findings of Linn and colleagues (1). As the authors noted, the bottom line is that the "significance of this tunnel enlargement is unknown and does not appear to adversely effect clinical outcome of allograft utilization."—J.S. Torg, M.D.

Reference

1. Linn RM, Fischer DA, Smith JP, et al: Achilles tendon allograft reconstruction of the anterior cruciate ligament-deficient knee. *Am J Sports Med* 21:825–831, 1993.

Risk Factors for Restricted Motion After Anterior Cruciate Reconstruction

Graf BK, Ott JW, Lange RH, Keene JS (Univ of Wisconsin, Madison)
Orthopedics 17:909–912, 1994   139-95-3–45

Background.—Intra-articular anterior cruciate ligament reconstruction is a common orthopedic procedure. Recently, attention has been focused on potential complications of this surgery. Restricted knee motion is a complication that is relatively frequent and significantly impairs knee function. Factors such as the extent of initial injury, timing of surgery, surgical technique, and rehabilitation protocol were examined to determine whether any could be correlated with restricted knee motion.

Methods.—Medical records of 373 patients were reviewed retrospectively to determine risk factors for restricted postoperative motion. All patients had undergone anterior cruciate ligament reconstruction using the central third of the patellar tendon. Stepwise logistic regression analysis determined factors that best predicted final range of motion.

Results.—Variables that were most strongly correlated with restricted final range of motion (flexion $\leq$ 125 degrees or flexion contracture $\geq$ 10 degrees) were open surgery and surgery performed 7 days or less after the injury. Range of motion was not significantly affected by age, meniscal repair, or associated collateral ligament injuries. Limited range of motion was significantly less likely to occur in a subgroup of 204 patients who underwent arthroscopic reconstruction more than 7 days after initial injury and started range-of-motion exercises within 2 days of surgery.

Conclusion.—Delayed arthroscopic anterior cruciate ligament reconstruction and aggressive early range-of-motion exercises and rehabilitation can help avoid postoperative motion problems.

▶ Numerous factors have been identified as being responsible for loss of joint motion after ACL reconstruction. They include improper tunnel placement, the "cyclops" lesion, and the infrapatellar contracture syndrome. It is interesting to note that all the patients in this study were placed in a knee immobilizer or similar splint for 6 weeks. Although the authors have ignored this factor, their conclusions were in keeping with those of Harner and associates (1), Shelbourne and colleagues (2), and Strum and co-workers (3) that a strong correlation exists between surgery performed within 1 week of injury and subsequent restriction of joint motion.—J.S. Torg, M.D.

References

1. Harner CD, Orrgamg KK, Paul JJ, et al: Loss of motion after anterior cruciate ligament reconstruction. *Am J Sports Med* 20:499–506, 1992.
2. Shelbourne KD, Wikkens JH, Mollabashy A, et al: Arthrofibrosis in the acute anterior cruciate ligament reconstruction: The effect of timing of reconstruction and rehabilitation protocol. *Am J Sports Med* 19:332–336, 1991.

3. Strum GM, Friedman MJ, Fox JM, et al: Acute anterior cruciate ligament reconstruction: Analysis of complications. *Clin Orthop* 253:184–189, 1990.

Infrapatellar Contracture Syndrome: Diagnosis, Treatment, and Long-Term Followup

Paulos LE, Wnorowski DC, Greenwald AE (Orthopedic Specialty Hosp, Salt Lake City, Utah)
Am J Sports Med 22:440–448, 1994   139-95-3–46

Purpose.—Infrapatellar contracture syndrome (IPCS) is associated with significantly reduced patellar mobility. Infrapatellar contracture syndrome may develop primarily as an exaggerated fibrous hyperplasia of the anterior soft tissues or secondarily after certain knee operations. The long-term outcome in patients who were operated on for IPCS was assessed.

Patients.—The study population consisted of 75 patients aged 12–63 years who had IPCS in 76 knees and who had been refractory to conservative treatment and had been referred for knee surgery to the Orthopedic Specialty Hospital in Salt Lake City, Utah. Twenty patients had primary IPCS and 55 had secondary IPCS. Secondary procedures performed included arthroscopic and open débridement, manipulation under anesthesia, and a DeLee proximal tibial osteotomy (Fig 3–20). The patients were divided into subgroups to examine the effects of various factors on clinical outcome. The average follow-up was 53.2 months after the index event. Only patients with at least 24 months of follow-up after the index event were included in the study.

Results.—The desired range of motion was achieved in most patients. However, residual symptoms, patellofemoral dysfunction, and activity-related pain and swelling were significant. The best results were obtained in younger patients with primary IPCS who had undergone fewer corrective procedures. The worst results were obtained in patients who had undergone acute anterior cruciate ligament (ACL) repair or reconstruction, had patellar tendon ACL autografts harvested, had patella infera, had multiple corrective procedures, and had undergone closed manipulation. The most common iatrogenic cause of IPCS was nonisometric ACL graft placement and graft impingement.

Conclusion.—Although the range of motion in patients with IPCS can be substantially increased with appropriate surgical procedures, many patients will have persistent residual functional morbidity.

▶ The observation of the authors that "The natural history of an anterior cruciate ligament–deficient knee appears to be more benign than the natural history of a knee that develops infrapatellar contracture syndrome" is noteworthy. Because prevention is the only way to avoid the morbidity associated

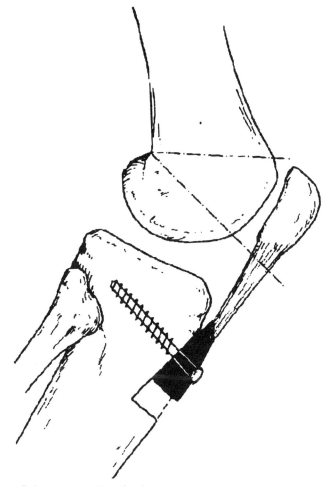

Fig 3–20.—DeLee osteotomy. Note that the osteotomy moves the affected attachment of the patellar tendon superiorly on the tibia as well as anteriorly. Not only does this osteotomy reduce the patella infera, but it also increases the distance between the patellar tendon and the anterior tibial complex, thus reducing the tendency for these structures to fibrose. (Courtesy of Paulos LE, Wnorowski DC, Greenwald AE: *Am J Sports Med* 22:440–448, 1994.)

with this problem, surgeons should refer to the original article for enumeration of 10 factors to be avoided.—J.S. Torg, M.D.

The Surgical Treatment of Arthrofibrosis of the Knee

Cosgarea AJ, DeHaven KE, Lovelock JE (Univ of Rochester, NY; Rochester Gen Hosp, NY)
Am J Sports Med 22:184–191, 1994   139-95-3–47

Introduction.—Arthrofibrosis of the knee is a common complication of knee surgery, especially ligament surgery. It significantly impairs the range of motion, which can result in progressive damage to the articular surface. The intermediate outcome of surgical treatment for arthrofibrosis of the knee was studied in patients who had undergone previous knee ligament surgery.

Methods.—Thirty-seven patients underwent lysis of adhesion procedures to treat arthrofibrosis of the knee caused by previous ligament surgery. Six of the patients required a repeat lysis of adhesion procedure. The precipitating surgeries were anterior cruciate ligament (ACL) reconstruction in 23 patients, ACL repair in 12, posterior cruciate ligament repair in 1, and medial collateral ligament repair in 1. All patients had functional impairment and a loss of flexion or of extension of at least 10 degrees that did not improve after 2 months of intense therapy. Follow-up averaged 3.6 years. A control group of 15 patients who had not had arthrofibrosis after ACL reconstruction surgery was also evaluated. This group was matched so patients could be studied for age, sex, ACL chronicity before reconstruction, and the incidence of associated ligament or meniscal lesions.

Results.—After lysis of adhesion procedures, the average flexion improved from 81% to 95% of contralateral flexion, and average flexion deficits improved from 14 to 3 degrees. Functional outcome was excellent in 9 patients, good in 14, fair in 10, and poor in 4. Of the 35 patients who were evaluated radiographically, 89% had osteophyte formation, 20% had narrowed joint space, 51% had soft tissue calcification, and 9% had patella infera. A comparison of range of motion, functional scores, and radiographic evaluations in the control patients revealed similar outcomes in patients undergoing lysis procedures less than 6 months after the ligament surgery and in patients with the localized intra-articular variant of arthrofibrosis.

Discussion.—Although patients undergoing surgical treatment for arthrofibrosis achieve significantly improved flexion and extension, they often have disappointing functional outcomes and radiographic degenerative changes. However, patients with the localized anterior intra-articular variant of arthofibrosis and those who undergo lysis of adhesion procedures within 6 months of the ligament surgery appear to have better outcomes.

Outpatient Surgical Management of Arthrofibrosis After Anterior Cruciate Ligament Surgery

Shelbourne KD, Johnson GE (Methodist Sports Medicine Ctr, Indianapolis, Ind)
Am J Sports Med 22:192–197, 1994   139-95-3-48

Introduction.—Arthrofibrosis, a complication of anterior cruciate ligament (ACL) surgery, usually results in an inability to straighten the leg, which causes functional difficulties. Several treatment strategies have been developed to manage severe flexion contractures, often using extensive resources. The results of a strategy that used outpatient surgery and physical therapy were examined.

Methods.—Nine patients with arthrofibrosis after ACL reconstruction that caused at least 15 degrees of flexion contracture and impaired gait were treated. While under general anesthesia, the patient underwent arthroscopy with tourniquet control. With the knee in full flexion, débridement of the adhesions in the suprapatellar pouch and in the medial and lateral gutters was performed. The knee was extended until the impinging scar in the notch was visualized. The impinging tissue was excised, and a notchplasty was performed if necessary. Persistent graft impingement was treated with resection of the anterior portion of the graft. The knee was placed in daily serial forced-extension casts during a period of 7–10 days and extension was maintained with nighttime splints. Patients underwent aggressive physical therapy with flexion exercises.

Results.—All patients reported decreased pain, including 7 who reported no pain postoperatively. Eight of the 9 patients could walk normally and participate in recreational sports. The range of motion improved significantly in all but 1 patient. Quadriceps and hamstring strength improved to an average of more than 80% of that of the contralateral leg.

Discussion.—The treatment strategy is based on the belief that anterior scar formation between the tibia and femur resulting from immobilization in flexion after ACL reconstruction allows flexion contracture to develop. Therefore, arthrofibrosis is best treated by prevention, which involves optimal timing of surgery after patients have regained full range of motion and postoperative rehabilitation protocols, including early extension. The treatment strategy for flexion contracture involving arthroscopic excision of mechanical blocks to extension and postoperative posterior capsular stretching was effective in restoring full hyperextension in most patients. The aggressive physical therapy also improved flexion. This program can be an effective and cost-efficient alternative to open arthrotomy.

▶ Although Cosgarea et al. (Abstract 139-95-3-47) emphasize that results are better with early intervention, they also point out that there are patients who "respond poorly to any type of treatment in the acute setting." These are patients who have a more intense inflammatory reaction and often have an overlying component of reflex sympathetic dystrophy (RSD). In this group, early aggressive motion or surgical intervention exacerbates the problem.

It would be interesting to know the results obtained in patients who have had their RSD successfully managed. It would appear that another factor to be considered is accurate tunnel and graft placement, an aspect that was not addressed in either (Abstract 139-95-3–47 or 139-95-3–48).—J.S. Torg, M.D.

Use of Allografts After Failed Treatment of Rupture of the Anterior Cruciate Ligament

Noyes FR, Barber-Westin SD, Roberts CS (Cincinnati Sportsmedicine and Orthopaedic Ctr, Ohio; Deaconess Hospital, Cincinnati, Ohio)
J Bone Joint Surg (Am) 76-A:1019–1031, 1994   139-95-3–49

Background.—Bone–patellar ligament–bone allografts have been used to reconstruct the anterior cruciate ligament in 66 knees that failed to respond to intra-articular or extra-articular surgeries. A total of 235 previous operations had been performed in these knees, including 81 for rupture of the anterior cruciate ligament.

Findings.—All but 1 patient returned for follow-up evaluation at a mean of 42 months after the operation. Substantial improvement of the anteroposterior displacement was noted in the majority of patients. Fifty-seven patients with unilateral conditions underwent arthrometric studies and pivot-shift tests. The results showed functional ligaments in 30 patients, partially functional ligaments in 12, and nonfunctional reconstructed ligaments in 15. An overall failure rate of 33% was noted when the 15 failures were considered together with an additional 10 failures that had occurred within 2 years after surgery. The subjective ratings of functional limitations and symptoms and overall rating scores were significantly improved, although there were significant differences between the scores of patients with normal-appearing articular cartilage surfaces at the index operation and those with notable fissuring and fragmentation or exposure of the subchondral bone. After rehabilitation, which included immediate motion of the knee, range of motion of 0 to 135 degrees was restored in all but 5 knees. Four of the 5 lacked only 5 degrees of this extent of flexion or extension.

Conclusion.—Bone–patellar ligament–bone allografts can be used when proper autogenous tissues are not available. The symptoms and abnormal displacement were decreased in most of the patients in this series.

▶ This 33% reconstruction failure rate is most disconcerting. Although it is commonly recognized that poorly placed femoral or tibial tunnels can result in graft failure, this issue was not really addressed other than the statement that 10 failures were "directly attributed" to this factor.

My experience has been that a staged bone grafting must be performed before the revision procedure if poor tunnel placement was responsible for the initial failure. The authors state that they avoided staged bone grafting in all of their patients, because many of these patients had already had multiple operations. Considering the high reconstruction failure rate, it appears that this approach deserves to be rethought. My experience with staged tunnel grafting before the definitive reconstruction has been most satisfactory.—J.S. Torg, M.D.

Graft Impingement After Anterior Cruciate Ligament Reconstruction: Presentation as an Active Extension "Thunk"
Lane JG, Daniel DM, Stone ML (Kaiser Permanente, San Diego, Calif)
Am J Sports Med 22:415–417, 1994   139-95-3-50

Introduction.—Although anterior cruciate ligament (ACL) reconstruction is designed to normalize knee motion, many complications can occur. A subset of patients who had a localized palpable sensation at the anterior aspect of the knee after surgery had a low-pitched "thunking" sound during the final 30 degrees of active knee extension that did not occur during passive extension.

Methods.—Of 215 ACL reconstructions performed, 12 patients had a postoperative thunking noise during active terminal extension of the reconstructed knee. The patients were followed up and the onset of noise was documented. Patients with this complication were treated as necessary with observation, arthroscopy, or notchplasty.

Results.—The noise occurred an average of 5 months after the reconstructive procedure (range, 1.5–13 months) and lasted for an average of 4 months (range, 1–9 months); 4 of the patients had concurrent effusion. The noise was associated with pain in only 1 patient. Resolution occurred without surgical treatment in 4 patients in an average of 3 months, although anterior laxity increased in 3 of these 4 patients after resolution of the noise. Seven of the 8 patients with persistent symptoms underwent arthroscopy an average of 5 months after the onset, which identified impingement of the graft in the notch in 6 patients. These 6 underwent notchplasties, during which partial tearing of the grafts was discovered in 3 patients. The remaining patient who underwent arthroscopy required débridement of the fat pad. The symptoms resolved in all 7 of these patients; the remaining patient declined arthroscopy and was lost to follow-up.

Discussion.—Several studies have documented the importance of the placement of the tibial tunnel in preventing graft impingement. When tibial tunnel placement is at the anterior edge of the insertion site of the ACL on the tibia, a superior notchplasty will be necessary. If a patient has a thunking noise during terminal active extension, the possibility of graft impingement should be evaluated with an arthroscopic examination. Graft impingement should be treated, because a delay could result in graft tearing.

▶ This paper emphasizes the importance of proper placement of the tibial tunnel in ACL reconstruction. This condition is similar to the "cyclops" syndrome reported by Jackson and Schaefer (1).—J.S. Torg, M.D.

Reference

1. Jackson DW, Schaefer RK: Cyclops syndrome: Loss of extension following in-
    tra-articular anterior cruciate ligament reconstruction. *Arthroscopy* 6:171–178,
    1990.

Reflex Inhibition of the Quadriceps Femoris Muscle After Injury or Reconstruction of the Anterior Cruciate Ligament

Snyder-Mackler L, De Luca PF, Williams PR, Eastlack ME, Bartolozzi AR III
(Univ of Delaware, Newark)
J Bone Joint Surg (Am) 76-A:555–560, 1994   139-95-3–51

Background.—Patients who have had anterior cruciate ligament reconstruction have substantial weakness of the quadriceps femoris muscle. Some have attributed this weakness to an inability to voluntarily activate the quadriceps femoris muscle fully. Whether patients with a
rupture of the anterior cruciate ligament can fully activate the quadriceps
femoris muscle before surgery and in the early phase of rehabilitation
after ligament reconstruction was investigated. It was hypothesized that
the failure of voluntary activation was associated with weakness of the
quadriceps femoris muscle in patients with a torn anterior cruciate ligament and in those with ligament reconstruction.

Methods and Findings.—The strength of the quadriceps femoris muscle was assessed by a burst-superimposition method in 3 patient groups.
Group 1 included 20 patients with a torn anterior cruciate ligament of
the knee and a reconstruction of the ligament 1–6 months after injury. In
group 2, 12 patients had a a torn anterior cruciate ligament for a mean
of 3 months (a subacute tear). Group 3 included 8 patients with a torn
anterior cruciate ligament for a mean of 2 years (a chronic tear). The patients in groups 2 and 3 had not had surgery for the torn ligament. The
patients in groups 1 and 3 showed no signs of failure of the activation of
the involved quadriceps. However, 9 of 12 patients in group 2 had reflex
inhibition of contraction of the muscle.

Conclusion.—In this series, most patients who had a torn anterior cruciate ligament for 6 months or less before testing and who had not undergone reconstruction were unable to fully activate the quadriceps muscle voluntarily. Therefore, such patients may not have responded well to
a rehabilitation program that relies on volitional exercise alone. If quadriceps inhibition is a direct result of capsular stress from joint laxity and
if irreversible atrophy occurs after a period of time, then patients with a
torn anterior cruciate ligament may be able to regain full function of the
quadriceps only if the reconstruction is done before such atrophy occurs.

▶ This article has a major ambiguity. The patients in group 3, those with a
chronic ACL tear, "demonstrated full voluntary activation" of the quadriceps

muscle. In light of this, it is difficult to understand how the authors could conclude that "a patient who has a torn anterior cruciate ligament may be able to regain full function of the quadriceps only if the reconstruction is done before such atrophy occurs."—J.S. Torg, M.D.

Complete vs Partial-Thickness Tears of the Posterior Cruciate Ligament: MR Findings

Patten RM, Richardson ML, Zink-Brody G, Rolfe BA (Univ of Washington, Seattle; Washington Orthopedics and Sports Medicine, Kirkland)
J Comput Assist Tomogr 18:793–799, 1994   139-95-3-52

Background.—Early diagnosis and surgical repair of tears of the posterior cruciate ligament (PCL) are important. Magnetic resonance imaging reliably demonstrates normal and abnormal PCLs. The MR appearance of complete and partial-thickness PCL tears was further defined in a large series, and patterns of injury and additional MR findings associated with these tears were described.

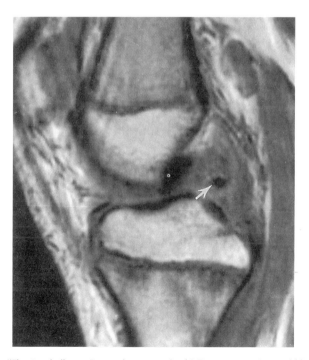

Fig 3–21.—"Floating dot" sign. Proton density–weighted MR image in a 13-year-old boy with complete PCL tear shows low signal intensity focus of meniscofemoral ligament (*arrow*) surrounded by intermediate signal intensity edema in the posterior joint space. (Courtesy of Patten RM, Richardson ML, Zink-Brody G, et al: *J Comput Assist Tomogr* 18:793-799, 1994.)

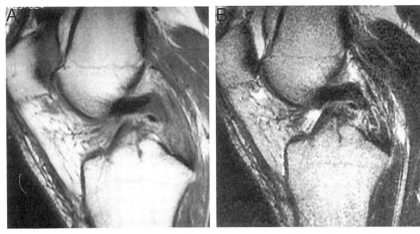

Fig 3–22.—Apparent focal ligamentous discontinuity in a 24-year-old man with surgically confirmed partial posterior cruciate ligament (PCL) tear. **A** and **B**, proton density- and T2-weighted MR images were interpreted as showing complete PCL disruption. (Courtesy of Patten RM, Richardson ML, Zink-Brody G, et al: *J Comput Assist Tomogr* 18:793–799, 1994.)

Methods.—The MR images and medical records of 32 patients with PCL tears were reviewed retrospectively by 3 radiologists. Magnetic resonance findings were correlated with the results of clinical testing and surgery.

Findings.—In 84% of the patients, the PCL had indistinct margins. In 78%, it was abnormally thickened. The torn PCL showed increased signal intensity on both T1- and T2-weighted pulse sequences in 97% of the patients. Seventy-five percent had all 3 signs of abnormality—abnormal thickness, indistinct margins, and abnormal signal intensity. In 56%, a focal bulge of heterogeneous signal intensity deformed the contour of the PCL at the tear site (Fig 3-21). Thickness, margination, and signal intensity of the PCL did not differ between patients with complete tears and those with partial tears. However, the MR images of patients with complete tears were more likely to show focal areas of ligamentous discontinuity. Associated knee injuries occurred in 66% of the patients, and they occurred more often in those with complete PCL tears. Also common were bony injury, which occurred in 34%; tears of the medial collateral ligament, in 41%; and menisci, in 31%. There was no identifiable, specific pattern of bony injury.

Conclusion.—Posterior cruciate ligament tears can be readily diagnosed by multiplanar MRI by morphologic and signal intensity characteristics. Differentiating between complete and partial-thickness PCL tears using MR criteria alone is more problematic. However, complete tears are more likely to show focal areas of discontinuity, whereas partial tears are more likely to show at least some intact fibers (Fig 3-22).

▶ As noted by the authors, this investigation lacked not only a control population but also a sufficient number of cases with surgical follow-up to draw any definitive conclusions. However, like many other reports, this study again documents that PCL tears can be differentiated from normal ligaments but that differentiation of complete from partial tears by MRI is elusive.—J.S. Torg, M.D.

Posterior Cruciate Ligament Allograft Reconstruction With and Without a Ligament Augmentation Device
Noyes FR, Barber-Westin SD (Cincinnati Sportsmedicine and Orthopaedic Ctr, Ohio; Deaconess Hosp, Cincinnati, Ohio)
J Arthro Rel Surg 10:371–382, 1994   139-95-3–53

Introduction.—Both primary repair and autogenous grafting have been used to reconstruct midsubstance or complete ruptures to the posterior cruciate ligament (PCL). A number of different allografts have been used successfully for repair of both acute and chronic PCL ruptures. In an effort to increase the success rate still more, a procedure involving arthroscopically assisted implantation of a combined allograft–ligament augmentation device (LAD) composite was developed.

Methods.—The records were reviewed of the results of 26 operations on 25 patients who had complete rupture of the PCL but an intact anterior cruciate ligament and lateral collateral ligament and were followed for at least 2 years postoperatively. Group 1 included 6 male and 4 female patients who underwent repair with allograft only. Of these 10 patients, 6 had surgery within 5 weeks of the injury and 4 had surgery 90–228 weeks after the injury. Group 2 included 9 male and 6 female patients who underwent repair with LAD. Of these 15 patients, 4 had surgery within 10 weeks after the injury, and 11 had surgery 24–192 weeks after the injury. The patients were evaluated with a comprehensive knee examination and questionnaires regarding symptoms, function, and sports and occupational activities. Knee displacement at 20 degrees and 70 degrees of knee flexion and muscle strength were tested.

Results.—There were no significant differences between the groups in anteroposterior (AP) displacement values at either 20 degrees or 70 degrees of flexion. At 20 degrees of flexion, all the knees with acute PCL rupture had 2.5 mm or less of increased AP displacement over the contralateral knee, as did 60% of the knees with chronic PCL ruptures. At 70 degree of flexion, there were more knees with either acute or chronic PCL ruptures that had more than 5.5 mm of increased AP displacement. There were no significant differences between the 2 groups in self-assessed symptoms, function, or sports and occupational activity level. Results in these areas were generally significantly better in patients with acute injuries than in those with chronic injuries.

Discussion.—The results demonstrated that there was no benefit associated with the use of the LAD. However, the outcome was significantly better for patients with acute injuries than for those with chronic injuries. Because all patients with acute injuries were able to return to sports activities, it was recommended that early operative treatment with an immediate knee motion postoperative program be considered for athletic patients.

▶ The authors indicate that this study was intended to compare the results of the use of allografts alone and the use of an LAD to reconstruct the PCL. Apparently, a combined allograft LAD was used to "increase the success rate" of PCL reconstructions. However, there was a lack of a "beneficial effect from the composite" compared with the results using the allograft. Interestingly, the authors also point out that "the qualifications of this study prevent definitive conclusions to be reached on the treatment of acute and chronic PCL ruptures." The authors also indicate that they "acknowledge that PCL reconstructive surgery is a multifactorial decision and stress to our patient that scientific data are still lacking for surgical and nonoperative treatment in isolated PCL ruptures."—J.S. Torg, M.D.

Office Operative Arthroscopy of the Knee: Technical Considerations and a Preliminary Analysis of the First 100 Patients
Small NC, Glogau AI, Berezin MA, Farless BL (Associated Arthroscopy Inst, Plano, Tex)
Arthroscopy 10:534–539, 1994   139-95-3–54

Objective.—The efficacy of surgical arthroscopy of the knee done as an office procedure under local anesthesia and light IV sedation was examined in 100 patients with 106 knees in 1989–1992. A total of 169 procedures were done.

Patient Selection.—Patients aged 16–65 years were accepted for office treatment. To be accepted for this office-based procedure, patients had to be in good general health and be psychologically able to have surgery under local anesthesia. Only patients who were thought not to have compromised ligaments or a repairable meniscal lesion were selected.

Results.—Two of the 100 patients were later taken to the hospital for additional arthroscopic treatment. Complications included 3 cases of hemarthroses and 1 case of reflex sympathetic dystrophy. All 4 complications were mild, and none led to permanent sequelae. All but 1 of 24 patients who had previously had arthroscopic surgery while hospitalized under general anesthesia preferred the office procedure.

Conclusion.—Surgical arthroscopy of the knee can be safely done as an office procedure under local anesthesia. It was cost-effective and well liked by patients.

▶ The statement that "the results of the first 100 patients undergoing office operative arthroscopy of the knee have led to the conclusion that this procedure is feasible, cost-effective, safe, and preferred by the patient" is not questioned. However, what is in question is whether the responsible orthopedic surgeon has the experience and the expertise to effectively use the emergency and monitoring equipment, which includes an ECG monitor with a defibrillator; crash cart; oxygen source; and appropriate medications for a potential cardiopulmonary event, including an assortment of laryngoscopes and endotracheal tubes. I believe that this is an anesthesiologist's domain, and there is no mention of one being present as part of the office operative arthroscopy scenario.—J.S. Torg, M.D.

Arthroscopic Drilling in Juvenile Osteochondritis Dissecans of the Medial Femoral Condyle

Aglietti P, Buzzi R, Bassi PB, Fioriti M (Univ of Florence, Italy)
Arthroscopy 10:286–291, 1994   139-95-3–55

Background.—In osteochondritis dissecans (OCD), a fragment of bone with overlying articular cartilage is separated from the surrounding normal bone. Juvenile OCD (JOCD) can be seen in young patients with open physes. The efficacy of arthroscopic drilling was studied in a selected series of symptomatic patients with JOCD of the medial femoral condyle who were not showing clinical and radiographic signs of healing.

Methods.—Fourteen children with JOCD of the medial femoral condyle in 16 knees underwent arthroscopic drilling of the lesion. The mean patient age at surgery was 12.8 years. All affected knees had open physes. In all patients, conservative treatment including restriction of activities had been tried unsuccessfully for an average of more than 1 year.

Findings.—Each lesion was found to have intact articular cartilage at surgery. All lesions progressed to healing. At a mean of 56 months after surgery, the patients were asymptomatic. Radiographic assessment demonstrated reconstitution of a normal or minimally flattened profile of the medial condyle.

Conclusion.—Arthroscopic drilling of the lesion in knees with JOCD and intact cartilage effectively promoted healing. In young patients who were unresponsive to conservative measures, this procedure was justified by its low morbidity and easy rehabilitation.

▶ The tendency for JOCD of the medial femoral condyle to heal without surgical intervention is well recognized. Although the authors report a healing rate of 95% with arthroscopic drilling, they do not deal with whether these results are superior enough to nonoperative management to justify surgical intervention.—J.S. Torg, M.D.

Anterior Cruciate Ligament Allograft Reconstruction in the Skeletally Immature Athlete

Andrews M, Noyes FR, Barber-Westin SD (Deaconess Hosp, Cincinnati, Ohio; Cincinnati Sportsmedicine and Orthopaedic Ctr, Ohio)
Am J Sports Med 22:48–54, 1994   139-95-3–56

Introduction.—An increasing number of nonosseous anterior cruciate ligament (ACL) injuries are being reported in sexually immature athletes. However, the natural history and optimal treatment of ACL injuries in this age group are unknown. The results of intra-articular ACL repair and allograft reconstruction in a highly selected group of skeletally immature patients were reported.

Methods.—The patients included 8 boys (average age 13½ years) who sustained ACL rupture during sports participation. Open growth plates were radiographically documented in every case. Surgical reconstruction was indicated because of the patients' desire to continue highly competitive athletics or the presence of significant symptoms. The patients underwent ACL repair and reconstruction with fascia lata or Achilles tendon allograft tissue. The grafts, which measured 7 mm, were placed centrally across the tibial physes and in an over-the-top position on the femur. After reconstruction, all patients were placed on an immediate knee motion and rehabilitation exercise program. At a mean follow-up of 58 months, the results were rated on a comprehensive evaluation system that included 20 variables.

Results.—The growth plates were closed in all patients at follow-up. There was a slight, nonsignificant difference in lower limb length, as measured by scanograms. KT-1000 arthrometer testing revealed less than 3 mm of increased anteroposterior displacement in 5 patients and no more than 5 mm in the other 3 patients. All patients could run normally or with only slight limitations, and 7 could jump and twist or cut without any or only slight limitations. All patients remained active in athletics, although some participated at a reduced level. The final results were considered excellent in 6 cases, good in 1, and fair in 1.

Conclusion.—The results of ACL allograft reconstruction in skeletally immature athletes were reported. The reconstructive procedure, when carefully performed, appears to carry minimal risk of growth disturbances. It will seldom be used, but the procedure appears to be of benefit in selected young athletes who do not want to modify their athletic activity or in those in whom associated meniscal repairs warrant consideration of reconstruction.

▶ The literature clearly indicates that expectant treatment of ACL-deficient knees in the skeletally immature athlete is associated with uniformly poor results. I think that early surgical reconstruction of the ligament is the most prudent approach. However, I have reservations about using allografts in this group of patients.

It should be noted that Lipscomb and Anderson (1) reported on the success in intra-articular reconstructions using the semitendinous and gracilis tendons in this age group. To date, there have been no reports of using autogenous infrapatellar bone tendon bone graft. I am not aware that growth plate disturbances have been noted by any authors who approached this problem surgically.—J.S. Torg, M.D.

Reference

1. Lipscomb AB, Anderson AF: Tears of the anterior cruciate ligament in adolescents. *J Bone Joint Surg* 68:19–28, 1986.

Cruciate Ligament Loading During Isometric Muscle Contractions
Zavatsky AB, Beard DJ, O'Connor JJ (Oxford Univ, England; Nuffield Orthopaedic Ctr Natl Health Service Trust, Oxford, England)
Am J Sports Med 22:418–423, 1994   139-95-3-57

Introduction.—There is no universally accepted postoperative rehabilitation regimen for reconstructive surgery for cruciate ligaments of the knee. Results of experimental and theoretical studies describing the optimal choice of knee flexion angles at which muscle contraction can be safely performed vary with the experimental setup and the loading conditions of the knee. Using the knee model of O'Connor (Fig 3–23), the reason the patterns of cruciate ligament loading depend not only on flexion angle but also on restraining load placement was determined.

Methods.—The O'Connor model is based on simple geometric representations of knee bones, ligaments, and muscles. Passive flexion-extension of the knee is represented by a 4-bar linkage, labeled ABCD. The linkage is formed by lines that represent the cruciate ligaments and lines joining their attachments on the tibia and femur. During simulated isometric quadriceps or hamstring contractions, the model is held fixed at a flexion angle of 0 degrees, 60 degrees, and 120 degrees by a restraining force applied to the tibia parallel to the tibial plateau, which prevents extension or flexion with an increase of leg muscle forces.

Results.—For each flexion angle, there is a proximal-distal position at which no ligament forces are required for equilibrium of the restraining load. The position of the restraining force needed for zero ligament force moves distally with knee flexion. At about 90 degrees flexion, this critical position reaches the ankle. Soft tissue forces are needed for equilibrium. The critical flexion angle depends on load placement and vice versa.

Conclusion.—Patients with newly reconstructed cruciate ligaments can safely perform maximum isometric quadriceps or hamstring contrac-

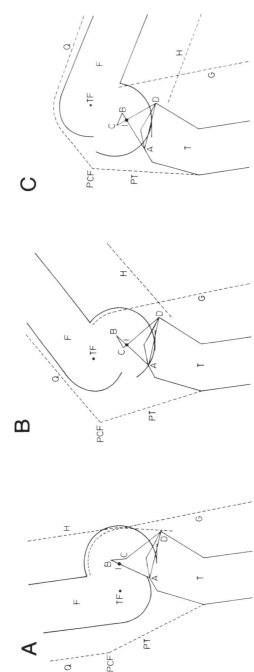

Fig 3-23.—The model knee drawn at 0 degrees (**A**), 60 degrees (**B**), and 120 degrees (**C**) of flexion. *Abbreviations: F*, femur; *T*, tibia; *AB*, anterior cruciate ligament link; *CD*, posterior cruciate ligament link; *AD*, tibial link; *BC*, femoral link; *I*, instantaneous center; *Q*, quadriceps; *PT*, patellar tendon; *PCF*, center of force of patella; *TF*, trochlear facet of femur; *H*, hamstrings; *G*, gastrocnemius. (Courtesy of Zavatsky AB, Beard DJ, O'Connor JJ: *Am J Sports Med* 22:418–423, 1994.)

tions. An optimal environment for rehabilitation can be provided and justified from a biomechanical standpoint.

▶ After an anterior cruciate ligament reconstruction, we want patients to exercise the hamstrings and quadriceps, but how do they do it without placing undue strain on the new ligament? These authors give us an answer using isometric contractions. Maximum isometric quadriceps contractions can be performed safely at any flexion angle selected.—Col. J.L. Anderson, PE.D.

Call Mosby Document Express at **1 (800) 55-MOSBY** to obtain copies of the original source documents of articles featured or referenced in the YEAR BOOK series.

---

4 Leg, Ankle, and Foot

Tendon Action of Two-Joint Muscles: Transfer of Mechanical Energy Between Joints During Jumping, Landing, and Running
Prilutsky BI, Zatsiorsky VM (Central Inst of Physical Culture, Moscow)
J Biomech 27:25–34, 1994   139-95-4–1

Background.—The function of 2-joint muscles during locomotion, including the transportation of mechanical energy between joints, is the subject of current speculation. "Tendon action" in 2-joint muscles has been studied with indirect experimental data, mathematical simulation, and observations of physical models of humans, but whether this action occurs in human movements has been unknown. The amount of mechanical energy transferred between leg joints by 2-joint muscles was measured during squat vertical jumps, jump landings from a height of 0.5 meters, and the jogging activity of human beings.

Methods.—Five healthy subjects participated; optical methods and a force platform were used to record the coordinates of the markers on the body and the ground reactions. The power developed by the joint movements and by each muscle was determined by solving the inverse problem of dynamics for a 2-dimensional, 4-link model of an 8-muscled leg. The time integration of the difference between the power effected at the joint by the joint moment and the total power of the muscles serving the joint was used to determine the energy transferred by 2-joint muscles to and from each joint.

Findings.—Mechanical energy is transferred from the proximal leg joints to the distal leg joints in the rectus femoris and gastrocnemius muscles during squat vertical jumps and in the push-off phase of running. Energy is transferred from the distal to the proximal joints of 2-joint muscles during landing and the shock-absorbing phase of running. During the squat vertical jump, the maximum amount of energy transferred from proximal to distal joints was 178.6 J; during landing, the maximum amount of energy transferred from distal to proximal joints was 18.6 J.

Conclusion.—The ability of the 2-joint muscles to distribute mechanical energy between joints allows the proximal 1-joint muscles to compensate for the deficiency in work production of the distal 1-joint muscles. A part of the mechanical energy generated by the proximal muscles during the push-off phase is transferred distally to help extend the distal joints. Similarly, the distal muscles are able to dissipate mechanical energy during the shock-absorbing phase by transferring it to the proximal muscles.

▶ This impressive study points out the great functional importance of the mechanism of energy transfer by 2-joint muscles. The authors point out that the muscles located on the proximal links of the lower extremity have considerably larger volumes than those of the muscles of the distal links. Others have explained that this is the result of longer fibers, relatively short tendons, and large cross-sectional areas of the proximal muscles. Such a distribution of muscle volume along the leg reduces its moment of inertia relative to the "suspension point," the hip joint. They say that this allows the leg to move with a lower consumption of energy.—Col. J.L. Anderson, PE.D.

Foot Biomechanics During Walking and Running

Chan CW, Rudins A (Mayo Clinic and Found, Rochester, Minn)
Mayo Clin Proc 69:448–461, 1994   139-95-4–2

Foot Functions.—The foot joins the body with the earth. During gait, it cushions the body, adapts it to uneven surfaces, provides traction for movement, and ensures awareness of joint and body position for balance. In addition, the foot allows the leverage needed for propulsion.

Basic Biomechanics.—The foot locks in place when it is about to leave the ground, becoming a rigid lever that propels the leg forward. The axis of the subtalar joint resembles an oblique hinge. Rotations that take place in the lower segment act on the talus, through the hinge at the subtalar joint, to transmit rotation to the foot. Any abnormal rotation in either the transverse tarsal joint or distal to this site may disrupt the entire gait pattern.

Walking.—At heel strike, the lower segment rotates internally until the foot is flat. The heel is everted at this point, and the flexible forefoot adapts to the ground. In midstance, the lower segment reverses into external rotation, and the heel is inverted. The longitudinal arch stabilizes progressively until toe-off. The posterior calf muscles and intrinsic foot muscles contract actively. As the foot is loaded, the talar head becomes firmly seated in the navicular, and the plantar fascia exerts force on the arch. Just before toe-off, the lower segment is maximally rotated externally, the heel is maximally inverted, and the axes of the transverse tarsal joint diverge.

Running.—The range of joint motion, muscle activity, and joint reaction forces during running all vary with speed, and often vary from one step to the next. Pronation-supination of the foot is one of the basic parts of the running cycle. Distance runners typically contact the ground heel first or with the foot flap, whereas sprinters frequently land on the midfoot. A number of forces, including vertical force, fore-aft and mediolateral shear forces, and torque, develop between the foot and the ground during running. The shear forces resemble those noted during walking, but they are larger. Trained runners may have a longer stride at a given speed. It remains unclear whether runners naturally adopt efficient running styles and what actually constitutes an efficient style. Those who run economically tend to have less vertical motion of the center of gravity, relatively small anteroposterior and vertical ground-reaction forces, a low impact peak of vertical force, and a rearfoot strike pattern.

▶ This report contains basic biomechanical information that explains the functions of walking and running. This information has received considerable attention over the past 10–15 years, with a proliferation of shoe manufacturers and the development of different shoes for almost every event. Of course, with the popularity of running, we are seeing more injuries to the lower extremities. In order to understand the roles running form, foot placement, and foot gear play in causing and preventing injuries, we need to understand something about the mechanics of running.

Here is some interesting information: walking gait is categorized as "stance phase (60%), which consists of two periods of double-limb support (each 12%) and one period of single limb support (35%), and a swing phase (40%)." Running gait differs from walking gait in that "a third phase—the nonsupportive float phase—develops." Running gait includes a stance phase (40%), a swing phase (30%), and 2 float phases (15% each).—Col. J.L. Anderson, PE.D.

Basic Kinematics of Walking: Step Length and Step Frequency: A Review
Zatsiorky VM, Werner SL, Kaimin MA (Pennsylvania State Univ, Pittsburgh; Central Inst of Physical Culture, Russia)
J Sports Med Phys Fitness 34:109–134, 1994   139-95-4–3

Background.—Variables such as step length, frequency, and the relationship between these variables have never undergone comprehensive study as part of the basic kinematics of walking. The published data on these 2 variables were reviewed and analyzed.

Method.—Terms such as double support, duty time, forced walk, free/preferred walk, stride, optimal walk, speed-controlled walk, step, step/stride frequency, step length, stride length, swing phase, and walking pattern are referred to in this review. Gait cycle or stride is illustrated in Figure 4-1.

Discussion.—Regardless of height, tall and short individuals walk with the same step frequency. The step frequency times the leg length is independent of body size. People choose their step length and frequency. Their preferred speed varies according to the circumstances. Energy output is minimal at a given walking speed at a given step frequency. Step time is consistent at normal speed, and step length is controlled by a kin-

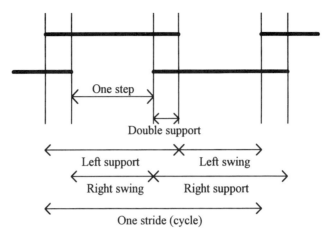

Fig 4–1.—Gait cycle (stride). (Courtesy of Zatsiorky VM, Werner SL, Kaimin MA: *J Sports Med Phys Fitness* 34:109–134, 1994.)

ematic chain of 7 segments with at least 12 degrees of freedom. Walking patterns are affected by the weight of the load carried and by sex differences. Treadmill walking is no different mechanically from walking on the ground. Women wearing high heels walk more slowly and with shorter steps than do women wearing low-heeled shoes.

▶ This is an excellent review of the literature on the basic kinematics of walking. A total of 176 studies were done by representatives of 2 fine biomechanics laboratories at Pennsylvania State University and the Central Institute of Physical Culture in Russia. The sections concerning sex, children, and the elderly are particularly good and should be useful to anyone studying these populations.—Col. J.L. Anderson, PE.D.

Variable Gearing During Locomotion in the Human Musculoskeletal System

Carrier DR, Heglund NC, Earls KD (Brown Univ, Providence, RI; Pharos Systems, Inc, South Chelmsford, Mass)
Science 265:651–653, 1994   139-95-4–4

Background.—Human feet and toes serve several purposes including providing traction, acting as tools and weapons, and maintaining balance. They may also improve locomotion because they can vary the velocity ratio between the ankle muscles and the center of force during running. Variable gearing may underlie the ability of individuals to move efficiently and quickly, accelerate rapidly, and jump high.

Method.—A lateral view of the foot of 3 male and 2 female subjects was photographed as the subjects ran over a Kistler 9281B force plate (Fig 4-2). Subjects ran at a constant speed and also accelerated to maxi-

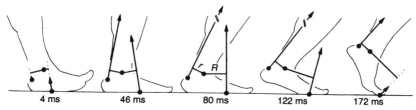

Fig 4–2.—Ground reaction force, force of the extensor muscles of the ankle, and the moment arms of these forces during foot support while running at a constant speed. The ground force moment arm (R) is the perpendicular distance from the ground reaction force to the ankle. The muscle force moment arm (r) is the perpendicular distance from the Achilles tendon to the ankle. The dot between the foot and the ground is the position of the center of force. (Courtesy of Carrier DR, Heglund NC, Earls KD: *Science* 265:651–653, 1994.)

mum speed from a standing position. The ground reaction force and the center of force were calculated. The force of the extensor muscles of the ankle was observed.

Results.—During running at a constant speed, the center of force was translated forward. In 4 subjects, the gear ratio was less than 1 at the start of the test, increasing to 3 or 4 by takeoff. When accelerating from a standing position, the gear ratio was higher early in the contact phase and lower in the later contact phase. During rapid acceleration, the gear ratio was low.

Discussion.—Variation in gear ratio is caused by a change in the length of the lever from the ankle to the center of force. The feet and toes of humans allow variation in the position of the center of force during running. Musculoskeletal gearing probably is a necessary adaptation.

▶ This concept of variable gearing is very interesting and certainly makes sense. It also helps to explain the importance of proper mechanics of locomotion. I have always assumed that proper mechanics of locomotion required that foot placement be such that the toes point directly along the line of movement. The calculations in this study would seem to support that belief.—Col. J.L. Anderson, PE.D.

Severe Obesity: Effects on Foot Mechanics During Walking
Messier SP, Davies AB, Moore DT, Davis SE, Pack RJ, Kazmar SC (Wake Forest Univ, Winston-Salem, NC; Duke Univ, Durham, NC)
Foot Ankle 15:29–34, 1994   139-95-4–5

Background.—Although walking would appear to be the exercise of choice for many obese individuals, carrying excessive mass significantly increases the metabolic cost of walking. Experimental studies have found that adding mass to various body segments does not cause global changes in gait mechanics. However, some evidence shows that severe obesity may adversely affect selected lower extremity gait parameters.

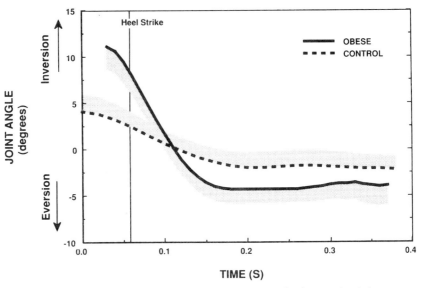

Fig 4–3.—Mean (± standard error) rearfoot angle vs. time curves for the control and obese groups. (Courtesy of Messier SP, Davies AB, Moore DT, et al: *Foot Ankle* 15:29–34, 1994.)

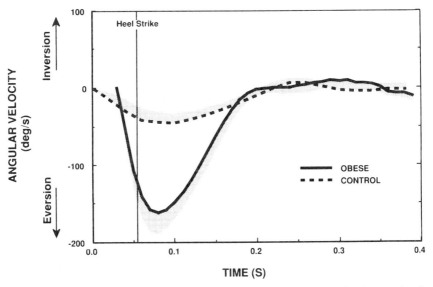

Fig 4–4.—Mean (± standard error) rearfoot angular velocity vs. time curves for the control and obese groups. (Courtesy of Messier SP, Davies AB, Moore DT, et al: *Foot Ankle* 15:29–34, 1994.)

The effects of severe obesity on the foot mechanics of women were studied.

Methods.—Twenty-nine women aged 20–48 years participated. Sixteen were severely obese, with a mean body mass index of 41, and 13 were of normal weight, with a body mass index of 21. Rearfoot movement during treadmill walking was recorded using a 100-Hz Locam camera positioned perpendicularly to the patients' posterior aspect.

Results.—The touchdown angle was significantly greater in the obese women. The obese group also showed more total eversion range of motion and a faster maximum eversion velocity (Figs 4–3 and 4–4). Analysis of dynamic foot angles showed that the obese group had significantly greater forefoot abduction. The obese women also had significantly greater Q angles than did the control group.

Conclusion.—Severe obesity appears to have some adverse effects on gait mechanics. Compared with normal-weight women, severely obese women have significantly increased rearfoot motion, foot angle, and Q angle values. The last factor may account for some of the variance in rearfoot motion observed in this study.

▶ None of us should be surprised that severe obesity appears to have adverse effects on gait mechanics. When we watch obese men and women walk, the toe-out foot placement is readily apparent. Many large linemen playing football—especially the slower ones who normally play on the offensive line—exhibit the same toe-out foot placement. Of course, we do not know the cause and effect of this, which is why biomechanical studies like this one are valuable. Of course, there are other adverse effects on the ankle, knee, and hip joints that are caused by the excess load and the poor gait mechanics. Is there any solution other than losing the weight?—Col. J.L. Anderson, PE.D.

Relationship Between Plantar Pressure Distribution Under the Foot and Insole Comfort

Chen H, Nigg BM, de Koning J (Univ of Calgary, Alta, Canada)
Clin Biomech 9:335–341, 1994   139-95-4-6

Background.—The definition and quantification of shoe comfort have not been determined. There may be a relationship between perceived comfort and measurable conditions such as force, pressure, and energy cost. Pressure distribution in the shoe is very important in the orthopedics and biomechanics of shoe comfort. In sports, safety and comfort may depend in part on plantar pressure distribution, which also may determine the suitability of a shoe for a specific activity. The relationship between plantar pressure distribution under the foot and the comfort of 4 different shoe insoles was investigated. Also, the relationship between plantar pressure distribution and running shoe comfort was studied.

Methods.—Fourteen male subjects were tested while walking and running on a treadmill. Subjects wore identically constructed running shoes and tested 4 pairs of insoles. The insoles were significantly different in shape, hardness, thickness, and flexibility to provide differences in comfort. Pressure at the plantar surface of the foot was measured by an EMED pressure-measuring insole.

Results.—For walking, there was significantly higher pressure and force in the midfoot area and significantly lower pressure in the medial forefoot and hallux area when wearing the most comfortable insole compared with the least comfortable insole. An even distribution of pressure at the plantar surface of the foot was provided by a shift of pressure from forefoot to midfoot with the most comfortable insole. With the most comfortable insole, the path of the center of force at the plantar surface of the foot shifted to the lateral aspect of the foot. For running, only the pressure in the medial forefoot was significantly lower with the most comfortable insole than with the least comfortable insole. The comfort of the insoles was rated differently by different subjects. In general, the most comfortable insoles were either made of polyethylene with a flat heel shape or made of ethylene vinyl acetate with a spherical heel shape. The least comfortable insole was made of cork with a flat heel shape.

Conclusion.—Ratings of shoe comfort differ from person to person. Pressure distribution between the plantar surface of the foot and the shoe can detect shoe comfort. Pressure measurement may be important in understanding shoe comfort. Comfortable running shoes should provide low and well-distributed pressures at the plantar surface of the foot.

▶ This study is an example of how researchers attempt to help shoe manufacturers and shoe wearers to agree. However, I have been surprised at the proliferation of the kinds of shoes now being manufactured, especially the different kinds of sports shoes. How did we ever get along in the 1950s and 1960s? Probably the most significant statement made by the authors of this study is that ratings of shoe comfort differ from person to person. That is probably why there is such demand for all of those different kinds of shoes.—Col. J.L. Anderson, PE.D.

Right to Left Differences in the Ankle Joint Complex Range of Motion
Stefanyshyn DJ, Engsberg JR (Univ of Calgary, Alta, Canada)
Med Sci Sports Exerc 26:551–555, 1994   139-95-4-7

Background.—After injury of the ankle joint complex (AJC), rehabilitation is assumed to be complete when the injured ankle shows the same strength and range of motion as the contralateral limb. No previous investigations to quantify differences in right and left ROM have been undertaken. Differences in AJC range of motion between right and left legs were, thus, investigated to determine whether this assumption is valid.

Participants and Methods.—Eleven men and 7 women were studied (mean age, 28.7 years). All participants were pain-free and had no history of previous major injuries that could have influenced AJC range of motion. Total right and left AJC range of motion was measured with an apparatus that permitted 6 degrees of freedom. Participants were seated on the apparatus with their knees bent at 90 degrees flexion. The shod foot rested flat on a horizontal foot plate and was secured with Velcro straps. The leg was positioned with C-clamps just above the malleoli, whereas the anterior aspect of the knee was pressed into a V-bar and secured with a Velcro strap around the posterior side. Active range of motion of the foot was measured while a constant compressive load was applied along the tibial axis. A 4-camera video system recorded all range-of-motion movements.

Results.—No significant differences between right and left legs were noted for total dorsiflexion-plantar flexion, eversion-inversion, or abduction-adduction range of motion, although separate abduction and adduction differences were observed. The right foot tended to abduct more than the left, whereas the left foot tended to adduct more than the right; however, these observed differences may have been inherent in the measuring device used.

Conclusion.—On the basis of these findings, the contralateral AJC can be used to determine restoration of total range of motion after injury.

▶ Although for years the unaffected knee joint has been successfully compared with the surgically repaired knee joint of the contralateral limb to measure the effects of the rehabilitation process, I would have bet that this comparison would not prove successful with the ankle joints. I say this because when I watch people run or walk, I often notice that their feet very often differ in foot placement, which could also be expected to exhibit a difference in the various range-of-motion tests. That these researchers appear to show that the contralateral AJC can be used to determine restoration of total range of motion after injury is helpful. Now, is there a practical way to make the measurements in physical therapy clinics and training rooms?—Col. J.L. Anderson, PE.D.

Spectral Signature of Forces to Discriminate Perturbations in Standing Posture
McClenaghan BA, Williams H, Dickerson J, Thombs L (Univ of South Carolina, Columbia)
Clin Biomech 9:21–27, 1994   139-95-4–8

Purpose.—Certain motor manifestations of neuromuscular disease may be evident before the clinical features become apparent. Spectral analysis has been suggested as a means of evaluating motor function in the preclinical assessment of patients who have neurologic impairments. The use of spectral analysis as a means of evaluating postural stability was studied to determine the reliability of the spectral signature of postural forces and the value of spectral analysis in identifying perturbations in standing posture.

Methods.—Healthy young volunteers were studied during normal standing and 3 conditions designed to perturb stability: a dark environment, conflicting visual feedback, and vestibular conflict. The research subjects stood on a force platform, and unique features of the spectral data created from each force vector—lateral, anteroposterior, and vertical—were extracted for creation of the spectral signature. The spectral signatures were analyzed primarily to identify those band widths and force directions that best discriminated between spectral data representing stable and unstable postures.

Results.—Significant differences in spectral data were found between subjects, suggesting that a unique spectral signature was identified for each. The spectral signatures were highly reliable within individual subjects and across different testing sessions. Spectral profiles obtained during full vision and visual conflict conditions were most similar; those created during the vestibular condition showed greater total energy distributed over the widest bandwidth. Discriminant analysis suggested that perturbations were appropriately classified according to postural sway/standing conditions, with an accuracy of 87% to 98%.

Conclusion.—Spectral analysis of posture can provide highly reliable spectral signatures that provide a sensitive indicator of postural stability. As such, spectral analysis may be clinically useful in the identification of impaired postural control, as in predicting which individuals are at high risk of falling. Before the clinical applications are studied, further research is needed to confirm the reliability of the spectral signature and assess its use in the study of additional motor patterns.

▶ After further data collection, these authors believe that the use of spectral signatures, obtained from ground reaction forces during standing, may be sensitive enough to changes in postural stability that they can be used to identify impaired postural control caused by aging or disease. Other researchers have shown that postural sway is higher among younger children, decreases during later adolescence, stays at a lower level until about the age of 60 years and then increases. The inability of the elderly to control postural sway plays an important part in their tendency to fall. There is some evidence that postural sway is greater in women of all ages. That may be one reason elderly women are more at risk of falling than elderly men. I wonder whether anyone has tried to use spectral signatures to identify alcohol intoxication.—Col. J.L. Anderson, PE.D.

Bilateral Performance Symmetry During Drop Landing: A Kinetic Analysis

Schot PK, Bates BT, Dufek JS (Univ of Wisconsin, Milwaukee; Univ of Oregon, Eugene)

Med Sci Sports Exerc 26:1153–1159, 1994   139-95-4–9

Objective.—The large number of unilateral injuries would appear to contradict the generally held view that bilateral lower extremity function is symmetrical. Performance variability suggests that the variability is either the cause or the effect of bilateral variability. Bilateral variability and bilateral asymmetry were evaluated to quantify bilateral functioning.

Methods.—Concurrent bilateral ground reaction force (GRF) and sagittal plane kinematic data were collected for 25 drop landings from 0.6 m on 3 consecutive days for each of 5 men and 5 women, aged 21 to 30 years. Landing patterns were analyzed as consistently symmetrical, consistently asymmetrical, single asymmetry, or reversed asymmetry.

Results.—Bilateral variabilities for GRFs were half as large as those for joint moment variables (12.8% vs. 25.3%). Although force asymmetries were much smaller than moment asymmetries, they occurred 3 times as frequently (52.5% vs. 16.7%).

Conclusion.—The magnitude of bilateral asymmetries was usually greater than the bilateral variability of the group. Bilateral asymmetries were unilaterally directed. These studies provide a good assessment of bilateral asymmetry that is clinically meaningful.

▶ Although these authors used both men and women as subjects, they do not indicate that the analysis considered the subjects as coming from more than 1 population. Data that we have collected at West Point over the past 20 years indicate that there are real physical performance differences between men and women in almost every physical activity. My observations concerning drop landing—albeit from greater heights and not as controlled—lead me to believe that there are significant differences between the landing patterns of men and women.—Col. J.L. Anderson, PE.D.

Electromyographic Analysis of Standing Posture and Demi-Plié in Ballet and Modern Dancers

Trepman E, Gellman RE, Solomon R, Murthy KR, Micheli LJ, De Luca CJ (Boston Univ; Yale Univ, New Haven, Conn; Harvard Med School, Boston)

Med Sci Sports Exerc 26:771–782, 1994   139-95-4–10

Background.—Choreographed movements and differences in training technique suggest that ballet and modern dancers may have different patterns of muscle use during similar movements. Fundamental dance movements were, thus, investigated in both types of dancers using electromyography to document lower extremity muscle activity.

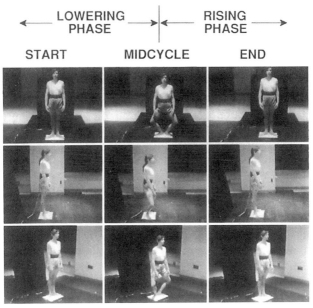

<--- LOWERING PHASE ---> | <--- RISING PHASE --->

START   MIDCYCLE   END

Fig 4–5.—Photographs of ballet dancer performing demi-plié in classic first position (turned out), as seen from the front (*top row*), side (*middle row*), and oblique (*bottom row*). The dancer is positioned upright just before the start of demi-plié (*left column*), proceeds through the lowering phase to midcycle (*middle column*), and then through the rising phase to complete the movement at the rising phase (*right column*). (Courtesy of Trepman E, Gellman RE, Solomon R, et al: *Med Sci Sports Exerc* 26:771-782, 1994.)

Participants and Methods.—Five female ballet and 7 female modern professional dancers were studied. Demographic characteristics and dance history were similar for both groups. Lower extremity muscle activity was recorded with surface electromyography during standard posture and demi-plié in first position with the lower extremities turned out. To facilitate analysis, movements associated with demi-plié were classified as lowering phase, during which the torso is lowered; rising phase, during which the torso rises to neutral; and midcycle, defined as the instant at which the torso is lowest, with the hips and knees at maximum flexion (Fig 4–5).

Results.—In all dancers, increased electromyographic (EMG) activity was noted most frequently at the medial gastrocnemius and tibialis anterior electrodes during standing posture. Compared with that of modern dancers, increased EMG activity in ballet dancers during standing posture was significantly less frequent at the medial gastrocnemius but more frequent at the tibialis anterior. All dancers had a discrete peak of EMG activity at the tibialis anterior during midcycle demi-plié. Midcycle EMG activity was also observed in the vastus lateralis and medialis in all dancers. At the end of the demi-plié rising phase, ballet dancers showed greater EMG activity in the vastus lateralis and medialis compared with midcycle findings. Conversely, modern dancers had a lower end-rising phase voltage at midcycle for the vastus lateralis and medialis. All ballet dancers, but not modern dancers, had genu recurvatum of 10 degrees or more at the beginning and end of the demi-plié. Marked variations of EMG activity were observed in the lateral and medial gastrocnemius, gluteus maximus, hamstrings, and adductors.

Conclusion.—Ballet and modern dancers have different patterns of muscle use in standing posture and demi-plié, which may be attributed to differences in genu recurvatum and turnout between groups. Additional studies are needed to clarify the role of these and other factors (foot arch structure, forward arm position, velocity of movement, shoewear, fatigue, and various lower extremity positions used in dance) in standing posture and demi-plié.

▶ Although I know little about dance, either ballet or modern, I found this study to be fascinating. The amount of biomechanical data generated from the study of 2 basic positions, standing posture and demi-plié, is impressive, and the authors still believe that further studies are necessary to clarify the role of foot turnout, genu recurvatum, training, and technique. They also specify other variables that must be included in future studies, which should include a nondancer control group. There is certainly enough research to be done, and the researchers who undertake it will find excellent ideas and help in this study.—Col. J.L. Anderson, PE.D.

Factors Associated With Hamstring Injuries: An Approach to Treatment and Preventative Measures
Worrell TW (Univ of Indianapolis, Ind)
Sports Med 17:338–345, 1994   139-95-4–11

Background.—Hamstring strain is a significant and complex injury in which the slow rate of recovery can be frustrating for both the athlete and the clinician. A hamstring rehabilitation model based on current understanding of the etiologic factors contributing to hamstring muscle strain was described.

Acute Phase.—Ice should be applied for 20–45 minutes 2–4 times per day to reduce inflammation until pain and limitation of daily activities function are resolved. During this acute phase, the athlete should retain a normal gait pattern with the help of a cane or single crutch on the side opposite the hamstring injury. After 20–45 minutes of ice application, gentle active knee extension and flexion can be performed while the athlete is seated for another 5–25 minutes.

Subacute Phase.—Once signs of inflammation have subsided and the athlete achieves full extension without pain, resistance exercises can begin. These include pain-free, multiple angle, submaximal hamstring isometric exercises (15- to 20-degree increments, 2 sets of repetitions, 5-second contraction). Stationary bicycle riding can also begin as tolerated

Summary of Hamstring Strain Rehabilitation

Phases	Goals	Treatment intervention
Acute	Control pain and edema Prevent muscle fiber adhesions Normal gait	Ice and compression Ice and electric stimulation Pain-free PROM (gentle stretching), AAROM, AROM Ambulatory aids
Subacute	Control pain and edema Full AROM Alignment of collagen Increase collagen strength	Ice and compression Ice and electric stimulation Pain free pool activities Pain free stretching Pain free submaximal isometrics Stationary bike
Remodeling	Control pain and edema Increase collagen strength Increase hamstring flexibility Increase eccentric loading	Ice and compression Ice and electric stimulation Prone concentric isotonic exercise Moist heat or exercise prior to anterior pelvic hamstring stretching Prone unilateral eccentrics, standing 'catch'
Functional	Return to sport without reinjury Increase hamstring flexibility Increase hamstring strength Control pain	Walk/jog/sprint, sport specific skills Anterior pelvic hamstring stretching Prone concentric and eccentric exercise, standing 'catch' Heat, ice, and modalities as needed

Abbreviations: AAROM, active-assistive range of motion; AROM, active range of motion; PROM, passive range of motion.
(Courtesy of Worrell TW: Sports Med 17:338–345, 1994.)

by the athlete. Swimming pool activities—including walking, progressive jogging with a walk vest, and use of a kickboard—help increase range of motion and strength. A jog and sprint progression should begin with caution to avoid increasing pain and inflammation.

Remodeling Phase.—Once multiple-angle hamstring isometrics can be performed at 100% effort, prone hamstring strengthening begins. These exercises begin unilaterally with ankle weights and are done on a knee table or on a variable-resistance exercise table. Initially, the hamstring strengthening program consists of high repetitions and low resistance to facilitate motor recruitment without increasing pain or inflammation. Isokinetic exercise follows when tolerated without pain. Stretching is a crucial part of rehabilitation and should be performed standing with the pelvis in an anterior pelvic tilt and the stretching leg on the table. Athletes are encouraged to maintain the head in a horizontal position while flexing forward as far as possible without pain for 15 seconds. Once athletes are comfortable with these exercises, they can progress to an eccentric strengthening exercise program and then to an aggressive eccentric one. One advanced eccentric exercise places the athlete parallel to a wall (using the upper extremity on the wall side as needed for stability) and simulating the swing phase of walking and running. The athlete performs a quick quadriceps contraction during the swing phase and then attempts to catch or stop the lower leg before reaching full knee extension. Ankle weights can be added later.

Functional Progression Phase.—Once normal gait is achieved, walking progression begins, helped by pool activities. When the athlete can walk for 20–30 minutes without pain, a walk and jog progression can be initiated that is then followed by a jog and sprint progression (table).

Conclusion.—Hamstring strain is a complex multiple-factor injury that involves strength imbalances, lack of flexibility, muscle fatigue, and insufficient warm-ups. Any rehabilitation program should, therefore, address all of these etiologic factors and involve pain-free progression of stretching, strengthening, and functional activity.

▶ This injury, "the hamstring pull," is, in my experience, one that has a very high recurrence rate. The author says that the slow rate of recovery can be very frustrating. Too often, athletes will attempt to return to participation before the injury is completely rehabilitated. These injuries often occur early in a season when everyone is trying to make the team. The athletes fear that if they don't participate, they may miss their opportunity to show the coaches what they can do. There are many factors to consider when treating a hamstring injury. Is it a new injury? Is there scar tissue present? Is a long-term weakness or muscle imbalance present? Is there sufficient flexibility present? This injury must be rehabilitated completely before the athlete returns to participation or that athlete will certainly return to the training room with a reinjury.—F.J. George, A.T.C., P.T.

The Piriformis Muscle Syndrome: A Simple Diagnostic Maneuver
Beatty RA (Univ of Illinois, Chicago)
Neurosurgery 34:512–514, 1994   139-95-4–12

Background.—Current methods of diagnosing piriformis syndrome are less than ideal. A new maneuver that brings a contraction of the muscle, rather than stretching, was done to facilitate diagnosis.

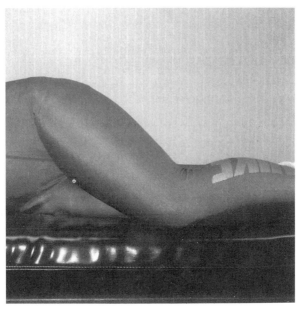

Fig 4–6.—The starting position with patient on his or her side, painful side up, hip flexed, knee resting on the table. (Courtesy of Beatty RA: *Neurosurgery* 34:512–514, 1994.)

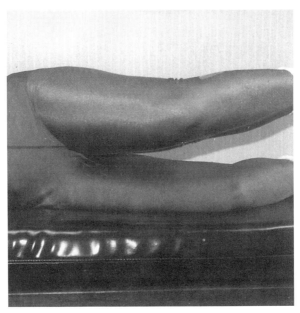

Fig 4–7.—The position in which pain is produced in the buttock by lifting and holding the knee several inches from the table. (Courtesy of Beatty RA: *Neurosurgery* 34:512–514, 1994.)

Method.—The maneuver was performed on 3 patients in the examining room. The patient was told to lie down with the painful side up, the painful leg flexed, and the knee resting on the table (Fig 4–6). Buttock pain was experienced when the patient lifted and held the knee several inches off the table (Fig 4–7). The first patient (a 55-year old man) had a history of buttock pain since age 21 years, after a 500-mile motor trip in a sports car with bucket seats. Another patient (a 16-year-old boy) was injured when a schoolmate pulled a chair out from under him. Symptoms included persistent buttock pain aggravated by sitting. The third patient was a 62-year-old woman who had bruised her buttock by sitting down hard on an icy ski slope. In all 3 patients, the reactions to maneuvers of Pace, Freiberg, and the one described above were positive.

Results.—The maneuver described above produced deep buttock pain in 3 patients who had convincing evidence of piriformis syndrome. All patients responded to conservative treatment and did not require imaging of the piriformis area. In 100 consecutive patients who had surgically diagnosed unilateral lumbar disk herniation, the maneuver often caused pain in the lumbar area and in the leg but not deep pain that occurred primarily in the fleshy part of the buttock. In 27 patients who had hip problems, pain was often experienced in the trochanteric area but not deep in the buttock.

Conclusion.—The maneuver described was found to be helpful in diagnosing piriformis syndrome. It is thought to rely on contraction rather than stretching, of the muscle, which appears to better reproduce the actual syndrome and offer a more complete diagnostic picture.

▶ There has been a good deal of controversy recently over the diagnosis of piriformis syndrome. This particular maneuver should give us another test to help make this evaluation. Whether the test will reduce the controversy surrounding this syndrome remains to be seen. However, because this is different from other tests we have used in that we are requiring a muscle contraction as opposed to the stretching of muscle tissue, this should be helpful.—F.J. George, A.T.C., P.T.

Effects of Stair-Stepping Exercise Direction and Cadence on EMG Activity of Selected Lower Extremity Muscle Groups
Zimmermann CL, Cook TM, Bravard MS, Hansen MM, Honomichl RT, Karns ST, Lammers MA, Steele SA, Yunker LK, Zebrowski RM (Univ of Iowa, Iowa City; Rehability Ctr, Urbandale, Iowa; Aberdeen Physical Therapy, SD; et al)
J Orthop Sports Phys Ther 19:173–180, 1994   139-95-4-13

Objective.—Stair-stepping exercises have become popular in health clubs and are being increasingly used in cardiovascular fitness and knee rehabilitation treatment. To maximize exercise tolerance and prevent injury, therapists are studying range-of-motion and muscle strengthening exercises in knee rehabilitation programs. Little information is available on the effects of stair-stepping on the muscles of the leg. The mean electromyographic (EMG) activity levels of leg muscles during knee extensions under 4 different exercise regimens were studied.

Methods.—Surface EMG measurements of leg muscles and electrogoniometer readings were performed throughout exercise on the right legs of 33 injury-free subjects aged 18–35 years. Subjects performed 20 cycles of 35 steps/min, 60 steps/min, 95 steps/min, and 60 retrograde steps/min, with 7-minute rests between tests. Each subject practiced for 30 minutes 1 week before testing. Maximum voluntary isometric contractions were measured for the gluteus maximus, rectus femoris, vastus medialis, semimembranosus/semitendinosus, and gastrocnemius.

Results.—There were significant differences in EMGs for all muscles at all cadences except for the semimembranosus/semitendinosus. The latter displayed a significantly different EMG between 35 and 95 steps/min only and was the only muscle to show a significantly different EMG for retrograde stepping. As cadence increased, the increase in EMG was greater in the rectus femoralis and vastus medialis than in the hamstring, indicating greater muscle stabilization during slower cadences. The duration of peak activity decreased as cadence increased.

Conclusion.—There is a significant difference in the EMG activity of muscles during the knee extension aspect of step exercising. The investigators caution that after anterior cruciate ligament injury or reconstruction, use of a lower stepping cadence may be appropriate because EMG activity of the rectus femoralis and vastus medialis increases with cadence more than does the EMG activity of the semimembranosus/semitendinosus.

The Differential Effects of External Ankle Support on Postural Control
Bennell KL, Goldie PA (La Trobe Univ, Victoria, Australia)
J Orthop Sports Phys Ther 20:287–295, 1994   139-95-4–14

Objective.—Ankle supports, while providing protection during sports participation, can have a detrimental effect on posture. The effects of tape and a brace on posture were evaluated, and the effects of tape, braces, and elastic bandages on ankle support were compared.

Methods.—Force along the mediolateral axis at the foot-force platform interface was measured in 24 normal, healthy volunteers, aged, 18–35 years, wearing strapping tape, commercial braces, or elastic bandages as ankle supports. With eyes closed and hands on hips, the participants balanced on 1 foot and posture control, foot force, and frequency of foot touchdowns were measured.

Results.—The elastic bandage had no significant effect on posture, but both the brace and the tape did. With the brace and the tape, instability and, therefore, the frequency of touchdowns increased, probably because of ankle movement restriction.

Conclusion.—Ankle supports that mechanically restrict ankle movement adversely affect posture.

▶ Ankle supports are used to prevent ankle sprains or to give support to athletes with previously sprained ankles. We are fairly confident in the results of studies that prove that ankle bracing reduces the frequency and severity of sprained ankles. We have all applied tape and braces to athletes with sprained ankles and have seen them participate when they normally would not have been able to do so. We have done this for different reasons, e.g., either increasing support or increasing proprioception or just because the athlete feels safer.

This study needs to be repeated with sprained ankles as well as healthy ankles, with different aspects of posture control, proprioception, joint stability, and performance being tested. We really need to know whether there is a scientific basis for using ankle supports. Clinically, they seem to work. The time has come to prove it scientifically. In my experience, a combination of taping and bracing provides the most support.—F.J. George, A.T.C., P.T.

Cushioning Effect of Heel Cups
Wang C-L, Cheng C-K, Tsuang Y-H, Hang Y-S, Liu T-K (Natl Taiwan Univ, Taipei, Republic of China)
Clin Biomech 9:297–302, 1994   139-95-4–15

Background.—Heel pain is one of the most common foot problems in orthopedic practice. The cushioning effect of heel cups from a biomechanical point of view was examined, and the mechanism of cushioning was defined. In addition, the differences in shock absorption of different materials and designs of heel cups were studied.

Method.—Sixteen volunteers without heel pain and 6 patients with heel pain were enrolled. Three types of heel cups were tested: Tender-Stride, Tuli's, and M-F. The first 2 were made of rubber with different designs. The Tender-Stride has numerous small circles, whereas the Tuli's has a waffle-like surface. The M-F is made of a special plastic material. The cushioning effect of the cups was assessed by plantar pressure measurement with a Computer Dyno Graphy system, pressure-sensitive films, pedobarography, and roentgenography. The Computer Dyno Graphy system was used for plantar force measurement. Eight load sensors were incorporated into the sole of each shoe, and the forces measured were transferred to a telemeter carried by the subject. Subjects were evaluated while walking and running on the floor and on a treadmill.

Results.—All 3 types of heel cups were found to increase the shock absorption of the heel pads. The amplitudes of the shock absorbency of the Tender-Stride (40.5%) and Tuli's (50.2%) were comparable to those of viscoelastic inserts (42%) reported in previous studies. The rigidity of the M-F plastic heel cups was seen to keep the heel pad from collapsing under weight-bearing by decreasing the contact area and increasing the thickness of the heel pad (Fig 4–8). Rubber caps lacked the rigidity for

A

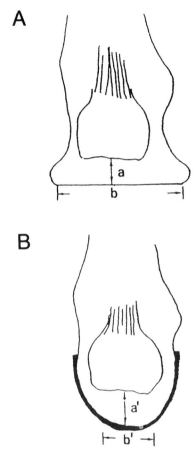

B

Fig 4-8.—*Abbreviations: a, a',* heel-pad thickness; *b, b',* contact area width. Plastic heel cup constrains heel pad under weight-bearing, decreasing contact area and increasing thickness of heel pad. **A,** barefoot. **B,** with plastic heel cup. (Courtesy of Wang C-L, Cheng C-K, Tsuang Y-H, et al: *Clin Biomech* 9:297–302, 1994.)

this confinement. The plastic cups also increased rear foot stability. Rubber caps increased shock absorbency principally at the calcaneal tuberosity, whereas plastic heel cups appeared to increase it over the whole heel area. Therefore, the ways in which rubber and plastic heel cups increase shock absorbency are different. The former acts as an external shock absorber; the latter increases the internal shock absorption of the heel pad.

Conclusion.—Rubber heel cups increase the external shock absorption of the heel pad through their viscoelastic material and cushioning designs. Plastic heel cups improve internal shock absorption of the heel through confinement of the heel pad and by increasing the stability of the hindfoot. Thus, the pathogenesis of the heel pain is the determining factor in choosing a heel cup: rubber cups are suitable for patients with inflammation, whereas plastic cups are more appropriate for those with atrophy of the heel pads.

▶ Evaluation of the cause of heel pain is very important and must be thorough before a protective device can be selected. In many cases, exercises may be prescribed to stretch a tight plantar fascia or Achilles tendon. The cause of the pain will determine the type of heel protection selected. We have used the plastic heel cup as a preventive device in all our high jumpers and long and triple jumpers to prevent the contusing of the heel pad that often occurs in these athletes. The heel cups are lightweight and inexpensive, and the athletes easily adapt to them. This study gives an excellent description of how and why different heel cups are effective.—F.J. George, A.T.C., P.T.

Athletic Footwear Affects Balance in Men
Robbins S, Waked E, Gouw GJ, McClaran J (Concordia Univ, Montreal; Montreal Gen Hosp; McGill Univ, Montreal)
Br J Sports Med 28:117–122, 1994   139-95-4–16

Objective.—Athletic footwear with thick, soft soles has been reported to affect the balance in older men and to contribute to falls. The effect of different types of athletic shoes on the balance in younger men was analyzed.

Methods.—An aluminum balance beam 9 m long, 7.8 cm wide, and 3.9 cm high was used to test the stability of 17 men aged 19–50 years during forward movement. The subjects were fitted with glasses that rendered them unable to see their feet and were tested barefoot and wearing 6 different types of athletic shoes with soles of various thickness and hardness. Falling off the beam constituted balance failure.

Results.—There was no significant correlation between falling frequency and age or weight, but there was a significant correlation between falling frequency and the subject's height and between falling frequency and being barefoot. There was a nonsignificant correlation between midsole thickness and hardness. Midsole hardness contributed to stability and midsole thickness contributed to instability. For comfort, all test subjects chose shoes with midsoles that were soft or medium; none chose the hard midsole shoes.

Conclusion.—Currently popular footwear with thick, soft soles destabilizes men. For maximum athletic performance, safety standards for footwear should be established to protect wearers from falls.

▶ A better, safer athletic shoe should be designed. Footwear plays an important role in athletic performance and injury frequency. The shoe must be comfortable, provide stability, and enhance performance. The shoe design or construction must never predispose the athlete to injury. Through the years, footwear has improved; however, like conditioning programs, footwear needs to be more sport-specific, which presents quite a challenge to shoe manufacturers.—F.J. George, A.T.C., P.T.

Kinetic Chain Dysfunction in Ballet Injuries
Macintyre J (Orthopedic Biomechanics Inst, Salt Lake City, Utah)
Med Probl Perform Art 9:39–42, 1994   139-95-4–17

Background.—Movements requiring the action of muscular forces on a series of rigid extremity segments joined by mobile linkages (commonly referred to as the "kinetic chain") are frequently performed in ballet. Optimum performance dictates that all segments of the kinetic chain be properly positioned to support the body's weight and permit movement. If normal joint mobility or stability are disrupted, increased compensatory stresses on other sites of the kinetic chain can occur. When the chain's capacity to compensate is exceeded, overt tissue breakdown and injury will occur. This failure may be at the site of the abnormality. However, the overt injury can occur at a distant site in the chain. To date, the role of kinetic chain dysfunction has been largely ignored in dance-related injuries, although this problem is commonly seen in injured dancers.

Patients and Methods.—The medical records of 16 female dancers aged 12–19 years were retrospectively reviewed for patterns of injury. At initial examination, the dancers were evaluated for functional asymmetries (the hallmark of kinetic chain dysfunction), including those of the low back and sacroiliac joint. Functional foot movement and mobility were also assessed.

Results.—Functional asymmetries were noted in 11 of the 16 dancers, including 9 of the 12 with overuse injuries and 2 of the 4 with acute injuries. Eight of the 9 dancers with overuse injuries had abnormal functional foot movements, and 7 of the 8 had reported previous injuries to the same region. In addition, sacroiliac joint dysfunction was observed in 4 of these 9 patients. Abnormal motion of the subtalar joint with a loss of supination was the most common abnormality of functional foot movement and was observed in 7 of the 8 dancers with lower leg injuries. Dysfunction of the sacroiliac joint was noted in the 2 dancers with acute injuries to the back, although abnormal functional foot movements were not observed.

Conclusion.—Kinetic chain dysfunction was common in this group of patients and may have been a cause of repeated injury. Untreated dysfunction at 1 site in the chain may lead to compensatory dysfunction at other sites. Thus, in dancers undergoing rehabilitation, the identification and treatment of kinetic chain dysfunction is important.

▶ This article was selected because its overall theory of evaluation and treatment applies not only to dancers' injuries, but to all athletic injuries. The injured site is a problem and must be treated. However, the dysfunction in the kinetic chain that caused the injury must also be identified and corrected. If this dysfunction is not corrected, the athlete will surely return with a similar injury. This happens all too often, and the time has come for us all to recognize and address the problem. Even if you never treat a dancer, this is an excellent article to use for guidance in treating athletic injuries. You must find the cause of the problem whether it be biomechanical or an error in the technique of training. The source of the problem must be addressed.

As K.R. Toburen states in her comments on this article, "athletic trainers must be able to recognize activity-specific movement relations. . .and view the unique movements of the entire kinetic chain (1)."—F.J. George, A.T.C., P.T.

Reference

1. Toburen KR: *Athletic Train: Sports Health Care Perspect* Vol. 1, No. 1, pp 90–91.

Tarsal Navicular Stress Fracture in Athletes
Khan KM, Brukner PD, Kearney C, Fuller PJ, Bradshaw CJ, Kiss ZS (Olympic Park Sports Medicine Centre, Alphington Sports Medicine Clinic, Sports Medicine Centres of Victoria, Australia; Private Radiology, Melbourne, Australia)
Sports Med 17:65–76, 1994   139-95-4-18

Background.—Stress fracture of the tarsal navicular bone, first described in 1970, is still considered to be underdiagnosed. However, without prompt diagnosis and definitive treatment, athletes can have prolonged disability.

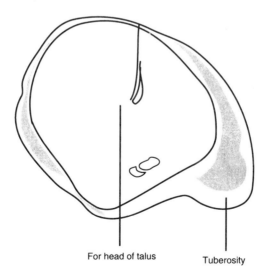

For head of talus   Tuberosity

Fig 4–9.—A typical site of the stress fractures in the navicular bone. (Courtesy of Khan KM, Brukner PD, Kearney C, et al: *Sports Med* 17:65–76, 1994.)

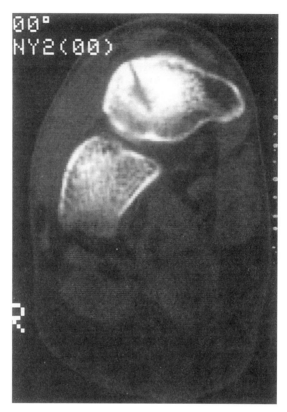

Fig 4–10.—Computerized tomographic scan of the right navicular bone taken in the plane of the talonavicular joint. A cortical defect extends plantarward. (Courtesy of Khan KM, Brukner PD, Kearney C, et al: *Sports Med* 17:65–76, 1994.)

Tarsal Navicular Stress Fracture in Athletes.—Most navicular stress fractures are partial fractures occurring in the sagittal plane (Fig 4-9). Track-and-field athletes are most commonly affected. Navicular stress fracture should be suspected in athletes reporting vague activity-related midfoot pain with associated tenderness over the dorsal proximal navicular or "N" spot. Because plain radiography often fails to show the fracture, radionuclide scanning is the investigation of choice for detecting navicular stress injury. The presence of the fracture can be confirmed by CT scanning (Fig 4-10). The treatment of choice for this injury is a minimum of 6 weeks of strict non–weight-bearing cast immobilization. After cast removal, another 6 weeks of rehabilitation with graduated return to activity, joint mobilization, and soft tissue massage are needed. If the initial therapy is appropriate, surgery for nonunion or delayed union is rarely required.

Conclusion.—Navicular stress fracture occurs more commonly than was once thought. Clinicians must maintain a high index of suspicion when evaluating athletes in sports involving sprinting and jumping. Persistent, activity-related vague foot pain and tenderness at the "N" spot are indications for radionuclide scan. If the scan demonstrates an area of increased focal uptake, CT scanning by an experienced radiologist is needed. Athletes with a positive CT scan must undergo at least 6 weeks of strict non–weight-bearing cast immobilization, followed by clinical monitoring. A gradual return to sports is allowed over 6–8 weeks.

▶ This is an excellent review and update of an entity that we originally reported on in 1982 (1). To be emphasized is the management of this problem with a minimum of 6 weeks of non–weight-bearing cast immobilization. Following this regimen and regardless of the time of its implementation, surgery is rarely required. However, it should be noted that cysts may persist, and complete obliteration of the fracture line may not occur before clinical healing.—J.S. Torg, M.D.

Reference

1. Torg JS, Pavlov H, Cooley LH, et al: Stress fractures of the tarsal navicular: A retrospective review of 21 cases. *J Bone Joint Surg* 64-A: 700–712, 1982.

Midfoot Sprains in Collegiate Football Players

Meyer SA, Callaghan JJ, Albright JP, Crowley ET, Powell JW (Univ of Iowa, Iowa City)
Am J Sports Med 22:392–401, 1994   139-95-4–19

Purpose.—Tarsometatarsal fracture dislocations have been well studied, but there is little information available on Lisfranc's midfoot sprains. The incidence, mechanisms, and injury patterns of lateral midfoot sprains and the disability resulting from them were examined.

Methods.—During a 5-year study, 23 men sustained 24 midfoot sprains while playing collegiate football. Follow-up questionnaires for assessing function and disability regarding activities of daily living and recreational and occupational activities were sent to all players, who were also asked to return for follow-up standing radiography of the foot. The mean follow-up was 30.8 months.

Results.—Nineteen players returned the questionnaire and 7 of them had follow-up weight-bearing radiography. The mechanism of injury was recognized and reported in 16 of the 24 cases (Fig 4–11). Analysis of the injuries by player position revealed that most of the lateral midfoot sprains occurred in offensive linemen and that none occurred in quarterbacks or tight ends. At physical examination, tenderness was localized medially in 8 players, mid-dorsally in 3, laterally in 11, and across the entire midfoot or globally in 2. The site of maximal tenderness to palpation was an important prognostic indicator of the time between injury and full healing. All injuries were treated with immobilization, and none required surgical intervention. An orthosis to relieve lateral weight-bearing was used on return to participation. The mean time away from prac-

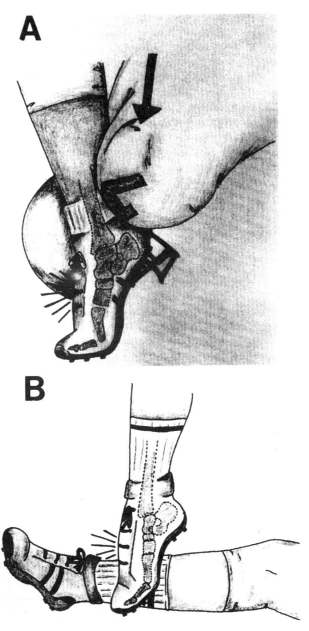

Fig 4–11.—One mechanism for a Lisfranc joint sprain may occur when a player's plantar flexed foot is driven into the ground by an opposing player falling on the hindfoot or leg (**A**). Another mechanism for this sprain may occur when a player's plantar flexed foot comes down on another player's leg during a pileup (**B**). (Courtesy of Meyer SA, Callaghan JJ, Albright JP, et al: *Am J Sports Med* 22:392–401, 1994.)

tice was 13.8 days, and the mean time until full healing was 40.5 days. Four players reported residual functional problems after returning to competition. The weight-bearing radiographs of 1 offensive lineman who had a recurrence revealed widening between the first and second metarsals and cuneiforms.

Conclusion.—Although midfoot sprains cause acute disability requiring prolonged restriction from athletic competition, they cause few long-term residual problems.

▶ This excellent paper not only brings to our attention the necessity for a high index of suspicion in view of the subtle radiographic changes, it also clearly delineates both short- and long-term prognosis. The original paper is recommended reading for those treating football players.—J.S. Torg, M.D.

"Snowboarder's Fracture": Fracture of the Lateral Process of the Talus
Nicholas R, Hadley J, Paul C, Janes P (Univ of Colorado, Denver; Vail-Summit Orthopaedics and Sports Medicine, Vail, Colo)
J Am Board Fam Pract 7:130–133, 1994   139-95-4-20

Background.—Fracture of the lateral process of the talus used to be uncommon, but it is increasingly recognized because of the growing popularity of snowboarding. The symptoms can mimic those of a simple inversion ankle sprain, and the diagnosis may be missed at first.

Case Report.—Man, 22, with pain and swelling of the left ankle, was seen within 1 hour after a fall while snowboarding. Physical examination revealed a swollen but stable ankle. Plain radiography of the ankle revealed a fracture of the lateral process of the talus that did not seem severe, and the foot was placed in a non–weight-bearing splint. However, CT of the ankle revealed a large comminuted fracture of the posterior inferolateral aspect of the talus (Fig 4–12). The fracture was treated by open reduction and internal fixation. At follow-up, the patient had good ankle function and only minimal residual discomfort.

Conclusion.—Because of its location, a fracture of the lateral process of the talus is easily missed on plain ankle radiographs. Computed tomography is recommended for all patients seen with ankle injuries that are sustained while snowboarding.

▶ Although in this case, because of the large comminuted and displaced fracture of the posterior inferior lateral aspect of the talus, the patient underwent open reduction and internal fixation, it should be pointed out that fractures that do not involve the articular surface can be treated conservatively with non-weight-bearing immobilization for a period of 4–6 weeks. Specifically, as the authors point out, "Appropriate treatment of this injury depends

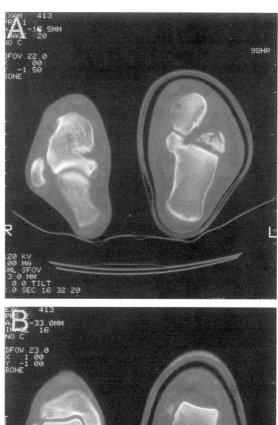

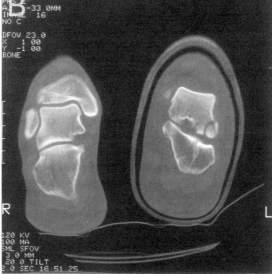

Fig 4–12.—Computed tomographic scan demonstrating comminuted fracture of the lateral process of the talus. (Courtesy of Nicholas R, Hadley J, Paul C, et al: *J Am Board Fam Pract* 7:130-133, 1994.)

on the finding of displacement and the severity of comminution."—J.S. Torg, M.D.

The Scientific Basis for the Use of Biomechanical Foot Orthoses in the Treatment of Lower Limb Sports Injuries: A Review of the Literature

Kilmartin TE, Wallace WA (Northampton School of Podiatry, England; Nottingham Univ, England)
Br J Sports Med 28:180–184, 1994   139-95-4-21

Introduction.—Although overuse injuries of the lower extremity are frequently alleviated by biomechanically designed foot orthoses, just how an orthosis functions remains uncertain. The biomechanical approach is based on identifying an abnormal position or abnormal function of the joints of the lower limb and foot. In-shoe orthoses (Fig 4–13) most often are used to resist excessive pronation of the foot and restore normal alignment to the extremity.

Clinical Effects of Orthoses.—A majority of runners with such complaints as anterior knee pain, foot pain, ankle sprain, and Achilles tendinitis reportedly have been relieved of symptoms by using a prescribed orthosis. Kinematic observations have indicated that foot orthoses significantly reduce foot motion in the transverse and frontal planes during heel strike and the midstance phase of walking without altering knee motion during the push-off phase of walking. Orthoses significantly reduce maximum pronation by reorienting the rear foot in relation to the running surface.

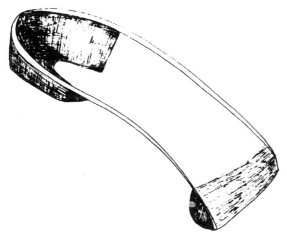

Fig 4–13.—An in-shoe biomechanical orthosis. The rearfoot and forefoot wedges or posts are intended to hold the foot close to its neutral position. (Courtesy of Kilmartin TE, Wallace WA: *Br J Sports Med* 28:180–184, 1994.)

Final Word.—Many injured athletes remain unaware of how they might benefit from using a biomechanical orthosis.

▶ Although the authors state that biomechanical foot orthoses have been shown clinically to be useful, they point out that the manner in which they work remains uncertain. They also conclude that "further research is necessary to justify and then, if indicated, promote their wider use."—J.S. Torg, M.D.

An Epidemiological Survey on Ankle Sprain
Yeung MS, Chan K-M, MPhil CHS, Yuan WY (Hong Kong Sports Inst; Chinese Univ of Hong Kong)
Br J Sports Med 28:112–116, 1994   139-95-4–22

Introduction.—Ankle sprain, an injury caused by stretching the fibers or the collagen of the ankle ligaments to the point of partial or complete disruption, occurs frequently and often recurrently among athletes. The prevalence of recurrent ankle sprain and residual symptoms among athletes in Hong Kong was studied.

Methods.—Athletes with a history of ankle sprain were asked to complete a questionnaire containing sections that addressed demographic information, information about the participant's sport, and information about the effects of the respondent's ankle sprain.

Results.—Of the 380 respondents, there were 271 males and 109 females (mean age, 24.57 years) participating in 19 different sports at various levels of expertise. Ankle injury was 2.4 times more common in the dominant than in the nondominant leg. Of the 563 sprained ankles, 73.5% had been sprained at least twice and 22% had been sprained at least 5 times. There was no significant difference in occurrence rates associated with level of expertise. Residual symptoms of ankle sprains included pain (30.2%), ankle instability (20.4%), crepitus (18.2%), and weakness (16.5%). Residual symptoms increased in association with increases in the number of recurrences. Recurrence rates also correlated significantly with the degree to which the athletes believed their performance was affected.

Discussion.—The prevalence of recurrent ankle sprain is high (73.5%) among athletes at all levels of regular play, and recurrent ankle injury is significantly associated with residual symptoms and impaired performance. Adequate medical attention and proper rehabilitation are important in injuries such as ankle sprain, which are common but are often assumed to be trivial.

The Efficacy of a Semirigid Ankle Stabilizer to Reduce Acute Ankle Injuries in Basketball: A Randomized Clinical Study at West Point
Sitler M, Ryan J, Wheeler B, McBride J, Arciero R, Anderson J, Horodyski MB (United States Military Academy, West Point, NY; Temple Univ, Philadelphia)
Am J Sports Med 22:454–461, 1994   139-95-4–23

Background.—Taping is traditionally used in an effort to prevent capsuloligamentous injuries of the ankle, although experimental and exercise studies have yielded conflicting data regarding its effectiveness in stabilizing the talocrural and subtalar joints. Ankle stabilizers offer a potential alternative to taping, but there have been few clinical studies of their effectiveness. The efficacy of a semirigid ankle stabilizer in reducing ankle injuries in basketball was assessed in a randomized clinical study.

Methods.—A total of 1,601 military academy cadets were studied over 6 intramural basketball seasons. The subjects had no clinical, functional, or radiographic evidence of ankle instability. All wore the same type of high-top athletic shoe and played on the same type of surface.

The cadets were stratified by history of previous ankle injuries and randomized into ankle stabilizer and control groups. The stabilizer used was the Aircast Sports Stirrup; ankle taping was not permitted. The subjects had a total of 13,430 athlete-exposures (A-E), including practices, during the 2 years of study. Any acute trauma to the ankle ligaments that made the athlete unable to participate in basketball the next day was considered an ankle injury.

Results.—Two thirds of the ligamentous injuries recorded occurred in the anterior talofibular ligament. The frequency of ankle injuries was 3.4/1,000 A-E overall, 5.2/1,000 A-E for the control group, and 1.6/1,000 A-E for the ankle stabilizer group. The ankle stabilizer group had a significant reduction in the total number of ankle injuries and in the number of single and combined anterior talofibular and calcaneofibular ligament injuries. However, the reduction depended on the nature of the injury: Contact injuries were less frequent among athletes who wore an ankle stabilizer, but there was no difference in the frequency of noncontact injuries. Use of an ankle stabilizer did not reduce the severity of the injury nor the frequency of knee injuries. The athletes' perceptions of stabilizer use became more positive during the season.

Conclusion.—The use of a semirigid ankle stabilizer appears to reduce the overall frequency of ankle injuries in basketball players. The difference is only significant in terms of contact injuries, however. Stabilizer wear does not reduce the severity of ankle injuries or the frequency of knee injuries.

▶ A conclusion to be drawn from these 2 papers (Abstracts 139-95-4–22 and 139-95-4–23) is that the Aircast Sports Stirrup may be indicated for those individuals with recurrent ankle sprains.—J.S. Torg, M.D.

A Fivefold Reduction in the Incidence of Recurrent Ankle Sprains in Soccer Players Using the Sport-Stirrup Orthosis

Surve I, Schwellnus MP, Noakes T, Lombard C (Univ of Cape Town, South Africa; Inst for Biostatistics, Parow, South Africa)
Am J Sports Med 22:601–606, 1994   139-95-4-24

Introduction.—Ankle sprain is the most common injury among soccer players. A history of ankle sprain is a highly important predictor of ankle sprain in this population. The effectiveness of prophylactic ankle taping has been questioned. The use of a semirigid orthosis has several advantages over taping, including lower expense and ease of application by the player without assistance. However, there are few prospective data documenting its efficacy. Therefore, the ability of the semirigid orthosis to prevent and minimize ankle sprains in soccer players was studied prospectively.

Methods.—After a detailed physical examination was performed and a history was taken, male soccer players at various skill levels were assigned to 1 of 2 groups: those with a history of ankle sprain (258 players) and those with no history of ankle sprain (246 players). The players in both groups were randomly assigned to play with or without a Sport-Stirrup orthosis for all practices and matches during the season. Ankle injuries that required the player to miss the next game or practice were recorded, as was the severity of ankle sprains.

Results.—Players with a history of ankle sprain who wore the Sport-Stirrup orthosis had a significantly lower incidence of ankle sprains than did players with a history of ankle sprain who did not wear the orthosis. Wearing the Sport-Stirrup orthosis did not significantly affect the incidence of ankle sprains in players with no previous history of ankle sprain, but its use did significantly reduce the incidence in players with such a history. Among players with a history of ankle sprain, the orthosis wearers had fewer severe ankle sprains in the previously injured ankles and no difference in severity of sprains in the previously uninjured ankles compared with the control group.

Discussion.—Using a semirigid ankle orthosis significantly reduced the incidence and severity of ankle sprains in previously sprained ankles among soccer players but did not change the incidence or severity of sprains in previously uninjured ankles. The orthosis may achieve its effects by improving proprioceptive function rather than by simply providing mechanical support.

▶ The recommendation that the orthosis be used by soccer players with a previous ankle sprain in conjunction with a comprehensive rehabilitation program to decrease the risk of recurrent injury is reasonable. It should be pointed out that the suggestion that the orthosis may achieve its effect by improving proprioceptive function is not supported by the data presented.

Although the efficacy of the Sport-Stirrup was not compared with ankle taping in this study, the authors claim that it has a "considerable advantage" over taping. That is, it is more cost-effective, does not require trained personnel for its application, and can be adjusted by the player during the game.—J.S. Torg, M.D.

Early Mobilization Versus Immobilization in the Treatment of Lateral Ankle Sprains
Eiff MP, Smith AT, Smith GE (Oregon Health Sciences Univ, Portland; David Grant USAF Med Ctr, Travis Air Force Base, Calif; Vacaville, Calif)
Am J Sports Med 22:83–88, 1994   139-95-4-25

Objective.—Ankle sprains are commonly seen in both the office and emergency department, yet no single method of treatment is accepted as best. Although several studies have compared immobilization and early mobilization for the conservative treatment of these injuries, they have failed to use standard diagnostic and assessment criteria and to control for previous ankle injury. Immobilization and early mobilization for mild-to-moderate, first-time inversion ankle sprains were compared.

Methods.—A total of 82 patients seen at a military medical center with lateral ankle sprains were studied. Half of the patients were randomly selected to receive early mobilization, in which an elastic wrap was placed around the joint for 2 days and a functional brace was used for 8 days. In this group, weight-bearing and ankle rehabilitation commenced 2 days after the injury. The other group of patients received immobilization, with non–weight-bearing plaster splinting for 10 days, followed by weight-bearing and the same rehabilitation program. Outcome assessment included time lost from work, recurrent sprains, and residual symptoms.

Results.—At 3 weeks, 87% of the immobilization group still had pain, compared with 57% of the early mobilization group. This was the only difference between the 2 groups in frequency of residual symptoms. Although most patients were asymptomatic by 6 weeks, one third still had a balance deficit. By 1 year, only 1 patient in each group was still symptomatic. There were 3 patients in each group who resprained their ankle. Fifty-four percent of the early mobilization group had returned to full work activity by 10 days, compared with just 13% of the immobilization group.

Conclusion.—For patients sustaining their first lateral ankle sprain, both immobilization and early mobilization can prevent late residual symptoms and ankle instability. However, earlier mobilization appears to permit a quicker return to full work activity and to be more comfortable for patients. Early mobilization may also be somewhat less expensive.

▶ It is important to note that patients having what are described as "grade III injuries" were excluded from this study. Thus, both the title and conclusions must be qualified by the term "mild" lateral ankle sprains.—J.S. Torg, M.D.

Comparison of Lateral Ankle Ligamentous Reconstruction Procedures
Liu SH, Baker CL (Hughston Sports Medicine Found, Columbus, Ga; Tulane Univ, New Orleans, La)
Am J Sports Med 22:313–317, 1994   139-95-4-26

Introduction.—The most commonly injured structure in sports is the lateral ankle ligament complex, with the anterior talofibular ligament being the most frequently injured ligament of the complex. Nonoperative management focuses on restoring stability. Ineffective treatment may lead to constant pain, swelling, recurrent injuries, instability, and degenerative arthritis. Surgical repair includes reconstruction using, usually, the peroneus brevis tendon. Although there are a variety of procedures that yield disparate results, direct comparisons of the procedures are few.

Methods.—Forty cadaveric ankles were divided into 5 groups: ankles with intact anterior talofibular and calcaneofibular ligaments, ankles with

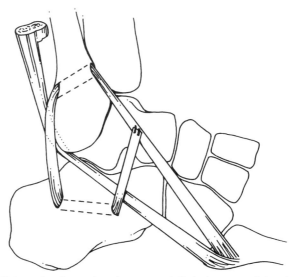

Fig 4–14.—In the Chrisman-Snook procedure, the anterior talofibular ligament and the calcaneofibular ligament are reconstructed using half of the peroneus brevis tendon. (Courtesy of Liu SH, Baker CL: *Am J Sports Med* 22:313–317, 1994.)

these ligaments incised, ankles with the Chrisman-Snook procedure (Fig 4–14), ankles with the Watson-Jones procedure, and ankles with the modified Broström procedure. Anterior drawer and inversion stress tests—at forces of 60, 120, and 160 newtons—were performed using the mechanical Telos apparatus. Anterior talar displacement and talar tilt angle were determined radiographically.

Results.—The talar tilt angle increased with increasing application of force. Ankles with incised ligaments showed the greatest talar tilt angulation, and ankles with intact ligaments showed the least, as expected. Of the procedures, the modified Broström best approximated the ankles with intact ligaments. Similar patterns were shown for the anterior drawer test.

Conclusion.—Surgical repair of ankle instabilities is still controversial. The ideal procedure would rectify talar tilt and anterior drawer–induced instabilities by repairing normal anatomy. The modified Broström procedure is a more anatomical repair and produces superior static restraints when compared with the other 2 procedures, which use the peroneus brevis tendon. There were no differences in angulation or anterior drawer between the procedures that used the peroneus brevis tendon. None of the procedures were as good as intact lateral ligaments. Normal anatomy, tendon preservation, and ankle motion are maintained in the Broström procedure and clinically produce a more stable tibiotalar joint.

▶ Although not necessarily the currently preferred method for lateral ankle ligamentous reconstruction, the Broström procedure has certainly withstood the test of time.—J.S. Torg, M.D.

Achilles Tendon Injuries in Athletes
Kvist M (Univ of Turku, Finland)
Sports Med 18:173–201, 1994   139-95-4–27

Background.—About 75% of all Archilles tendon ruptures and most partial tendon ruptures are related to sports activities, usually from abrupt repetitive jumping and sprinting motions. Athletes in running sports have a high incidence of these injuries. Most Achilles tendon injuries resulting from sports occur in men. Surgery is required in 25% of athletes with Achilles tendon overuse injuries; 70% to 90% of these athletes can successfully return to sports after surgery, 20% require a second surgery, and 3% to 5% must abandon their sports career. Marked forefoot varus occurs in athletes with Achilles tendon overuse injuries, which reflects the predisposing role of ankle joint overpronation. Athletes whose major stress is in the lower extremities can have limited range of motion in the passive dorsiflexion of the ankle joint and total subtalar joint mobility, which may be a predisposing factor.

Cause.—Several factors are involved in overuse injuries. These injuries are usually associated with unusual movements, resumption of work after absence, and repetitive movements. In competitive athletes, as many as 90% of overuse injuries result from repetitive microtraumas over months or years; in recreational athletes, these injuries usually result from acute overloading. Other factors include training errors, malalignments and biomechanical faults, insufficient strength and flexibility, improper footwear, and traumas. The most common error in training is excessive intensity or duration. A change in training schedule has been reported by 22% to 56% of individuals with running injuries. Fatigue can also lead to injury because fatigued muscles lose their ability to absorb shock and provide dynamic stability for the joints.

Discussion.—The best treatment for patients with exertion injuries is said to be prevention. The following could help prevent Achilles tendon injuries: regular flexibility and resistance training exercises; correction of muscle imbalance; correction of structural defects of lower extremities with orthoses; proper shoes, insoles, and training surfaces; and proper training.

▶ This is an excellent review paper with an exhaustive bibliography of 358 references.—J.S. Torg, M.D.

Surgical Management of Achilles Tendon Overuse Injuries: A Long-Term Follow-Up Study

Schepsis AA, Wagner C, Leach RE (Boston Univ Med Ctr/Univ Hosp)
Am J Sports Med 22:611–619, 1994   139-95-4–28

Introduction.—Overuse injuries are becoming increasingly frequent as more Americans take up running and as sports training becomes more intensive. Runners in particular are at risk of overuse injury of the Achilles tendon.

Series.—Seventy-six patients had surgery on 92 extremities for overuse injuries of the Achilles tendon that had failed to respond to conservative measures. Sixty-six patients with 79 injured tendons were followed for a mean of 6.5 years. The patients, with a mean age of 33 years, had been symptomatic for an average of 15 months before surgery. Eight percent of patients were runners and most of these ran competitively, averaging 40–120 miles per week. The most frequent operative findings were retrocalcaneal bursitis, paratenonitis, and partial rupture or degeneration of the tendon.

Management.—Preoperative MRI is very helpful for delineating regions of tendon degeneration or rupture. Involved areas of tendon were split longitudinally and foci of degeneration were excised. In cases of partial rupture, scar tissue was excised and the tendon reapproximated by side-to-side suturing. Retrocalcaneal bursitis was treated by totally excising the bursa and removing the posterosuperior angle of the os calcis. In cases of insertional tendinitis, a small splitting incision was made within the insertion, spurs removed, and areas of degeneration débrided. Only patients having extensive tendon débridement were casted.

Results.—Sixty-two patients (79%) had good-to-excellent results and were able to return to sports activity at the desired level with no more than mild or intermittent discomfort. Four patients with tendinosis, all of them older men with extensive degeneration, required reoperation. Six patients with retrocalcaneal bursitis had an unsatisfactory outcome.

Conclusion.—Operative management is a useful option for runners and other athletes who have overuse injuries of the Achilles tendon that have failed to respond to conservative measures. Older men with degenerative changes in the tendon should be aware that symptoms may recur, especially if the men continue to run competitively.

▶ It is important to note that the authors state that "Nonoperative management is usually successful in alleviating most symptoms of Achilles tendon overuse injuries."—J.S. Torg, M.D.

Immediate Free Ankle Motion After Surgical Repair of Acute Achilles Tendon Ruptures
Sölveborn S-A, Moberg A (Uppsala Univ, Sweden)
Am J Sports Med 22:607–610, 1994   139-95-4--29

Introduction.—Opinions vary about the best way to treat ruptured Achilles tendons. Currently, athletes and young, active patients with this injury are often treated with surgical repair followed by ankle immobilization for 4-6 weeks. However, studies have shown healing benefits associated with early mobilization. A new cast, used after surgical repair of the Achilles tendon, which allows free ankle movement, was studied.

Methods.—Seventeen patients who had undergone surgical repair of acute and complete rupture of the Achilles tendon were followed for 1 year. After surgery, a patellar tendon–bearing cast with a metal frame passing under the foot was put on the affected leg (Fig 4–15), and a platform for the contralateral shoe equaled the distance from frame to foot. The patients wore this arrangement for 6 weeks; they could move the ankle in the pain-free range and could put weight on the frame. The patients were evaluated clinically and by subjective questionnaire at 6 weeks, 3 months, and 1 year postoperatively.

Results.—There were no complications. Fourteen of the 17 patients reported no subjective feeling of adhesion between skin and tendon at 6 weeks and at 3 months, although clinical evaluation identified slight adhesion in 6 patients at 6 weeks and 3 months and in 5 patients at 1 year. Isokinetic muscle strength, strength in dorsal extension, and range of motion were nearly the same as that in the contralateral side, although

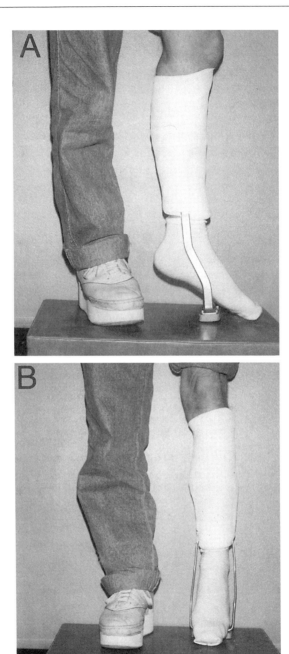

Fig 4–15.—Side (**A**) and front (**B**) view of the patellar tendon–bearing plaster cast with the protecting metal frame attached, allowing weight-bearing and free ankle motion. (Courtesy of Sölveborn S-A, Moberg A: *Am J Sports Med* 22:607–610, 1994.)

plantar flexion was slightly weaker in most patients at 1 year. Thirteen patients reported full recovery at a mean of 6 months. At 1 year, 15 patients had excellent ratings (6 at 3 months) and 2 had good ratings (11 at 3 months) on the Arner-Lindholm rating scale. No patients had poor ratings at any time.

Discussion.—The patients achieved good or excellent results with this cast arrangement allowing free ankle motion immediately postoperatively. A randomized, prospective study that compares this arrangement with traditional postoperative immobilization is justified.

Surgical Repair of Achilles Tendon Ruptures Using Polypropylene Braid Augmentation
Giannini S, Girolami M, Ceccarelli F, Catani F, Stea S (Rizzoli Orthopaedic Inst, Bologna, Italy; Rizzoli Research Ctr, Bologna, Italy)
Foot Ankle Int 15:372–375, 1994   139-95-4–30

Introduction.—There are several surgical procedures for correcting ruptures of the Achilles tendon. However, they often involve long postoperative immobilization, which prolongs rehabilitation. An augmentation technique was developed involving tendon reinforcement with polypropylene braid, which does not require prolonged joint immobilization.

Technique.—With the use of general anesthesia and the surgical area under tourniquet control, a winding posteromedial incision through the subcutaneous tissues and deep fascia exposes the Achilles tendon. The proximal and distal stumps of the tendon are split longitudinally, and the polypropylene braid augmentation device is positioned in a sagittal position into the tendon and sutured to the distal stump. With the foot in a slight equinus, the device is sutured to the proximal stump. The area is covered with dry padding and elastic bandage. Postoperatively, the leg is elevated and the knee flexed 40 degrees. Active and continuous passive motion between 40 degrees of plantar flexion and 5 degrees of dorsiflexion begin the next day, with the patient on non–weight-bearing crutches. Gradual weight-bearing occurs over 4–5 weeks. Swimming can begin after wound healing and sport activities after 3 months.

Patients.—Fifteen patients with unilateral, acute, spontaneous ruptures underwent the procedure within 6 days of the injury. They were followed with isokinetic assessment every 3 months for up to 18 months.

Results.—All the patients returned to their preinjury activity level and reported excellent results. There was no incidence of rerupture or healing impairment. At 1 year, the injured leg had a 1.1-cm reduction in calf circumference, a nonsignificant difference. There were no significant differences between the surgically treated and contralateral legs for strength, work time, or ankle range of motion.

Discussion.—The isokinetic results of the polypropylene braid augmentation procedure for repair of Achilles tendon rupture were similar to those reported with other surgical techniques. However, this procedure, because it does not require immobilization, resulted in an early return to work and to preinjury activity levels.

➤ We have recently completed a clinical study using an unbraided, absorbable polylactic acid suture device followed by an accelerated rehabilitation program for the management of acute Achilles tendon ruptures. Our results were similar to those reported in Abstracts 139-95-4–29 and 139-95-4–30. It should be noted, however, that both of these studies lack an appropriate control group. It appears that the important factor in the surgical management of Achilles ruptures is minimal immobilization and early aggressive rehabilitation.—J.S. Torg, M.D.

Medial Tibial Stress Syndrome: The Location of Muscles in the Leg in Relation to Symptoms
Beck BR, Osternig LR (Univ of Oregon, Eugene)
J Bone Joint Surg (Am) 76–A:1057–1061, 1994   139-95-4–31

Introduction.—The condition popularly called "shinsplints" is better termed "medial tibial stress syndrome," which accurately reflects the site of the symptoms along the distal half to one third of the medial border of the tibia. Among the etiologic theories regarding its occurrence is muscle and/or fascial traction on the periosteum causing tibial bending. Several structures have been implicated: the tibialis posterior, soleus, flexor digitorum longus, and the deep crural fascia. The origins of these structures were investigated to determine their potential for causing traction stress at the characteristic symptom sites.

Methods.—One leg from each of 50 cadavers was dissected to reveal and measure the attachment sites of the fibers of the tibialis posterior, the soleus, the flexor digitorum longus, and the deep crural fascia to the tibia. The mean measurements for the superior and inferior attachment sites were calculated. The tibia was divided into 6 segments, and the segment corresponding to each origin was noted; the most common site of origin was calculated. The data were compared with composite diagrams derived from descriptions in anatomy texts.

Results.—With an average inferior attachment site at 48% and 35% of the length of the tibia, respectively, the soleus and the flexor digitorum longus muscles attached at the characteristic site of the symptoms of medial tibial stress syndrome. Some fibers of both of these muscles arose from sites other than the medial border of the tibia—including medial, intermediate, and lateral sites—with the greatest variability seen with the flexor digitorum longus. However, in no legs did the tibialis posterior attach to the distal half of the medial border of the tibia. The deep crural fascia attachment was consistently found along the entire length of the medial border. The average origins of each structure were similar to those seen in standard anatomy texts.

Discussion.—Although the tibialis posterior has been most frequently implicated, these data and standard anatomy texts indicate that this muscle is not involved in medial tibial stress syndrome. The origins of the soleus and flexor digitorum longus muscles and the deep crural fascia support their potential for causing traction stress, resulting in medial tibial stress syndrome.

▶ Here is an interesting paper with virtually no clinical relevance.—J.S. Torg, M.D.

Lowered Motor Conduction Velocity of the Peroneal Nerve After Inversion Trauma
Kleinrensink GJ, Stoeckart R, Meulstee J, Sukul DMKSK, Vleeming A, Snijders CJ, Van Noort A (Erasmus Univ Rotterdam, The Netherlands; Univ Hosp, Rotterdam, The Netherlands)
Med Sci Sports Exerc 26:877–883, 1994   139-95-4-32

Background.—Inversion trauma to the ankle is very common. Motor conduction velocity was measured to determine the effect of inversion trauma on peroneal nerve function.

Methods and Findings.—Eighteen men and 4 women aged 17–45 years were included in the study. Four to 8 days after trauma, motor nerve conduction velocity in the knee–caput fibulae segment of the superficial peroneal nerve was significantly smaller in the injured leg than in the contralateral leg or in control subjects. Five weeks after the injury, these values were normal again. Four to 8 days after trauma, the motor conduction velocity was significantly decreased in 3 segments of the deep peroneal nerve compared with control group values. In the caput-ankle and knee-ankle segment, motor conduction velocity was still significantly reduced 5 weeks after injury. Amplitudes of the compound motor action potentials of the extensor digitorum brevis muscle were reduced 4–8 days after injury. Motor nerve conduction velocities and subjective clinical tests were uncorrelated.

Conclusion.—These findings support the hypothesis that inversion trauma is often associated with lesions of the peroneal nerve. Motor conduction velocity measures can be useful in the objective assessment of functional instability of the ankle joint induced by inversion injury.

▶ As stated by the authors, this study "focuses on the short-term effects of inversion trauma (without clinical signs of peroneal nerve palsy) on motor nerve conduction velocity of the superficial and deep peroneal nerve." The purpose of this study, however, is "to contribute to a better understanding of persistent instability of the ankle and. . .create an objective way of quantifying effects of inversion trauma." In that there is no correlation between the motor conduction velocity changes and function, it does not appear that this latter goal was accomplished.—J.S. Torg, M.D.

5 Other Injuries

Stimulation of Bone Growth Through Sports: A Radiologic Investigation of the Upper Extremities in Professional Tennis Players
Krahl H, Michaelis U, Pieper H-G, Quack G, Montag M (Alfried Krupp von Bohlen und Halbach Krankenhaus, Essen, Germany)
Am J Sports Med 22:751–757, 1994   139-95-5–1

Introduction.—Bone increases in density and diameter in response to continuous mechanical stress. The influence of mechanical factors on epiphyseal plates has not been well defined. Ossification of the distal epiphyseal plates in the forearm occurs at the end of the second decade of life, making it an excellent area in which to investigate the influence of high strain on bone growth. Tennis players become professional at the age of 15 or 17 years, with professional practice beginning at about age 10 years. An investigation was conducted to determine the influence of the constant strain of training and competition on bone growth in 20 nationally and internationally ranked tennis professionals.

Methods.—The age range of the subjects was 13 to 26 years (mean age, 20.1 years). Twelve players were male and 8 were female. All had had at least 5 years of training and competition, with all of them starting serious training by age 11 years. Daily practice time was a minimum of 2 hours. Radiographic measurements were taken of the stroke arm and contralateral arm in each player. Measurements were also taken in a control group of 12 research subjects in the same age range.

Results.—An obvious difference in bone structure was noted between the stroke arm and the contralateral arm on visual inspection of the radiographs. The following were significantly different in the stroke arm of all players compared to the contralateral arm and arms of the controls: ulnar diameter was larger, ulnar length was longer (Fig 5–1), and the second metacarpal showed increased bone density and cortical thickness (Fig 5–2). The mean length differences between stroke and contralateral arm were 3% for the ulna and 3.7% for the second metacarpal. No significant differences were found for player age, sex, or handedness.

Conclusion.—Increases were seen in bone density, thickness, and length in response to continuous mechanical stress. The stimulation of longitudinal growth has never been reported.

▶ It is generally understood that all bone growth is determined by functional forces. The potential for growth is directly proportional to local stress effects. German researchers have reported that bone will grow axially as long

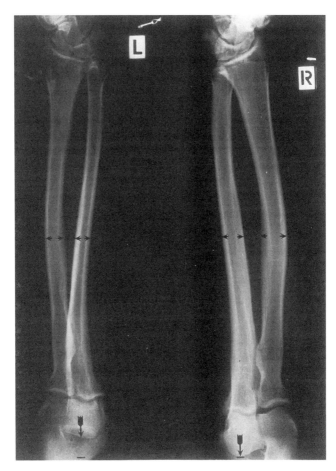

Fig 5–1.—The forearms of a tennis professional (right-handed) with a hypertrophy of the right arm (widening of 4.4 mm, lengthening of 13 mm). (Courtesy of Krahl H, Michaelis U, Pieper H-G, et al: *Am J Sports Med* 22:751–757, 1994.)

as stress is placed on the full width of the epiphyseal plate. Obviously, the dominant forearm and hand absorb the strain of tennis. These authors believe that the mechanical vibration from the racket to the hand over many hours of practice and many years is the stress that causes the hypertrophy of the bones in the dominant arm and hand of tennis players. They also report that there seems to be a temporary hyperemia of the muscular system of the dominant arm in tennis players that is induced by this sports-specific strain. The authors report, however, that the exact size, direction, and duration of the effective forces and the exact increase in vascularization have not, as yet, been determined.—Col. J.L. Anderson, PE.D.

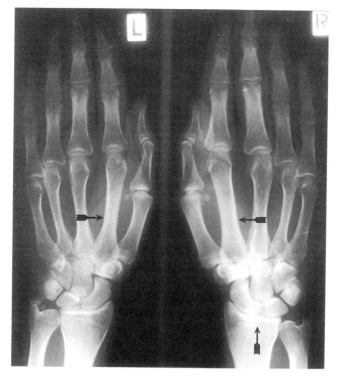

Fig 5–2.—Hands of a tennis professional (right-handed) with significant changes of the right as compared with the left second metacarpals (widening of 1.6 mm, lengthening of 4.1 mm). (Courtesy of Krahl H, Michaelis U, Pieper H-G, et al: *Am J Sports Med* 22:751-757, 1994.)

A Prospective, Double-Blind Trial of Electrical Capacitive Coupling in the Treatment of Non-Union of Long Bones

Scott G, King JB (Royal London Hosp)
J Bone Joint Surg (Am) 76–A:820–826, 1994   139-95-5–2

Background.—Although encouraging clinical studies have been published, the proper clinical role of electric stimulation in the treatment of established nonunion of long bones is unknown. A capacitively coupled bone-stimulating device was used in a double-blind, randomized study of the treatment of long bones with established nonunion.

Methods.—Twenty-three adult patients whose time since injury had been at least 9 months and whose fracture had shown no clinical or radiographic signs of progress toward healing for at least 3 months were entered into the study. The form of external support was a continuation of what had been used during the preceding 3 months, but holes were cut into any plaster cast to allow application of surface electrodes. The commercially available Orthopak bone-growth stimulator was used. It consisted of 2 stainless steel disks, 1 disk applied to each side of the limb, that continuously delivered a 5–10 volt peak-to-peak sine wave at 60 kHz. The initial treatment period was 6 months.

Results.—Twenty-one patients completed the study; 10 were actively treated and 11 were treated with a placebo unit. Six of the 10 patients who were actively treated had a healed nonunion at 6 months, compared with none of the 11 patients who had used the placebo units. The statistical difference in healing between the 2 groups was highly significant. In the 6 patients who healed, the mean duration of capacitive coupling was 21 weeks. By chance, all of the femoral fractures had been assigned to the actively treated group, so a separate analysis of only the tibial fractures was done. Three of the 5 tibial fractures in the actively treated group healed, compared with none of the 10 tibial fractures in the placebo group. This was still a statistically significant difference.

Conclusion.—A capacitively coupled bone-stimulating device is beneficial in the treatment of an established nonunion of a long bone. These commercially available devices are noninvasive and completely portable.

▶ This study appears to demonstrate that electrical capacitive coupling is highly effective in the treatment of patients with nonunion of long bones. This randomized, double-blind study was done at the Royal London Hospital in England. It was a surprise to me that in a preliminary study done in 1985 by other researchers, the researchers believed they could not do a double-blind, randomized study in the United States because they thought patients would not accept the possibility of being treated with a placebo unit for as long as 6 months.—Col. J.L. Anderson, PE.D.

Cervical Spinal Stenosis and Stingers in Collegiate Football Players
Meyer SA, Schulte KR, Callaghan JJ, Albright JP, Powell JW, Crowley ET, El-Khoury GY (Univ of Iowa, Iowa City)
Am J Sports Med 22:158–166, 1994   139-95-5–3

Background.—The "stinger syndrome," a common injury in collision sports, is thought to be caused by trauma to the brachial plexus and/or nerve roots. There is uncertainty as to the primary location of the injury along the nerve, although it is well documented that the C5 and C6 nerve distributions are most commonly involved with stingers. The relationship of cervical spinal stenosis to the stinger syndrome was evaluated.

Methods.—A retrospective record review was conducted of collegiate football players who played at the study institution during the years 1987 through 1991. The study group consisted of only those players for whom preparticipation standard cervical spine radiographs were available. Each radiograph was evaluated for evidence of degenerative changes, instability, and congenital abnormalities, and the Torg ratio was measured.

Results.—Two hundred sixty-six players' records and radiographs were obtained and evaluated. Forty players sustained stinger injuries, 31 had time-loss neck pain injuries, and 195 were asymptomatic. In the stinger group, 34 had extension-compression mechanisms and 6 had brachial plexus stretch mechanisms. More than 1 stinger in a season was incurred by 10 of the 40 players. There was no significant difference in the occurrence of radiographic abnormalities among the 3 groups. The mean sagittal canal diameter at each cervical level was narrower in the stinger group compared with the other 2 groups. For the stinger group compared with the neck pain group, the mean Torg ratio was smaller at all vertebral levels. The mean Torg ratio of the stinger group was significantly smaller compared with the asymptomatic group at levels C4, C5, and C6, but not at C3 or C7.

No interaction was found between position played and the incidence of stingers when analyzed by Torg ratio at each vertebral level. The risk of being in the stinger group was 2.98 times greater for a player with cervical stenosis, as indicated by a Torg ratio of less than 0.8, than for a player without stenosis.

Conclusion.—Cervical spine stenosis increases the risk for stingers caused by an extension-compression mechanism.

▶ Kelly et al. (1) and Warren et al. (2) have also recognized an association between the "stinger syndrome" and developmental narrowing of the cervical spinal canal. The possible explanation for this association is that a decreased canal diameter may be associated with a narrow intervertebral foramen. This concept is supported by the fact that a narrow cervical spinal canal was found only in those players with stingers caused by an extension-compression mechanism rather than brachial plexus traction. The assumption here is that symptoms are caused by compression of the spinal nerve root in the foramen.—J.S. Torg, M.D.

References

1. Kelly JD, Clancy M, Marchetto PA, et al: The relationship of transient upper extremity paresthesias and cervical stenosis, *Orthop Trans* 16:732, 1992–1993.
2. Warren R, et al: *Orthop Trans* 16:733, 1992–1993.

Sagittal Measurements of the Cervical Spine in Subaxial Fractures and Dislocations: An Analysis of Two Hundred and Eighty-Eight Patients With and Without Neurological Deficits
Kang JD, Figgie MP, Bohlman HH, (Case Western Reserve Univ, Cleveland, Ohio)
J Bone Joint Surg (Am) 76–A:1617–1627, 1994   139-95-5–4

Background.—The relationship of the sagittal diameter of the spinal canal before an injury to the severity of an injury in patients with a cervical fracture or dislocation appears to be controversial. Three factors involved in fractures and dislocations of the cervical spine and their relationship to the degree of spinal cord injury were investigated.

Methods.—The space available for the spinal cord at the level of the injury, the sagittal diameter of the spinal canal at the uninjured levels, and the Pavlov ratio at the uninjured levels were assessed in 288 patients. Eighty-three had a complete injury of the spinal cord, 92 had an incomplete injury of the spinal cord; and 30 had an isolated nerve-root injury. Eighty-three had no neurologic deficit.

Findings.—The mean space available for the spinal cord at the level of injury differed significantly among groups, except between patients with an isolated nerve-root injury and patients with no neurologic deficit. The mean sagittal diameter of the canal at the uninjured levels did not differ significantly between patients with a complete injury of the spinal cord and those with an incomplete injury or between patients with an isolated nerve-root injury and those with no neurologic deficit. However, patients with a complete injury of the spinal cord and those with an incomplete injury differed significantly from patients with an isolated nerve-root injury and those with no neurologic deficit. There was a nonsignificant difference in mean Pavlov ratio at the uninjured levels between patients with a complete injury of the spinal cord and those with an incomplete injury and between those with an isolated nerve-root injury and those with no neurologic deficit. The patients with a complete injury of the spinal cord and patients with an incomplete injury did differ significantly from patients with an isolated nerve-root injury and those with no neurologic deficit.

Conclusion.—The severity of the injury of the spinal cord is partly associated with the space available for the cord after the injury, as measured on plain lateral radiographs. Also, patients with a permanent cord injury have a narrower sagittal diameter of the spinal canal before the injury. Patients with a large sagittal diameter of the canal may be less likely to sustain permanent injury of the spinal cord after a fracture or dislocation of the cervical spine than are patients with a narrow canal.

▶ It is important to note, as pointed out by the authors, that "The degree of damage to the spinal cord in patients who sustain a cervical fracture or dislocation, or both, probably depends on several factors. Important factors may be the characteristics of the injury itself, such as the total energy absorbed by the spinal cord during the injury and the degree of displacement of the osseous elements causing mechanical deformation of the spinal cord." We believe that this partially explains our observation that with regard to tackle football, there was no correlation between canal diameter and neurologic sequelae.—J.S. Torg, M.D.

Posture and the Compressive Strength of the Lumbar Spine

Adams MA, McNally DS, Chinn H, Dolan P (Univ of Bristol, England)
Clin Biomech 9:5–14, 1994   139-95-5-5

Background.—It is generally assumed that a lumbar lordosis can protect against compressive injury of the spine, although this protective action has never been demonstrated at the high load levels encountered in heavy labor. Even when bending the knees, most individuals flex the lumbar spine when lifting objects from the ground. Unless the presumed advantages of a lordotic lifting technique can be demonstrated clearly, the typical advice to "keep the back straight" when lifting may be unwise. A series of cadaveric experiments was performed to study the effects of posture on spinal compressive strength.

Methods and Results.—Compression was applied to lumbar "motion segments," consisting of 2 vertebrae with their intervening disk and ligaments, with the segments in various angles of flexion and extension (Fig 5–3). The first experiment, based on measurements of intradiskal pressure, suggested that the load was shared between the disk, the apophyseal joint surfaces, and the intervertebral ligaments. With extension, the apophyseal joints became load bearing and were vulnerable to damage at

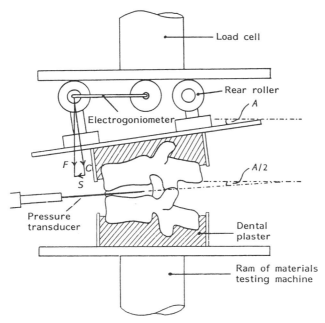

Fig 5–3.—Apparatus used to apply bending and compression to the specimens. The height of the rear roller is adjustable, allowing the specimens to be flexed to various angles of flexion and extension. The low-friction bearings of the rollers transmit only a vertical force F between load cell and specimen. The compressive force C is defined as $C = F \times \cos (A/2)$ where A = flexion angle. (Courtesy of Adams MA, McNally DS, Chinn H, et al: *Clin Biomech* 9:5–14, 1994.)

compressive loads as low as 500 newtons. When flexion angles exceeded approximately 75% of the full range of flexion, as defined by the posterior ligaments, the result was high tensile forces in these ligaments and substantial increases in intradiskal pressure. Optimal resistance to compression was observed in the range of 0% to 75% flexion.

A second experiment compared distribution of compressive stress within the disk at 0% and 75%. At the low end of this range, many disks showed high stress concentrations in the posterior annulus; at the high end, stress was usually distributed evenly. A third experiment found no significant difference in compressive strength between motion segments positioned in 0% and 75% flexion.

Conclusion.—These findings, in comparison with the range of flexion/extension movements in vivo and in vitro, suggest that moderate flexion of the lumbar spine is preferred when the spine is subjected to high compressive forces. During heavy lifting, flexion of about 80% is recommended to optimize compressive and tensile stresses in the annulus fibrosus.

▶ This paper was selected as the Clinical Biomechanics Award Paper for 1993, for best full paper, under the auspices of the International Society of Biomechanics. That speaks to the excellence of the authors' work and earns the paper a right to be included in the YEAR BOOK OF SPORTS MEDICINE. It also deals with one of the most difficult injuries in sports medicine, injuries to the back, especially the low back.—Col. J.L. Anderson, PE.D.

Passive Stiffness of the Lumbar Torso in Flexion, Extension, Lateral Bending, and Axial Rotation: Effect of Belt Wearing and Breath Holding
McGill S, Seguin J, Bennett G (Univ of Waterloo, Ontario)
Spine 19:696–704, 1994   139-95-5–6

Objective.—Data on the stiffness properties of the intact torso are needed for human impact studies, for the design of torso braces and stabilization hardware, and for use in biomechanical models to estimate spinal loads. Information on torso stiffness is also important in clarifying the role of abdominal belts—as worn by some industrial workers and weight lifters—and breath holding. Most research of the bending properties of the spine has been performed in cadaveric spines. The passive bending properties of the intact torso about its 3 principal axes and the effects of an abdominal belt and breath holding on trunk stiffness were investigated in healthy volunteers.

Methods.—The research subjects were 22 young men and 15 young women who had no disabling low back pain. Each individual was held "floating" in a frictionless jig and subjected to passive bending movements with isolated torso bending measured with a magnetic device. The passive bending properties of the torso were measured about the 3 principal axes of flexion-extension, lateral bending, and axial rotation. Passive resistance of the lumbar torso was measured during torque application in the principal planes of motion, and a relationship suitable for inclusion of total torso passive stiffness into a biomechanical model was constructed. The effects of wearing an abdominal belt and of holding the breath in full inhalation were studied as well.

Results.—Wearing an abdominal belt and holding the breath appeared to stiffen the torso in the lateral bending and axial rotation axes. The flexion-extension axis was unaffected, however. In the lateral bending axis, the torsos were stiffer and stored more elastic energy. The research subjects were able to tolerate much higher torques in lateral bending than in any other axis; men generally tolerated higher bending torques than women. Compared with previously reported data in osteoligamentous spine preparations, the intact torso was stiffer over a more moderate range of motion; thus, passive tissue, other than ligaments and disks, contributed to stiffness. However, tissues lacking ligamentous contact with the spine—such as viscera and skin—did not appear to contribute significant torque to the spine.

Conclusion.—Abdominal belt wearing and breath holding appear to stiffen the torso in the coronal and transverse planes but not in the sagittal plane. This finding might suggest that belt wearing is advantageous; however, most lifting tasks are dominated by the extensor moment, and stiffness is only 1 factor that should be considered in prescribing a belt. The regression equations calculated to define stiffness and energy stored will be useful in biomechanical models for examining low back function and in the design of stabilization or bracing hardware.

▶ This is an excellent study that all doctors should read before prescribing torso belts for protecting workers with low back pain who have to do heavy lifting as a part of their jobs. These authors point out that whereas belt wearing and breath holding appear to stiffen the torso in the coronal and transverse planes, they are not effective in the sagittal plane. They also report that other factors—biomechanical, physiologic, and psychological—should be considered in the decision regarding belt prescription.

The authors recognize that there are limitations that restrict the relevance of their data to the population as a whole. For instance, the subjects were all young undergraduates with no history of low back pain. Also, only leather belts were tested, and they were of the type usually used by athletes.—Col. J.L. Anderson, PE.D.

Identification of Dynamic Myoelectric Signal-to-Force Models During Isometric Lumbar Muscle Contractions

Thelen DG, Schultz AB, Fassois SD, Ashton-Miller JA (Univ of Michigan, Ann Arbor)
J Biomech 27:907–919, 1994   139-95-5--7

Background.—Measures of the load on the lumbar spine during task performance may improve the understanding of the causes of low back pain. However, lumbar spine load cannot be measured directly. Therefore, several models that measure lumbar myoelectric signals (MES) during light-to-moderate sagittal loading have been developed. An isometric lumbar MES-to-force prediction model that differs from previous models was developed and evaluated.

Method.—Nine healthy men ranging in age from 21 to 31 years participated in this study. They had a mean height of 175.8 cm and a mean body weight of 73.2 kg. Each subject performed 22 separate tasks that evaluated trunk flexion and extension, right and left lateral bend, and counterclockwise and clockwise twist (Fig 5-4). A model was constructed that related the normalized root mean square MES to the measured moments about the spine at the L3–L4 level. Myoelectric signals

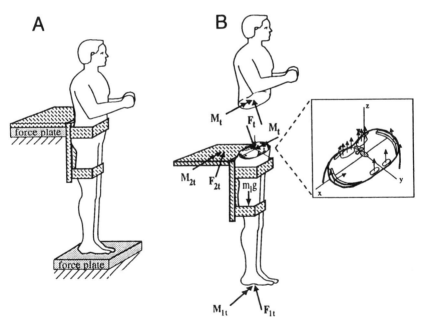

Fig 5-4.—A, schematic representation of the experimental set-up. Padded restraints were placed around the upper body during attempted exertions. **B,** free body diagram used to calculate the net forces and moments at the L3–L4 level of the trunk. Moments about the lumbar spine were assumed to be generated by the 14 muscles included in the model of the transverse cross-section of the lumbar trunk. (Courtesy of Thelen DG, Schultz AB, Fassois SD, et al: *J Biomech* 27:907–919, 1994.)

from 14 lumbar muscles were recorded with electrodes placed on each side of the trunk. The model was evaluated by comparing measured and MES-predicted moments during the tasks.

Results.—The mean peak moments were 65.6 newton meters (N-m) in attempted flexion, 95.4 N-m in attempted extension, 80.7 N-m in attempted lateral bending, and 40.5 N-m in attempted twist. Measured and predicted moments correlated during slow and rapid trunk flexion and extension, lateral bending, and twisting. Moment prediction errors of 25% occurred with trunk flexion-extension movements; 30% with lateral bends; and 40% with axial twisting movements. Reproducible MES-stress models were obtained.

Conclusion.—This calibration method can be used to predict the lumbar muscle and spine loads exerted for specific individuals during certain physical tasks.

▶ The authors of this study demonstrate how a calibration method involving system identification techniques can be used to estimate dynamic MES-driven lumbar muscle force prediction models for individual subjects. They state that this type of approach, coupled with a thorough assessment of model performance, should improve the accuracy with which muscle forces can be estimated using MES.—Col. J.L. Anderson, PE.D.

Sagittal Plane Rotation of the Pelvis During Lumbar Posteroanterior Loading

Lee M, Lau H, Lau T (Univ of Sydney, Australia)
J Manipulative Physiol Ther 17:149–155, 1994   139-95-5–8

Purpose.—Clinicians may apply manual posteroanterior (PA) force in the assessment and treatment of low back disorders. Understanding which tissues are the likely sources of symptoms produced by PA movements or which tissues might be affected by PA force treatments requires knowledge of the bone movements that occur with the application of PA force. Sagittal plane rotation of the pelvis during PA loading of the lumbar spine was measured in normal subjects.

Methods.—The subjects were 10 men and women with no recent history of significant low back pain. A mechanical device was used to apply PA force to the L3 spinous process, and biomechanical data were collected during slow cyclical loading (Fig 5–5). Measurements included the stiffness of the PA movement at the point of loading, the sagittal plane rotation of the pelvis, and the resistance to rotation provided by the bed on which the subject was lying.

Findings.—All 10 subjects had measurable anterior sagittal rotation of the pelvis during PA loading. For each 100 newtons of PA force applied, the mean pelvic rotation was 2.1 degrees. The mean value for PA stiff-

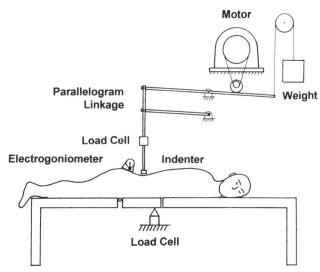

Fig 5–5.—Schematic diagram of mechanical mobilizing device. (Courtesy of Lee M, Lau H, Lau T: *J Manipulative Physiol Ther* 17:149–155, 1994.)

ness was 13.4 newtons/mm, and the mean resistance to pelvic rotation was 2.71 newton meters/degree of pelvic rotation.

Conclusion.—The pelvic rotation that occurs during midlumbar PA force application may be clinically significant. This rotation averages about 2 degrees per 100 newtons of force applied at the L3 level. In patients who show abnormalities during lumbar PA force application, the abnormalities may originate in tissues caudad to the lumbar spine itself.

▶ These investigators developed their own mechanical device to apply measured PA force to the L3 spinous process and measure the pelvic rotation. As with any measuring device, this one needs to be used and tested numerous times to validate the reliability of the measurements. A large number of subjects must be tested to establish norms for the measurements.—Col. J.L. Anderson, PE.D.

The Geometry of the Psoas Muscle as Determined by Magnetic Resonance Imaging
Reid JG, Livingston LA, Pearsall DJ (Queen's Univ, Kingston, Ontario; Wilfrid Laurier Univ, Waterloo, Ontario)
Arch Phys Med Rehabil 75:703–708, 1994   139-95-5–9

Introduction.—The psoas muscle, a major flexor of the hip, is not amenable to detailed examination in living patients. Morphometric data on the psoas and its moment arms are important in the study of spinal mechanics and in models for investigating low back pain. Much of the

$$C_x = \frac{[(y_1 - y_n)(x_n^2 + x_n x_1 + x_1^2) + \sum_{i=1}^{n-1} (y_{i+1} - y_i)(x_i^2 + x_i x_{i+1} + x_{i+1}^2)]}{6 \times \text{Area}} \qquad (2)$$

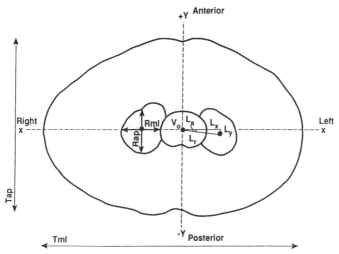

Fig 5–6.—Outline of an MRI (as viewed from the inferior aspect). Variables derived for analysis are shown. This drawing represents the L4–L5 level. (Courtesy of Reid JG, Livingston LA, Pearsall DJ: *Arch Phys Med Rehabil* 75:703–708, 1994.)

knowledge regarding the geometry of the psoas has been gained from cadaveric dissections. With the advent of MRI and CT, the psoas and other trunk muscles can now be studied in vivo. An MRI study was performed to provide a more detailed profile of its geometry.

Methods.—Fifteen physically active, asymptomatic men (mean age, 21.5 years) were studied. Magnetic resonance imaging data were obtained from 9 vertebral and/or intervertebral levels from L2 to S1 (Fig 5–6).

Findings.—The psoas tended to increase in size as it descended the trunk, moving anteriorly and slightly laterally in relation to the vertebral column. The maximal cross-sectional area of the psoas (16 cm²) was seen at the L4–L5 level. The psoas muscle showed right-left symmetry in the anteroposterior (Y) dimension but not in the mediolateral (X) diameter. From L3 to S1, the X moment arm was significantly longer for the right than for the left psoas, with length increasing as the psoas descended the trunk. This trend was not observed in the Y moment arm, in which the noted values were relatively small throughout the course of the muscle.

Conclusion.—This MRI study suggests that more than just anthropometric measures must be considered in predicting psoas dimensions. The findings indicate that the psoas muscles are not necessarily symmetric in cross-sectional area and X moment arms. At different vertebral levels, the flexion and extension tendency of the psoas varies. The new data will be useful in studying the onset of low back pain and in designing appropriate rehabilitation interventions.

▶ These investigators, using MRI to study the psoas muscle, found that their data differed significantly from data of other investigators using either CT or MRI equipment. Although it is generally agreed that these 2 measuring techniques are the most accurate methods available today, other variables must be taken into consideration before the accurate measurements may make any sense. Studies of the psoas muscle are important because it is most often mentioned when someone experiences low back pain. Is it a coincidence that these investigators found the largest cross-sectional area of the psoas muscle to be at the L4–L5 level, which also seems to be the level at which a high percentage of low back pain is diagnosed?—Col. J.L. Anderson, PE.D.

Physiological and Subjective Responses to Maximal Repetitive Lifting Employing Stoop and Squat Technique
Hagen KB, Hallén J, Harms-Ringdahl K (Norwegian Forest Research Inst, Ås, Norway; Natl Inst of Occupational Health, Oslo, Norway; Karolinska Inst, Stockholm)
Eur J Appl Physiol 67:291–297, 1993   139-95-5-10

Background.—Lifting tasks are common in occupations requiring manual handling of materials. To determine safe levels for physical strain in occupational repetitive lifting, specific maximal working capacity was investigated.

Participants and Methods.—Ten male forestry workers (mean age, 30.6 years) participated. All participants were healthy and free of back pain. Power output, oxygen consumption, heart rate, and ventilation were measured during maximal squat lifting and stoop lifting. Both modes of lifting were further compared with maximal treadmill running. Electromyographic activity was also recorded in 4 muscles, and perceived central, local low back, and thigh exertion were evaluated during the lifting procedures.

Results.—No significant differences in power output were observed between the 2 lifting procedures, although mean oxygen consumption was significantly increased during maximal squat lifting, at 38.7 compared with 32.9 mL/kg per minute for maximal stoop lifting. Oxygen consumption during maximal treadmill running was not significantly associated with maximal stoop lifting but was highly correlated with maximal squat lifting. Maximal heart rates among the 3 exercises significantly differed, although differences were not observed in the central rated perceived exertions. Perceived low back exertion during squat lifting was rated significantly lower than it was during stoop lifting. Higher activity was observed for the vastus lateralis muscle on electromyographic recordings, with lower activity noted for the biceps femoris muscle during squat lifting than during stoop lifting. The highest maximal voluntary contraction activity was observed in the erector spinae muscle, regardless of lifting mode.

Conclusion.—Additional studies are needed to determine the influence of lifting mode on various physiologic and perceptual responses to repetitive lifting at submaximal levels.

▶ These authors studied the effect of the squat and stoop lifting techniques on various muscle groups. Because lifting of heavy loads is probably the most frequent cause of low back pain, it should not be a surprise that the erector spinae muscle produced the highest electromyographic activity levels for both lifting techniques. The erector spinae muscles are among the most difficult muscles to exercise and in which to develop strength and muscular endurance. However, it can be done, and the frequency of low back pain can be greatly reduced through prevention. (See also Abstract 139-95-5–11.)
—Col. J.L. Anderson, PE.D.

Electromyographic Median Frequency Changes During Isometric Contraction of the Back Extensors to Fatigue
Mannion AF, Dolan P (Univ of Bristol, England)
Spine 19:1223–1229, 1994   139-95-5–11

Background.—Although electromyography is widely used to monitor muscle fatigue, its relationship to endurance time is not well established. The changes in median frequency of the erector spinae muscle group were investigated during a clinical test of back endurance to determine the relationship between such changes and endurance time to fatigue.

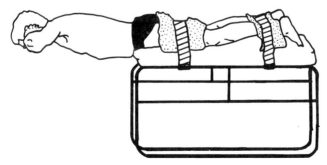

Fig 5–7.—Test position used for determining back extensor endurance. (Courtesy of Mannion AF, Dolan P: *Spine* 19:1223-1229, 1994.)

Participants and Methods.—Two hundred twenty-nine healthy volunteers participated. There were 21 men and 209 women (mean ages, 27.7 and 26.2 years, respectively). Skin-surface electrodes were used to record electromyographic signals from thoracic (T10) and lumbar (L3) regions of the erector spinae during an isometric exercise test. Participants were placed in a prone position on an examination couch. The lower body, from the superior border of the iliac crest downward, was strapped to the couch (Fig 5–7). The unsupported upper body was then maintained in a horizontal position until participants could no longer overcome the force of gravity as a result of fatigue. The rate of change in median frequency of the electromyographic power spectrum (MF_{GRAD}) was calculated.

Results.—The MF_{GRAD} was significantly higher at L3 compared with T10. The greater MF_{GRAD} observed at either region provided the best prediction of endurance time. When calculated during a submaximal period (50% total time or 60 seconds), MF_{GRAD} was also significantly associated with endurance time. Women had a significantly longer endurance time and lower MF_{GRAD} than men.

Conclusion.—Endurance is limited by the most fatigable region of the muscle group. The MF_{GRAD} technique is suitable for monitoring back muscle fatigue, even when evaluated during a submaximal period. The back extensors of women are less fatigable than those of men when the same exercise is undertaken.

▶ This is an excellent bit of research regarding the fatigability of the erector spinae muscles of male and female subjects. Although the procedures used by these researchers appear to show that the back extensors of women fatigue less quickly than those of men when the same back extension exercise is done, that is not what intrigued me most. We are all aware that low back pain is a very extensive and expensive medical problem. It is generally accepted that over 80% of low back pain is the result of muscular imbalance or poor muscular endurance.

Here at West Point, we have been using back extension exercises successfully to treat low back pain for the past 10 years. We started with the Back-Mate procedure, which required the use of a partner. More recently, however, I have found that back extension exercises on weight machines, such as the Life Circuit Back Extension machine, are very effective for strengthening and conditioning the erector spinae muscles and, thus, helping prevent low back pain.—Col. J.L. Anderson, PE.D.

Passive Stiffness of the Human Neck in Flexion, Extension, and Lateral Bending

McGill SM, Jones K, Bennett G, Bishop PJ (Univ of Waterloo, Ontario)
Clin Biomech 9:193–198, 1994   139-95-5–12

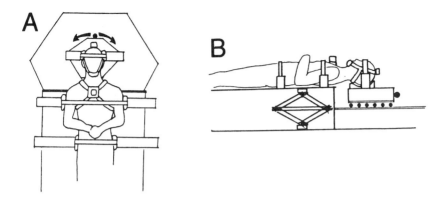

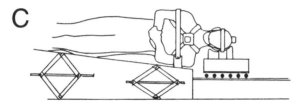

Fig 5–8.—Lateral bending (**A, B**) and flexion-extension (**C**) bending moment was applied with a cable attached to the head/neck, which rotated in a plar.ar bearing system. Angular displacement was measured with a 3-SPACE ISOTRAK with the magnetic modules attached to the sternum and the top of the head. Spines were aligned along their full length with a scissor-jack system, which independently elevated the upper and lower parts of the body. (Courtesy of McGill SM, Jones K, Bennett G, et al: *Clin Biomech* 9:193–198, 1994.)

Objective.—Biomechanical studies of the neck frequently use a modeling method to estimate tissue loads because in vivo measurements are problematic. The ability to quantify the passive stiffness of the intact neck will enhance the biological validity of physical and analytical models of the cervical spine.

Methods.—Passive bending stiffness was quantified in 59 university students (40 men and 19 women) together with the ability to store elastic energy and the maximum tolerated level of bending moment. Bending moments were applied to the neck as the subject lay on a frictionless jig (Fig 5–8). Angular displacement of the skull relative to the rib cage was recorded at the same time. The subjects were taught to relax their sternocleidomastoid and splenius capitis muscles by listening to amplified myoelectric signals. Studies were repeated twice in each of 3 positions: flexion, extension, and lateral bending.

Findings.—The maximum level of bending moment tolerated in all positions averaged less than 10 newton meters. The participants tolerated greater moment during flexion than during either extension or lateral bending and stored more elastic energy in the cervical tissues. Energy storage was greatest during flexion. Men tolerated greater moments than women, were more stiff, and stored more energy under all loading conditions. Men had greater stiffness than women at all angles.

Summary.—These data provide a first approximation to values of dynamic bending stiffness that may be included in biomechanical models of the cervical spine.

▶ These authors recognize that there are some limitations to this study. The subjects were young undergraduates in good health with no history of disabling spine pain or injury. Also, the loading of the cervical spine was pure bending moment through the application of a shear load. That did not allow for a comprehensive preload, and the stiffnesses measured in these experiments are probably lower than those developed during head-first loading situations such as American football and ice hockey. The authors decided that given the low magnitude of applied moment that was tolerable at the low loading rates used, it would appear that the human neck must have substantial viscoelastic properties to dissipate energy and to allow it to tolerate much higher applied moments when rapid loading takes place over a very brief period, as in impact loading. Also, the authors believe that preparatory muscle activation would act to both stiffen the neck and to absorb energy through eccentric contraction.—Col. J.L. Anderson, PE.D.

The Sequential Scrum Engagement: A Biomechanical Analysis
Milburn PD, O'Shea BP (Univ of Wollongong, Australia; Australian Inst of Sport)
Aust J Sci Med Sport 26:32–35, 1994   139-95-5–13

Background.—During scrum engagement in rugby, techniques are sometimes used that are potentially hazardous to the players. There is a high incidence of scrum-related cervical spine injuries in front-row players during scrum engagement. A 4-stage engagement sequence of scrum formation has been adopted by the International Rugby Board for universal application. Since the application of these modified scrummaging laws in all Australian matches in 1988, there has not been a scrum-related serious cervical spine injury in an Australian rugby union. The resultant forces experienced in sequential scrum engagement were analyzed and compared with the forces experienced in traditional scrummaging techniques.

Methods.—Data on the forces carried by front-row players were collected using 3 force plates incorporated into a scrum machine. Each player pushed against a section of the scrum machine. Data on each player could be simultaneously obtained under all test conditions.

Results.—There was a risk of front-row players being exposed to potentially dangerous forces on engagement with all variations of scrum formation. The 2 variations of sequential or staggered engagement that were examined did not substantially reduce the forces experienced by individual players. The hooker is exposed to the greatest force of all front-row players. Front-row players are most vulnerable to serious cervical spine injury during the formation of the scrum, especially when players charge inward at engagement, when the scrum collapses, or when a head is popped out of a scrum when the 2 front rows come together. The sequential scrummaging technique decreased scrum stability.

Conclusion.—The risk of injury can be more readily reduced through coaching strategies and good management by referees than through changing scrummaging techniques and laws. Because the hooker is the most vulnerable to serious cervical spine injury, he should determine the timing of the engagement.

▶ These authors studied rugby scrummaging techniques to develop ways to reduce the incidence of scrum-related cervical spine injuries. I am impressed by their use of biomechanical techniques to study ways to make rugby safer rather than to call for the abolition of the game. Too often, a person's first reaction is to say "abolish the sport" rather than undertake studies to find ways to make the sport safer. I apply this same argument to the sport of boxing. I truly believe that we can make that sport safer if we set out to do so, rather than to attempt to abolish it.—Col. J.L. Anderson, PE.D.

Evaluation of Muscle Force Prediction Models of the Lumbar Trunk Using Surface Electromyography
Hughes RE, Chaffin DB, Lavender SA, Andersson GBJ (Univ of Michigan, Ann Arbor; Rush-Presbyterian-St Luke's Med Ctr, Chicago)
J Orthop Res 12:689–698, 1994   139-95-5-14

Background.—Optimization-based models for predicting muscle forces in the lumbar region of the torso are used to gauge forces that act on spinal motion segments, particularly for asymmetric tasks. Four torso model formulations—including the sum of cubed muscle stresses, the sum of squared muscle stresses, the minimum stress compression, and the eigenvector-synergy model—were evaluated to determine which best predicted electromyographic data. Each model predicts muscle forces from net reaction moments at L3–L4. In addition, the difference in muscular contribution to spinal compression force was determined for the 4 models, as was the effect of using the lowest possible muscle stress bound in the muscle formulation.

Methods and Findings.—An approach for the assessment of competing optimization model formulations was developed and illustrated with electromyographic data from static asymmetric loading conditions. The method was based on the selection of experimental conditions in which models predict decisively different muscle forces and the ability to ensure that the experimental conditions were such that the minimum number of assumptions concerning force-electromyogram associations were made in order to choose among competing model predictions. Of the 4 models, only the formulation with an objective function that was the sum of cubed muscle stresses provided acceptable prediction of the electromyographic data. The muscle contribution to spinal compression force predicted by each model differed by as much as 160% for certain experimental conditions. Use of the lowest possible muscle stress bound did not appear to predict muscle forces that corresponded to the electromyographic data.

Conclusion.—Three of the 4 models analyzed were inconsistent with the empirical data. The sum of cubed stresses model appears to be the most promising and should be investigated further.

▶ Getting accurate, reliable electromyographic data is difficult by itself. When using optimization-based models to best predict electromyographic data, how can we be certain the predicted data are accurate? If the predicted data are compared with the measured data, how do we know that the measured electromyographic data are accurate?—Col. J.L. Anderson, PE.D.

Electrically Evoked Myoelectric Signals in Back Muscles: Effect of Side Dominance

Merletti R, De Luca CJ, Sathyan D (Boston Univ)
J Appl Physiol 77:2104–2114, 1994   139-95-5-15

Objective.—Studies of muscle fatigue have used myoelectric signal variables and fatigue indices. The effect of hand dominance on these measurements and the repeatability of such measurements were studied.

Methods.—Longissimus dorsi muscles were stimulated in 5 left-handed and 5 right-handed men aged 20–33 years. Rectangular current pulses, 25-Hz frequency, lasting 0.2 ms were applied to elicit a maximal M wave or a pain threshold. Two 30-second contractions, 1 on each side, were applied 5 minutes apart, 5 times per subject on 5 separate days. Muscle fiber conduction velocity was estimated and fatigue indices were calculated.

Results.—Fatigue indices were significantly related to side dominance in right-handed but not in left-handed subjects. This difference can be attributed to the preferred use of nondominant back muscle groups to compensate for periodic activity demands placed on the dominant back muscles.

Conclusion.—Nondominant muscles on the right side in right-handed individuals are more easily fatigued than are dominant muscles; they are also more easily fatigued than muscles on either side of left-handed individuals.

▶ Why would fatigue indices be significantly related to side dominance in right-handed but not in left-handed subjects? Nothing in this study made the answer intuitively obvious to me.—Col. J.L. Anderson, PE.D.

Emergency Removal of Football Helmets
Patel MN, Rund DA (Ohio State Univ, Columbus)
Physician Sportsmed 22:57–59, 1994   139-95-5–16

Background.—The National Collegiate Athletic Association (NCAA) has developed guidelines for the removal of football helmets when a player has a suspected head or neck injury. These guidelines differ from the protocol followed by emergency medical technicians and paramedics, who are trained to remove motorcycle helmets early in the assessment and before patient transport. Special factors characteristic of football equipment, however, make the NCAA protocol preferable.

Characteristics of the Football Helmet.—A football helmet is custom-fitted and secured more tightly than a motorcycle helmet. The cheek pads make it extremely difficult to pry the helmet away from the head, and such an attempt may cause further injury. In addition, the football player's shoulder pads elevate the shoulders so that helmet removal might cause difficulties in immobilizing the cervical spine in a neutral position. The plastic loops that attach the face mask to the helmet can be

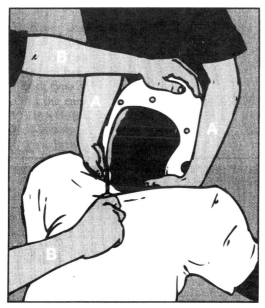

Fig 5–9.—Removal of cheek pad. (Courtesy of Patel MN, Rund DA: *Physician Sportsmed* 22:57–59, 1994.)

cut away if resuscitation is required. The head, neck, and spine can be stabilized during transport by using a spine board and leaving the helmet and shoulder pads on until the player arrives in the emergency department.

Helmet Removal.—The NCAA protocol should be followed after the patient arrives at the emergency department. If trained personnel are not present, the helmet can be left in place during initial skull and cervical radiographs. The removal method requires a 2-member medical team. Person A, positioned at the top of the patient's head, places an arm on each side of the head and uses the hands to hold the patient's neck stable. Person B removes the face mask, cuts the chin strap, and removes the cheek pads from the helmet by slipping the flat blade of a screwdriver or bandage scissor between the pad snaps and the helmet's inner surface (Fig 5–9). Person B then deflates the air inflation system and takes over in-line immobilization of the head by grasping the patient's mandible with one hand and placing the other under the occiput. Person A places a thumb inside each ear hole of the helmet and positions the fingers along the bottom edge of the helmet, pulling in line with the head and neck so that the helmet can be eased off. With care to avoid moving the head, the shoulder pads are then removed and a cervical collar applied. Standard implementation of these guidelines would help to prevent further injuries to the head and neck.

▶ There were 2 very enlightening abstracts on this subject in the 1994 *Year Book of Sports Medicine* (1). I will repeat some of my comments on these 2 abstracts and make some new observations. Yes, there is controversy between emergency medical technicians and athletic trainers regarding the removal of an injured football player's helmet. The authors of this article stress that the differences between a football helmet and a motorcycle helmet should eliminate any controversy occuring over helmet removal. They say the NCAA protocol should be followed and the football helmet should not be removed until the athlete is in the hospital. Face masks can be removed and airways may be established with and without face mask removal. A protocol must be established and practiced, and practiced, and practiced.—F.J. George, A.T.C., P.T.

Reference

1. 1994 YEAR BOOK OF SPORTS MEDICINE, pp 30–32.

Magnetic Resonance Imaging of Iliotibial Band Syndrome
Ekman EF, Pope T, Martin DF, Curl WW (Wake Forest Univ, Winston-Salem, NC)
Am J Sports Med 22:851–854, 1994   139-95-5–17

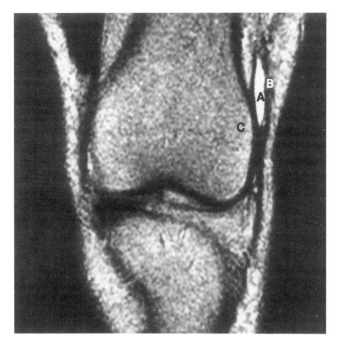

Fig 5–10.—Coronal MRI scan of a patient with iliotibial band (*ITB*) syndrome. A, a signal consistent with fluid deep to the ITB; B, ITB; C, lateral femoral epicondyle. Scan parameters: T2-weighted; repetition time (TR), 2,250; echo time (TE), 80. (Courtesy of Ekman EF, Pope T, Martin DF, et al: *Am J Sports Med* 22:851–854, 1994.)

Background.—Iliotibial band (ITB) syndrome, a common cause of lateral knee pain, is observed most often in distance runners. Traditionally, the diagnosis of this syndrome has been based on clinical examination. Magnetic resonance imaging findings in ITB syndrome were presented.

Methods.—Seven patients with ITB syndrome underwent MRI. The findings in these patients were compared with MR findings in 10 age- and sex-matched control knees with no evidence of lateral knee pain. Cadaveric dissections were also performed in 10 nondiseased knees to further investigate the pathoanatomical correlation between ITB syndrome and the corresponding MR findings.

Findings.—On MR scans, signal consistent with fluid was seen deep to the ITB in the region of the lateral femoral epicondyle in 5 of 7 patients (Fig 5–10). Compared with the control group, patients with ITB syndrome had a significantly thicker ITB over the lateral femoral epicondyle. The mean thickness of the ITB was 5.49 mm in the patients and 2.52 in the control group. The cadaveric dissection study showed a potential space—a bursa—between the ITB and the knee capsule.

Conclusion.—Magnetic resonance imaging provides objective evidence of ITB syndrome and can be useful for establishing a definitive diagnosis when necessary. Correlated with anatomical dissection, MRI identifies this as a problem within a bursa beneath the ITB rather than in the knee joint.

▶ The authors have very nicely demonstrated the pathophysiology of ITB syndrome using MRI. However, they state that ". . .we do not suggest that MRI scans be obtained anytime a problem is suspected." I would question another suggestion: that MR imaging may be indicated in the competitive athlete desiring early return to activity. Clearly, for the experienced clinician, MRI is not necessary for establishing a diagnosis to implement early treatment. Perhaps there is a relative indication for MRI if surgery is being considered or if the pain is more diffuse in nature to rule out other causes of pain.—J.S. Torg, M.D.

Chronic Groin Injuries in Athletes: Recommendations for Treatment and Rehabilitation
Karlsson J, Swärd L, Kälebo P, Thomée R (Univ of Göteborg, Sweden)
Sports Med 17:141–148, 1994   139-95-5–18

Introduction.—From 2% to 5% of all sports injuries are groin injuries. Although acute injury can occur from direct trauma, groin injuries are most commonly caused by overuse of a muscle and strain at the tendinous insertion to the bone, particularly involving the adductor longus tendon, the rectus femoris, and the rectus abdominis muscles and tendons. The clinical management of groin injury was examined.

Differential Diagnosis.—Diagnosis is frequently delayed because symptoms of groin injury are often uncharacteristic. Differential diagnoses include stress fractures of the femoral neck or the inferior ramus of the pubic bone, prostatitis, bone and joint diseases (e.g., arthritis, osteoarthrosis, epiphyseal slipping, Perthes' disease), hernias, referred pain from the spine or abdominal viscera, tumors, and nerve entrapment.

Diagnostic Imaging.—Magnetic resonance imaging is generally useful in visualizing both macroscopic injuries and microruptures (with T2-weighted spin-echo images or fat-suppressed images). Computed tomography is more useful for detecting calcified tendinitis or bony abnormalities at tendon insertion sites. Ultrasonography is also useful, especially in the diagnosis of chronic injuries.

Treatment.—Nonsurgical treatment designed to restore full range of motion, muscle strength, endurance, balance, and coordination is usually indicated. Exercises are restricted in the acute phase to pain-free, high-repetition, low-loading activities and are progressively adjusted to allow higher loads and greater range of motion. Exercises that promote coordinated movements are added to the rehabilitation program after strength returns. If the muscle and tendon unit is completely torn or if a partial tear causes intramuscular hematoma, surgery should be considered (either longitudinal splitting of the tendon or tenotomy), followed by a similar program of progressive rehabilitation.

Conclusion.—Because the symptoms of groin injury are often uncharacteristic, diagnosis requires a multidisciplinary approach. Management of a groin injury may require 3-6 months of rehabilitation. Chronic groin injury should be prevented with adequate warm-up, stretching, preseason training programs, and prompt treatment of minor groin strains.

▶ This is a comprehensive, but somewhat superficial, review of chronic groin injuries in the athlete. Not emphasized is the presence of an inguinal hernia as a cause of refractory "groin injury." This is of significance today because of success in both diagnosing and remedying the problem with endoscopic repair of the indirect inguinal hernia.—J.S. Torg, M.D.

Avulsion of the Anterior-Superior Iliac Spine in Athletes: Case Reports
Veselko M, Smrkolj V (Univ Med Centre, Ljubljana, Slovenia)
J Trauma 36:444–446, 1994   139-95-5–19

Background.—Avulsion of the anterior-superior iliac spine appears to result from a sudden pull of the sartorius muscle. Although common in competitive athletes, the condition is infrequently seen in adolescents. Conservative treatment, which consists of bed rest, immobilization in a Brown splint, and a period of walking on crutches, can last up to 12 weeks. Two adolescents who sustained avulsion of the anterior-superior

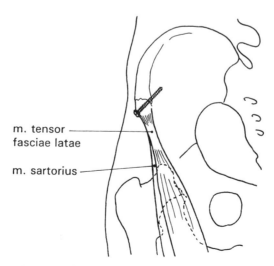

m. tensor
fasciae latae

m. sartorius

Fig 5–11.—Surgical technique for fixation of anterior-superior iliac spine. (Courtesy of Veselko M, Smrkolj V: *J Trauma* 36:444-446, 1994.)

iliac spine underwent open reduction and internal fixation, allowing them to resume active training within 3–4 weeks.

Case Report.—Boy, 15 years, had sudden pain in the left groin during training. Examination at the hospital within an hour of the injury revealed swelling and hematoma in the area of the anterior-superior iliac spine. The pain radiated along the sartorius muscle, and the hip joint could not be flexed when the knee was extended. Avulsion was confirmed by roentgenograms that also showed dislocation of a loose fragment. At surgery 2 days later, the fragment was found 3 cm distal to the avulsion site. Screw fixation maintained reduction of the apophysis (Fig 5–11). The patient was walking with crutches 2 days after surgery and was able to resume sports activities 3 weeks later. Three months postoperatively, the fixation screw was removed.

Discussion.—Both young patients with avulsion of the anterior-posterior iliac spine were successfully treated by open reduction and internal fixation. With only a short period of convalescence, they were able to return to competitive sports with no significant decrease in strength of the thigh muscles. Surgical treatment of this injury need not be reserved for cases of severe dislocation and grossly displaced fragments.

▶ This anecdotal report does not demonstrate surgical management to be preferable to nonsurgical management. Also, the statement "Treatment by open reduction and internal fixation is. . .indicated. . .in patients requiring a short convalescent period" is not supported by the data.—J.S. Torg, M.D.

Hip Arthroscopy Utilizing the Supine Position
Byrd JWT (Vanderbilt Univ, Nashville, Tenn)
Arthroscopy 10:275–280, 1994   139-95-5–20

Introduction.—The techniques for performing arthroscopy about the hip have advanced, and the indications for its use have expanded in recent years. A technique of operative arthroscopy about the hip, with the patient in the supine position, was reported.

Methods.—Over a period of 40 months, 20 arthroscopic procedures were performed for intractable mechanical hip pain. The patients had an average age of 44 years (range, 17–76 years), had relatively little radiographic evidence of deterioration, had a relatively recent onset of symptoms, and had not improved with conservative treatment.

Technique.—Under general anesthetic, the patient is placed in the supine position on the fracture table with the peroneal post lateralized to the operative side (Fig 5–12). The operative hip is placed in extension, with 25 degrees of abduction, in neutral rotation. The image intensifier is positioned between the legs, and the contralateral leg is abducted to accommodate it, keeping the foot anchored to provide a slight counterforce during distraction. Distraction is accom-

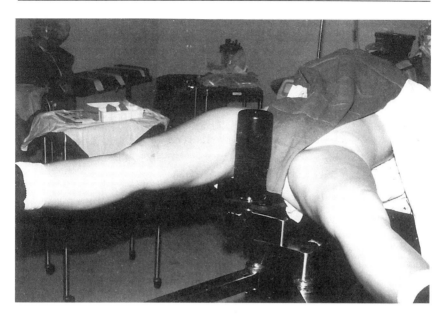

Fig 5–12.—The patient is positioned on the fracture table so that the peroneal post is placed as far laterally as possible toward the operative hip resting against the medial thigh. (Courtesy of Byrd JWT: *Arthroscopy* 10:275–280, 1994.)

plished with 25–50 pounds of traction and confirmed by fluoroscopic examination. Three arthroscope cannulas are placed in anterior, anterolateral, and posterolateral portals under fluoroscopic control, allowing systematic examination and operative arthroscopy by interchanging the instruments and arthroscope among the cannulas, while rotating the hip.

Results.—All hips were well visualized including the superior weight-bearing portion of the acetabulum; the fovea; the ligamentum teres; and the anterior, posterior, and lateral aspects of the acetabular labrum. All but 2 patients with avascular necrosis reported significant pain relief. None had major complications.

Discussion.—Operative arthroscopy about the hip with the patient in the supine position allows effective visualization and instrumentation, uses common operating room equipment, and is a familiar position for orthopedic surgeons experienced in the management of fractures of the proximal femur.

▶ Hip arthroscopy utilizing the supine position as described by the author differs from that described by Glick and associates, who used the lateral position (1). Both approaches appear to be both effective and reproducible. Of interest would be stated indications for hip arthroscopy; they were not included in the paper.—J.S. Torg, M.D.

Reference

1. Glick J, Sampson T, Gordon R, et al: Hip arthroscopy by the lateral approach. *Arthroscopy* 3:4–12, 1987.

Hamstring Injuries in Sprinters: The Role of Concentric and Eccentric Hamstring Muscle Strength and Flexibility
Jönhagen S, Németh G, Eriksson E (Karolinska Hosp, Stockholm)
Am J Sports Med 22:262–266, 1994   139-95-5-21

Introduction.—Athletes, particularly sprinters, have a high incidence of hamstring strains. Previous studies have reported an important role for eccentric muscular work and muscle tightness in the development and prevention of sports injuries. The causes of hamstring strains and possible differences in eccentric and concentric hamstring and quadriceps torques and in hamstring muscle tightness were evaluated in sprinters who had had hamstring injuries and in uninjured sprinters.

Methods.—Eleven sprinters, all men with recent hamstring injuries, and 9 sprinters who had never sustained a hamstring injury were studied. Hamstring muscle tightness was evaluated by observing the angle of straight-leg flexion in the supine position without warm-up. All participants warmed up with knee bends and stretching exercises before muscle torque testing in a muscle dynamometer. Concentric muscle torques were tested at velocities of 30, 180, and 270 degrees per second, and eccentric torques were tested at velocities of 30, 180, and 230 degrees per second, with contractions made at angles of 0–180 degrees.

Results.—The uninjured sprinters had significantly less tightness in their hamstrings, with an average range of motion of 74.1 degrees, compared with 67.2 degrees in the injured sprinters. Concentric torques of the hamstrings and quadriceps were significantly higher in the uninjured than in the injured sprinters at a velocity of 30 degrees per second, but they were similar in the 2 groups at higher angular velocities. Eccentric contraction of the hamstring muscles had a significantly higher peak torque in the uninjured than in the injured sprinters at all angular velocities.

Discussion.—The uninjured sprinters had more flexible hamstrings and greater hamstring and quadriceps strength in concentric contractions at slow velocities and in eccentric contractions at all velocities when compared with sprinters who had sustained hamstring injuries. The overall greater strength in eccentric contractions among the uninjured sprinters was, therefore, not explained by greater concentric strength. Reduced eccentric hamstring strength may contribute to the tendency for hamstring injuries to recur.

▶ The crucial unanswered question regarding these findings is whether the hamstring tightness and relative muscular weakness observed in the injured group were caused by, or were the cause of, the injury.—J.S. Torg, M.D.

Femur Fractures in Alpine Skiing: Classification and Mechanisms of Injury in 85 Cases
Sterett WI, Krissoff WB (Univ of California, Davis–Tahoe Forest Hosp, Truckee, Calif)
J Orthop Trauma 8:310–314, 1994   139-95-5-22

Background.—Among the more than 12 million skiers in the United States, approximately 600,000 injuries occur in 1 winter season. There are correlations between the lack of skiing expertise and ski injuries. In 1 study, the injury ratio of beginning to expert skiers was 5:1. Cases of femur fractures sustained in alpine skiing were reviewed retrospectively to determine the incidence, severity, and mechanisms of injury.

Methods.—Eighty-five cases of femoral fracture treated in the north Lake Tahoe area were reviewed. Data were collected on the type of fracture; difficulty of the terrain; ability, age, and sex of the skier; and the time of day when the accident occurred.

Results.—The study population was 60% male and 40% female. The mean age of the skiers was 30.2 years. The highest incidence of injuries was in skiers aged 30–40 years. Among the 85 injuries, 14% were femoral neck fractures, 21% were peritrochanteric fractures, 60% involved the shaft of the femur, and 5% involved the supra/intercondylar region. The comminuted femoral shaft and trochanteric fractures from high-energy impact usually occurred in advanced skiers under firm or icy conditions. The low-energy impact and minimally comminuted femur fractures occurred mainly in skeletally immature skiers younger than age 18 years. These injuries resulted from an indirect, torsional, or bending mechanism, and they typically occurred while skiing fast and then catching the tip of a ski in wet or heavy snow. Fifty-five percent of fractures occurred in skiers aged 18–45 years, and most of these injuries resulted from a high-energy, direct-impact fall or collision that led to a severely comminuted femoral shaft and trochanteric fractures. Nineteen percent of injuries occurred in skiers older than age 45 years, and more than two thirds of these persons had fractures about the hip. These injuries were typically a simple fracture from low-impact falls on a hard or icy surface. There were no fractures to the femoral shaft in skiers older than age 52 years.

Conclusion.—Femoral fractures in alpine skiing seem to be a function of day-to-day variability in snow conditions and seasonal totals. There are reports on the rarity of femoral fractures in the Rocky Mountains, where the slope conditions are more consistent because temperatures are less likely to go above freezing. Ski lessons and an increased number of days of skiing in a season help protect against injuries from alpine skiing.

▶ It is interesting to note that femur fractures are one of the few injuries in which the advanced, expert skier is more susceptible than the beginner.—J.S. Torg, M.D.

Stress Fractures of the Femoral Shaft in Athletes: More Common Than Expected: A New Clinical Test
Johnson AW, Weiss CB Jr, Wheeler DL (Lafayette College, Easton, Pa)
Am J Sports Med 22:248–256, 1994   139-95-5–23

Purpose.—Most stress fractures in athletes and military recruits are tibial fractures; femoral stress fractures are fairly uncommon. The results of a prospective study of stress fractures in varsity athletes were examined.

Methods.—A total of 914 athletes from 20 Division I AA varsity sports and 1 club sport were followed during 2 consecutive academic years. All sports-related injuries were recorded by sport and by year of competition. Athletes with suspected stress fractures were assessed by plain radiography and bone scans. A new clinical test, the fulcrum test, was used to identify stress fractures of the femoral shaft.

Technique.—The examiner places 1 arm proximally under the distal thigh of the involved leg and applies gentle pressure with the free hand to the dorsum of the knee (Figs 5–13 and 5–14). In case of a femoral shaft stress fracture, even slight pressure on the knee will produce pain and instill apprehension. The uninvolved leg is used as a negative control.

Results.—During the 2-year study, 34 stress fractures were diagnosed in 24 athletes; 7 (20.6%) were in the femoral shaft, 7 (20.6%) in the metatarsals, and 13 (38.2%) in the tibia. Sixteen stress fractures occurred in women and 12 occurred in men. The overall annual incidence of stress fractures was 3.7%. The fulcrum test accurately identified each femoral shaft stress fracture. The test was also useful in monitoring fracture healing as pain induced by the test gradually diminished over time.

Conclusion.—Stress fractures of the femoral shaft are more common than previously recognized. The fulcrum test aids significantly in the clinical diagnosis and management of these fractures.

▶ In this era of extraordinarily expensive, high-tech imaging techniques, it is both encouraging and refreshing to find a clinical observation that is reliable, noninvasive, and inexpensive. However, it must be pointed out that a positive femoral fulcrum test does not differentiate between stress fracture and stress reaction of bone. This is an important distinction if the athlete is to be precluded from sports participation until the test is completely negative. This takes an average of 7 (range, 3–12) weeks.—J.S. Torg, M.D.

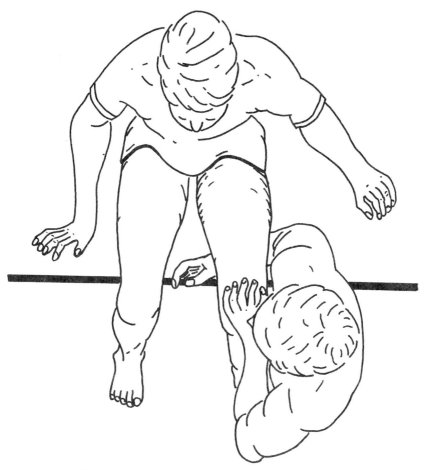

Fig 5–13.—The fulcrum test starts with the examiner's arm (fulcrum) under the distal thigh, as gentle pressure is applied to the dorsum of the knee. (Courtesy of Johnson AW, Weiss CB Jr, Wheeler DL: *Am J Sports Med* 22:248–256, 1994.)

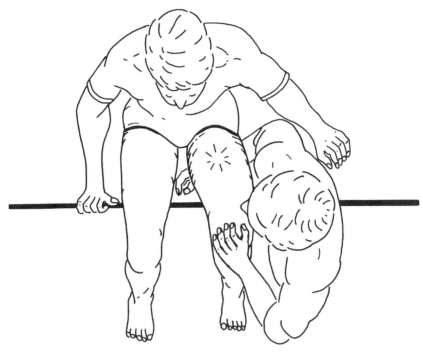

Fig 5–14.—The fulcrum test with the examiner's arm (fulcrum) moved proximally under the thigh. Pain develops when the arm is placed directly under a stress fracture of the femoral shaft and gentle pressure is applied to the dorsum of the knee. (Courtesy of Johnson AW, Weiss CB Jr, Wheeler DL: *Am J Sports Med* 22:248–256, 1994.)

Influence of Hamstring Length on the Standing Position and Flexion Range of Motion of the Pelvic Angle, Lumbar Angle, and Thoracic Angle

Gajdosik RL, Albert CR, Mitman JJ (Univ of Montana, Missoula)
J Orthop Sports Phys Ther 20:213–219, 1994   139-95-5–24

Background.—An understanding of the relationship between the length of the hamstring muscle and certain pelvic and trunk postures may be useful when developing therapeutic interventions. The length of the hamstring muscle in relation to the pelvic angle, the lumbar angle, and the thoracic angle was studied. Standing measurements were compared with those taken in the toe-touch position.

Method.—The passive straight-leg raising test was used to divide 30 male subjects into 3 groups according to hamstring length. All subjects were healthy, nonobese men with no history of hamstring disorder. None of the subjects had low back pain during the study. The pelvic angle, the lumbar angle, and the thoracic angle were determined with surface markers and platform pointers. The angles were measured from photographs taken of the subjects while in a standing position and in a toe-touch position. The flexion range of motion was also evaluated. Data were analyzed with *F*-ratios and Tukey's post hoc analyses. The intraclass correlation coefficient and the standard error of measurement were also calculated.

Results.—When patients were in a standing position, no significant differences among groups were found for the 3 angles measured. Significant differences were found between the short and medium hamstring groups and the short and long hamstring groups for the pelvic angle in the toe-touch position. There was a significant difference between the lumbar flexion range of motion for the short hamstring group (54 degrees) and the long hamstring group (64 degrees). The pelvic angle and lumbar angle both showed decreased flexion range of motion with shorter hamstring length. In subjects with shorter hamstring length, a decrease in the flexion range of motion was associated with an increased flexion angle and an increased thoracic flexion range of motion.

Conclusion.—Therapeutic interventions that affect posture must consider the relationship in the toe-touch position between hamstring length and the pelvic angle and the flexion range of motion, the lumbar angle flexion range of motion, and the thoracic angle and flexion range of motion.

▶ Hamstring muscles have always held a fascination for me, probably because I have what have always been called "tight hamstrings." Now I may call them "short hamstrings." For the past 40 or so years, I have tried to stretch my hamstrings, using all of the standard exercises, but I still cannot touch my toes when my knees are straight. Some questions I would like to have answers for are the following:

1. How much can a person with short hamstrings expect to lengthen them through exercise, and how long would it normally take?

2. Are short hamstrings more a genetic trait or are they the result of poor conditioning because of poor exercise habits?

3. Is the sit-and-reach test a valid fitness test when national norms are used, given that the length of the hamstrings appears to correlate highly with performance on this test?—Col. J.L. Anderson, PE.D.

6 Training, Performance, and Environment

Physically Active Commuting to Work: Testing Its Potential for Exercise Promotion
Vuori IM, Oja P, Paronen O (Urho Kaleva Kekkonen Inst for Health Promotion Research, Tampere, Finland)
Med Sci Sports Exerc 26:844–850, 1994   139-95-6–1

Background.—Physical activity such as walking or cycling while commuting to work may have considerable health-enhancing potential. Several studies were undertaken to determine whether physically active commuting to work (PACW) is an effective and feasible means of providing basic exercise to nontrained individuals. The main results of these investigations are summarized.

Methods and Findings.—Three successive mail inquiries were sent to 2,014 individuals representing the 20- to 64-year-old population of Tampere, Finland, to determine the length, mode of commuting, and perceived safety of work trips. Physically active commuting to work provided habitual exercise for one third of the employed urban population.

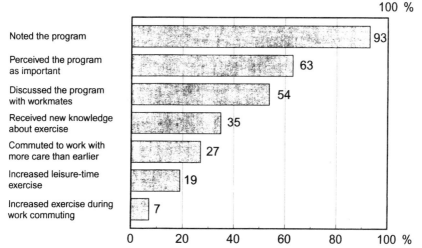

Fig 6–1.—Reception and self-reported effects of the program in postprogram survey, percent of respondents. (Courtesy of Vuori IM, Oja P, Paronen O: *Med Sci Sports Exerc* 26:844–850, 1994.)

In addition, more than one fifth of the respondents indicated a willingness and ability to increase PACW. The lack or poor condition of pedestrian and cycling routes were cited by 40% of the respondents as factors limiting their ability to participate in PACW. A 10-week, randomized, controlled trial was also undertaken to determine the effects of PACW on physical fitness and blood lipids. Sixty-eight inactive middle-aged men and women responding to the survey participated. Of these, 35 participated in 1 hour of daily PACW and 33 served as passive controls. After 10 weeks, PACW increased maximum oxygen consumption by 4.5%, maximal treadmill time by 10.3%, and high-density-lipoprotein cholesterol by 5%. The final study consisted of a 6-month demonstration project in a large industrial plant, undertaken to assess the acceptability, efficacy, and feasibility of promoting PACW in a work site setting. Program promotion was accomplished using low-cost measures. Evaluations done via inquiries and interviews showed a positive response. More than 90% of the respondents had noticed the program, and 63% indicated that the program was important (Fig 6–1).

Conclusion.—Physically active commuting to work has the potential for enhancing health and fitness substantially, provided that it can be practiced safely.

▶ Canadian health promotion experts are increasingly recognizing that the focus of their activity programs should be on the incorporation of physical activity into daily living rather than reliance on organized fitness or sports programs. There are a number of reasons for such advocacy. Costs are much lower, both for the community and for the participant. Perhaps more importantly, the time commitment is much smaller. It does not make much sense to spend an hour driving each way in order to spend 30 minutes in a gymnasium! Nor is it surprising that compliance with such a recommendation is poor. The "opportunity cost" is high, and the patient will explain that "lack of time" prevents exercise. In contrast, if commuting to work is the recommended source of activity, the time commitment can be quite small, and there is a strong likelihood that such activity will continue 5 days a week for many years.

This study by Vuori and associates was conducted in the medium-sized town of Tampere, Finland. As much as one third of the population was already adopting the tactic of walking or cycling to work, and there were suggestions that improvements to sidewalks and cycle paths might increase this number further. Perhaps most importantly, the intensity of such activity was sufficient to improve aerobic power and high-density-lipoprotein cholesterol over a period as short as 10 weeks. More prominence should be given to such programs in North America, with increasing adaptation of urban streets to the needs of cyclists.—R.J. Shephard, M.D., Ph.D., D.P.E.

Hypervolemia and Cycling Time Trial Performance

Luetkemeier MJ, Thomas EL (Univ of Utah, Salt Lake City)
Med Sci Sports Exerc 26:503–508, 1994   139-95-6-2

Introduction.—The practical significance of exercise-induced hypervolemia (ExH) on endurance performance during a maximal effort has not been previously defined. Three simulated time trial performances of 10 experienced cyclists were run to determine whether hypervolemia was associated with improvements in exercise performance.

Methods.—All cyclists were actively engaged in bicycle training of greater than 80 km per week. A 13-day exercise protocol was used. It consisted of the following: day 1, work capacity test; days 2–4, short-term training program; day 5, ExH time trial; days 6–8, no exercise; day 9, euvolemic time trial; days 10–12, no exercise; and day 13, dextran-induced hypervolemic (DxH) time trial. Time trials were approximately 90 minutes in length. Body composition measurements, food intake, resting blood volume, plasma volume, red blood cell volume, rectal temperature, and mean sweat rates were determined at appropriate intervals.

Results.—Compared with the euvolemic time trial, the ExH and DxH time trials indicated significantly greater resting blood volume and plasma volume, better performance times, and higher average power output (Fig 6–2). No significant difference between ExH and DxH was noted in resting blood or plasma volumes, performance times, or average power output. No significant between-trial differences were noted in red blood cell volume, body mass, lean body mass, fat mass, total body water, food intake, sweat rates, or rectal temperatures.

Conclusion.—Exercise- and dextran-induced hypervolemia each had beneficial effects on performance time and average power output during 90-minute time trials. Because there were no selective differences between training and dextran-induced hypervolemic conditions, it is likely that hypervolemia was responsible for the additional performance advantages.

▶ Plasma volume has an increasing impact on athletic performance as the duration of an activity is extended and fluid is lost from the circulation by a combination of sweating and exudation into the active tissues. Thus, we might anticipate that plasma volume expansion by either a brief period of training or dextran infusion would increase sustained power output, enhance sweating, and improve thermoregulation. However, previous experiments have not always demonstrated such a response (1, 2); Luetkemeier and Thomas suggest that others did not see the anticipated benefits because in these previous trials, not all subjects were able to complete the full experiment under dehydrated conditions.

The gain in power output from dextran infusion seems to depend on the volume infused: Large volumes not only increase stroke volume but also decrease hemoglobin concentrations, neutralizing any potential improvement in

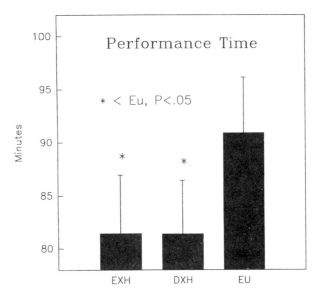

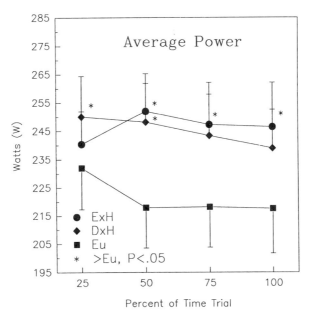

Fig 6–2.—Mean performance times and average power during the simulated cycling time trials. (Courtesy of Luetkemeier MJ, Thomas EL: *Med Sci Sports Exerc* 26:503–508, 1994.)

performance. The increase selected for this experiment (300–400 mL) was probably optimal from this viewpoint. The enhanced plasma volume may increase endurance performance not only by boosting stroke volume, but also by a glycogen-sparing effect (3).—R.J. Shephard, M.D., Ph.D., D.P.E.

References

1. Montain SJ, Coyle EF: *J Appl Physiol* 73:903–910, 1992.
2. Sawka MN, et al: *Eur J Appl Physiol* 51:303–312, 1983.
3. Green HJ, et al: *J Appl Physiol* 66:622–631, 1989.

Spironolactone Administration and Training-Induced Hypervolemia
Luetkemeier MJ, Flowers KM, Lamb DR (Ohio State Univ, Columbus)
Int J Sports Med 15:295–300, 1994   139-95-6-3

Introduction.—The expansion of plasma volume that occurs at the start of physical training and persists until training ceases has been linked to changes in hormone concentrations (vasopressin or the renin-aldosterone system) or to increased plasma protein concentrations (either an influx of lymphatic proteins or newly synthesized proteins). To determine the extent of involvement of aldosterone in plasma volume expansion, subjects trained for 3 days while taking spironolactone. It was theorized that if aldosterone participates in the process, individuals taking spironolactone should not experience the training-induced hypervolemia.

Methods.—Twelve men 18–45 years of age were randomly assigned to a control or a spironolactone group. Diet was controlled for 4 days before and during the 3 days of training. Three days before training, maximal oxygen consumption was determined. The drug group took doses of spironolactone (25 mg 4 times per day) for the next 7 days. The subjects trained on a cycle ergometer for 2 hours per day at 65% of maximum oxygen consumption. Plasma volume, sodium, osmolarity, protein, albumin, renin, aldosterone, and vasopressin were determined from blood samples obtained before and after each exercise session.

Results.—Control subjects significantly increased their plasma volume by an average of 500 mL, whereas the increase in the drug-treated subjects (163 mL) was not statistically significant. Increases in plasma volume, sodium, and osmolarity were attenuated by spironolactone. Similar increases in protein and albumin occurred in both groups (Fig 6–3).It is unknown why the drug-treated group had less of an increase in plasma volume than would be expected from the increase in plasma proteins.

Summary.—It was estimated that 40% of the expansion in plasma volume from training was attributable to aldosterone activity. The remaining 60% was caused by an increase in the mass of plasma proteins. Because the rise in oncotic pressure caused by the increased plasma protein

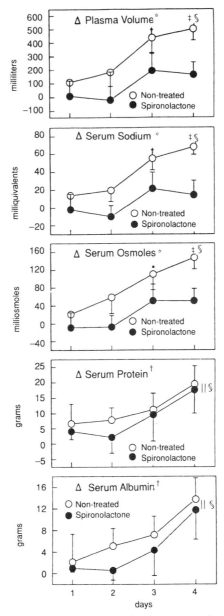

Fig 6–3.—Changes in plasma volume and total serum contents of sodium, osmoles, protein, and albumin. * $P < 0.05$ significant interaction between days and treatment groups. † $P < 0.05$ main effect of days. ‡ $P < 0.05$ significant difference between treatment groups isolated to one day. § $P < 0.05$ significant difference from baseline isolated to one treatment group. || $P < 0.05$ significant difference from baseline, no interaction between groups. (Courtesy of Luetkemeier MJ, Flowers KM, Lamb DR: *Int J Sports Med* 15:295–300, 1994.)

concentration did not yield all of the expected increase in plasma volume, a third, unidentified factor remains to be determined.

▶ The increase of maximal oxygen intake that occurs with regular aerobic training is caused in large measure by an expansion of plasma volume. This report examines how the expansion of plasma volume is brought about. In essence, there must be an influx of osmotically active molecules into the circulation; these could be minerals, regulated by the aldosterone system, or plasma proteins.

In seeking to distinguish between these two possibilities, Luetkemeier et al. administered spironolactone, a potassium-sparing diuretic that competes with aldosterone for receptor sites on the distal tubules of the kidneys. When this drug was given, plasma expansion dropped from 501 mL to 163 mL and the training-increased gain in serum sodium was reduced by 79%. Total plasma protein still increased by 10%, and this in itself should have yielded a plasma expansion of 290 mL rather than 163 mL. Possibly, the reason for the discrepancy was that the spironolactone stimulated an increase of renin/angiotensin II secretion; this could have increased capillary pressures and, thus, the filtration of fluid from the circulation for a given osmotic pressure. Also, because of the diuretic action of spironolactone, it seemed that the total body water content decreased.

All of this may seem to be rather abstract physiology and biochemistry, but an understanding of the effects of training on plasma sodium and blood volumes also has practical relevance to the treatment of moderate hypertension by exercise programs.—R.J. Shephard, M.D., Ph.D., D.P.E.

Echocardiographic Findings in Endurance Athletes With Hypertrophic Non-Obstructive Cardiomyopathy (HNCM) Compared to Non-Athletes With HNCM and to Physiological Hypertrophy (Athlete's Heart)

Dickhuth H-H, Röcker K, Hipp A, Heitkamp HC, Keul J (Univ of Tübingen, Germany; Univ of Freiburg, Germany)
Int J Sports Med 15:273–277, 1994   139-95-6–4

Objective.—Hypertrophic nonobstructive cardiomyopathy (HNCM) is one of the most common causes of sudden death among young athletes, but it is difficult to diagnose noninvasively. Echocardiographic parameters were compared in HNCM-diagnosed patients with no activity, HNCM-diagnosed patients with regular endurance training, and normal subjects during endurance training.

Methods.—Subjects in the retrospective study were 9 patients with HNCM and no regular physical activity; 9 patients with HNCM participating in regular, intensive endurance training for at least 3 years; and 9 healthy athletes participating in regular, intensive endurance training for at least 3 years.

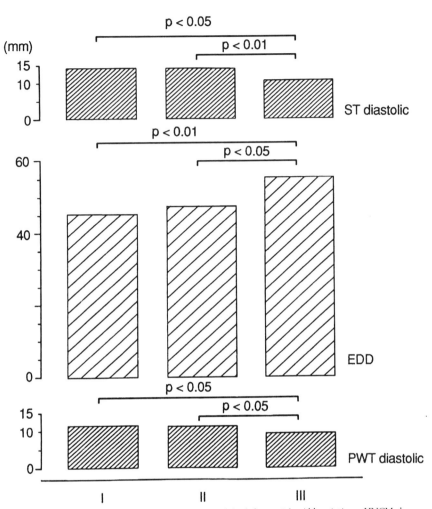

Fig 6–4.—Echocardiographic diastolic dimensions of the left ventricle. *Abbreviations: HNCM,* hypertrophic nonobstructive cardiomyopathy; *ST,* septum; *EDD,* end-diastolic left ventricular diameter; *PW,* posterior wall. Group I = HNCM, Group II = HNCM + endurance sport, and Group III = endurance sport. (Courtesy of Dickhuth H-H, Röcker K, Hipp A, et al: *Int J Sports Med* 15:273–277, 1994.)

Results.—One patient in the first group and 2 patients in the second group were asymptomatic. Echocardiograms were not significantly different between the first 2 groups. (Fig 6–4). Increased wall thickness, especially in the septum, is usually observed in echocardiograms of patients with HNCM, along with atypical hypertrophy. Whether exercise exacerbates this hypertrophy is unknown.

Conclusion.—Intensive endurance exercise does not appear to make much difference in the echocardiograms of patients with HNCM. Conventional echocardiography is an effective noninvasive diagnostic tool for detecting HNCM, although the technique may not give unequivocal results in all cases.

▶ Regular and intensive endurance sports increase the volume and muscle mass of all 4 cardiac chambers. But this "athlete's heart" is a benefit, not a detriment. In contrast, the pathologic hypertrophy known as hypertrophic nonobstructive cardiomyopathy is, according to a recent review (1), "the most common congenital cardiac abnormality found in most studies of sudden death in athletes." It is vital, then, to diagnose HNCM early. The most sensitive noninvasive method of diagnosing HNCM is the echocardiogram.

The question is whether endurance sports in the face of HNCM enhance the hypertrophy or shape the cardiac geometry to frustrate the diagnosis of HNCM. According to this study, the answer is "no." Endurance exercise in the face of HNCM had little influence on the echocardiographic measurements. In contrast, "athlete's heart" was distinguishable from HNCM (with or without a background of endurance exercise) by its greater end-diastolic left ventricular diameter and lesser thickening of the septum and posterior wall.

The echocardiogram, of course, cannot pinpoint the correct diagnosis in every case. A recent article reports that familial HNCM can be caused by mutations in the genes for beta cardiac myosin heavy chain, alpha tropomyosin, or cardiac troponin T (2).—E.R. Eichner, M.D.

References

1. Winget JF, et al: *Sports Med* 18:375, 1994.
2. Watkins H, et al: *N Engl J Med* 332:1058, 1995.

Is a Decrease in Arterial Pressure During Long-Term Aerobic Exercise Caused by a Fall in Cardiac Pump Function?
Ketelhut R, Losem CJ, Messerli FH (Ochsner Clinic and Alton Ochsner Med Found, New Orleans, La)
Am Heart J 127:567–571, 1994   139-95-6-5

Background.—Recent studies demonstrate that prolonged strenuous exercise may lead to impaired left ventricular function. Whether decreases in arterial pressure seen with prolonged aerobic exercise are caused by a decrease in cardiac pump function and whether such decreases can occur during moderate training were examined.

Methods.—Ten untrained, normotensive volunteers (2 women, 8 men) with established cardiovascular health exercised in the sitting position on a bicycle ergometer for 5 minutes. After they rested for 30 minutes, the exercise continued for 60 more minutes. Workloads were adjusted to maintain constant heart rates of 130–140 beats per minute. The heart rate was monitored by continuous ECG recording, and 2-dimensional

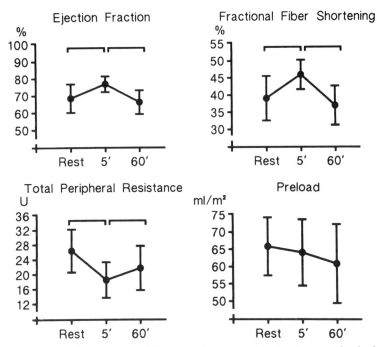

Fig 6–5.—Ejection fraction, fractional fiber shortening, total peripheral resistance, and preload in 10 healthy normotensive subjects before, after 5 minutes, and after 60 minutes of aerobic exercise. (Courtesy of Ketelhut R, Losem CJ, Messerli FH: *Am Heart J* 127:567–571, 1994.)

guided M-mode echocardiography of the left ventricle was performed at rest before exercise and after 5 and 60 minutes of exercise.

Results.—Significant increases in blood pressure occurred from rest to after 5 minutes of exercise. During the 60-minute period of before exercise, there was a continuous, significant decrease in both systolic and diastolic pressure from the fifth minute to the sixtieth minute. Significant decreases in systolic dimensions were shown by echocardiography from before exercise to the fifth minute of exercise, whereas after 60 minutes of exercise, a significant increase was observed. The same trend in end-systolic volume was demonstrated. From 5 minutes of exercise to 60 minutes of exercise, diastolic dimension and end-diastolic volume did not change significantly. Stroke volume increased significantly from before exercise to the fifth minute of exercise, whereas a significant decrease was noted after 60 minutes of exercise. Although showing increases after 5 minutes of exercise, ejection fraction, fractional fiber shortening, and contractility index decreased to the point at which preexercise levels were obtained after 60 minutes (Fig 6–5). Total peripheral resistance decreased after 5 minutes of exercise but gradually increased throughout the 60-minute exercise period. Preload, as estimated by end-diastolic volume, showed no significant changes during either of the test periods.

Conclusion.—One hour of moderate-to-severe aerobic exercise leads to continuous reduction in arterial pressure in normotensive patients. This is associated with an increase in total peripheral resistance and a fall in cardiac output and left ventricular pump function indices, all of which indicate possible cardiac fatigue.

▶ This study supports the idea of "cardiac fatigue" during endurance exercise, as proposed earlier to explain why, in triathletes at the grueling Ironman Triathlon in Hawaii, global ejection fraction, gauged by 2-dimensional echocardiographic imaging, fell from 51% at rest to 46% at the end of the race but recovered within 24 hours to 54% (1). The mechanism for cardiac fatigue is unclear but may be related to regional metabolic abnormalities.

Two caveats in interpreting such studies are as follows: noninvasive assessment of contractility indices has well-documented limitations, and a decreased contractility index does not necessarily imply a decreased inotropic state of the heart because these indices depend on preload and afterload. In fact, in this study, subjects lost a mean of 0.9 kg, and so may have been expected to have a decrease in preload. However, the authors argue against a change in preload because end-diastolic dimensions did not change.—E.R. Eichner, M.D.

Reference

1. Douglas PS, et al: *Circulation* 82:2108, 1990.

Rating of Perceived Exertion and Heart Rate as Indicators of Exercise Intensity in Different Environmental Temperatures

Potteiger JA, Weber SF (Univ of Kansas, Lawrence)
Med Sci Sports Exerc 26:791–796, 1994   139-95-6–6

Background.—Exercise intensity can be monitored by measuring the blood concentration of lactate. However, assessing concentrations of lactate in the field is impractical. The rating of perceived exertion (RPE) scale is one suggested alternative for monitoring training intensity. The validity of the RPE and the heart rate (HR) values observed during an incremental exercise test as indicators of exercise intensity during constant-load exercise in different environmental conditions was investigated.

Methods.—Nine male cyclists performed an incremental exercise test, and RPE and HR at the onset of blood lactate accumulation (OBLA) were determined. Three constant-load exercise work bouts at OBLA were completed in an environmental chamber at randomly assigned temperatures. The HR and the RPE were recorded every 5 minutes.

Findings.—There were no significant differences across the temperature conditions for the RPE and the HR. The RPE obtained at OBLA during incremental exercise differed significantly from the ratings ob-

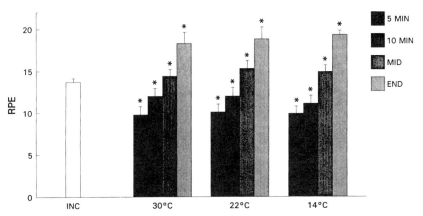

Fig 6–6.—The rating of perceived exertion (RPE) values in comparing incremental exercise to constant load exercise in 3 environmental temperatures (means ± standard deviation). *Indicates significant difference from incremental exercise. (Courtesy of Potteiger JA, Weber SF: *Med Sci Sports Exerc* 26:791–796, 1994.)

tained at 5 minutes, 10 minutes, midpoint, and at the end of the constant-load exercise in all temperatures (Fig 6–6). The HR measures at OBLA during incremental exercise were significantly higher than at 5 minutes of constant load for all temperatures, but did not differ significantly from constant-load exercise at 10-minute, midpoint, or end measures.

Conclusion.—It is not always practical to measure a variety of metabolic responses during exercise to monitor the intensity of activity. In these situations, the HR values obtained from an incremental exercise test appear to be more valid than those obtained by using the RPE scale.

▶ Although there are still many people who believe that the RPE can be used to monitor the intensity of individual training sessions, the variation in the relationship between oxygen consumption and the perception of exertion is such that a common recommendation (somewhat hard exercise, RPE = 13 units) can correspond to under 50% of maximal oxygen intake for 1 patient and over 90% of maximal effort for another (1). The precision of effort production can be improved somewhat if a "calibration curve" is constructed for a particular individual, but even then one is often trying to extrapolate responses perceived during a brief incremental test to the production of a sustained, steady bout of exercise, and—as this paper by Potteiger and Weber shows—HR is then a more useful index than RPE. Another possibility, particularly useful for patients, is to specify the time needed to cover a fixed walking or jogging distance.

Other investigators have described a reduction of RPE with substantial cooling of the environment (2, 3). It is, thus, a little surprising that in the present study, neither the HR nor the RPE was influenced by environmental temperatures that ranged from 14°C to 30°C. Further tests are needed with concomitant changes·in radiant heating and a wider spread of temperatures and humidities. It may also be important to see whether HR remains a useful index if the patient does not have an ECG or a "Sport-tester" to make the necessary measurements.—R.J. Shephard, M.D., Ph.D., D.P.E.

References

1. Shepard RJ, et al: *Med Sci Sports Exerc* 24:566, 1992.
2. Horstman DH: *Med Sci Sports Exerc* 9:52, 1977.
3. Toner MM, et al: *Percept Mot Skills* 62:211, 1986.

Cardiac Patients' Perception of Work Intensity During Graded Exercise Testing: Do They Generalize to Field Settings?

Brubaker PH, Rejeski WJ, Law HC, Pollock WE, Wurst ME, Miller HS Jr (Wake Forest Univ, Winston-Salem, NC)
J Cardiopulmon Rehabil 14:127–133, 1994   139-95-6-7

Background.—Ratings of perceived exertions (RPEs) are often used in association with target heart rates (HRs) or specific metabolic levels to regulate exercise intensity in cardiac rehabilitation programs. How cardiac patients' estimates of exertion at a given HR during a graded exercise test (GXT) would correspond to HR responses that occurred when patients were asked to produce specific RPEs during daily exercise training was examined.

Methods.—In study I, 15 patients (mean age, 54 years; mean post–cardiac event period, 14 weeks) estimated RPEs during a symptom-limited treadmill GXT. In a gymnasium 1 and 2 weeks later, they were asked to produce 3 different levels of work using RPEs taken from the GXT. In study II, 25 patients who had been exercising in a cardiac rehabilitation program for an average of 21 weeks underwent symptom-limited GXT. The RPEs were collected after a specified period of work (estimation), in contrast to study I, in which patients used RPEs to control their exercise intensity (production). The estimated RPEs of study II patients were compared during a GXT and during an exercise training session.

Results.—In study I, for each of the 3 levels of exertion, the mean HRs were significantly higher during GXT than during exercise training in the gym (low RPE, 106 vs. 90; moderate RPE, 119 vs. 95; hard RPE, 131 vs. 103) (Fig 6–7). In study II, at matching HRs, the patients' RPEs were significantly higher during the exercise training session than during GXT.

Conclusion.—Patients with cardiac disease perceive exercise to be more difficult during exercise training than during GXT. This may ex-

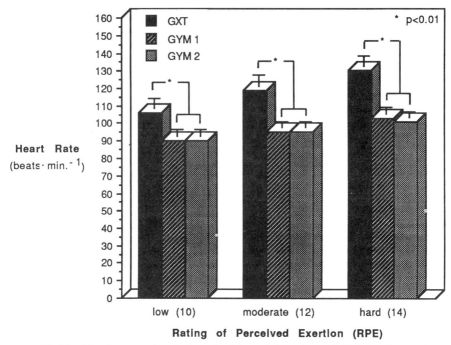

Fig 6–7.—Mean heart rates (standard error bars) for graded exercise test (GXT), 1-week gymnasium scores (GYM 1), and 2-week gymnasium scores (GYM 2) at low (approx. 10), moderate (approx. 12), and hard (approx. 14) ratings of RPE for 15 patients. Heart rates during GXT were significantly higher than during GYM 1 and GYM 2 for all 3 levels (low, moderate, hard) of RPE (P < 0.01). (Courtesy of Brubaker PH, Rejeski WJ, Law HC, et al: *J Cardiopulmon Rehabil* 14:127–133, 1994.)

plain why many patients with cardiac disease have difficulty attaining the intensity of exercise established for their exercise prescriptions.

▶ Although there are still a substantial number of authors who advocate the RPE scale as a means of regulating the intensity of exercise prescription (1), we have argued that interindividual differences in effort production are too broad for this approach to have great practical value as a means of regulating exercise prescriptions (2). Not only is there a wide variation in personal perceptions of exercise intensity within a given environment, but (as this paper by Brubaker and associates emphasizes) the response is situational, perceptions of an appropriate level of HR being much greater when exercise takes place away from the test laboratory (3).—R.J. Shephard, M.D., Ph.D., D.P.E.

References

1. Noble BJ: *Med Sci Sports Exerc* 14:406–411, 1982.
2. Shephard RJ, et al: *Med Sci Sports Exerc* 24:556–567, 1992.
3. Ceci R, Hassmen P: *Med Sci Sports Exerc* 23:732–738, 1991.

Development of a Scale for Use in Monitoring Training-Induced Distress in Athletes

Raglin JS, Morgan WP (Indiana Univ, Bloomington; Univ of Wisconsin, Madison)
Int J Sports Med 15:84–88, 1994   139-95-6–8

Purpose.—Staleness in endurance athletes is the inability to train at customary levels, coupled with worsened performance, after a period of overtraining. Overreaching or training-induced distress is a milder form of staleness. A psychometric scale that can identify distressed athletes before the staleness syndrome occurs was developed.

Methods.—The Profile of Mood States (POMS)—a 65-item questionnaire that assesses the mood states of tension, depression, anger, vigor, fatigue, and confusion—was used for the study. During a 4-year period, 70 female swimmers and 100 male swimmers (mean age, 19.6 years) routinely completed the POMS on a monthly basis throughout the competitive training season. Athletes with performance losses of 5% or greater were classified as stale. Athletes whose performance had dropped for several days or more or whose performance was maintained with increased difficulty were classified as distressed. The collected POMS scores were used to construct a psychometric scale.

Results.—On the average, 32.1% of the swimmers became distressed each season and 45.9% became distressed in more than 1 training season. Seven POMS items were most effective in identifying distressed

Profile of Mood States Items Most Commonly Appearing in the
Men and Women Discriminant Function Analyses for the
Classification of Distress

Rank	Number	Item	Scale
1	58	Worthless	Depression
2	36	Miserable	Depression
3	57	Bad-tempered	Anger
4	62	Guilty	Depression
5	23	Unworthy	Depression
6	12	Peeved	Anger
7	14	Sad	Depression

(Courtesy of Raglin JS, Morgan WP: *Int J Sports Med* 15:84–88, 1994.)

swimmers (table). A validation test was carried out in a sample of 33 male swimmers, of whom 9 were considered distressed by the coach. The mean prediction rate of distress with the 7-item scale was 69.1%, which was 37% above the chance rate of prediction. A cross-validation test of the 7-item scale in 29 collegiate track-and-field athletes yielded a prediction rate of 66.7%.

Conclusion.—A 7-item scale developed from POMS data can effectively identify distressed swimmers and other distressed endurance athletes.

▶ Earlier work from our laboratory (1) demonstrated that the POMS scale was the most effective simple method of detecting overtraining. This paper extends this work; by using 7 simple items, the score gives a better prediction than either the total POMS score or the depression subscale.—R.J. Shephard, M.D., Ph.D., D.P.E.

Reference

1. Verde T, et al: *Br J Sports Med* 26:167–175, 1992.

Relationships Between Self-Efficacy and Mood Before and After Exercise Training
Stewart KJ, Kelemen MH, Ewart CK (Johns Hopkins School of Medicine, Baltimore, Md; Columbia Med Plan, Md; Johns Hopkins School of Hygiene and Public Health, Baltimore, Md)
J Cardiopulmon Rehabil 14:35–42, 1994   139-95-6–9

Introduction.—Psychological benefits are thought to result from physiologic and function improvements associated with exercise. However, studies have shown inconsistent results, with only some showing favorable effects. It has been suggested that study results may be affected by self-efficacy or one's own judgment regarding capabilities in performing specific physical tasks. Exercise programs that have a positive effect on self-efficacy may be accompanied by beneficial psychological effects, whereas little psychological benefit may be gained from programs that do not alter self-efficacy. The effect of exercise training on self-efficacy and on improving positive and reducing negative affects were assessed. Patients participating in an antihypertensive study and receiving drug therapy (propranolol) that could potentially limit the full benefits of exercise training were evaluated during a 10-week physical training program.

Methods.—Fifty-two subjects participating in a hypertension control trial were included in the study. Participants who had mild hypertension were randomized to receive either diltiazem (360 mg daily), propranolol (240 mg daily), or placebo. Physical and psychological evaluations were performed at baseline, after a placebo washout, after 2 weeks of drug therapy, and after 10 weeks of exercise training. The 10-week training program consisted of circuit weight training and walking, jogging, or cycling. Physiologic measurements included maximal oxygen uptake and maximal strength for arm and leg exercises. Heart rate and blood pressure were also monitored. Self-efficacy scales were used to measure the subject's perceived ability to perform arm and leg tasks before and after training, and the Profile of Mood States (POMS) was used to identify 6 affective states.

Results.—A total of 51 participants completed the study. Maximal oxygen uptake was decreased in the propranolol group at 2 weeks ($P <$ 0.05). Those in the diltiazem and placebo groups had an increase in maximal oxygen uptake after exercise ($P < 0.05$). Maximal oxygen uptake increased in the propranolol group after training as compared with the 2-week value ($P < 0.05$), but it did not exceed baseline measurement. All groups had an increase in strength after arm and leg exercises ($P < 0.0001$). Mean baseline blood pressures were reduced after training in all groups ($P < 0.05$), with drug therapy showing no additional antihypertensive benefit over exercise. Participants in all 3 groups showed significant increases in self-efficacy for leg and arm tasks after training, as compared with baseline ($P < 0.05$). Based on the POMS subscales, total mood disturbance was improved for all groups; gains in vigor and decreases in tension were similar in all groups. The gains seen in maximal oxygen uptake and strength were not related to changes in mood or self-efficacy. Changes in the POMS subscales of tension, depression, and total mood disturbance correlated negatively with changes in arm and leg self-efficacy. Additionally, changes in the POMS subscale of confusion also correlated negatively with changes in leg self-efficacy.

Conclusion.—As determined by this study, psychological changes were not related to changes in physical ability (maximal oxygen uptake and strength). As would be expected from the pharmacologic effects of the drug, those receiving propranolol did not show increases in aerobic power (maximal oxygen uptake); arm and leg strength had similar increases in all groups. However, all groups experienced positive psychological changes as shown by reduction in the POMS tension and total mood disturbances and a gain in vigor, showing that changes in self-efficacy are not totally dependent on physiologic improvements.

▶ We all know that exercise makes us feel better, but how? Are changes in mood caused only by changes in physiology? This study explores possible links between changes in physiology and changes in mood and "self-efficacy." Self-efficacy, a gauge of confidence in one's ability to perform physical tasks, usually increases after exercise training. This study-evaluated relationships between self-efficacy, emotion, aerobic capacity, and muscle strength before and after exercise training in men with hypertension who were also randomly assigned to diltiazem, propranolol, or placebo.

The training increased self-efficacy independent of physiologic measures, suggesting that self-efficacy comes from a variety of external and internal clues. Gains in self-efficacy also correlated with decreases in negative moods. The flip side of this coin is that athletes who injure themselves often experience "self-diminution" (1) and often show greater depression and anxiety and lower self-esteem soon after injury than do controls (2). See Abstract 139-95-6–10 for the mechanism of reduction in the state of anxiety by exercise and Abstract 139-95-6–11 for running and mood in women.—E.R. Eichner, M.D.

References

1. McGowan RW, et al: *J Sports Med Phys Fitness* 34:299, 1994.
2. Leddy MH, et al: *Res Q Exerc Sport* 65:347, 1994.

State Anxiety Reduction and Exercise: Does Hemispheric Activation Reflect Such Changes?
Petruzzello SJ, Landers DM (Univ of Illinois, Urbana-Champaign; Arizona State Univ, Tempe)
Med Sci Sports Exerc 26:1028–1035, 1994   139-95-6-10

Introduction.—Reductions in both acute and chronic anxiety have been linked with aerobic exercise, with a number of hypotheses proposed to explain this finding. Available evidence appears to support the cerebral lateralization hypothesis, which proposes that the degree of activation influenced by exercise may differ between the 2 cerebral hemispheres. A reduction of activation in the right hemisphere (an increase in alpha power) could account for the positive affect associated with exercise. Although studies that evaluate electroencephalogram (EEG) activity after exercise have reported an increase in alpha activity, methodological failings have made interpretation of results difficult. The cerebral lateralization hypothesis was tested, as well as whether resting EEG asymmetry could predict affective responses to exercise.

Methods.—Nineteen individuals participating in an aerobic exercise program were studied. Anxiety was measured using a 10-item state anxiety questionnaire. The EEG was recorded from both hemispheres at the frontal and anterior temporal sites. Maximum aerobic capacity ($\dot{V}O_{2max}$) was determined using a maximal treadmill exercise test according to 1 or more of the following criteria: plateau in oxygen consumption; respiratory exchange ratio greater than 1; and heart rate greater than age-predicted maximum. The workload for submaximal exercise was established using this $\dot{V}O_{2max}$. After EEG recording, individuals underwent submaximal exercise (intensity at 75% of $\dot{V}O_{2max}$) using a treadmill. The EEG was recorded again after submaximal exercise. The 10-item anxiety questionnaire was completed before submaximal exercise, and at 5, 10, 20, and 30 minutes after exercise.

Results.—Anxiety was found to be significantly lowered at 10, 20, and 30 minutes after exercise compared with values before exercise

($P < 0.05$). A strong inverse relationship ($P < 0.05$) was found for only the frontal region when mean anxiety and mean EEG asymmetry were computed for each time point in the frontal and temporal areas. This indicated that the frontal area of the left hemisphere became more active, relative to the right, as anxiety decreased from preexercise to postexercise levels, primarily because of increased alpha activity in the right frontal region. The left frontal EEG showed alpha activity to decrease slightly from before exercise to 5 minutes after exercise ($P = 0.088$). Alpha power was found to be greater in the frontal areas than in the temporal areas ($P < 0.001$). At 30 minutes post exercise, alpha activity in the right frontal area was greater than at 10 minutes after exercise ($P = 0.004$), indicating a decrease in activation. Variance (30%) in postexercise anxiety at 10 minutes was predicted by preexercise EEG asymmetry ($P = 0.008$), whereas only 15% of the variance was accounted for by preexercise anxiety ($P = 0.11$)

Conclusion.—Based on these findings, the cerebral lateralization hypothesis is a rational explanation for the reduction in anxiety associated with exercise. The significant increase in activation observed in the left frontal area from preexercise levels to 5 minutes after exercise, along with the nonsignificant change in right frontal alpha activity, is indicative of lower activation of the anterior right hemisphere as compared with the left. Anxiety was found to be significantly lowered after exercise compared with preexercise evaluations. However, studies using a larger sample size and evaluating individuals experiencing higher levels of anxiety or other negative affects are needed to confirm these results.

➤ The study in Abstract 139-95-6–9 shows that exercise training improves mood and "self-efficacy." This EEG study suggests *how* exercise may improve mood. Compared with preexercise values, state anxiety was reduced at 10, 20, and 30 minutes after exercise (running 30 minutes at 75% $\dot{V}O_{2max}$). The decline in anxiety was associated with relative activation of the left frontal area of the brain. This study included men only (and men who were only "low anxious" at baseline) and it lacks a nonexercise control group, but at least it gives us food for thought. See Abstract 139-95-6–11 for information on running and mood in women.—E.R. Eichner, M.D.

Qualitative and Quantitative Effects of Running on Mood
Morris M, Salmon P (Univ of College, London)
J Sports Med Phys Fitness 34:284–291, 1994   139-95-6–11

Background.—An understanding of how exercise affects mood may give insight into why some individuals exercise and others do not. Both an increase in positive mood and a decreased negative mood have been described after a period of exercise, but in neither case is the evidence convincing.

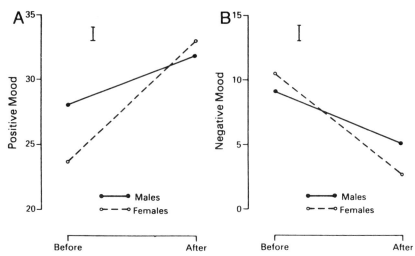

Fig 6–8.—Mean component-based scale scores for positive mood (**A**) and negative mood (**B**) before and after running. *Bars* show SED for comparisons between the 2 occasions for each sex. (Courtesy of Morris M, Salmon P: *J Sports Med Phys Fitness* 34:284–291, 1994.)

Study Design.—The effects of strenuous road running on mood were studied in 173 members of a running club who participated in a 3-mile "fun run" that was completed in 15–30 minutes. All the participants regularly ran 3 or more times per week. A questionnaire containing items from the Profile of Mood States and a mood adjective checklist was administered shortly before and after the run. Both parts of the study were completed by 165 runners, 98 men and 67 women (average age, 34 years).

Results.—Positive mood increased after running (Fig 6–8), particularly in women, whose prerun scores were lower than those for men. Negative mood decreased at the same time, and this effect also was more evident in men than in women. The men appeared to be more sociable than the women before the run and also were more relaxed. Women were less depressed after the run and scored higher for vigor.

Conclusion.—These results may help explain why vigorous exercise has particular significance for women.

▶ This study explored how exercise acutely alters mood—both positive and negative mood—in men and women. The subjects were members of the London Road Runners' Club, who filled out questionnaires just before and after a 3-mile fun run in Hyde Park. Rather than use the Profile of Mood Scores, which the authors think keys too much on negative moods, they had the subjects rate a broad set of mood adjectives—41 in all—chosen to cover a wide range of moods, from annoyed to affectionate, bad-tempered to bored, calm to carefree, sad to sorry, sluggish to suspicious, and sympathetic to spiteful. The most intriguing finding, shown in Figure 6–8, was that improvements in mood after the race were greater for women than for men: Women increased more in positive mood and decreased more in negative mood, largely because their moods were worse before the race began. For women, especially, exercise is a bad-mood–buster and a good-mood–booster. For more on exercise and mood, see Abstracts 139-95-6–9, 139-95-6–10, and 139-95-6–12.—E.R. Eichner, M.D.

Psychological Monitoring and Modulation of Training Load of World-Class Canoeists

Berglund B, Säfström H (Karolinska Hosp, Stockholm; Swedish Canoe Federation, Farsta, Sweden)
Med Sci Sports Exerc 26:1036–1040, 1994   139-95-6–12

Background.—Overtraining in world-class athletes may produce staleness and mood disturbances. Based on psychological indices, canoeists' training loads were varied to determine whether adjusting the training load would maximize it. The Profile of Mood States (POMS) was used to identify markers of distress in these athletes.

Methods.—Fourteen world-class canoeists aged 20–30 years were administered a modified POMS questionnaire several times during low–training load and high–training load periods. The POMS measures tension, depression, anger, vigor, fatigue, and confusion. The training load was adjusted based on the POMS results. Participants completed a questionnaire with a visual analogue scale giving their impression of using the POMS to titrate training. Unpaired *t*-tests and analysis of variance were used to evaluate data.

Results.—Values of the POMS decreased with the first competition (122 ± 23.1) from the POMS values at the start of the study (130 ± 15.7). During heavy training, the POMS values increased. The increase was followed by a decrease in values as the training load was adjusted. Athletes were at risk of experiencing staleness at the end of heavy training. Although mood disturbances were indicated for 57% of the athletes at some time during training, no athlete reported sleep disturbances or decreased appetite. The athletes were positive about the use of the POMS to adjust their training loads.

Discussion.—Athletes were in favor of using POMS scores to increase and decrease their training loads. In the majority of athletes, the POMS values led to significant changes in their training schedules.

▶ In this study, as in many prior studies, mood waxed and waned inversely with the training load: The harder the training, the worse the mood. Although this study is mainly descriptive, it suggests that monitoring the POMS and adjusting training accordingly can help prevent staleness or overtraining. Training was increased when mood was good and decreased when mood deteriorated. In all but one case, mood disturbances returned to acceptable levels within 1 week.

Some say that the best gauge of overtraining is how the athlete feels, i.e., whether the athlete is tired, sore, or sad. And mood changes rapidly with overtraining. In both male and female swimmers, for example, mood changes within 3 days of increased training (1). Monitoring the POMS has also helped predict athletic success and/or prevent overtraining in speed skaters, rowers, and track-and-field athletes (2). Overtraining also affects male reproductive status (3).—E.R. Eichner, M.D.

References

1. O'Conner PJ, et al: *Med Sci Sports Exerc* 23:1055, 1991.
2. Eichner ER: *J Sports Sci* in press, 1955.
3. 1994 YEAR BOOK OF SPORTS MEDICINE, pp 342–343.

Imagery Interventions in Sport
Murphy SM (United States Olympic Committee, Colorado Springs, Colo)
Med Sci Sports Exerc 26:486–494, 1994   139-95-6-13

Objective.—Imagery is a technique used by some athletes to enhance performance. The research in this area covering mental practice (MP), precompetition preparation, psychological comparisons of successful vs. unsuccessful athletic performance, and mediating variables was studied, and discrepancies in the findings were discussed.

Definitions.—Imagery is the conscious, unstimulated visualization or sensing of an imaginary experience. Two aspects of imagery are as follows: Imagery rehearsal involves repeating in the mind the steps of an athletic skill, and mental practice involves silent psychological development of the proper mental attitude.

Empirical Research on Imagery and Mental Practice.—Surveys show that 90% of athletes and 94% of coaches use imagery for training. Mental practice has long been used to learn and maintain skills, and it has been found to be effective in influencing athletic ability. However, studies found no consistent effect of "psyching up" on athletic performance. The "mental practice model" for studying imagery has created confusion.

An Analysis of the Mental Practice Model.—The "mental practice model" breaks down for several reasons. First, mental practice is not a single method; it means different things to different athletes. Second, there are no objective measurements of outcome. Third, there is no way to determine how much mental practice is going on or how often it occurs.

Future Research Suggestions.—Researchers must have descriptive methods of past studies, they must verify that athletes' experiences are those desired by investigators, individual variables must be evaluated, psychophysiologic measurements must be developed, and researchers need to be trained in the techniques of measurement.

Conclusion.—Imagery is a cognitive function that is used by athletes to learn and maintain skills. Additional research needs to be done to understand the mechanism of this performance mastery technique.

▶ Will techniques taught by sport psychologists help me be a better athlete? Will they help my team win more games? These are questions asked by many athletes and coaches. Some think they know the answers and rely heavily on the teachings of a sport psychologist. Some athletes and coaches practice their own brand of psychological techniques and wouldn't compete without them. There are still others who believe these techniques are not for them and they compete very successfully. I suspect that everyone uses some type of mental preparation before competition. As this article suggests, more studies need to be done to label and test the effects of this mental preparation.—F.J. George, A.T.C., P.T.

Exercise and Self-Esteem: Validity of Model Expansion and Exercise Associations

Sonstroem RJ, Harlow LL, Josephs L (Univ of Rhode Island, Kingston; Healthsouth Rehabilitation Ctr, Alexandria, Va)
J Sport Exerc Psychol 16:29–42, 1994   139-95-6–14

Background.—In 1989, Sonstroem and Morgan developed an Exercise and Self-Esteem Model (EXSEM) to trace the manner in which physical training activities influence self-esteem. The model is based on contemporary theory stipulating that self-concept is best assessed as a collection of self-perceptions organized on hierarchic levels of specificity vs. generality. Expansion of the EXSEM to include 2 levels of perceived physical competence as operationalized by the Physical Self-Perception Profile (PSPP) was tested.

Methods.—Two hundred sixteen female aerobic dancers (mean age, 38.4 years) completed a self-esteem scale and the PSPP to assess general physical self-worth and more specific subdomains of perceived sport competence, physical condition, attractive body, and strength. The women also completed self-efficacy scales for jogging, sitting, and aerobic dancing.

Findings.—Confirmatory factor analysis supported model measurement as hypothesized. Structural equation modeling supported EXSEM component relationships. In addition, structural equation modeling correlating 2 exercise self-reports with the EXSEM again showed satisfactory fit indices, explaining up to 27.6% of exercise variance.

Conclusion.—Exercise in female aerobic dancers is associated with positive assessments of their physical condition and with negative assessments of their bodies. The reliability and validity of the PSPP for use with women were documented. The internal structure of the EXSEM was also validated.

▶ Many women are involved with aerobic dance programs for social reasons, for enjoyment, for exercise, for health, for weight loss, because their friends do, because they want to look better, and for many more reasons. One underlying factor of this study is that many of these women have a negative assessment of their bodies and a positive assessment of their physical condition. In this study, there was a reverse relationship between age and the women's perception of their bodies and their physical condition. Younger women believed they were more fit but had a negative assessment of their bodies; older women believed they were less fit but had a more positive assessment of their bodies. Education aimed toward improving the way these women perceive their bodies should be a part of every dance aerobics program.—F.J. George, A.T.C., P.T.

Psychological Skills for Enhancing Performance: Arousal Regulation Strategies
Gould D, Udry E (Univ of North Carolina, Greensboro)
Med Sci Sports Exerc 26:478–485, 1994   139-95-6–15

Background.—An athlete's ability to regulate his or her level of emotional arousal is often thought to positively or negatively affect athletic performance. The literature on this subject, however, is divergent. There is a need to integrate and summarize it. Current empirical and theoretical research on arousal regulation strategies for enhancing athletic performance was reviewed.

Arousal Regulation Strategies.—The literature emphasizes the need to view arousal as a multifaceted construct made up of both cognitive and physiologic components. It is also important to understand arousal-performance relationship theories that are more complex than the simple inverted-U notion. Categories of arousal regulation strategies include arousal energizing techniques, biofeedback methods, relaxation response strategies, cognitive behavioral interventions, and mental preparation routines. Although these techniques could effectively influence arousal and facilitate performance, more research is needed using more rigorous methods to determine how and why certain interventions work, to identify personality and situational factors influencing arousal regulation efficacy, and to establish the most effective way to teach arousal regulation.

Conclusion.—Knowledge of arousal regulation has increased markedly during the past 20 years. Current research demonstrates that arousal regulation strategies can be used to influence an athlete's arousal and enhance performance. Additional research is now needed to better explain how, when, and with whom these strategies are most effective.

▶ Many athletes and teams have benefited from techniques taught by sport psychologists. Coaches and athletic trainers have used some of these techniques to improve an athlete's performance and team dynamics. Athletic trainers are also using some of these teachings in our treatment and rehabilitation programs. With more research and education, we will become more effective in using these techniques.—F.J. George, A.T.C., P.T.

Hyperhydration Effect on Endurance Trained Subjects' Capacity for Maximum Physical Exercise After Exposure to Hypokinesia
Zorbas YG, Matveyev IO, Federenko YF (European Inst of Environmental Cybernetics, Athens, Greece)
Sports Train Med Rehabil 5:145–156, 1994   139-95-6–16

Introduction.—A previous report from the study institution demonstrated that body rehydration through the additional daily intake of fluid and salt can effectively increase an individual's capacity for maximum physical exercise after a prolonged restriction of muscular activity. In this study, the effect of chronic hyperhydration on the exercise capacity of endurance-trained male athletes after a year's restriction of muscular activity was evaluated.

Methods.—The 30 study participants had a mean age of 24 years and had competed in long-distance running for 3–5 years. Ten runners

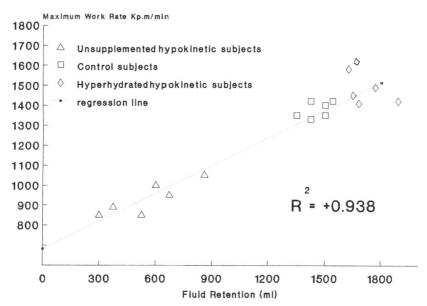

Fig 6–9.—Increase in physical capacity in 30 endurance-trained volunteers in response to a maximum physical exercise test, as a function of the amount of fluid retained in the body after exposure to prolonged restriction of muscular activity (mean ± standard error of mean). (Courtesy of Zorbas YG, Matveyev IO, Federenko YF: *Sports Train Med Rehabil* 5:145–156, 1994.)

served as controls and continued training in long-distance running (averaging 14.9 km/day), and 20 were placed on a regimen that restricted their muscular activity to 2.7 km/day. Ten of the runners whose activity was restricted followed their usual diet (hypokinetic group) and 10 consumed daily supplemental amounts of fluid and salt to increase or maintain the level of circulating blood volume (hyperhydrated group). All the study subjects performed graded physical exercise tests, and their cardiovascular responses, blood biochemical changes, and fluid balance were measured at regular intervals.

Results.—During the period of restricted activity, body mass increased significantly in the hyperhydrated group and decreased significantly in the hypokinetic group. The hyperhydrated volunteers also had an increase in body fat and a decrease in lean body mass. The hypokinetic volunteers experienced significant decreases in lean body mass and body fat, compared with the control and hyperhydrated groups. The hyperhydrated men significantly increased their capacity to perform maximal physical exercise with a daily intake of fluid and salt supplementation, compared with unsupplemented hypokinetic men after exposure to hypokinesia. Their mean heart rate decreased and their stroke volume, blood pressure, and fluid retention increased. Decreases in hematocrit, hemoglobin, plasma osmolality, plasma protein, and sodium and potassium concentrations also accompanied hyperhydration, whereas plasma volume increased. The hypokinetic-only group exhibited the opposite pattern of change. The amount of fluid retention differed significantly between the hypokinetic group and the hyperhydrated group (Fig 6–9). The greatest reductions in maximum physical ability were associated with the lowest fluid retention levels, and the most pronounced increases in maximum physical ability was associated with the highest fluid retention levels.

Conclusion.—A daily intake of fluid and salt supplementation during a long period of hypokinesia allowed these athletes to significantly increase their capacity to perform maximal physical exercise. The beneficial effects of fluid and salt supplementation appeared to be related to increases in circulating blood volume.

▶ The subjects of this study were quite fit (with a maximal oxygen intake of 65 mL/kg per minute), and it is intriguing that the investigators were able to persuade them not to exercise seriously for a whole year! What is even more remarkable is that at the end of the year during which running had been limited to 2.7 km/day, aerobic power was marginally increased if extra salt and fluid had been provided, whereas without such supplementation, aerobic power dropped to 52 mL/kg per minute.

This certainly points to the importance of maintaining fluid and mineral intake if an athlete is obliged to reduce training because of injury. However, the amount of hyperhydration adopted was substantial (a fluid retention of 300 to 1,950 mL). Moreover, the fluid supplements did not prevent an accumulation of fat and a loss of lean tissue in the subjects as a result of their inactivity, so drinking dilute salt solutions cannot be recommended as a standard method for the improvement of overall aerobic capacity without the need for physical effort.—R.J. Shephard, M.D., Ph.D., D.P.E.

Jogging or Walking: Comparison of Health Effects

Suter E, Marti B, Gutzwiller F (Univ of Zurich, Switzerland; Federal Office of Public Health, Bern, Switzerland)
Ann Epidemiol 4:375–381, 1994   139-95-6–17

Introduction.—Controversy surrounds the intensity of physical activity required to achieve desired health benefits. To improve cardiovascular fitness, a high exercise intensity of 60% to 86% maximum oxygen uptake ($\dot{V}O_{2max}$) has been previously recommended. However, it has recently been confirmed that to improve cardiovascular fitness, lower intensity activity performed over a longer duration is as effective as higher intensity activity over a shorter period.

Methods.—To compare the health effects of jogging and walking over a 6-month period, 75 nonsmoking, sedentary men were divided into 2 groups: 28 jogged in a home-based, unsupervised exercise program of 4 times a week for 30 minutes at an intensity of 75% $\dot{V}O_{2max}$, and 28 walked at an intensity of 50% $\dot{V}O_{2max}$ 6 times a week for 30 minutes. Changes in endurance capacity, body fat, serum lipid levels, exercise adherence, and injuries related to exercise training were evaluated.

Results.—Results of a maximal bicycle ergometer test showed that after 6 months, joggers and walkers had a similar increase in $\dot{V}O_{2max}$ (2.9 $\pm$ 4.1 mL/kg per minute and 2.5 $\pm$ 5.7 mL/kg per minute, respectively). In joggers, a significant association was seen between the amount of training (kilometers exercised) and the increase in high-density-lipoprotein cholesterol levels. In walkers, the amount of exercise, the decrease in the sum of skinfolds, and the waist–hip ratio were significantly associated. Changes in blood lipid levels were not significant in either group. The joggers trained for an average of 90 $\pm$ 41 min/wk, and the walkers trained for an average of 121$\pm$ 72 min/wk. The incidence of injuries was 25% for joggers and 21% for walkers.

Conclusion.—With respect to changes in endurance capacity and body fat, brisk walking at 50% $\dot{V}O_{2max}$ is as effective as a higher intensity training program. Fewer injuries occur with walking than with jogging. Walking is a valuable exercise for promoting health. A submaximal-intensity training program should be more effective than a higher intensity training program if reduction in body fat is the main goal. A significant relationship between the amount of training and a decrease in the sum of skinfolds and the waist–hip ratio was found only among the walkers. However, the distance run and the increases in high-density-lipoprotein cholesterol levels were significantly associated in joggers but not in walkers.

▶ What type of fitness program should I undertake to improve my . . . ? The answer lies within the question. Recent studies indicate that if you want to increase your longevity, a more vigorous type of exercise program may be required. If the goal is to reduce body fat or lower blood pressure, the exercise program may not have to be as vigorous. This becomes confusing because reducing body fat and lowering blood pressure are certainly considered healthy goals for many people. Each individual's goal for exercise should determine the type of program in which that individual participates. This holds true from the sedentary person to the elite athlete.—F.J. George, A.T.C., P.T.

Upper Extremity Proprioceptive Training
Stone JA, Partin NB, Lueken JS, Timm KE, Ryan EJ III (US Olympic Committee, Colorado Springs, Colo; Nacogdoches, Tex; Indiana Univ, Bloomington; et al)
J Athletic Train 29:15–18, 1994   139-95-6-18

Objective.—Although proprioceptive rehabilitation is standard for patients who have lower extremity injuries, use of such training in athletes who had upper extremity injuries has not been evaluated. The use of proprioceptive training was examined in athletes who had upper extremity injuries, and additional proprioceptive exercises not heretofore found in the literature were suggested. The differences in such training programs for athletes in open kinetic chain activities—such as throwing—vs. athletes in closed kinetic chain activities—such as gymnastics, swimming, and rowing—were also studied.

Exercises.—Proper rehabilitation requires that proprioceptive exercises be specific to the type of sport in which the athlete engages. The exercises proposed progress from open to closed chain kinetic exercises. Proprioceptive rehabilitation should emphasize rhythmic stabilization, mirroring upper extremity positions by passive movements, having the athlete actively duplicate passive upper extremity movements, and having the athlete engage in double- and single-arm balancing activities on various surfaces (Fig 6–10). Other beneficial exercises include having the athlete balance on the hands on a rocking platform and engage in single- or double-arm balancing on 1 or more balls.

Conclusion.—Proprioceptive exercises develop range of motion, muscular endurance, and muscle strength.

▶ Sport-specific rehabilitation is a must for any athlete with an upper extremity injury. Proprioceptive rehabilitation should be included in all upper extremity rehabilitation programs. The authors have described a unique

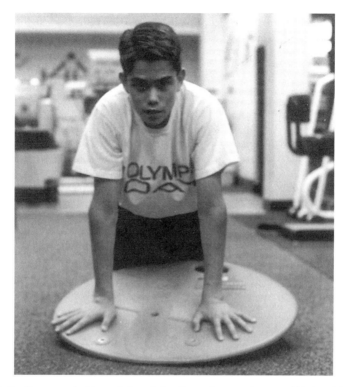

Fig 6–10.—Eyes open, double-arm balance in kneeling push-up position on wobble board. (Courtesy of Stone JA, Partin NB, Lueken JS, et al: *J Athletic Train* 29:15–18, 1994.)

group of exercises, some of which should be included for all athletes with shoulder injuries. We have become very specific in rehabilitation programs for our throwing athletes. This specificity should carry over to all athletes with shoulder injuries. A good reference on this subject is an article titled "Biomechanical Differences of Open and Closed Chain Exercises With Respect to the Shoulder"(1).—F.J. George, A.T.C., P.T.

Reference

1. Dillman CJ: *J Sport Rehabil* 3:228–238, 1994.

The Effects of Athletic Massage on Delayed Onset Muscle Soreness, Creatine Kinase, and Neutrophil Count: A Preliminary Report
Smith LL, Keating MN, Holbert D, Spratt DJ, McCammon MR, Smith SS, Israel RG (East Carolina Univ, Greenville, NC; Duke Univ, Durham, NC; Martha Jefferson Hosp, Charlottesville, Va)
J Orthop Sports Phys Ther 19:93–99, 1994   139-95-6–19

Objective.—Delayed-onset muscle soreness (DOMS) usually results from eccentric muscle action. Typically, muscle and connective tissue are injured and inflammation can occur. If DOMS is caused by acute inflammation reaction as the result of swelling, massage could reduce the intensity of the inflammation by disrupting the process of margination and emigration of neutrophils to the site of trauma. Whether massage, given within 2 hours of injury, can significantly reduce DOMS by affecting the levels of circulating neutrophils was studied.

Methods.—Fourteen healthy men performed 20 submaximal and 5 maximal eccentric, isokinetic contractions of the biceps and triceps of the nondominant arm followed, after a 2-minute rest, by 4 or 5 sets of 35 eccentric muscle actions, maintaining the same force, if possible. After 2 hours, 7 subjects received 30 minutes of massage, and 7 received none. The DOMS and creatine kinase (CK) were determined before exercise and at 8, 24, 48, 72, 96, and 120 hours after exercise. Neutrophils and cortisol levels were measured before and after exercise and every 30 minutes for 8 hours.

Results.—The massage group reported significantly less DOMS and, over time, reduced levels of CK, a slight increase in neutrophils, and less reduction in cortisol levels.

Conclusion.—Sports massage within 2 hours of eccentric injury appears to reduce DOMS and CK, possibly because of reduced neutrophil emigration and/or higher levels of cortisol.

▶ The authors state that previous studies have indicated that massage does not reduce DOMS. The difference between these previous studies and this study is the timing of the administration of the massage. The authors quote a Soviet theory of "restorative massage" in which the massage is administered between 1 and 3 hours after strenuous exercise. This study indicates that the type and timing of the massage is very important. More studies need to be done following this protocol, with larger numbers of subjects, and the controls should receive a "sham" type of massage.—F.J. George, A.T.C., P.T.

Acute Rhabdomyolysis Due to Body Building Exercise: Report of a Case
Bolgiano EB (Univ of Maryland, Baltimore)
J Sports Med Phys Fitness 34:76–78, 1994   139-95-6–20

Objective.—Rhabdomyolysis is commonly associated with excessive physical exertion, such as long-distance running, rigorous training of military recruits, and contact sports. Rhabdomyolysis associated with weight lifting and bodybuilding is relatively infrequent, possibly because many cases go unrecognized and are diagnosed as simple muscle strain.

Case Report.—Man, 40, had severe biceps pain and inability to fully extend his elbows after weight lifting. He had also started a program of "negative curls" for the first time. He denied the use of anabolic steroids in the previous 3 years or any change in urine volume or color. Laboratory findings included total serum creatine kinase (CK) levels of 76,080 IU/L, with a CK-MB fraction of 23.4 ng/mL. The urine was strongly positive for blood on dipstick, but microscopic examination revealed no red blood cells. A diagnosis of rhabdomyolysis was made, and the patient was treated with IV sodium chloride solution, sodium bicarbonate, and mannitol. Renal failure did not ensue, and his symptoms resolved after 2 weeks.

Discussion.—Previous reports of rhabdomyolysis associated with bodybuilding involved patients new to the sport. This report indicates that rhabdomyolysis can occur in otherwise physically well-conditioned and active persons, particularly during excessive weight loads or new, extreme exercise routines. There is a need for a high degree of vigilance in making the diagnosis. Treatment for rhabdomyolysis associated with weight lifting or bodybuilding is essentially the same as for rhabdomyolysis resulting from other causes.

▶ The point is that any new, strenuous, especially *eccentric* muscle action (in which the muscle exerts force as it lengthens), as in this case of "negative curls," can cause acute rhabdomyolysis. Repeatedly stepping down off of a box causes more damage than stepping up onto it. Doing 100 consecutive deep knee bends, or "squats," can cause severe rhabdomyolysis (1). Most reports of acute rhabdomyolysis in bodybuilders (or weight lifters) involve unaccustomed eccentric exercise (2, 3). The authors surmise that many cases of rhabdomyolysis in bodybuilders are misdiagnosed as muscle strain. Last year, we abstracted articles suggesting that, in rare athletes with sickle cell trait, "heroic" exercise bouts in adverse climes can evoke a vicious cycle of sickling in working muscles, fulminant rhabdomyolysis, lactic acidosis, shock, collapse, acute renal failure, hyperkalemia, and death (4).—E.R. Eichner, M.D.

References

1. Frucht M: *N Engl J Med* 330:1620, 1994.
2. 1989 YEAR BOOK OF SPORTS MEDICINE, pp 326–327.
3. 1993 YEAR BOOK OF SPORTS MEDICINE, pp 203–204.
4. 1994 YEAR BOOK OF SPORTS MEDICINE, pp 413–415.

Exercise-Induced Muscle Pain, Soreness, and Cramps
Miles MP, Clarkson PM (Univ of Massachusetts, Amherst)
J Sports Med Phys Fitness 34:203–216, 1994   139-95-6-21

Background.—Exercise-related pain includes pain experienced during or immediately after exercise, delayed-onset muscle soreness, and pain induced by muscle cramps. The time course and proposed causes for each type of pain were described.

Discussion.—To date, no single causative factor for pain experienced during exercise has been identified. Lactic acid is commonly implicated, although a combination of acids, ions, proteins, and hormones may also be responsible. Delayed-onset muscle soreness occurs 24–48 hours after strenuous exercise that is geared toward eccentric muscle actions or intense endurance events. Simultaneous prolonged loss of strength, reduced range of motion, and elevated levels of serum creatine kinase are also noted. These are considered to be indirect indicators of muscle damage. Examinations of biopsy specimens have shown damage to the contractile elements. Although the exact cause of the soreness response is not clear, an inflammatory reaction to muscle damage may be involved. Muscle cramps are sudden, acute, electrically active contractions evoked by motor neuron hyperexcitability. Cramps during exercise are presumed to be the result of fluid electrolyte imbalance induced by sweating, although 2 studies have failed to support this assumption. Furthermore, individuals in professions not associated with profuse sweating but who require long-term use of a muscle, such as musicians, frequently experience cramps. In hot environments, fluid electrolyte imbalance may cause cramps if associated profuse and prolonged periods of sweating occur. Pharmaceutical treatment and stretching of the affected muscles may prove effective in individuals who frequently experience muscle cramps.

Conclusion.—Although exercise-related pain is common, the exact cause of such pain remains to be determined.

▶ This is a very good review article with an extensive list of references on exercise-induced muscle pain, soreness, and cramps. This is an area of sports medicine research that is still in the investigatory stage. There are many theories, some with a good scientific basis and others with less evidence supporting them. In doing these studies, the level of the subject's fitness is a very important factor to consider.

Clinically, we use many methods and modalities to treat these pains and cramps. Some of our treatments have a scientific basis and others do not. We have used every method available to us—heat, cold, electricity in all forms, acupressure, flexibility and stretching, curtailment of exercise, and increased exercise. You name it, we've tried it—with inconsistent results. When we know the cause of the pain, we will find the best method of treating patients who have it.—F.J. George, A.T.C., P.T.

Twitch Analysis as an Approach to Motor Unit Activation During Electrical Stimulation

Heyters M, Carpentier A, Duchateau J, Hainaut K (Université Libre de Bruxelles, Brussels, Belgium)

Can J Appl Physiol 19:451–461, 1994   139-95-6–22

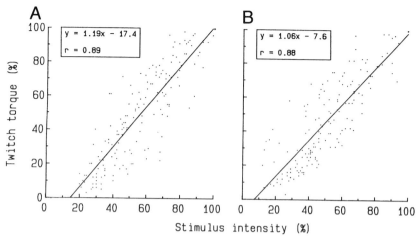

Fig 6–11.—Relationship between twitch torque and stimulus intensity in soleus (**A**) and lateral gastrocnemius (**B**) in response to electrical stimulation at the motor point. Data were obtained from 10 subjects and expressed as a percentage of maximum twitch torque and corresponding stimulus intensity. Data best fitted by linear regression lines. Sloped and ordinate intercepts were significantly different ($P < 0.05$) in the 2 muscles. (Courtesy of Heyters M, Carpentier A, Duchateau J, et al: *Can J Appl Physiol* 19:451–461, 1994.)

Introduction.—Neuromuscular electrical stimulation (ES) has been widely used in physical therapy; in the treatment of paralyzed patients; and, more recently, to augment muscle strength in normal individuals. High-frequency ES is claimed to increase muscle force, whereas lower frequencies chiefly promote endurance.

Objective and Methods.—The relationship between twitch time-to-peak and stimulus intensity during ES was studied in 12 healthy men and 1 woman (aged 20–37 years) to learn whether a homogeneous muscle, the soleus, exhibits a less curved relationship than a heterogeneous muscle, e.g., the gastrocnemius. In addition, the effects of ES were compared when delivered at the muscle motor point and along the nerve trunk in 2 hand muscles, the first dorsal interosseous (FDI) and the adductor pollicis (AP). The soleus and gastrocnemius were stimulated only at their motor points.

Results.—A positive linear relationship between the intensity of ES and twitch torque was observed in all muscles (Fig 6–11). In the FDI and AP, the relationship was similar, regardless of whether ES was applied at the motor point or over the nerve. At lower levels of activation, ES produced larger twitch torques in the lateral and medial parts of the gastrocnemius, which contains roughly equal parts of slow and fast motor units, than in the soleus, which consists mainly of slow-type fibers. The relation between ES intensity and twitch time-to-peak was best described by a power curve having a greater range of time-to-peak twitch in its initial portion for muscles containing larger proportions of fast motor units.

Conclusion.—These observations suggest that the sequence of motor unit activation is the reverse of the sequence of voluntary contractions.

▶ This is interesting information, but I'm not certain what it means in relationship to the use of ES to produce powerful muscular contractions for either rehabilitation or athletic strength development purposes.—Col. J.L. Anderson, PE.D.

Voluntary and Neuromuscular Electrical Stimulation-Induced Torque Production in the Elderly

Hooker SP, Morley SD, Simmons MD (Univ of Southern California, Los Angeles)
Sports Med Train Rehabil 5:121–130, 1994   139-95-6–23

Introduction.—Tension developed in muscle has a direct effect on muscle strengthening, suggesting that cutaneous neuromuscular electric stimulation (NMES)—alone or combined with maximal voluntary isometric contraction (MVC)—has important implications for physical rehabilitation. The combination of MVC and NMES is of potential benefit for the elderly, who may be unable to achieve complete motor unit activation in large muscle groups such as the quadriceps and hamstrings. The peak and average isometric and isokinetic torque produced by these muscle groups during voluntary effort alone and during voluntary effort plus NMES were assessed in healthy, sedentary older adults.

Methods.—The study included 5 women and 4 men (age range, 62–82 years). After habituation, the participants performed voluntary isometric and isokinetic quadriceps and hamstring contractions—1.05, 1.57, and 2.09 rad/sec—with and without NMES on a Kin-Com dynamometer. The tests, conducted on 4 separate days, were randomized for muscle group, contraction velocity, and NMES application. Cutaneous NMES was applied at the maximal tolerable level—with a symmetric biphasic waveform of 0.250 ms and a duration of 50 pps—using 2 pairs of electrodes placed over motor points of the 2 muscle groups.

Results.—The mean quadriceps peak torque was 67 to 110 newton meters. With NMES alone, peak torque was only 1% to 20% of isometric MVC. Neither muscle group showed any significant differences in either isometric or isokinetic torque between voluntary effort with and without NMES. With a few exceptions, there was no absolute pattern of benefit or detriment according to subject, muscle group, or velocity of contraction.

Conclusion.—Isometric and isokinetic quadriceps and hamstring MVC supplemented with NMES does not result in additional recruitment of motor units in healthy elderly subjects. The lack of benefit may result from poor tolerance of NMES in elderly individuals or from adequate ability to recruit motor units during voluntary effort alone.

▶ This study reminds me that several years ago, a colleague of mine went to the Soviet Union while it was still the Soviet Union and while they still had sports medicine organizations training their world-class athletes. At one of their training centers, my colleague volunteered to be a subject in a demonstration on the use of NMES for increasing muscular strength. He was surprised at the amount of electrical stimulation that was administered. He said that the entire procedure was uncomfortable and even painful. From my discussions with him on the use of electrical stimulation, I cannot imagine our using that technique in this country. However, my colleague said there was no doubt that the technique would be effective if the electrical stimulation were strong enough. What is the maximum level of electrical stimulation that any of us, young or elderly, would find tolerable?—Col. J.L. Anderson, PE.D.

The Influence of Electrostimulation on Mechanical and Morphological Characteristics of the Triceps Surae
Martin L, Cometti G, Pousson M, Morlon B (Université de Bourgogne, Dijon, France)
J Sports Sci 12:377–381, 1994   139-95-6–24

Introduction.—The physical preparation of athletes has included increasing use of electrostimulation of muscle (EMS); training with EMS is believed to modify the contractile qualities of muscle. To show how muscles adapt to this training technique, muscular contractility in both static and dynamic conditions was evaluated using isokinetic ergometry.

Methods.—Twelve individuals participated in the study as either experimental (6) or control (6) subjects. The EMS sessions were conducted with a "Compex"-type stimulator using flexible elastomer electrodes placed on the belly of the triceps surae. The knee was fully extended and the ankle was positioned at full dorsiflexion. Sessions for each muscle lasted for 10 minutes and consisted of 15 seconds of rest time and 5 seconds of contraction time with symmetrically alternating pulses of 200 μs duration delivered at a frequency of 70 Hz. Training continued for 4 weeks with 3 sessions given per week. Torque-angle and torque-velocity relationships were used to evaluate the contractile qualities of ankle extensors; a CT technique was used to measure the cross-sectional area (CSA) of the triceps surae.

Results.—After EMS training, the torque-velocity relationship shifted significantly upward. Greater absolute gains in strength were observed in the torque-angle relationship in dorsiflexion than in plantar flexion. The gain in strength decreased as angular velocity increased for the torque-velocity relationship. No changes were found in the torque-angle and peak torque-velocity relationships for the control group, and no variation was reported for the 2 groups in muscle CSA.

Discussion.—The use of EMS in strength training can be justified because EMS—unlike voluntary training in which gains are specifically related to training conditions—allows the contractile qualities of muscle to be developed in both static and dynamic conditions. The morphological results lend credence to the assumption that EMS induces neural adaptation; EMS training may improve motor control and muscle contractility without affecting hypertrophy. This adaptation could be the result of enhanced activation of the motor units and preferential work of type IIb muscle fibers by EMS.

▶ These authors used EMS in strength training because they found that the contractile qualities of muscle can be developed in static as well as dynamic conditions. They also support the concept that EMS may improve motor control. (Please refer to Abstract 139-95-6–23 concerning electrical stimulation and a colleague's experience in the Soviet Union.)—Col. J.L. Anderson, PE.D.

Maximum Rate of Force Development Is Increased by Antagonist Conditioning Contraction
Grabiner MD (Cleveland Clinic Found, Ohio)
J Appl Physiol 77:807–811, 1994   139-95-6–25

Introduction.—Conditioning contractions involve standardizing the state of at least 1 element of the neuromotor system. It is largely accepted that training using antagonist conditioning contractions improves strength, although force potentiation with this strategy has not been clearly established. The effects of graded conditioning contractions with the knee flexor muscles on the maximum performance of the quadriceps femoris as measured by maximum force, work, and maximum rate of change in force were studied. In addition, it was determined whether the effects of the conditioning contractions were similarly distributed to the components of the quadriceps femoris.

Methods.—Six healthy men and 3 healthy women participated. The participants performed 3 trials of maximum isometric contraction with the knee flexors on an isokinetic dynamometer, and the mean was calculated. Then 3 trials for each of 5 knee extensor conditioning contraction intensities were performed at 0%, 25%, 50%, and 75% of the mean maximum isometric knee flexion force value. Distribution of the effects to the components of the quadriceps femoris was assessed with electromyography.

Results.—Unexpectedly, maximum knee extension force and work were not improved with the antagonist conditioning contractions. However, the maximum rate of change in force did increase significantly. There was a significant general increase in the activation level of the components of the quadriceps femoris.

Discussion.—These results indicate a relationship between the intensity of antagonist conditioning contractions and the enhancement of agonist activation, possibly because conditioning contractions may increase the amount of large-threshold motor units available for activation. However, the increased maximum rate of change in force may suggest the presence of a motor unit recruitment scheme for activation unrelated to size or increased maximum discharge rate in the involved motor units. Contrary to other reports, the activation levels of the quadriceps femoris components were similar, which restricts the conditions under which selective nervous system activation may occur.

▶ Any researcher has experienced problems when trying to replicate the results of past research, especially if the procedures are not exactly the same. This author was aware that previous research reported potential agonist force and enhanced agonist activation when preceded by a maximum isometric contraction of the antagonist muscle. However, his study did not find an increase in the maximum knee extension or the isokinetic knee extension work after conditioning contractions with the antagonist muscles. He wonders whether the difference in results between his work and the work of others could be caused by the differences in the isokinetic velocity at which the knee extension contractions were performed, because of different subject pools, or because of the nature of the conditioning contraction. I believe the logical respective responses would be "Yes," "Certainly," and "Absolutely." There are also other reasons differences might be observed.—Col. J.L. Anderson, PE.D.

Ballistic Movement: Muscle Activation and Neuromuscular Adaptation

Zehr EP, Sale DG (McMaster Univ, Hamilton, Ontario)
Can J Appl Physiol 19:363–378, 1994   139-95-6–26

Background.—Movements performed with maximal velocity and acceleration are considered ballistic actions. Ballistic movements are believed to be preprogrammed and run off closed-loop; in contrast, slower ramp movements are executed in open-loop fashion and involve peripheral sensory feedback. The muscle activation associated with ballistic movement and the neuromuscular adaptations occurring as a result of ballistic movement training were examined.

Ballistic Movement.—Ballistic movements are characterized by extremely high maximal motor-unit firing rates, brief contraction times, and high rates of force development. During ballistic movement, there is a triphasic agonist/antagonist/agonist electromyographic burst pattern, in which the amount and intensity or antagonist coactivation is variable. During low-grade tonic muscular activity, a premovement electromyographic depression, or a premovement silence, can occur in agonist muscles before ballistic contraction. The period of agonist premovement depression may potentiate the force and velocity of the subsequent contraction. A selective activation of fast-twitch motor units may occur in ballistic contractions under certain movement conditions. High-velocity ballistic training causes specific neuromuscular adaptations that are a function of underlying neurophysiologic mechanisms that subserve ballistic movement.

Discussion.—Ballistic movements have many characteristics that distinguish them from other types of movement. The neurophysiologic mechanisms and anatomical loci underlying agonist premovement depression, as well as the physiologic adaptations responsible for specific neuromuscular training effects after ballistic training, are not understood.

▶ That there is a specific effect of high-velocity training on strength or muscular adaptation has been shown by a number of authors going back to the early 1980s. Some studies have shown that high-velocity or ballistic training will produce greater improvement in fast-force production than in strength. It has been concluded that explosive ballistic training can cause significant neural and selective muscular adaptations, resulting in improved explosive performance. The authors of this study have stated that the physiologic adaptations responsible for specific neuromuscular training effects subsequent to ballistic training are not clearly understood and must await further study.—Col. J.L. Anderson, PE.D.

Respiratory Effects of Low-Level Photochemical Air Pollution in Amateur Cyclists
Brunekreef B, Hoek G, Breugelmans O, Leentvaar M (Univ of Wageningen, The Netherlands)
Am J Respir Crit Care Med 150:962–966, 1994   139-95-6-27

Introduction.—Respiratory responses to ozone exposure are accentuated with exercise. Ozone exposure can lead to large decrements in forced expiratory volume in 1 second (FEV_1) and vital capacity; these

Estimated Odds Ratios Expressing the Relative Change in Symptom Score
Associated with a 100-$\mu g/m^3$ Difference in Ozone Exposure During
Exercise, After Adjustment for Absolute Air Humidity

Symptom	Estimated Odds Ratio (95% CI)
Shortness of breath	2.45 (1.05–5.74)*
Chest tightness	2.27 (0.87–5.93)†
Cough	1.06 (0.54–2.09)
Eye irritation	0.75 (0.32–1.72)
Wheeze	5.21 (0.99–27.39)†

Note: Ratios are per 100-$\mu g/m^3$ difference in ozone exposure during exercise.
* $P < 0.05$.
† $P < 0.10$.
(Courtesy of Brunekreef B, Hoek G, Breugelmans O, et al: *Am J Respir Crit Care Med* 150:962–966, 1994.)

persist after exercise but slowly return to normal with time. The respiratory responses of highly trained cyclists who had been exposed to ambient ozone over a training season and in competition were studied.

Methods.—Twenty-three amateur cyclists (average age, 25 years) were examined a minimum of 4 times. Lung function tests were performed before and after training sessions and races that were conducted in rural Holland. Training and competition occurred in the late afternoon. Information on air quality was obtained from the National Air Quality Monitoring Network.

Results.—The ozone concentration averaged 87 μg/m³, the temperature averaged 17.9°C, and the humidity averaged 14.7 mbar. Exercise averaged 75 minutes per session. During training, the heart rate averaged 161 beats/min, whereas the heart rate averaged 176 beats/min during competition. Preexercise lung volumes were forced vital capacity, 6.15 L; FEV_1, 4.95 L; peak expiratory flow, 12.55 L/sec; and forced expiratory flow after 25% to 75% of vital capacity had been expelled, 4.66 L/sec. The difference in lung function between preexercise and postexercise measurements was inversely related to ozone concentrations. This held even at the lowest ozone concentrations. Midsummer ozone exposure caused a greater decrease in pulmonary function than did late summer ozone exposure. The odds ratio for selected symptoms (table), corrected for humidity, suggested that ozone exposure during exercise resulted in significant symptoms of shortness of breath, chest tightness, and wheeze.

Conclusion.—Low photochemical air pollution has a significant effect on lung function and respiratory symptoms in well-trained cyclists. The relationship was stronger in midsummer than in late summer. Effects on lung function at low ozone concentrations were demonstrated.

▶ Because vigorous exercise causes air to be inspired through the mouth rather than the nose (1), the toxic effects of a number of air pollutants are observed at substantially lower ambient concentrations during exercise. This paper shows that even the relatively low levels of ozone encountered in a rural area of Holland (< 120 μg/m³) are enough to exert immediate adverse effects on pulmonary function in athletes who are exercising hard.

In large cities, ozone levels are likely to be several times higher than this. What is less clear is whether such immediate changes of lung volumes betoken an increased risk of subsequent chronic obstructive lung disease. Given that ozone accelerates the aging process, there is certainly a need for caution in circumstances in which there is an acute decrease in lung volume.

This paper is also interesting in that it confirms the work of Hackney and associates (2) showing that the response to ozone diminishes as exposure to this gas is repeated. The mechanism of adaptation is unclear; perhaps increased mucus production neutralizes the ozone or perhaps there is an increased production of antioxidant enzymes.—R.J. Shephard, M.D., Ph.D., D.P.E.

References

1. Niinimaa V, et al: *Respir Physiol* 42:61, 1980.
2. Hackney JD, et al: Responses of selected reactive and non-reactive volunteers to ozone exposure in high and low pollution seasons, in: Schneider T, et al (eds): *Atmospheric Ozone Research and Its Policy Implications.* Amsterdam, Elsevier, 1989, pp 311–318.

Pre-Exposure to Ozone Does Not Enhance or Produce Exercise-Induced Asthma

Weymer AR, Gong H Jr, Lyness A, Linn WS (Univ of California, Los Angeles; Rancho Los Amigos Med Ctr, Downey, Calif)
Am J Respir Crit Care Med 149:1413–1419, 1994   139-95-6–28

Background.—Ozone is known to have acute pulmonary effects in healthy individuals. The effects of acute ozone exposure in asthmatic patients with and without exercise-induced asthma (EIA) were investigated.

Methods.—Twenty-one otherwise healthy asthmatic patients aged 19–40 years were studied. All had a forced expiratory volume in 1 second (FEV_1) above 70% of predicted and methacholine hyperresponsiveness. They underwent 3 exposures of 1 hour each on separate days to 0.10 ppm of ozone in filtered air (FA), 0.25 ppm of ozone in FA, and FA

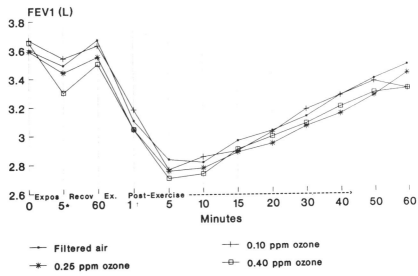

Fig 6–12.—Mean values of forced expiratory volume in 1 second (FEV_1) at pre-exposure baseline (zero), at 5 and 60 minutes after exposure, and at 1, 5, and 10–60 minutes after exercise challenge. The exposures consisted of 1-hour exposures to zero (filtered air), 0.10, 0.25, and 0.40 ppm of ozone. *Time after exposure. †Time after conclusion of exercise challenge. (Courtesy of Weymer AR, Gong H Jr, Lyness A, et al: *Am J Respir Crit Care Med* 149:1413-1419, 1994.)

Moving?

I'd like to receive my *Year Book of Sports Medicine* without interruption.
Please note the following change of address, effective:

Name: _____

New Address: _____

_____

City: _____ State: _____ Zip: _____

Old Address: _____

_____

City: _____ State: _____ Zip: _____

Reservation Card

Yes, I would like my own copy of *Year Book of Sports Medicine*. Please begin my subscription with the current edition according to the terms described below.* I understand that I will have 30 days to examine each annual edition. If satisfied, I will pay just $68.95 plus sales tax, postage and handling (price subject to change without notice).

Name: _____

Address: _____

City: _____ State: _____ Zip: _____

Method of Payment
○ Visa   ○ Mastercard   ○ AmEx   ○ Bill me   ○ Check (in US dollars, payable to Mosby, Inc.)

Card number: _____ Exp date: _____

Signature: _____

LS-0909

*Your *Year Book* Service Guarantee:

When you subscribe to the *Year Book*, we'll send you an advance notice of future volumes about two months before they publish. This automatic notice system is designed to take up as little of your time as possible. If you do not want the *Year Book*, the advance notice makes it quick and easy for you to let us know your decision, and you will always have at least 20 days to decide. If we don't hear from you, we'll send you the new volume as soon as it's available. And, of course, the *Year Book* is yours to examine free of charge for 30 days (postage, handling and applicable sales tax are added to each shipment.).

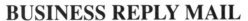

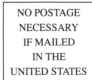
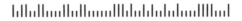

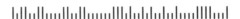

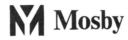 **Mosby**

Dedicated to publishing excellence

alone. In addition, 12 subjects underwent exposure to 0.40 ppm of ozone in FA. The subjects performed intermittent light exercise in an environmentally controlled chamber. After each exposure, they rested for 1 hour in a clean-air environment and performed serial postexposure spirometry. A standardized exercise challenge in clean air was then performed, followed by serial spirometry for 1 hour.

Findings.—There were no significant changes in FEV_1 or forced vital capacity (FVC) after 1-hour exposures to 0, 0.10, and 0.25 ppm of ozone. The 12 subjects who underwent all 4 exposures had a significant excess decrease in FEV_1 after a 1-hour exposure to 0.40 ppm of ozone, regardless of the EIA status. Within 1 hour, postexposure FEV_1 returned to baseline levels. The postexposure changes in FVC had a similar magnitude and time course, but they were not statistically significant across exposure conditions or EIA status. Increasing the levels of ozone did not produce significant differences in the FEV_1 response to postexposure exercise challenges (Fig 6–12).

Conclusion.—One-hour preexposure to ozone does not enhance or produce EIA in patients with mild asthma. The acute effect of 0.40 ppm of ozone on FEV_1 did not sensitize the airways to produce greater exercise-induced airflow obstruction. The ozone-induced effects on airway mechanics do not appear to be additive or synergistic with exercise-related responses in patients with asthma.

▶ Exposure to the concentrations of ozone encountered in many large cities can induce a sensation of tightness in the chest, a decrease of forced expiratory volumes, and a limitation of exercise ventilation, with an associated decrease in maximal oxygen intake and physical performance. At the cellular level, there is also a recruitment of neutrophils to the bronchial tract and a release of prostaglandins. Thus, some interaction between ozone and asthma might be anticipated. Our research has, in fact, suggested that subjects with asthma show slightly greater pulmonary function and airway resistance changes than do healthy individuals when they exercise vigorously during ozone exposure (1), although the interaction between asthma and ozone response is relatively small.

Presumably, whether an interactive effect is detected depends on the severity of the asthmatic condition, the intensity of the ozone exposure, and the ventilation reached during exposure. In the study by Weymer et al., the FEV_1 of the asthmatics was normal, although the subjects with EIA had an enhanced response to methacholine; furthermore, the subjects performed only very mild exercise (walking at 2.4 km/hr) while they were exposed to the ozone; in consequence, the ventilation (20–30 L/min) remained below the threshold for mouth breathing. This is in contrast to our experiments, in which the subjects performed vigorous exercise in the exposure chamber.—R.J. Shephard, M.D., Ph.D., D.P.E.

Reference

1. Folinsbee L: Exercise and air pollution, in: Torg J, Shephard RJ, (eds): *Current Therapy in Sports Medicine, ed. 3.* Philadelphia, Mosby, 1995.

Sickle Cell Trait Performance in a Prolonged Race at High Altitude

Thiriet P, Le Hesran JY, Wouassi D, Bitanga E, Gozal D, Louis FJ (Natl Inst for Youth and Sports of Yaoundé, Cameroon; Université, Lyon 1, France; Organisation de Coordination pour la Lutte Contre les Endémies en Afrique Centrale, Yaoundé, Cameroon; et al)
Med Sci Sports Exerc 26:914–918, 1994   139-95-6–29

Background.—Among individuals of African descent, sickle cell trait is a frequent genetic abnormality. Physiologic studies conducted during either aerobic or anaerobic exercise have failed to support the implication of sickle cell trait as a risk factor for increased morbidity and mortality related to exertion. The aerobic exercise capacity of athletes with sickle cell trait was evaluated in naturally occurring, hypobaric hypoxic conditions.

Methods.—The performance of African runners with sickle cell trait was evaluated in the International Mount Cameroon Ascent race. The 34.1-km race is run over difficult terrain with slopes ranging from 7% to 40% and altitudes varying from 615 to 4,095 m above sea level.

Results.—Thirty-three of the 266 Cameroonian runners had sickle cell trait. Overall, mean performance times were higher for runners with sickle cell trait compared with non–sickle cell trait runners, but the differences were not statistically significant. Runners with sickle cell trait had significantly lower performance times measured after reaching the third portion of the race, that is, after arrival at an altitude of 3,800 m, including the peak crossing, and returning to 3,800 m (T3). This difference remained when athletes with sickle cell trait were matched with non–sickle cell trait athletes for performance times in the first portion of the race (to 2,700 m). Three runners with sickle cell trait were among the first 50 racers to reach T3, but no runners with sickle cell trait were among the first 50 runners to complete T3.

Conclusion.—Sickle cell trait is probably associated with an inherent susceptibility to hypoxia that may induce significant reductions during prolonged aerobic performance, particularly under hypobaric conditions. Further studies are needed to confirm these preliminary findings.

▶ Although rare athletes with sickle cell trait (SCT) are prone to sickling and collapse during heroic exercise when new to altitude (1), debate continues as to whether SCT limits endurance performance. Young athletes in Cameroon have the expected prevalence of SCT, suggesting that it does not limit performance (2). Champion runners in the Ivory Coast also have the expected prevalence of SCT, but runners with SCT seem to be underrepresented among winners of the longest races (3). Similarly, typical runners in an Ivory Coast semimarathon have the expected prevalence of SCT, but internationally ranked runners tend not to have SCT (4).

This study also suggests that, at least at altitude, SCT limits racing performance. In the Bakoueri tribe, where winning races confers social status, runners with SCT are underrepresented. Also, in the altitude part of the race (and *only* in the altitude part) runners with SCT slow down more than do non-SCT runners. Probably, in rare athletes in rare settings—especially at altitude—SCT limits performance and poses a risk of sickling, collapse, and death.—E.R. Eichner, M.D.

References

1. 1994 YEAR BOOK OF SPORTS MEDICINE, pp 413–415.
2. Thiriet P, et al: *Med Sci Sports Exerc* 23:389, 1991.
3. Le Gallais D, et al: *Int J Sports Med* 12:509, 1991.
4. Le Gallais D, et al: *Int J Sports Med* 15:399, 1994.

Mechanisms of Reduced Pulmonary Function After a Saturation Dive

Thorsen E, Segadal K, Kambestad BK (Norwegian Underwater Technology Centre A/S, Ytre Ladsevåg, Norway)
Eur Respir J 7:4–10, 1994   139-95-6–30

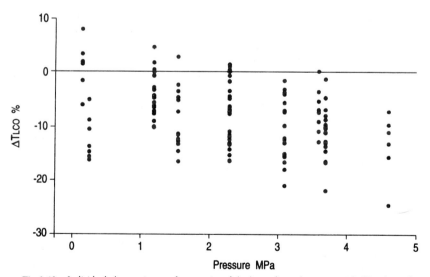

Fig 6–13.—Individual changes in transfer capacity of the lungs for carbon monoxide (T_{LCO}) in relation to maximal pressure of the dives. (Courtesy of Thorsen E, Segadal K, Kambestad BK: *Eur Respir J* 7:4–10, 1994.)

Objective.—Seventeen different saturation diving operations to depths of 5–450 m of sea water were studied to assess the relative contributions of various factors to the effects of such dives on pulmonary function. Divers using the saturation technique are compressed to the pressure correponding to the working depth in a hyperbaric chamber complex.

Methods.—Four to 15 divers participated in each operation, descending to pressures of 0.15 to 4.5 MPa. In all dives to pressures of 1.2 MPa or more, the atmospheres were helium and oxygen mixtures. The dive to 0.25 MPa used a mixture of helium, nitrogen, and oxygen, and the dive to 0.15 MPa used a mixture of nitrogen and oxygen. The partial pressure of oxygen never exceeded 21% of total pressure. The duration of the isopression phase ranged from 3.5 to 27.75 days, and that of the decompression phase from 0.25 to 18 days. The 90 divers had a median age of 32 years and a median body mass of 79 kg. Measurements obtained included static and dynamic lung volumes and flows, transfer factor of the lungs for carbon monoxide (TLCO), and closing volume.

Results.—The dives caused a significant reduction in TLCO and carbon monoxide transfer coefficient (KCO), together with an increase in static lung volume and closing volume. The mean reduction in TLCO after the dives was 8.3% (Fig 6–13), a change that correlated with cumulative hyperoxic exposure and load of venous gas microembolism, independently of each other. Increases in closing volume and reductions in forced midexpiratory flow rate correlated with culmulative hyperoxic exposure. A correlation was also observed between increases in total lung capacity and cumulative hyperbaric exposure. Changes in lung function variables showed no correlation with any of the divers' characteristics.

Conclusion.—Saturation diving exposes the diver to various factors that are potentially harmful to the lungs. The exposure variables, cumulative hyperoxic and hyperbaric exposure, and load of venous gas microemboli all exhibited a strong correlation with maximal pressure. The strongest correlation was that between the change in lung function variables and the hyperoxic exposure. There is a need for hyperoxic exposure and decompression stress to be reduced in the diving procedure.

▶ Many years ago, I worked at the Royal Air Force Institute of Aviation Medicine. The military aircraft were only lightly pressurized, if at all, and the aircrew breathed pure oxygen over many hours on long bombing missions. It was soon appreciated that far from being an innocuous aid to flight, the oxygen was leading to collapse of the lungs and a decrease of pulmonary diffusing capacity.

In the saturation dives discussed here, the percentage of oxygen is relatively low; however, because of the high ambient pressures underwater, the partial pressure of oxygen reaching the lungs can be as high as 100% oxygen at sea level. As in our aviators of many years ago, the lung reaction seems to involve a collapse of the airways (shown by a high closing volume) and a decrease of diffusing capacity. The authors express the toxic dose of oxygen as an integral above the normal ambient pressure of 21 kPa. Typically, an exposure of 300–600 kPa/day causes a 10% loss of resting diffusing capacity, although the threshold pressure for an adverse response is an excess pressure of only 30–40 kPa (1). When breathing compressed air, this threshold for oxygen toxicity is reached at a depth of only 15–20 m, although the recreational diver does not usually remain at this depth long enough for manifestations of oxygen damage to build up. A further factor that may contribute to the impairment of gas exchange in the divers is a trapping of small gas bubbles in the pulmonary circulation.—R.J. Shephard, M.D., Ph.D., D.P.E.

Reference

1. Harabin AL, et al: *J Appl Physiol* 63:1130, 1987.

Role of Cardiorespiratory Abnormalities, Smoking and Dive Characteristics in the Manifestations of Neurological Decompression Illness
Wilmshurst P, Davidson C, O'Connell G, Byrne C (St Thomas' Hosp, London)
Clin Sci 86:297–303, 1994   139-95-6–31

Background.— The most serious manifestations of decompression illness are neurologic. A group of amateur divers in whom neurologic symptoms developed within 5 minutes of surfacing were investigated for the role of cardiopulmonary abnormalities, including a history of smoking, in the etiology of their decompression illness.

Methods.— During a 4-year period and using a variety of outreach methods, a group of amateur divers who had experienced decompression illness were recruited. All were evaluated, under blinded conditions, using contrast echocardiography and spirometry.

Results.— One hundred twenty-nine divers were evaluated. Of those without intracardiac shunts, pulmonary abnormalities were significantly more frequent than in those divers with shunts. Smoking also tended to be more common among those without shunts (55% vs. 15%, not significant). Those divers without intracardiac shunts had cerebral, as opposed to spinal, symptoms after dives that were significantly more shallow and had significantly lower tissue nitrogen loads. Clinical manifestations in divers with shunts resembled those observed after rapid ascent with missed decompression stops.

Conclusion.— Systemic gas embolism caused by occult lung disease or paradoxical gas embolism may be responsible for early-onset neurologic symptoms among divers having decompression illness. Smoking may contribute to this pathology, and smokers at risk for decompression illness should be tested for small airway disease.

▶ Classic decompression sickness relates to the liberation of dissolved nitrogen as bubbles in the tissues. However, a further source of pathology is overdistention of the lungs, with a rupture of the pulmonary vessels that allows entry of air into the vasculature during a rapid ascent (1). If gas enters directly into the venous circulation, there is a potential for death resulting from cerebral gas embolism. If there is a right-to-left intracardiac shunt, a level of nitrogen bubble formation that would otherwise have been filtered out by the lungs may also cause fatal complications.

In this study by Wilmshurst and colleagues, 36 of 129 cases of decompression sickness developed within 5 minutes of surfacing. In 12 of these patients, the cause seemed to be pulmonary barotrauma with too rapid a rate of ascent, and among the remaining 24 cases, 13 had intracardiac shunts. Lung function tests were performed on 10 of the final 11 subjects, and they proved abnormal in 5 cases. It is on this somewhat slender basis that the authors suggest the etiologic role of small airway disease in predisposing to pulmonary barotrauma.—R.J. Shephard, M.D., Ph.D., D.P.E.

Reference

1. Shephard RJ: *Physiology and Biochemistry of Exercise.* New York, Praeger Publications, 1982.

Marine Injuries: Prevention and Treatment
Frey C (Univ of Southern California, Los Angeles)
Orthop Rev 23:645–649, 1994   139-95-6-32

Purpose.—Common sources of seaside foot injuries were reviewed, together with methods of prevention and treatment of the most common injuries.

Foreign Body Injuries.—Fishing hooks, splinters, glass, sharp stones, and tar can be encountered on beaches and be the source of an injury. The most common foreign body is a wood splinter, and it most often is easily removed with a fine-pointed forceps. Asymptomatic foreign bodies need not be removed but should be if they are acute or become problematic. Locating the object may be difficult, requiring an image intensifier, radiographs, or a metal detector. No matter the type of foreign body, tetanus immunization status should be assessed and a tetanus shot given if the immunization is not current. Prophylactic antibiotics should be given if indicated.

Sea Urchin Wounds.—Stepping on the spines of a sea urchin can result in painful ulceration and erythema, sometimes accompanied by neurotoxic symptoms of weakness and paralysis of the lips, tongue, and face lasting for a few hours. Treatment should be supportive and directed toward the symptoms. Surgery is recommended if the spines remain in the skin.

Coral Wounds.—Many species of coral cause painful stings because of the microscopic nematocysts they contain. More serious wounds are caused by abrasions from the sharp skeleton. Coral wounds should be cleansed immediately with copious amounts of water to promptly and completely débride the wound.

Fish and Stingray Stings.—Over 200 venomous species of marine fish are known, and most are found inshore or in shallow-water reefs. General principles of treatment are those for any poisonous sting or bite: alleviate pain, combat the effects of venom, and prevent secondary infection. Stingray injuries are the most serious because the wound may be extensive and may result in significant bleeding. The venom affects the cardiovascular, respiratory, and neurologic systems, resulting in a range of symptoms including peripheral dilation, cardiac arrhythmias, convulsions, and respiratory depression. Wounds inflicted by venomous fish should be treated immediately with thorough irrigation with saline solutions, excision of any stingers, and soaking of the injured limb in hot water for 30 minutes to 1 hour. Intravenous calcium gluconate may be needed to relieve muscle spasms, and local infiltration of 0.5% to 2% procaine may provide pain relief. Tetanus immunizations should be current, and surgical excision of necrosed tissue may be necessary.

Infection.—A puncture wound from marine life or an abrasion in contaminated water may result in infection with *Mycobacterium marinum*. This atypical acid-fast bacillus may be sensitive to ethionamide, ethambutol, rifampin, or cycloserine but is resistant to the usual antituberculin drugs.

Conclusion.—Prevention through education regarding the possible hazards and the wearing of proper beach footwear—reef walkers, sandals, or sneakers—is the best treatment for marine foot injuries.

▶ This is a comprehensive review dealing with penetrating wounds, stings, and venom inoculation that commonly occur to unwary sand and sea walkers during the summer season. The recommendation that beach walkers wear sandals or sneakers seems to be simply a matter of common sense.—J.S. Torg, M.D.

Heat Exhaustion in the Sun-Herald City to Surf Fun Run
Lyle DM, Lewis PR, Richards DAB, Richards R, Bauman AE, Sutton JR, Cameron ID (NSW Health Dept, North Sydney, Australia; NSW Health Dept, Newcastle, Australia; Westmead Hosp, Australia; et al)
Med J Aust 161:361–365, 1994   139-95-6–33

Objective.—The incidence of exercise-induced heat exhaustion and potentially fatal heat stroke in "fun runs" is higher in less-experienced racers. Medical organizers of the 14-km Sun-Herald City to Surf fun run in Sydney, Australia, reported that the runners in whom heat exhaustion develops are more likely to be amateur male athletes, aged 20–39 years, who are not conditioned for the competition. The motivational reasons and the physiologic factors leading to heat exhaustion were examined.

Methods.—Attitudinal questionnaires were mailed to 79 runners who experienced heat exhaustion and 310 control racers within 3 days after the race. Response rates were 81% for those with heat exhaustion and 71% for controls.

Results.—Major risk factors for heat exhaustion included high motivation, failure to acclimatize, failure to drink fluids during the race, and a history of heat exhaustion. More than 1 risk factor accounted for 52% of heat exhaustion cases and 1 risk factor accounted for 36%. In the control group, the corresponding figures were 17% and 42%.

Conclusion.—The incidence of heat exhaustion can possibly be decreased by identifying those runners with high-risk behavior and appropriately modifying that behavior.

▶ The American College of Sports Medicine states that those especially prone to heat exhaustion are the obese, the unfit, the young, the old, the dehydrated, those not acclimatized to the heat, those with a previous history of heat exhaustion, and anyone who runs while ill. But at races like the one studied here, most victims of heat exhaustion are young men who try too hard and take chances. Fortunately, the attack rate of heat exhaustion in this race tends to be low, about 0.14%. This study explores attitudes and habits that predispose to heat exhaustion. Unlike findings in some other studies, novice runners were not especially prone to heat exhaustion; nor were alcohol, lack of sleep, or recent viral infection clear risk factors here. Rather, the 4 major risk factors were a history of heat exhaustion, urge to improve, not acclimatizing, and not drinking fluids during the race (see Abstract 139-95-6–34). It seems that these young men know the risks for heat exhaustion but ignore them. They're immortal, of course.—E.R. Eichner, M.D.

Hematological, Electrolyte, and Biochemical Alterations After a 100-km Run

Rama R, Ibáñez J, Riera M, Prats MT, Pagés T, Palacios L (Univ of Barcelona)
Can J Appl Physiol 19:411–420, 1994   139-95-6–34

Objective.—Little information is available regarding the physiologic effects of long-distance races. The hematologic and enzymatic effects of ultra–long-distance running were measured.

Methods.—Seven experienced male long-distance runners 27–41 years of age were studied before and after a 100-km race. Runners were weighed, venous blood samples were taken, and plasma volume was calculated. Potassium, sodium, plasma glucose, urea, and creatinine concentrations were determined.

Results.—The runners' body weight decreased significantly after the race. The only hematologic parameter to change significantly was hematocrit, which was increased after the race. Leukocytes, neutrophils, lymphocytes, and monocytes increased significantly. Sodium and potassium

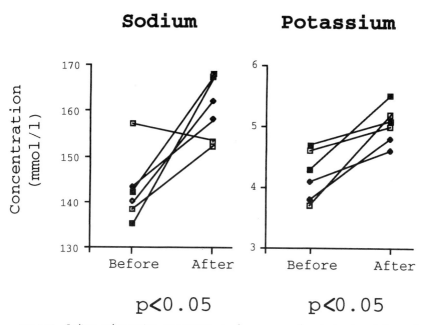

Fig 6–14.—Sodium and potassium concentration in plasma expressed as single values, before and after the 100-km race. (Courtesy of Rama R, Ibáñez J, Riera M, et al: *Can J Appl Physiol* 19:411-420, 1994.)

levels (Fig 6–14) increased significantly (13% and 22%, respectively), whereas plasma volume decreased by only 5.7%. Plasma lactate concentrations tripled. The creatinine concentration increased by 60% and urea increased by 37% (Fig 6–15). Creatine kinase increased significantly.

Conclusion.—Of all the changes observed after ultra–long-distance running, the increase in extracellular potassium is the most worrisome because hyperkalemia has been shown to inhibit the sodium channels of heart muscle.

▶ This study shows what well-trained runners can get away with, even if it is not prudent. They raced 100 km on a warm day, with a mean racing time of 10 hours. Yet they drank barely more than 3 L of fluid on average and lost a mean of nearly 5% of body weight. Figure 6–14 shows that, just as drinking too much water can cause hyponatremia (see Abstract 139-95-6–35), drinking too little can cause hypernatremia. The hyperkalemia immediately after the end of the race is not as ominous as the authors seem to suggest. As they point out, an increase in plasma potassium during exercise is well known and related to the intensity of the exercise; contracting muscles are likely the main source of this potassium. When exercise ends, plasma potassium rapidly—within minutes—declines to normal, because of re-uptake of released potassium by potassium-depleted muscles.—E.R. Eichner, M.D.

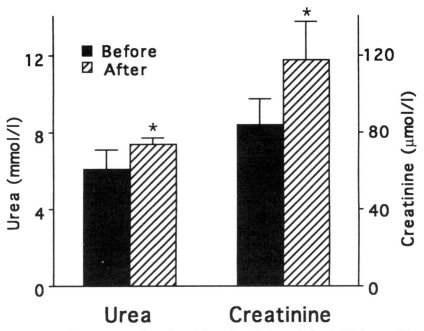

Fig 6–15.—Plasma concentrations of creatinine and urea before and after the 100-km race. *P < 0.05. (Courtesy of Rama R, Ibáñez J, Riera M, et al: *Can J Appl Physiol* 19:411–420, 1994.)

Clinical and Biochemical Characteristics of Collapsed Ultramarathon Runners
Holtzhausen L-M, Noakes TD, Kroning B, De Klerk M, Roberts M, Emsley R (Univ of Cape Town, South Africa; Univ of Stellenbosch, South Africa)
Med Sci Sports Exerc 26:1095–1101, 1994   139-95-6–35

Introduction.—Exercise-associated collapse (EAC) occurs frequently in endurance events lasting more than 2 hours. It is not in itself a diagnosis; rather it describes a main complaint characterized by the inability to stand or walk unaided as a result of light-headedness, faintness, dizziness, or syncope. The true nature of this condition is unknown.

Objectives.—During a 56-km ultramarathon footrace run on a cool day in Cape Town, South Africa, the clinical and biochemical characteristics of runners with EAC were studied, and the roles of dehydration, postural hypotension, and hypoglycemia in its pathogenesis were examined.

Methods.—The time of onset of collapse, rectal temperature, cardiovascular status, and the incidence of readily identifiable medical conditions were compared in male athletes who collapsed and those who did not who were running in the same race. Weight changes during recovery were studied in a subgroup of runners.

Results.—Forty-six male runners experienced EAC, including 38 who collapsed after they had completed the race. Identifiable medical conditions were present in all 8 runners who collapsed before finishing the race (100%), significantly more often than in runners who collapsed at the race's finish (34%). Among the runners who collapsed after the finish line, the rectal temperature (mean, 38.5°C) and supine heart rate (mean, 87.5/min) were only modestly elevated. There was a high but equal incidence of abnormal biochemical and clinical findings in runners experiencing EAC and control runners. The postrace concentrations of sodium and changes in plasma volume and mass during recovery did not differ significantly between groups. Although serum concentrations of urea and creatinine were higher in runners who collapsed after the race, there were no distinguishing biochemical characteristics that indicated the likely nature of this condition.

Discussion.—The majority of runners in endurance events who collapse do so after finishing the race, and all runners who collapse before finishing the race have identifiable medical conditions. Because runners collapse more frequently near cutoff times for medals and race closure, it is possible that extreme physical effort, perhaps beyond the capabilities and training status of the participants, may play a role in the etiology of EAC. It is likely that EAC is a syncopal episode resulting from postural hypotension caused by a sudden cessation of exercise and loss of the skeletal muscle pump in the lower extremities. Other factors—such as mild dehydration, excessive racing effort, and a training-induced reduction in the vasoconstrictor response to any hypotensive stress—may contribute to EAC.

▶ This study shows that, in a very long race on a cool day, most (85%) of the runners who collapse do so after crossing the finish line, often having made a supreme effort to make a cutoff time. They tend to have normal cardiovascular status while supine and are not notably dehydrated or hyperthermic. They seem "benign" medically and respond to leg elevation and oral fluids. The thesis is that this form of EAC is syncope from venous pooling after the cessation of running. The authors are probably right, but they exaggerate the risk of giving 1–2 L of IV normal saline solution (NSS).

In a prior study by this group, runners with EAC (who *were* slightly more dehydrated than controls) were randomized to receive either oral fluids or IV D5 NSS. Although the IV fluid caused temporary hyponatremia and hyperglycemia, there were no adverse clincal results (1). In fact, most reported cases of grave hyponatremia seem to stem from the massive amounts (up to 12 L) of water or other hypotonic fluids the racers drink *on the course*, not from the 1–2 L of NSS they get intravenously *in the tent*. The upshot: In a very long race on a cool day, most runners with EAC may not need IV fluids, but in a shorter race on a very hot day, beware of dehydration and heat stroke, and be ready to use IV NSS for EAC.—E.R. Eichner, M.D.

Reference

1. 1992 YEAR BOOK OF SPORTS MEDICINE, pp 143–145.

Sport-Specific Conditioning
Kibler WB, Chandler TJ (Lexington Clinic Sports Medicine Ctr, Ky)
Am J Sports Med 22:424–432, 1994   139-95-6–36

Introduction.—Conditioning programs for enhancing sports performance are widely used, but the basic principles of conditioning are commonly misunderstood or misapplied. Sport-specific conditioning programs seek to prepare the athlete for the unique stresses, metabolic demands, and injury risks of the athlete's particular sport. The objectives, components, and basic physiology of sport-specific conditioning programs, including the principles of the periodization model—the most scientifically based framework for effective sport-specific conditioning—were reviewed.

Objectives of Sport-Specific Conditioning.—To optimize athletic fitness for a particular sport, the conditioning program should meet several objectives in sequential order, from general to specific: attainment of general athletic fitness, refinement of the general fitness components to achieve sport-specific athletic fitness, and development of the level of aerobic or anaerobic endurance needed for the particular sport (Fig 6-16). Each goal must be met to avoid problems in the conditioning process. Today's conditioning programs emphasize preventing or reducing injury, especially repetitive microtrauma or overload injuries, more

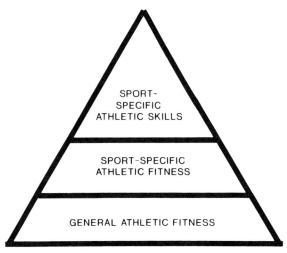

Fig 6–16.—General athletic fitness as the base on which sport-specific athletic fitness and skills are built. (Courtesy of Kibler WB, Chandler TJ: *Am J Sports Med* 22:424–432, 1994.)

than improving athletic performance. The development of smaller antagonistic muscle groups is emphasized to provide force regulation or balance around a joint. The most effective way to meet the goals of sport-specific conditioning is the periodized conditioning program. The athlete's entry level of fitness, determined by the preconditioning evaluation, determines the best course of conditioning for sport-specific athletic fitness.

Periodization.—The concept of periodization is based on manipulating the volume and intensity of work performed during various periods of the athletic season. The length of the phases varies from sport to sport, but each phase includes different amounts of general fitness, sport-specific fitness, and skill work. In the active rest phase, which takes place immediately after the competitive season, the athlete rests completely for 1 or 2 days and then participates in physical activities not directly related to the primary sport. In the off-season, or general preparation, phase, the body is prepared for more intense training. The focus is on general athletic fitness, with general flexibility exercises, heavy weight training, and running or other appropriate aerobic work. This is followed by the preseason, or specific preparation, phase, in which the athlete follows a course of high-intensity, sport-specific work. General fitness drills continue at a reduced volume while sport-specific skills are practiced and refined. Conditioning for sports with a long season may include an early in-season, or early competitive, phase in which conditioning remains high but not maximal. The late in-season, or peaking, phase aims at maximal efficiency of performance for intense competition. Condititoning work is minimized to focus on sport-speccific flexibility and light weight training.

Summary.—Well-designed sport-specific conditioning programs can achieve the twin goals of optimizing performance and minimizing injury risk. The soundest scientific basis for these programs is the periodization model, in which the goals of conditioning change according to the phase of the athletic season.

▶ This is a very good article describing sport-specific conditioning. An ideal program can and should be designed to optimize performance and decrease injuries. The program must be adhered to and monitored closely.

R.I. Moss, in his comments on this article, makes some very timely and important observations. He does not believe that sport-specific conditioning programs are properly utilized. Coaches resort to programs they are familiar with and, in fact, some may become "overzealous proponents of the doctrine 'if a little sports-specific conditioning is good then a megadose is better.' Typical overuse injuries can occur very easily in such an environment (1)."

A good scientific basis for conditioning programs that improve performance and decrease injuries has been designed. These programs must be monitored closely and changed when necessary to meet the goals that have been set. This is not an easy task, especially with large teams and large groups of athletes. Programs must be individualized and supervised constantly for safety and improvement of performance.—F.J. George, A.T.C., P.T.

Reference

1. Moss RI: *Athletic Train: Sports Health Care Perspect* Vol. 1, No. 1, pp 80–81.

Call Mosby Document Express at **1 (800) 55-MOSBY** to obtain copies of the original source documents of articles featured or referenced in the YEAR BOOK series.

---

7 Women and Aging

Peak Torque Occurrence in the Range of Motion During Isokinetic Extension and Flexion of the Knee

Kannus P, Beynnon B (Univ of Vermont, Burlington)

Int J Sports Med 14:422–426, 1993   139-95-7–1

Introduction.—Peak torque, the most frequently used variable in the measurement of muscular performance, refers to the single highest torque output of a joint produced by muscular contraction as a limb moves through its range of motion. During isokinetic movement, the maximum torque position may be affected by the movement's angular velocity. The knee angles of hamstring and quadriceps peak torques at the 2 most commonly used isokinetic velocities were characterized to determine if the increment in velocity has a quantitative transfer effect on the knee angles of extension and flexion peak torques. Whether the results were affected by the participants' gender, age, or muscular strength was also examined.

Results.—Participants included 143 healthy men and 106 healthy women. The Cybex II dynamometer (Lumex, Inc., Ronkonkoma, NY) was used to record the measurements. Hamstring mean peak torque occurred at 33 degrees for men and 37 degrees for women at a velocity of 60 degrees/sec and at 40 degrees for men and 44 degrees for women at a velocity of 180 degrees/sec, an increase of 7 degrees in both groups. The peak torque angle of the quadriceps was 54 degrees for both men and women at a velocity of 60 degrees/sec, but at 180 degrees/sec the angle occurred significantly later in both men and women (11 and 10 degrees later, respectively). The effect of subject age was not significant. Sex proved significant only in that the hamstrings of women displayed peak torque angles that occurred later in the range of motion when muscle strength was decreased.

Conclusion.—Increasing angular velocity did cause hamstring and quadriceps peak torques to occur later in the range of motion. This occurs to a greater extent when testing less powerful muscle groups, such as the hamstrings of women; this may explain the difference observed between the peak torque angles of the hamstring in men and women. A problem may occur in isokinetic testing at high angular velocities because the limb may pass the optimal joint position for muscular performance, and the peak torque recorded may not represent the subject's maximal torque capacity.

▶ Again, the differences in results between women and men do not surprise me. Over 20 years or more, our testing here at West Point has produced more differences than likenesses when we have compared physical performance between men and women. These authors used only young, healthy subjects in this research. They state that further research is needed to measure the findings in different states of knee pathology, especially in knee ligament instabilities and patellofemoral pain states.—Col. J.L. Anderson, PE.D.

Sex Differences in Surface EMG Interference Pattern Power Spectrum

Cioni R, Giannini F, Paradiso C, Battistini N, Navona C, Starita A (Univ of Siena, Italy; Univ of Pisa, Italy)
J Appl Physiol 77:2163–2168, 1994   139-95-7–2

Objective.—Sex differences in maximal voluntary contraction have been observed in the surface electromyelogram power density spectrum. An attempt was made to verify those results and to establish normative data for men and women.

Methods.—The maximal voluntary contraction of the tibialis anterior muscle of 15 healthy men and 15 healthy women, aged 24–42 years, was determined from electromyelographic measurements.

Results.—The mean torque values for women were 33.9% lower than for men. There was a nonlinear increase in median power frequency

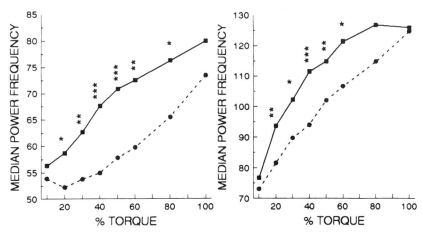

Fig 7–1.—Median power frequency (in Hz) in women (*solid circles*) and men (*solid squares*) for different torque values. An electromyographic signal was recorded with unipolar (**left**) and bipolar (**right**) leads. Significant difference between male and female study subjects: *P < 0.05; **P < 0.01; ***P < 0.001. (Courtesy of Cioni R, Giannini F, Paradiso C, et al: *J Appl Physiol* 77:2163–2168, 1994.)

with an increase in torque using both leads, although this increase was smaller for women (Fig 7–1).

Conclusion.—The significantly lower median power frequency seen in women is probably caused by the smaller muscle fiber size.

▶ The fact that these authors found differences in motor performance between male and female subjects is no surprise to me. Other authors have shown that women have a lower total number of muscle fibers of smaller size than do men, whereas the number of fast-twitch fibers is the same; in women, these fibers are distributed mainly on the ventral surface of the muscle. These authors also reveal significant differences in the spectral parameters of the sexes, which are probably correlated with anatomical differences reported by other researchers.—Col. J.L. Anderson, PE.D.

The Accuracy of the ACSM and a New Cycle Ergometry Equation for Young Women

Latin RW, Berg KE (Univ of Nebraska, Omaha)
Med Sci Sports Exerc 26:642–646, 1994   139-95-7–3

Background.—Many methods have been developed for estimating oxygen uptake during exercise. One method, the metabolic equations of the American College of Sports Medicine (ACSM), is widely used for exercise prescription and fitness evaluation. The ACSM cycle ergometry equation, used to predict the oxygen cost of cycle exercise, is $\dot{V}O_2$ (mL/min) = kg/min $\times$ 2 mL/kg + (3.5 mL/min $\times$ kg of body weight). However, no studies have examined the precision of this equation for

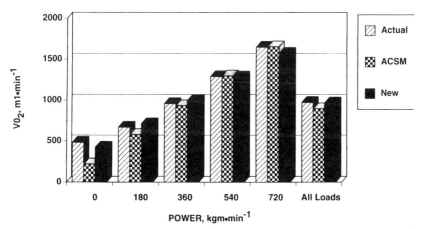

Fig 7–2.—Histogram of mean actual American College of Sports Medicine (ACSM) and a new equation predicted oxygen uptake ($\dot{V}O_2$) at each power load. (Courtesy of Latin RW, Berg KE: *Med Sci Sports Exerc* 26:642–646, 1994.)

women. The accuracy of the ACSM cycle ergometry equation was tested in healthy young women.

Methods.—The 60 research subjects, whose mean age was 26 years, underwent a 5-stage submaximal cycle ergometry test. The test progressed until the women reached 85% of their predicted maximum heart rate, using the formula of 220 minus the subject's age, or until they finished the final stage of the test. Steady-state oxygen consumption was measured to assess the accuracy of the ACSM equation and, if necessary, to develop a new equation based on an actual oxygen uptake–power relationship. The results were cross-validated in another sample of 40 similar young women.

Results.—The standard error of estimate for predicted oxygen consumption ranged from 79–156 mL/min. Total error ranged from 167 to 275 mL/min. The range of Pearson correlations between actual and predicted values was $r = -0.22$ to $r = 0.38$; only 1 correlation was significant. Regression analysis was used to develop a new equation, which was applied to the data. The associated correlations were almost identical to those from the ACSM equation. For all stages combined, the correlation of $r = 0.96$ between actual and predicted oxygen uptake remained the same, whereas the mean difference of -7 mL/min was lower. In the validation sample, all of the standard error of estimate and total error values were lower and all of the correlations were higher at each power load (Fig 7–2).

Conclusion.—A new cycle ergometry equation provides for more accurate depiction of the oxygen uptake–power relationship for women. The revised equation, which is based on an actual oxygen uptake–power relationship is $\dot{V}O_2$ (mL/min) = kg/min $\times$ 1.6 mL/kg + ((3.5 mL/kg/min $\times$ kg of body weight) + 205 mL/min). The revised equation includes 205 mL/min added to the intercept of the oxygen uptake estimate for resting metabolism.

▶ Perhaps the ACSM metabolic equations were based on the assumption that expressing oxygen uptake in milliliters per kilogram per minute and adding body weight to the prediction equation offset any differences in the response of men and women. According to these authors, the equation can be improved for both men and women. Actually, Figure 7–2 suggests the ACSM equation was quite accurate at all except the lowest loads and the new equation is not as accurate as the ACSM equation at the highest-power load. It will be interesting to see whether the "improved" equation works as well with older women, the group with whom it is most likely to be used.—B.L. Drinkwater, Ph.D.

Body Composition Assessment in Women: Special Considerations for Athletes

Oppliger RA, Cassady SL (Univ of Iowa, Iowa City; St Ambrose Univ, Daven-

port, Iowa)
Sports Med 17:353–357, 1994

139-95-7–4

Health Issues.—Many new methods are now available for evaluating body composition, but clinicians must remain aware of how the athlete or coach may interpret the findings and what the implications may be for the athlete's health. Areas of significant concern for young female athletes include menstrual dysfunction, which may include delayed puberty; osteoporosis; and eating disorders. The risk of disordered eating increases when an athlete becomes preoccupied with reaching a target weight or a certain level of body fat.

Clinical Interpretation.—Female athletes generally have below-average body fatness, but this is especially the case for those who engage in sports such as distance running and gymnastics where excess fat weight compromises performance. Published fatness values should not be arbitrarily accepted when evaluating a particular athlete, because of inherent measurement error and also the considerable variability among individual athletes. Muscle mass, as well as fat, is lost during extreme dieting, and this may adversely affect the athlete's performance. Summing skinfold thicknesses at multiple sites is a change-sensitive parameter, but it provides minimal normative information. However, it has the advantage of avoiding the psychological overtones associated with reporting fatness.

Measurement Issues.—Research is needed to explore differences in fat patterns between athletic populations as well as racial or ethnic differences. Bone is a significant part of the body's fat-free mass, and, as a result, altered bone mass may influence the density composition of the body. Prediction equations tend to err in the direction of the mean. For athletes who tend toward below-average fatness, these equations will tend to overestimate relative fatness.

Recommendations.—In general, body fatness should be maintained above a level of 12% to 14%. Body composition should be interpreted with reference to optimal performance rather than arbitrary criterion values. Standardized test protocols should be used.

▶ The misuse of body composition measures is all too frequent in some sports. Setting a standard percentage body fat target for all athletes on a team, as some coaches have done, ignores not only measurement error but individual variability as well. One athlete may be healthy and perform well at 14% body fat, whereas her teammate achieves her personal best at 20% body fat. Trying to "fool Mother Nature" and bring the body fat down to 14% could precipitate disordered eating, or even a serious eating disorder, in this young athlete. The authors review issues relating to measurement techniques and warn against a misuse of the results, which could put the athlete's health at risk.—B.L. Drinkwater, Ph.D.

Physiological and Physical Performance Changes in Female Runners During One Year of Training

Berg K, Latin RW, Hendricks T (Univ of Nebraska, Omaha)
Sports Med Train Rehabil 5:311–319, 1995   139-95-7–5

Objective.—Because few studies of trained female runners are available and most of them have been of limited duration, 7 women on a university cross-country and track team (average age, 19 years) were monitored physiologically over 1 year of training and competition.

Physiologic and Performance Changes During 1 Year of Training ($n = 7$)

Variable[a]	First Season			Second Season			Change %	*t* Ratio	p Level
	Mean	SD	Range	Mean	SD	Range			
Weight (kg)	52.7	6.5	45.7–64.0	53.3	6.6	46.3–63.7	1.1	1.36	0.22
Fat (%)	17.4	3.6	13.6–24.8	15.9	3.4	11.9–21.1	8.6	−0.48	0.65
VO_{2max} (mL·kg^{-1}·min^{-1})	53.4	4.1	47.8–60.0	53.9	3.8	50.4–60.3	0.9	0.53	0.62
Peak grade (%)	3.9	2.3	0.1–8.0	4.4	3.0	1–10.0	12.8	1.83	0.12
Speed at VT (mph)	8.1	0.4	8.0–9.0	8.2	0.3	7.5–8.5	1.2	0.14	0.89
Elapsed time at VO_{2max} (min)	1.7	0.8	2.0–3.0	2.6	1.3	1.0–4.0	52.9	2.79	0.03†
Economy (VO_2 at 201 m·min^{-1})	41.4	3.9	34.8–46.4	40.3	2.1	37.6–42.7	2.7	−1.02	0.35
5 km time (min)	22.1	1.3	19.6–24.0	21.1	1.6	19.1–23.2	4.5	−2.61	0.04†

[a]VO_{2max} represents maximal oxygen uptake.
†Significant at P ≤ 0.05.
(Courtesy of Berg K, Latin RW, Hendricks T: *Sports Med Train Rehabil* 5:311–319, 1995.)

Methods.—The training year extended from the end of 1 cross-country season to the end of a second season, when the athletes were likely to be in top condition. All participants trained indoors in the winter. Each year there were seven 5-km cross-country races, 7 indoor track meets, and 7 outdoor meets. The subjects ran distances ranging from 400 to 5,000 m. Running economy was estimated during peak aerobic power testing on a treadmill. Physical performance was based on the time needed to complete the same 5-km course at the same time each year.

Results.—The only significant changes that occurred were in elapsed time at peak aerobic power, which increased 5.3%, and the 5-km performance time, which improved 4.5% (table). Percentage of body fat, peak work rate, and peak aerobic power tended to improve but not to a significant degree. Physical performance correlated significantly with the peak treadmill grade and the speed at ventilation threshold. The percentage of body fat correlated with peak aerobic power, and running performance increased as body fat decreased.

Conclusion.—Cross-country running performance improves as body fat declines, but it does not require adaptations in peak aerobic power or ventilation threshold.

▶ One has to be very cautious these days in associating decreases in body fat or body weight with improvements in performance, as studies on eating disorders demonstrate. In this instance, there was a nonsignificant decrease in percentage of body fat, which amounted to 0.7 kg, and an increase of 1.3 kg in lean body mass. It is possible that the increase in lean mass rather than the decrease in fat mass was responsible for the improved performance? In this study, as well as others reviewed in this chapter, the sample size is small (n = 7). Although there are certainly occasions in which only a small number of subjects are available for a study, it would be helpful to the reader to know the statistical power of the test to put the results in perspective.—B.L. Drinkwater, Ph.D.

Effects of a 10-Week Step Aerobic Training Program on the Aerobic Power and Body Composition of College-Age Women

Porcari JP, Chapek CL, Huntley EL, Brice GA, Price S (Univ of Wisconsin, La Crosse)

Sports Med Train Rehabil 5:321–329, 1995   139-95-7–6

Background.—Step aerobics—stepping on and off a bench or platform as music plays—is an increasingly popular fitness activity. Often, it begins as a way of rehabilitating the knee and promoting quadriceps strength while, at the same time, maintaining cardiovascular function.

Objective and Methods.—The effects of 10 weeks of step aerobics training on aerobic power and body composition were examined in 66 women 18–25 years of age. Thirty enrolled in a university step aerobics class that met 3 times per week and involved exercising at 70% to 85% of the maximal predicted heart rate, as estimated by treadmill testing. The remaining 36 students served as a control group.

Results.—Final results were available for 21 exercising subjects and 28 controls. On average, 76% of maximal heart rate was maintained during aerobic training. Changes in body weight, lean body mass, fat weight, body fat, and body density were comparable in the exercising and control groups. Body fat decreased 0.6% in exercising research subjects and increased 0.4% in controls. Treadmill running time increased significantly more in the trained research subjects, who also had significant post-test increases in peak aerobic power and maximal minute ventilation.

Discussion.—The lack of change in body composition with aerobic step training in these women may reflect their initially low percentage of body fat (25.6%). The 12% increase in peak aerobic power is similar to that found in other studies of young women who engage in aerobic training, running, or cycling.

▶ The young women in this study must have been rather active before their participation in this study considering their $\dot{V}O_{2peak}$ values of 51.8 and 48.6 mL/kg/min for the control and experimental groups, respectively. Asking women with a $\dot{V}O_{2peak}$ of 51.8 ml/kg/min not to change their normal activity during the 10-week study does not ensure that they were less active than the control group. With a percentage body fat averaging 22.3% and 25.6% for the control and experimental groups, respectively, one might wonder why any decrease in body fat would be desirable. All of us these days have to be very careful in discussing exercise in relation to percentage body fat when obesity in not a problem. The primary purpose of an aerobics program is to increase aerobic power, which this program did. That is where the emphasis should be.—B.L. Drinkwater, Ph.D.

Postexercise Oxygen Consumption in Trained Females: Effect of Exercise Duration

Quinn TJ, Vroman NB, Kertzer R (Univ of New Hampshire, Durham)
Med Sci Sports Exerc 26:908–913, 1994   139-95-7–7

Background.—Many studies have reported the long-lasting elevation of metabolism after exercise. However, little is known about the impact of duration and intensity on this phenomenon. The effects of a constant walking intensity on the treadmill at various levels of duration on 3-hour recovery of oxygen uptake were investigated.

Method.—Eight healthy, well-trained women participated in the study. All had regular menstrual cycles and had trained for at least 1 year before the study. The women were requested to chart basal temperature on a

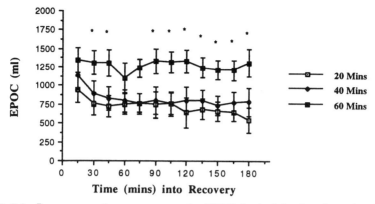

Fig 7–3.—Excess postexercise oxygen consumption (EPOC) for the 3 durations during the 3-hour postexercise recovery period. All 3 durations were significantly elevated compared with the preexercise period. *$P < 0.05$ (60-minute duration is significantly higher than those for 40 and 20 minutes). (Courtesy of Quinn TJ, Vroman NB, Kertzer R: *Med Sci Sports Exerc* 26:908–913, 1994.)

daily basis. The graphs provided the investigators with temperature information so that all testing could be performed during the follicular phase of the menstrual cycle at the lowest body temperature. The women reported to the laboratory for a maximal oxygen consumption test and returned on 4 additional occasions in random fashion. Treadmill speed and grade were measured to yield the appropriate intensity for each subject. After exercise, the women sat quietly for a 3-hour period. Variables measured every 15 minutes of recovery included maximal oxygen uptake ($\dot{V}O_{2max}$), minute ventilation ($\dot{V}_E$), respiratory exchange ratio (RER), heart rate (HR), systolic blood pressure (SBP), diastolic blood pressure (DBP), and core (rectal) temperature (T_c). Excess postexercise oxygen consumption (EPOC) was calculated by subtracting the resting $\dot{V}O_2$ from the absolute $\dot{V}O_2$ and summing the individual EPOCs during each 3-hour postexercise session and comparing these values with the preexercise values.

Results.—The EPOC was significantly increased in each of the 3 durations compared with the control (sitting) and preexercise periods (Fig 7–3). The total EPOC was significantly higher for the 60-minute duration (15.2 L) compared with the 20-minute duration (8.6 L) or 40-minute duration (9.8 L). This was seen without significant changes in $\dot{V}_E$, RER, HR, SBP, DBP, or T_c. Moreover, there were no differences during exercise across the 3 durations in $\dot{V}O_2$, $\dot{V}_E$, RER, HR, SBP, DBP, or T_c.

Conclusion.—There is a nonlinear relationship between exercise duration and excess postexercise oxygen consumption in endurance-trained females after moderate-intensity treadmill exercise. The EPOC is not accounted for by an increased rate of fat metabolism or an increased body temperature during the postexercise period. Further studies should examine circulating levels of catecholamines and cortisol and their impact on EPOC after bouts of exercise of varying intensity and duration.

▶ There remains a good deal of confusion regarding the type, intensity, and duration of exercise that is optimal for those who want to alter their body composition by decreasing body fat. One part of the equation is how best to elicit increased metabolic activity after cessation of activity. According to this study, walking 60 minutes rather than 20 or 40 minutes almost doubles the postexercise oxygen consumption. However, before recommending a 60-minute walk at 70% $\dot{V}O_{2max}$ to obese women, keep in mind that the subjects in this study were trained athletes with 16% body fat. Also, the results apply only during the follicular phase of the menstrual cycle. Although one can understand the scientific reasoning behind standardizing the phase of the cycle, limiting a study to 1 phase is not too helpful to women who progress through all phases each month. Perhaps the authors will repeat this protocol during the luteal phase so that we will learn whether cycle phase has any effect on the metabolic response.—B.L. Drinkwater, Ph.D.

Maximal Aerobic Capacity and Total Blood Volume in Highly Trained Middle-Aged and Older Female Endurance Athletes

Stevenson ET, Davy KP, Seals DR (Univ of Colorado, Boulder)
J Appl Physiol 77:1691–1696, 1994   139-95-7–8

Background.—Maximal aerobic capacity, as shown by the maximal rate of oxygen consumption ($\dot{V}O_{2max}$), is known to decline with age and results in a reduction in the maximal work rate that can be achieved during dynamic exercise performed with large muscle groups. The hypothesis that, relative to age-matched sedentary controls, highly trained middle-aged and older female Masters endurance athletes show similar levels of $\dot{V}O_{2max}$ to those previously reported in highly trained male endurance athletes was investigated. Whether the high levels of $\dot{V}O_{2max}$ observed in female athletes are associated with correspondingly greater levels of total blood volume was also studied.

Method.—Thirty healthy women participated in the study. Thirteen were endurance-trained athletes, aged between 49 and 67 years, and 17 were age-matched, nonobese sedentary-to-minimally active controls who did not follow any program of regular exercise. Twenty-nine of the women were postmenopausal, and 1 of the runners was premenopausal. The active women had been training for approximately 18 years, running around 31 miles per week, and most performed at least 1 hour of high-intensity exercise daily. The $\dot{V}O_{2max}$ was measured during a constant-speed protocol: controls walked at a brisk pace, and runners ran at 75% to 85% of their 10-km race pace. For both groups, the treadmill grade was increased 2.5% every 2 minutes; the test continued until volitional exhaustion. Plasma volume was measured in all the runners and in 14 of the 17 controls after a 12-hour fast using a modified Evans blue dye

Maximal Exercise Responses

	$\dot{V}O_{2\ max}$		$ml \cdot kg\ FFM^{-1} \cdot min^{-1}$	RER_{max}	HR_{max}, beats/min	$\dot{V}E_{max}$ BTPS, l/min
	l/min	$ml \cdot kg^{-1} \cdot min^{-1}$				
Runners	2.70±0.08*	48.6±1.9*	58.0±1.8*	1.19±0.02	167±3†	116.4±3.7*
Controls	1.74±0.06	26.5±0.8	38.8±1.2	1.19±0.01	177±2	81.1±2.9

Note: Values are means ± standard error for 13 runners and 17 controls.
* $P < 0.001$ vs. controls.
† $P < 0.01$ vs. controls.
Abbreviations: $\dot{V}O_{2\ max}$, maximal rate of O_2 consumption; RER_{max}, respiratory exchange ratio at maximal exercise; HR_{max}, maximal heart rate; $V_{E\ max}$, minute expired ventilation at maximal exercise; FFM, fat-free mass.
(Courtesy of Stevenson ET, Davy KP, Seals DR: *J Appl Physiol* 77:1691–1696, 1994.)

technique. Body fat was assessed by using the sum of skinfolds measured at 5 body sites.

Results.—The runners were found to have lower body weight, body mass index, and estimated body fat than the controls. The $\dot{V}O_{2max}$ was 55%, 83% and 49% higher for the runners than the controls expressed in liters per minute, milliliters per kilogram per minute, and milliliters per kilogram of fat-free mass (FFM) per minute, respectively (table). The maximal heart rate was lower for the runners compared with controls (1% greater than age-predicted maximal heart rate for the runners vs. 8% greater for the controls). No significant differences in maximal respiratory exchange ratios were found between the 2 groups. The absolute blood volume was 14% higher in the runners than the controls, whereas levels of total blood volume expressed relative to body weight and to estimated FFM were 39% and 10% higher, respectively. The higher total blood volume in runners was attributed to both higher plasma and erythrocyte volumes. Overall $\dot{V}O_{2max}$ correlated significantly with total blood volume, plasma volume, and erythrocyte volume when all were expressed relative to body weight. The runners also demonstrated higher hemoglobin concentrations than the controls.

Conclusion.—Relative to age-matched sedentary controls, highly trained middle-aged and older female endurance athletes are capable of attaining levels of $\dot{V}O_{2max}$ similar to those of middle-aged male athletes. Moreover, the high levels of $\dot{V}O_{2max}$ in these trained women are significantly related to their total blood volumes. Further studies are required to define the mechanisms responsible for the high levels of $\dot{V}O_{2max}$ in these women and to establish the role these levels of $\dot{V}O_{2max}$ play in their superior performance.

▶ There are probably as many myths about the physical capabilities of older men and women as there were about women some years ago. Supposedly, women were unable to cope with distance running, tolerate exercise in the heat, climb at altitude, etc. In the case of women, the primary factor turned out to be cardiovascular fitness, not sex. I suspect that a lack of physical fitness and/or medical problems explain much of the decrement in physical abilities of older individuals rather than chronological aging. As more men and women continue their competitive careers as Masters athletes, we will have a better understanding of how lifelong training affects the aging process in healthy adults.—B.L. Drinkwater, Ph.D.

Comparison of Whole and Split Weight Training Routines in Young Women

Calder AW, Chilibeck PD, Webber CE, Sale DG (McMaster Univ, Hamilton, Ont, Canada)

Can J Appl Physiol 19:185–199, 1994   139-95-7-9

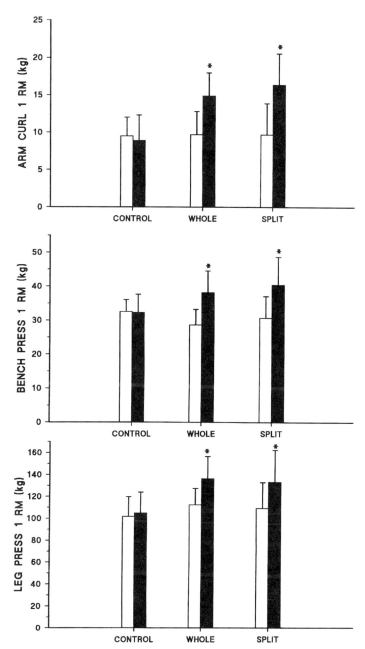

Fig 7–4.—Arm curl (**top**), bench press (**middle**), and leg press (**bottom**) 1 repetition maximum (RM) before (*unfilled bars*) and after training (*filled bars*) (mean ± SD) in control, whole, and split routine training groups. All 3 measures had a significant Group × Time interaction, $P < 0.001$. *Asterisks* indicate $P < 0.05$, increase with training. (Courtesy of Calder AW, Chilibeck PD, Webber CE, et al: *Can J Appl Physiol* 19:185–199, 1994.)

Introduction.—Athletes often use split routine weight training; the exercises are divided into 2 groups and each group is done on separate days. This practice is thought to avoid significant cumulative fatigue that might diminish the value of the exercises at the end of the session. However, some evidence suggests that anabolic hormone response relates directly to the amount of muscle mass used in a single session. The relative effectiveness of whole and split routine training in improving strength was compared.

Methods.—Thirty young, active, healthy women were assigned to 3 groups: a control group, a whole routine training group, and a split routine training group. The 3 groups were matched for age, height, body mass, and physical activity backgrounds. The women had two 10-week training periods separated by 2 weeks. The training regimen included upper body exercises (bench press, pulldown, arm curl, and triceps extension) for 5 sets of 6–10 repetitions and lower body exercises (leg press, knee extension, and knee flexion) for 5 sets of 10–12 repetitions. The split routine group did the upper and lower body exercises in separate sessions twice per week each. The whole routine group did the upper and lower body exercises together twice per week. Measurements of single maximal lift and body composition (measured by dual-energy x-ray absorptiometry) were taken before and after the training period.

Results.—The control group did not have significant changes in either single maximal lift or body composition. Both the whole and split routine training groups had significant post-training increases in single maximal lift with the arm curl, bench press, and leg press exercises (Fig 7–4), and in arm and whole-body lean tissue mass. The magnitude of these changes was not significantly different in the 2 groups. Leg lean tissue mass increased significantly only in the whole routine training group.

Discussion.—The training changes seen confirm other reports of the ability of young women to substantially increase strength and muscle mass with resistance training. In general, the same training response was achieved with either the whole or split routine training program, although the whole routine group had greater increases in leg lean tissue mass, and the split routine group had greater increases in single maximal lift with the arm curl exercise. Although these women exercised each muscle group twice a week, athletic training is more typically done 3 times a week, which may produce different results. The separation between the 2 training periods did not reduce the training progress. More study of periodization with advanced athletes in either a whole or a split routine program is required.

▶ Having some flexibility in planning weekly workouts is important for people with busy schedules. The results of this study will provide encouragement for women who cannot spend more than an hour per day working out and also for those who can spend more time per session but only for 2 or 3 days per week. In both cases, women can be assured of benefit from their strength-training program. With the increase in interest in strength training for older women and men, more studies may be forthcoming in which both young and older men and women are subjects in the same protocol. It may be that what is effective in the young person is not as effective in an older individual. If so, we need to find out what is the most effective way to increase strength in the older population, as it plays such an important role in their ability to maintain an independent lifestyle.—B.L. Drinkwater, Ph.D.

Routine Use of External Weights During a Low-Impact Aerobic Dance Conditioning Program: Training Benefit

Engels H-J, Bowen J, Wirth JC (Wayne State Univ, Detroit)
Sports Med Train Rehabil 5:283–291, 1995   139-95-7–10

Background.—Aerobic dancing is an increasingly popular mean of achieving and maintaining cardiovascular fitness, but its effects on body composition remain uncertain. Whether adding external weight to the body will enhance the effects of training was studied.

Study Plan.—Twenty college women participated in a low-impact aerobic dance program but avoided other formal exercise. Three 50-minute exercise sessions were held each week for 10 weeks at a level of 60% to 90% of maximal heart rate. The weight-training group wore two 1.5-lb clip-on ankle weights and carried 3-lb hand weights for 60% to 80% of each exercise session.

Results.—Most participants exercised close to the upper limit of the prescribed training level. There were no training-related injuries. Aerobic power and maximum ventilatory volume increased significantly after

---

Pretraining and Post-Training Responses to Maximal Treadmill Exercise

	Group	Pretraining	Post-Training
$\dot{V}O_{2max}$ (L·min^{-1})	WT	1.93 ± 0.14	2.16 ± 0.26[†]
	NWT	1.88 ± 0.20	2.06 ± 0.30[†]
$\dot{V}O_{2max}$ (mL·kg^{-1}·min^{-1})	WT	29.23 ± 4.84	32.50 ± 5.10[†]
	NWT	28.81 ± 4.63	31.92 ± 6.39[†]
RER_{max}	WT	1.12 ± 0.07	1.15 ± 0.08
	NWT	1.11 ± 0.04	1.14 ± 0.07
$\dot{V}_{Emax}$ (l·min^{-1})	WT	64.31 ± 6.56	73.49 ± 10.19[†]
	NWT	66.93 ± 10.84	78.01 ± 13.85[†]
HR_{max} (beats/min)	WT	188.63 ± 4.03	185.75 ± 3.85
	NWT	193.75 ± 13.59	192.25 ± 11.83
RPE_{max}	WT	17.88 ± 1.13	17.62 ± 1.30
	NWT	18.38 ± 0.74	18.13 ± 0.64

°For 16 research subjects. Values are mean ± standard deviation
†Significantly different from pretest ($p \leq 0.05$).
Abbreviations: $\dot{V}O_{2max}$, maximum oxygen consumption; RER_{max}, maximum respiratory exchange rate; $\dot{V}_{Emax}$, maximum minute ventilation; HR_{max}, maximum heart rate; RPE, rate of perceived exertion; WT, low-impact aerobic dance group; NWT, regular low-impact aerobic dance group.
(Courtesy of Engels H-J, Bowen J, Wirth JC; *Sports Med Train Rehabil* 5:283–291, 1995.)

training, but there were no significant differences between the weight training and the control groups (table). Body weight was unaltered, but both fat weight and the percent of body fat decreased significantly, and fat-free weight increased in both groups.

Conclusion.—The use of ankle and hand weights during low-impact aerobic dance training is no more effective than training without weights in increasing aerobic power or decreasing body fat.

▶ Although the authors state that "the routine carriage of weights by a participant practicing a low-impact training regimen does not increase the training benefit," that statement can apply only to the variables measured: aerobic power and body composition. Complaints from some of the women training with weights regarding muscular fatigue in arms, legs, and hips suggest that the weights might have had more effect on the muscles than on aerobic power and body composition. Considering the limited amount of time some women have to fit an exercise program into their busy schedules, it would be interesting to know whether muscular strength and endurance could be improved during an aerobic dance conditioning program by adding leg and hand weights.—B.L. Drinkwater, Ph.D.

Eating Disorders in Female Athletes
Sundgot-Borgen J (Norwegian Univ of Sport and Physical Education, Oslo, Norway)
Sports Med 17:176–188, 1994   139-95-7–11

Background.—Weight and eating disorders are common conditions with potentially long-lasting physical and psychological effects. Women and girls who are athletes are more likely to have symptoms of eating disorders than female nonathletes. The definitions and diagnostic criteria, prevalence, and risk factors for eating disorders in female athletes were reviewed, together with some practical considerations in the identification and treatment of these disorders.

Definitions.—Patients with eating disorders have gross disturbances in eating behavior. Clinical diagnoses in the athletic population include anorexia nervosa, bulimia nervosa, eating disorders not otherwise specified; pica (a craving for unnatural types of food), rumination disorder (regurgitation of food in infancy), and binge-eating disorder. Athletes who have significant symptoms of eating disorders but do not meet the diagnostic criteria for the above conditions are classified as having the subclinical eating disorder anorexia athletica. The classic feature is intense fear of getting fat in an athlete who is already lean (table). These patients lose weight by reducing their energy intake, often combining this with extensive or compulsive exercising. They usually report that they have to lose weight because of their sport or because they have been told to do so by a coach. If these patients are identified and treated early, it may be possible to prevent a full eating disorder from developing.

Diagnostic Criteria for Anorexia Athletica

Weight loss (>5% of expected bodyweight)	+
Delayed puberty [no menstrual bleeding at age 16 (primary amenorrhoea)]	(+)
Menstrual dysfunction (primary amenorrhoea, secondary amenorrhoea and oligomenorrhoea)	(+)
Gastrointestinal complaints	(+)
Absence of medical illness or affective disorder explaining the weight reduction	+
Distorted body image	(+)
Excessive fear of becoming obese	+
Restriction of food (<1200 kcal/day)	+
Use of purging methods (self-induced vomiting, use of laxatives and diuretics)	(+)
Binge eating	(+)
Compulsive exercise	(+)

Symbols: +, absolute criteria; (+), relative criteria.
(Courtesy of Sundgot-Borgen J: *Sports Med* 17:176–188, 1994.)

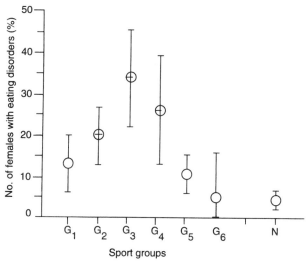

Fig 7–5.—Prevalence of eating disorders in female elite athletes representing the following sports groups: technical (G₁), endurance (G₂), aesthetic (G₃), weight-dependent (G₄), ball games (G₅), and power sports (G₆). The *shaded band* indicates the prevalence of eating disorders in nonathletes (N), for comparison. (Courtesy of Sundgot-Borgen J: Sports Med 17:176–188, 1994.)

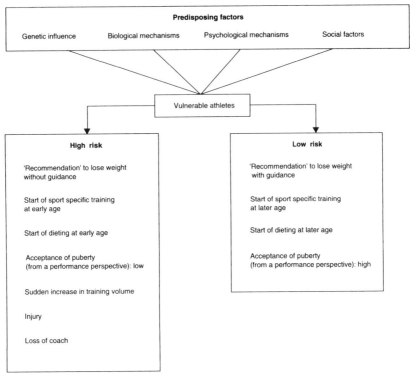

Fig 7–6.—General and sport-specific factors that can contribute to the development of eating disorders in athletes. (Courtesy of Sundgot-Borgen J: *Sports Med* 17:176–188, 1994.)

Prevalence.—Reported prevalences of eating disorders among athletes range from 1% to 39%. Whatever the true prevalence, eating disorders are more common in athletes than in nonathletes, especially in sports in which leanness or a specific weight are considered important (Fig 7–5). Athletes underreport eating disorders, often because they fear losing their place on a team. Those who admit to having an eating disorder say they have anorexia nervosa, whereas most actually have bulimia nervosa or subclinical eating disorders.

Risk Factors.—The additional stresses of athletics appear to make female athletes more vulnerable to eating disorders. One hypothesis is that sport or specific sports may attract individuals who are anorexic, at least in attitude. They may be attracted to sports that will help them to hide their illness. This hypothesis would not appear to apply to elite gymnastics, for which high-level training begins as young as 6 years of age, 10 years before eating disorders develop. Some risk factors are assumed to be intensified in elite athletes, although it would be difficult to compete at this level with an eating disorder. As a result, athletes who fail to stay at an elite level may have an even higher prevalence of eating disorders.

Other key risk factors may involve increased training load, early start of sport-specific training, dieting and body-weight cycling, personality factors, traumatic events, and input from coaches and trainers (Fig 7–6).

Prevention.—Coaches should be aware of their powerful influence on athletes and understand that requiring weight loss without offering further guidance can lead to unhealthy eating behaviors. Coaches and others who work with athletes should be aware of behaviors that may signal an eating disorder, the consequences of such disorders, and the available treatment options. Early intervention is critical. Preventive measures to follow include identifying realistic weight goals; periodic monitoring of weight, preferably in private; nutritional guidance; awareness of the symptoms; seeking professional help; and assisting and supporting the athlete during treatment.

Summary.—Eating disorders are a common and important health problem in female athletes. Further research is needed in several key areas, including the risk factors and causes of eating disorders among athletes at different competitive levels and in different sports, and the short- and long-term effects of eating disorders on health and athletic performance.

▶ The emphasis on low body weight or percentage of body fat in weight-dependent and aesthetic sports has placed many young female athletes at risk for the morbidity and mortality associated with eating disorders. Strict adherence to the *Diagnostic and Statistical Manual of Mental Disorders,* ed IV-R, criteria in determining prevalence rates has probably resulted in an underestimation of the problem among athletes. In this excellent review, the author suggests another term, "anorexia athletica," which recognizes the unique pressures on the female athlete and the need to recognize and treat the subclinical precursor of eating disorders at a time when appropriate intervention may prevent more serious problems in the future.—B.L. Drinkwater, Ph.D.

Risk and Trigger Factors for the Development of Eating Disorders in Female Elite Athletes

Sundgot-Borgen J (Norwegian Univ of Sport and Physical Education, Oslo, Norway)

Med Sci Sports Exerc 26:414–419, 1994   139-95-7–12

Objective.—Athletes are more likely to have eating disorders than are nonathletes, and female athletes who compete in sports that put a premium on leanness are especially at risk. Risk factors for eating disorders and the factors that may trigger the onset or worsening of such disorders were examined in a series of 603 elite female Norwegian athletes 12–35 years of age. The participants engaged in technical, endurance, aesthetic, weight-dependent, ball game, and power sports. All of them trained 8 or more hours per week and continued competing for at least 6 months.

Table 1.—Characteristics of the Eating-Disordered Athletes Representing the Different Sports Groups and Athletic Controls

Sport Groups	N	Age (yr)	BMI	Training Volume	% with High EDI*	% with ED**
Technical sports	13	19 (14–30)	21 (17–26)	14 (12–19)	21	14
Endurance sports	24	22 (15–28)	20 (15–22)[b]	21 (19–26)[c]	20	20
Aesthetic sports	22	17 (12–24)[a]	18 (15–21)[b]	18 (17–23)[c]	40[d]	35[c]
Weight-dependent sports	11	21 (15–23)	21 (17–23)	14 (11–16)	37[d]	29[c]
Ball game sports	21	20 (17–27)	21 (19–27)	15 (12–17)	14	12
Total sample	92	20 (13–28)	21 (15–27)	17 (12–26)	22	18
Athletic controls	30	20 (13–28)	22 (18–24)	15 (10–22)		18

Note: Values for age, body mass index (BMI), and training volume are given as means with ranges in parentheses.

*Percent of total sample (n = 522);

**Percent of total sample (minus those with high Eating Disorder Inventory [EDI] scores who did not have the clinical interview [n = 14]).

a. Significantly different from all other sports groups and controls (P < 0.05).

b. Significantly different from technical, weight dep, ball game sports, and controls (P < 0.05).

c. Significantly different from all other sports groups and controls (P < 0.05).

d. Significantly higher prevalence than in endurance and ball game sports (P < 0.05).

e. Significantly higher prevalence than in endurance, technical, and ball game sports (P < 0.05).

(Courtesy of Sundgot-Borgen J: Med Sci Sports Exerc 26:414–419, 1994.)

Table 2.—Reasons for Dieting

	ED Athletes* (%)	Athletic Controls* (%)
To enhance performance	100	100
Recommended by coach	67	75
Recommended by parents	15	38
Recommended by friends	8	50
To improve physical appearance	40	25

Note: Multiple answers were allowed.
*Athletes with eating disorders (ED) and athletic controls who reported dieting.
(Courtesy of Sundgot-Borgen J: Med Sci Sports Exerc 26:414-419, 1994.)

Methods.—A questionnaire on eating disorders was completed by 86% of those contacted. Of 117 athletes whose scores on the Eating Disorder Inventory (EDI) identified them as being at risk, 103 were interviewed, together with 30 controls matched for age, sport, and site of residence. The at-risk athletes had increased scores on the Drive for Thinness and Body Dissatisfaction subscales of the EDI.

Results.—Athletes engaging in aesthetic and endurance sports were the leanest and had relatively high training volumes. Eating disorders were most prevalent in those competing in aesthetic and weight-dependent sports (Table 1). Fully 85% of the athletes with eating disorders—those who met criteria for anorexia nervosa, bulimia nervosa, or anorexia athletica—were dieting, compared with 27% of controls. Most of the athletes dieted to improve their performance, and the majority had been told by their coach to diet (Table 2). Factors associated with the development of eating disorders included a prolonged period of dieting or weight change; traumatic personal, school-related, or work-related events; a loss of or a change in the coach; and an increase in training volume.

Conclusion.—Elite female athletes are at increased risk of having eating disorders. Athletes who diet at an early age and those whose diet is unsupervised are particularly at risk. When no specific reason is apparent, increased training accompanied by a significant weight loss may be responsible.

▶ This study confirms a general impression gained from previous reports that eating disorders are most prevalent in sports in which low body weight is deemed essential for success. Although no sport is immune, health professionals should be particularly alert to indications of problems among athletes in weight-dependent and aesthetic sports. The recognition of dieting as the number 1 trigger factor for serious eating disorders emphasizes the importance of avoiding pressure on athletes to lose weight and ensuring that they have access to good nutritional counseling.—B.L. Drinkwater, Ph.D.

The Prevalence and Consequences of Subclinical Eating Disorders in Female Athletes

Beals KA, Manore MM (Arizona State Univ, Tempe)
Int J Sport Nutr 4:175–195, 1994   139-95-7–13

Background.—In certain subgroups of female athletes, the prevalence of eating disorders and excessive concerns about body weight appears to be increasing. For some of these women, the pressure to achieve and maintain a low body weight results in potentially harmful patterns of restrictive eating or chronic dieting. Anorexia athletica, a recently identified subclinical eating disorder in female athletes, was discussed.

Criteria for Subclinical Eating Disorders.—In the continuum hypothesis of eating and dieting behavior, dieting is thought to result in disordered eating behaviors that, in turn, may lead to anorexia nervosa. A subclinical form of anorexia is one possible point along this continuum. One researcher has proposed "athletic anorexia" as a name for the subclinical form of anorexia in athletes. Certain features distinguish a subclinical eating disorder, but the number of these that must be present to be classified as anorexia athletica has not been determined. The criteria for subclinical eating disorder include preoccupation with food, calories, body shape, and weight; distorted body image; intense fear of gaining weight or becoming fat despite being moderately or extremely underweight; below-normal body weight maintained for at least 1 year; absence of medical illness or affective disorder explaining the weight loss or maintenance of low body weight; gastrointestinal symptoms; menstrual dysfunction; frequent use of purging methods; and binging.

Energy Intake in Amenorrheic and Eumenorrheic Athletes.—Research has shown that amenorrheic runners generally have lower energy intakes than eumenorrheic runners, despite similar body weights and body composition and training regimens (table). These women may simply underreport energy intake, or suboptimal energy intakes may be the result of physiologic adaptations—specifically an increased energy efficiency—which permits some female athletes to function normally and maintain energy balance on fewer calories than would be expected on the basis of body size and activity level.

Possible Consequences of Anorexia Athletica.—Chronic energy restriction or inadequate micronutrient intake combined with excessive exercise could theoretically reduce athletic performance. Psychological consequences also occur. Dieting has been associated with depression, feelings of failure, and lowered self-esteem. Dieting predicts stress, whereas stress does not predict dieting. Concerns about excessive body weight and severe dieting practices may predispose susceptible athletes to an increased risk for development of more pathologic weight loss behaviors or even clinical eating disorders.

Conclusion.—Research suggests that subclinical eating disorders do exist and may be more common in women participating in sports that

Summary of Studies on Mean Energy Intakes of Amenorrheic and Eumenorrheic Runners

Study	Amenorrheic				Eumenorrheic				kcal difference	p†
	kcal/day	kcal/kg FFM/day	Miles/week	% BF*	kcal/day	kcal/kg FFM/day	Miles/week	%BF*		
Baer & Taper‡	1,911	44.0	40	16.2 ± 1.0	1,644	39.0	20	17.3 ± 1.3	+268	NS
Brooks et al.‡	1,991	48.0	45	17.2 ± 0.9	2,279	51.0	47	17.2 ± 0.9	−288	—
Deuster et al.§	2,151	49.0	~70	11.9 ± 0.3	2,489	54.3	~70	11.9 ± 0.3	−338	NS
Drinkwater et al.§	1,623	35.6	42	15.8 ± 1.4	1,965	41.0	25	16.9 ± 0.8	−342	NS
Kaiserauer et al.§	1,582	36.0	39	11.8 ± 1.5	2,490	52.0	31	10.7 ± 1.4	−908	<.02
Marcus et al.§	1,272	28.5	58	11.1 ± 2.0	1,715	36.0	58	10.0 ± 1.1	−443	NS
Myerson et al.||	1,731	39.5	53	14.6 ± 2.2	1,935	41.0	52	15.0 ± 1.4	−204	NS
Nelson et al.§	1,730	38.3	35	21.6 ± 1.7	2,250	50.6	40	19.7 ± 0.8	−520	<.05
Wilmore et al.§	1,781	39.1	~60¶	10.8 ± 4.4	1,690	36.3	~60¶	10.3 ± 3.6	+91	NS

*Body fat as measured by skinfolds or hydrostatic weighing and reported as mean ± SE (except for studies by Brooks et al. and Wilmore et al., in which body fat was measured as mean ± SD).

‡ Indicates whether groups statistically significantly differed for mean energy intakes.

‡ 7-day diet record.

§ 3-day diet record.

|| 6-day diet record.

¶ Study did not mention mileage, only that the participants were elite distance runners and that elite distance runners typically run 50–70 miles per week.

Abbreviations: BF, body fat; FFM, fat-free mass.

(Courtesy of Beals KA, Manore MM: *Int J Sport Nutr* 4:175-195, 1994.)

emphasize a low body weight or thin body build. Some female athletes may engage in restrictive eating or obsessive weight control behavior to improve their appearance or performance, or both. More research on anorexia athletica is needed.

▶ There appears to be a growing acceptance of the concept that many female athletes have a subclinical form of an eating disorder. That is, they do not meet the strict *Diagnostic and Statistical Manual of Mental Disorders,* ed IV-R, criteria but still use some forms of pathologic weight control. Although not diagnosed as a clinical disorder, this behavior can lead to both impaired health and poor performance. The reported incidence of eating disorders in the athletic population will underestimate the problem if women with subclinical problems are not identified. The problem may be more prevalent than current data suggest.—B.L. Drinkwater, Ph.D.

The Role of Physical Activity in the Development and Maintenance of Eating Disorders
Davis C, Kennedy SH, Ralevski E, Dionne M (Toronto Hosp)
Psychol Med 24:957–967, 1994   139-95-7–14

Background.—The finding of psychological similarities between individuals described as excessive exercisers and patients with eating disorders suggests a link between the 2 behaviors. These behaviors can exist independently or jointly, and both appear to be motivated by a strong element of perfectionism. Some investigators describe undereating and overexercise as mutually reinforcing behaviors that are self-perpetuating

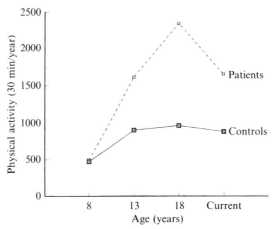

Fig 7–7.—Physical activity participation levels for eating-disordered patients and normal controls from 8 years of age to current age. (Courtesy of Davis C, Kennedy SH, Ralevski E, et al: *Psychol Med* 24:957–967, 1994.)

and resistant to change. The interrelated dynamics of exercise and starvation were investigated in 2 studies.

Methods.—Research subjects in the first study were 51 women aged 18–27 years who were randomly assigned to 1 of 3 experimental conditions. All were volunteers and none had a history of anorexia nervosa or bulimia nervosa. The first condition used memory aids at both testing sessions; the second used memory aids at 1 of the 2 testing sessions; and the third did not use memory aids at either session. The purpose of study 1 was to test the reliability of historical physical activity data collected retrospectively and to estimate the typical degree of physical activity in a nonclinical sample of young women. The second study included 45 consecutive women younger than 35 years of age who were hospitalized for eating disorders. At admission, anorexia nervosa had been diagnosed in 32 patients and bulimia nervosa in 13, 10 of whom had previously met criteria for anorexia nervosa. Physical activity data were collected as in the first study, except that memory aids were used at both testing sessions. Patients also took part in a semistructured interview and were asked to complete a symptom checklist.

Results.—Physical activity scores of controls and patients were similar at 8 years of age but differed significantly at 13 and 18 years of age and at their current ages (Fig 7–7). Analysis of responses from patient interviews revealed that 78% of patients engaged in excessive exercise, 60% had been competitive athletes before the onset of their eating disorder, 60% reported that sport or exercise had predated dieting, and 75% indicated a relationship between periods of increased physical activity and those of decreased food intake and weight loss.

Conclusion.—Among these young women hospitalized for eating disorders, participation in sports and excessive exercise often predated dieting and the development of eating disorders. In some cases, the end of training led to a strong fear of weight gain. Social influences affecting these women include the quest for a slender body and the current fitness craze. In many women who are anorexic or bulimic, overactivity appears to be integral to the pathogenesis and maintenance of the eating disorder.

▶ The suggestion that sport/exercise has the potential to "create a psychological predisposition to an eating disorder . . ." and contribute to its progression will not be a popular hypothesis. The battle for gender equity on the playing field will not be helped if there is a perception that physical activity can precipitate an eating disorder. Fortunately, this report does not present convincing evidence that sport/exercise per se is the culprit. The pressure on female athletes to maintain a low body weight in some sports is not inherent in the activity itself but in the perception of what is required of the athlete for optimum performance. However, this caveat does not negate the possibility that the biochemical consequences of a severe energy deficit play an important role in the pathogenesis of an eating disorder. This places even more responsibility on those who work with young athletes to avoid comments or actions that might initiate the cycle of decreased caloric intake and increased energy expenditure.—B.L. Drinkwater, Ph.D.

Exercise-Induced Menstrual Cycle Changes: A Functional, Temporary Adaptation to Metabolic Stress

Bonen A (Univ of Waterloo, Ont, Canada)
Sports Med 17:373–392, 1994

139-95-7–15

Effect of Intense Exercise on Menstrual Function in Individuals Who Were Permitted to Lose Body Weight ($-4 \pm .3$ kg), and in Those on a Body Weight Maintenance Diet (-1 ± 0.2 kg) During 2 Months of Training

Group	Clinical disorders			Hormonal disturbances	
	no disorders	abnormal bleeding	delayed menses	abnormal luteal function	Loss of LH surge
Bodyweight maintenance (n = 12)	3 (25%)	7 (58%)	1 (8%)	8 (66%)	5 (42%)
Bodyweight loss (n = 16)	1 (6%)	7 (44%)	12 (75%)	10 (63%)	13 (81%)
Significance	NS	NS	<0.005	NS	<0.05

Abbreviations: LH, luteinizing hormone; NS, nonsignificant.
(From Bonen A: *Sports Med* 17:373–392, 1994. Adapted from Bullen BA, Skrinar GS, Beitins IZ, et al: *N Engl J Med* 312:1349–1353, 1985.)

Introduction.—Although chronic exercise alters the menstrual cycle, exercise alone does not easily induce secondary amenorrhea; it seems to require other metabolic stressors. Change in the menstrual cycle that is exercise-related can be viewed as a functionally adaptive response, rather than a maladaptive dysfunction, and could be an energy-conserving strategy to protect more important biological processes. There is a practical need to know what it is about exercise that prompts the changes and whether women in general are at risk of changes in their menstrual cycle when they exercise, especially women who are trying to conceive. Evidence is presented that shows (1) there is little known about the predisposing factors that can change the menstrual cycle, (2) the estimates of change induced by exercise are probably overestimated, (3) some transient changes may occur with recreational exercise, (4) the severity of exercise-related changes probably represents the additive effects of several metabolic factors, and (5) exercise-related change is a form of metabolic arrest and a functional adaptive response.

Metabolic Arrest.—Although the mechanisms of metabolic arrest are complex, it appears that there is a gynecologic arrest mechanism. To support this, it must be shown that maintaining a normal menstrual cycle is metabolically more costly than reducing the menstrual cycle. The factors that support this are (1) an increased energy cost during the normal menstrual cycle, (2) a markedly reduced metabolic rate in amenorrheic women, (3) a lower caloric intake in amenorrheic athletes than in eumenorrheic athletes, and (4) women with anorexia are amenorrheic and have a lower basal metabolic rate. There seems to be a very strong link between gynecologic function and metabolic stress. Exercise appears to be just another metabolic stressor, which induces changes in the menstrual cycle much like other metabolic disturbances such as reduced food intake. Schematically, metabolic arrest and gynecologic arrest are correlated with each other.

Conclusion.—It is not known how many women will be affected by exercise, but it is important to establish an "energy drain" index to provide some predictability. Simply maintaining body weight is a good strategy to decrease the risk of secondary amenorrhea (table). Change in the menstrual cycle associated with exercise is a normal adaptive phenomenon and a good example of metabolic arrest designed to conserve energy.

▶ Not all readers will agree with the author that "changes in the menstrual cycle associated with training are a normal adaptive phenomenon. . . ." There is good evidence that oligomenorrhea, as well as amenorrhea, is associated with bone loss that may be irreversible. New data from our laboratory show that women who were amenorrheic/oligomenorrheic 10 years ago and had low bone density at that time have not regained a significant amount of bone even though they have been eumenorrheic or have received hormone replacement during most of the intervening 10 years. Rather than accepting menstrual irregularities as a benign condition, it would seem more prudent to concentrate on tracking down the etiology of these disruptions in the reproductive cycle in order to avoid the sequelae.—B.L. Drinkwater, Ph.D.

Clinical Consequences of Athletic Amenorrhoea
Constantini NW (Wingate Inst, Netanya, Israel)
Sports Med 17:213–223, 1994   139-95-7–16

Background.—Reports of the effects of strenuous training on the reproductive system and the consequent deleterious effect on the skeletal system have raised concerns about the long-term effect on the health of female athletes. The clinical consequences of athletic amenorrhea were reviewed, with an emphasis on skeletal problems.

Skeletal Problems.—The most serious effect of athletic amenorrhea is that on the skeleton. Amenorrheic athletes may fail to reach peak bone mass; lose bone; fail to mineralize weight-bearing bones with stress; and have increased rates of stress fractures, primarily as a result of prolonged periods of hypoestrogenism. Pubertal stage, sex-steroids milieu, weight, and height appear to be the most important factors predicting bone mineral density in adolescents. Reduced spinal bone mineral density is consistently found in amenorrheic athletes (Table 1). Athletes with oligomenorrhea or asymptomatic ovulatory disturbances also have decreased spinal bone mineral density. In most studies, cortical densities do not appear to be decreased, in contrast to trabecular bone.

In amenorrheic athletes, hormonal milieu is not the only cause of decreased bone mineral density. Other risk factors for osteopenia—such as

TABLE 1.—Differences in Bone Mineral Density Between Amenorrheic and Eumenorrheic Athletes

Reference	Sport	Amenorrhoeic age (no. of athletes)	Eumenorrhoeic age (no. of athletes)	Difference (%)
Ding et al. (1988)	Mixed*	26.8 (19)	30.1 (35)	17
Drinkwater et al. (1984)	Runners	24.9 (11)	25.5 (16)	14
Drinkwater et al. (1990)	Mixed†	30.0 (21)	25.2 (21)	17
Jonnavithula et al. (1993)	Dancers	20.4 (5)	23.5 (12)	16
Marcus et al. (1985)	Runners	20.0 (11)	23.8 (6)	17
Nelson et al. (1986)	Runners	25.2 (11)	29.2 (17)	8
Myerson et al. (1992)	Runners	29.5 (13)	30.3 (13)	10
Warren et al. (1991)	Dancers	19.2 (22)	22.1 (29)	13
Wolman et al. (1992)	Mixed†	24.2 (25)	25.1 (27)	20

* Primarily runners.
†Rowers, runners, and dancers.
(Courtesy of Constantini NW: *Sports Med* 17:213–223, 1994.)

TABLE 2.—Risk Factors for Osteoporosis in
Female Athletes

Hormone milieu

Estrogen exposure

Low levels of estrogens (estradiol and estrone)

Delayed puberty (menarche and telarche)

Duration of amenorrhoea (present and past history)

Low use of oral contraceptives (or other estrogens)

Other hormones

Anovulation/short luteal phase (i.e. low progesterone)

Low androgen levels

High cortisol levels

Nutrition

Low bodyweight

Low percentage body fat

Eating disorders

Low caloric intake

Low calcium intake

High protein intake

High fibre intake

Others

Family history of osteoporosis

Lack of mechanical load

(Courtesy of Constantini NW: *Sports Med* 17:213-223, 1994.)

low body weight and body fat, low energy intake with negative caloric balance, pathologic eating behavior, and low calcium intake—are also common in such women (Table 2). The combination of estrogen deficiency with any of these probably increases the risk for bone loss. Calcium supplements and hormone replacement treatment are recommended to prevent bone loss in amenorrheic athletes.

Exercise does appear to constitute an important factor in maintaining bone mass. Studies have found that amenorrheic runners have higher bone mineral density than less active amenorrheic women and that amenorrheic lightweight rowers do not have reduced bone mineral content compared with nonathletes. Another study on anorectic women showed that very active individuals had significantly higher cortical bone densities than less active ones.

Infertility.—Infertility can occur in regularly menstruating athletes who have a shortened luteal phase or anovulation as well as in amenorrheic and oligomenorrheic athletes. Infertility associated with exercise is usually reversible by reducing training or weight gain.

Conclusion.—Decreased bone mass in amenorrheic athletes can reflect both inadequate acquisition of peak bone mass during adolescence and excessive bone loss later in life. This osteopenia exposes female athletes to an increased risk for skeletal fragility, fractures, vertebral instability, and curvature. Early treatment with estrogen replacement and calcium supplements may be useful for preventing irreversible bone loss and osteoporosis and for positively affecting the lipid profile.

▶ It is certainly better to be active and amenorrheic than sedentary and amenorrheic, but it is much better to be active and eumenorrheic. Even though physical activity appears to modulate the negative consequences of amenorrhea on bone in some cases, amenorrheic athletes generally have a lower bone density than their eumenorrheic teammates. Some of the young women in our studies have bone mineral density similar to that of women in their 70s and 80s. One might also wonder whether the apparent protective effect of intense mechanical loading will disappear if these women become less active.—B.L. Drinkwater, Ph.D.

Induction of Low-T_3 Syndrome in Exercising Women Occurs at a Threshold of Energy Availability
Loucks AB, Heath EM (Ohio Univ, Athens)
Am J Physiol 266:R817–R823, 1994   139-95-7–17

Objective.—Athletic women often have dietary energy intakes similar to those of sedentary women. The dietary intakes of the athletic women are therefore less than expected for their activity level. This has led investigators to suspect that the reproductive disorders occurring among women involved in competitive aerobic sports have a nutritional basis. Amenorrheic athletes have low 3,5,3'-triiodothyronine (T_3) levels—a sign of energy deficiency—whereas regularly menstruating athletes do not. If this low T_3 syndrome occurs abruptly in women who exercise at a threshold of energy availability, then partially compensating for exercise energy expenditure through diet might be enough to avoid reductions in T_3 levels. This issue has important implications for diet and exercise programs in women. The functional relationship between energy availability and thyroid metabolism was assessed.

Methods.—The study included 27 healthy, regularly menstruating, sedentary young women. All kept prospective diet records for 7 consecutive days to estimate their habitual energy intake and underwent a modified Balke treadmill test to measure their aerobic capacity. The women were assigned to 1 of 4 groups for experimental manipulation of energy availability, which was defined as dietary energy intake minus energy expenditure during exercise (Fig 7–8). All groups expended about 30 kcal/kg of lean body mass (LBM) of energy on 4 consecutive days, beginning on days 2, 3, 4, or 5 of the menstrual cycle. The women received a liquid clinical dietary product as their only food source for the 4 treatment

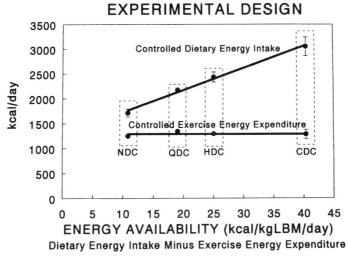

Fig 7–8.—The experimental design. All women performed approximately 30 kcal/kg lean body mass $(LBM)^{-1}/day^{-1}$ of supervised aerobic exercise for 4 days, receiving no dietary compensation (NDC), one quarter dietary compensation (QDC), one half dietary compensation (HDC), or complete (CDC) dietary compensation for the energy expended during exercise. (Courtesy of Loucks AB, Heath EM: *Am J Physiol* 266:R817–R823, 1994.)

days. At one extreme, for women receiving complete dietary compensation for the energy cost of exercise, energy availability was 40 kcal/kg of LBM per day; at the other extreme, for women who received no dietary compensation, energy availability was 11 kcal/kg of LBM per day. Those in the intermediate groups had energy availability of 25 and 19 kcal/kg of LBM per day (table). Blood samples were obtained at 8 AM for 9 days, beginning 2 days before the treatments. Radioimmunoassays were used to measure thyroid hormones.

Results.—Pretreatment thyroid hormone levels were not significantly different among the 4 groups and were within the normal range. Assessment of the effects of energy availability on T_3 found that models of proportionality and threshold relationships were both significant. However, the threshold model explained a much greater proportion of the variance in data (61% vs. 39%). Similarly, the threshold model explained more of the variance in free T3 (29% vs. 19%). Both of these T_3 levels were reduced below a threshold of energy availability between 19 and 25 kcal/kg of LBM per day (Fig 7–9). For the 2 groups above this threshold, treatment effects on T_3 and free T_3 levels were indistinguishable from 0.

Conclusion.—When exercising women receive the dietary energy intake of sedentary women, the low-T_3 syndrome is induced within 4 days. A diet that replaces one half of the energy cost of exercise prevents the low-T_3 syndrome, but a diet that replaces one fourth of the cost does not. The T_3 levels decline in energy-deficient women, even though T_4 is adequate as a precursor, suggesting that energy availability influences the

Descriptive Information About the Research Subjects

Treatments	Energy Availability Groups, kcal/kg LBM				P Value
	10.8 ± 0.5	19.0 ± 0.6	25.0 ± 0.6	40.4 ± 1.2	
n	6	8	8	5	
Daily exercise					
%VO$_{2max}$	70	70	70	70	
%HR$_{max}$	86 ± 1.2	85 ± 1.2	82 ± 1.0	83 ± 1.4	0.18
HR, beats/min	170 ± 4	166 ± 4	162 ± 3	162 ± 4	0.40
RPE	16 ± 0.5	14.5 ± 0.6	14.4 ± 0.6	15.2 ± 1.5	0.48
Duration, min/day	169 ± 7	172 ± 4	177 ± 7	166 ± 6	0.62
Daily energy					
Dietary intake					
kcal	1,714 ± 79	2,180 ± 66	2,433 ± 99	2,960 ± 173	$<10^{-5}$
kcal/kg LBM	39.5 ± 1.2	48.6 ± 0.7	53.4 ± 1.7	68.4 ± 1.2	$<10^{-5}$
Exercise expenditure					
kcal	1,244 ± 64	1,332 ± 55	1,293 ± 69	1,217 ± 101	0.68
kcal/kg LBM	28.7 ± 1.0	29.6 ± 0.4	28.3 ± 1.1	28.0 ± 1.0	0.64
Availability					
kcal	470 ± 23	850 ± 17	1,140 ± 31	1,743 ± 84	$<10^{-5}$
kcal/kg LBM	10.8 ± 0.5	19.0 ± 0.6	25.0 ± 0.6	40.4 ± 1.2	$<10^{-5}$

Note: Values are means ± standard error; n, number of research subjects. The achieved significance levels (P) estimate the likelihood that the treatment groups experienced similar treatments.
Abbreviations: HR$_{max}$, maximal heart rate; RPE, Borg scores of perceived exertion.
(Courtesy of Loucks A, Heath EM: Am J Physiol 266:817R-823R, 1994.)

peripheral activity of 5'-deiodinase in converting thyroxine to T_3. The results suggest that women on weight control diets should be carefully advised to avoid combinations of caloric control and physical activity that would result in subthreshold levels of energy availability.

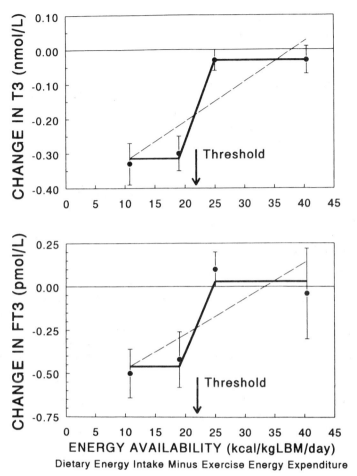

Fig 7–9.—Effects of energy availability on 3,5,3'-triiodothyronine (T_3) and free T_3 (fT_3). For T_3 (**top**), the regression (proportionality) model (*dashed line*), P < 0.001 and the analysis of variance (threshold) model (*solid line*, P < 0.00001) were both statistically significant but the threshold model explained much more variance ($R^2_{proportionality}$ = 39%; $R^2_{threshold}$ = 61%). For fT (**bottom**), the proportionality (P = 0.02) and threshold model (P = 0.004) were also both significant, with the threshold model again explaining more variance ($R^2_{proportionality}$ = 19%; $R^2_{threshold}$ = 29%). For both T_8 and fT_3, the threshold was detected between 10 and 25 kcal/kg lean body mass $(LBM)^{-1}/day^{-1}$. (Courtesy of Loucks AB, Heath EM: *Am J Physiol* 266:817R–823R, 1994.)

▶ Although the hypoestrogenic status of most amenorrheic athletes has been associated with osteopenia and increased risk of musculoskeletal injuries, research into the etiology of this condition has decreased as the cost and complexity of the research has increased. However, the work of Loucks and her colleagues appears to be headed down a very productive path: the deficit between energy intake and energy expenditure. If their further work can demonstrate that weight can be safely lost or controlled by maintaining an energy availability above a critical threshold, it will be a significant contribution to the health of athletes and nonathletes alike.—B.L. Drinkwater, Ph.D.

Dietary Restriction Reduces Luteinizing Hormone (LH) Pulse Frequency During Waking Hours and Increases LH Pulse Amplitude During Sleep in Young Menstruating Women

Loucks AB, Heath EM (Ohio Univ, Athens)
J Clin Endocrinol Metab 78:910–915, 1994   139-95-7–18

Purpose.—A great deal of experimental evidence suggests that the functional integrity of the female mammalian reproductive system relies on energy availability rather than body size or composition. This energy availability hypothesis was tested in young eumenorrheic women by assessing the effects of dietary energy restriction on luteinizing hormone (LH) pulse frequency and amplitude.

Methods.—Seven healthy, regularly menstruating young women, with a mean gynecologic age of 8 years, participated in the study (Table 1). Samples for measurement of LH and follicle-stimulating hormone (FSH) were drawn at 10- and 60-minute intervals, respectively, over 24 hours on days 9, 10, or 11 of 2 menstrual cycles. Samples collected at 30-minute intervals were used to measure cortisol. Measurements of estradiol (E_2) were made every 6 hours. Twenty-four–hour transverse means for LH, FSH, and E_2 were calculated, and LH pulse frequency and amplitude were determined. On the 4 days before and on the day of sampling, the women received a dietary energy intake of 45 or 10 cal/kg of lean body mass in random order (Table 2). They followed their normal sedentary habits throughout the study. Starting 2 days before treatment,

TABLE 1.—Demographic Characteristics of the Research Subjects

Characteristics	Units	Mean $\pm$ SE
N		7
Calendar age	yr	21 $\pm$ 1.3
Age of menarche	yr	13.2 $\pm$ 0.2
Gynecological age	yr	7.7 $\pm$ 1.2
Menstrual cycle length	days	29.8 $\pm$ 0.8
Ht	cm	165.8 $\pm$ 1.6
Wt	kg	58.6 $\pm$ 2.1
Body fat	%	24.6 $\pm$ 1.3
LBM	kg	43.8 $\pm$ 1.3
V_{O_2max}	mL O_2/kg BW·min	39.8 $\pm$ 1.4
Dietary intake	Cal/day	2000 $\pm$ 90
Dietary intake	Cal/kg LBM·day	45.7 $\pm$ 2.2

(Courtesy of Loucks AB, Heath EM: *J Clin Endocrinol Metab* 78:910–915, 1994.)

TABLE 2.—Effects of Dietary Restriction on Metabolic Hormones

Hormone	Units	Baseline conc.	Treatment effect	P
T_3	nmol/L	1.7 ± 0.04	-0.3 ± 0.1	<0.01
IGF-I	ng/ml	373 ± 47	-196 ± 31	<0.001
Insulin	pmol/L	60 ± 4	-31 ± 6	<0.001
Cortisol				
24-h mean	nmol/L	230 ± 20	20 ± 10	0.13
0300-1100 h	nmol/L	310 ± 20	20 ± 20	0.18
1100-1900 h	nmol/L	230 ± 10	20 ± 20	0.14
1900-0300 h	nmol/L	130 ± 30	20 ± 20	0.13

Note: Values are expressed as mean $\pm$ standard error. Treatment effects are paired differences within individuals. (Courtesy of Loucks AB, Heath EM: *J Clin Endocrinol Metab* 78:910-915, 1994.)

daily blood samples were taken at 8 AM on 3 consecutive days and assayed for triiodothyronine (T_3), insulin-like growth factor-I (IGF-I), E_2, and insulin.

Results.—When they were receiving balanced dietary treatment, the women showed no significant differences in their controlled dietary energy intake and recorded 24-hour energy expenditure. However, when dietary intake was restricted, the recorded 24-hour energy expenditure was much greater than the controlled dietary energy intake. The research subjects lost 1.5 kg of body weight during the dietary restriction period.

LH PULSATILITY

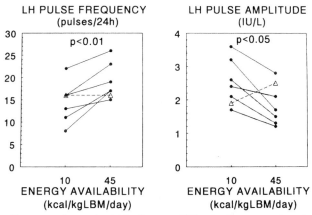

Fig 7–10.—Treatment effect on luteinizing hormone (*LH*) pulse frequency and amplitude. One research subject with elevated estradiol levels did not respond in the same way as the others. *Abbreviation: LBM,* low body mass. (Courtesy of Loucks AB, Heath EM: *J Clin Endocrinol Metab* 78:910-915, 1994.)

This was accompanied by a 20% reduction in T_3, a 58% reduction in IGF-I, and a 54% reduction in insulin. There was no increase in serum cortisol. Dietary restriction was also associated with a 23% reduction in LH pulse frequency and a 40% increase in LH pulse amplitude (Fig 7-10). The LH pulse frequency slowed significantly during sleep when the women were receiving an energy-balanced diet but not when they were receiving a restricted diet. There was a significant increase in LH pulse amplitude during sleep when the women ate the energy-balanced diet; this effect was even greater when dietary intake was restricted.

Conclusion.—A restricted energy intake causes the LH pulse frequency to decrease, mainly during the day, and the LH pulse amplitude to increase, mainly at night. These compensatory changes maintain the 24-hour transverse mean LH level. The findings in normal young women resemble those reported for women with hypothalamic amenorrhea. As a result, as in other mammalian females, LH pulsatility in women appears to depend on energy availability. A similar experimental design is being used to determine whether LH pulsatility also depends on energy availability in exercising women.

▶ The carefully crafted series of studies from this laboratory suggest an important role for "energy deficit" in precipitating that cascade of events leading to the disruption of the hypothalamic-pituitary-ovarian axis. If this line of investigation can be expanded to demonstrate a cause-and-effect relationship with changes in ovarian function, the "energy availability" theory will become an important tool in helping active and athletic women to exercise and train without the risk of interruption of the normal menstrual cycle. It also explains why women with normal dietary habits may become amenorrheic if the energy cost of their training exceeds the caloric intake of what would be an adequate diet for a less active woman.—B.L. Drinkwater, Ph.D.

Clinical Tests Explain Blunted Cortisol Responsiveness But Not Mild Hypercortisolism in Amenorrheic Runners

De Souza MJ, Luciano AA, Arce JC, Demers LM, Loucks AB (Univ of Connecticut, Farmington; Pennsylvania State Univ, Hershey; Ohio Univ, Athens)
J Appl Physiol 76:1302–1309, 1994   139-95-7-19

Introduction.—Amenorrheic runners have a mild hypercortisolism, which suggests hypothalamic-pituitary-adrenal axis mediation in the disruption of the hypothalamic-pituitary-ovarian axis. To investigate the mechanisms involved in the reduced adrenocortical responsiveness to exercise and the mild hypercortisolism in amenorrheic runners, the responses to a dexamethasone suppression test and adrenocorticotropic hormone (ACTH) stimulation test in amenorrheic and eumenorrheic runners and eumenorrheic sedentary women were compared.

Methods.—Healthy adult women with a consistent menstrual status were chosen in the following categories: 9 eumenorrheic runners, 9

TABLE 1.—Urinary Free Cortisol (24 Hours) at Rest and During Hard Training Days in Eumenorrheic Sedentary Women and Eumenorrheic and Amenorrheic Runners

	Groups			
Test Conditions	ES (*n* = 6)	ER (*n* = 9)	AR (*n* = 9)	*P*
Rest days (mean of 2 days)	202±25	228±12	360±19*	<0.001
Hard training days (mean of 2 days)		224±19	346±28*	<0.001
Change (hard training days − rest days)		−4	−6	
P		>0.8	>0.8	

Abbreviations: ES, eumenorrheic sedentary women; *ER*, eumenorrheic runners; *AR*, amenorrheic runners.
Note: Values are means ± standard error in mmol/24 hr.
* Significantly different from other group(s).
(Courtesy of De Souza MJ, Luciano AA, Arce JC, et al: *J Appl Physiol* 76:1302–1309, 1994.)

amenorrheic runners, and 6 eumenorrheic sedentary women. Baseline serum cortisol levels were determined. All participants underwent 2 ACTH-stimulation tests, with and without dexamethasone, with cortisol responses measured in blood samples taken at 15 minutes and then every 30 minutes for 3 hours. Twenty-four hour urines were collected on resting and training days for verification of cortisol status.

Results.—The 2 groups of runners had similar training levels. Compared with the eumenorrheic sedentary women, the eumenorrheic runners had shorter luteal phases and longer follicular phases. The estradiol and progesterone levels in the amenorrheic runners were consistent with chronic ovarian suppression. Amenorrheic runners had significantly higher levels of 24-hour urinary free cortisol excretion than the eumenorrheic groups (Table 1). Amenorrheic runners also had substantially greater cortisol plasma levels in the absence of dexamethasone but similar low levels of cortisol in response to the dexamethasone challenge (Table 2). Stimulation with ACTH resulted in similar peak cortisol response levels in all 3 groups with and without dexamethasone suppression. However, the area under the cortisol response curve with dexamethasone suppression was smaller for the amenorrheic vs. the eumenorrheic women and faster without dexamethasone in the amenorrheic runners.

Discussion.—Because the training levels in the 2 runner groups were similar, the mild hypercortisolism seen in the amenorrheic runners is likely to be associated with amenorrhea rather than with exercise. The suppressed cortisol levels after low-dose dexamethasone in the amenorrheic group suggest that neither a central defect in cortisol feedback nor a peripheral anomaly of the adrenal cortex is involved. Extrapituitary fac-

TABLE 2.—Effects of Dexamethasone on Cortisol in Eumenorrheic Sedentary Women and Eumenorrheic and Amenorrheic Runners

| | Group | | | | | |
Condition	ES (n = 6)	ER (n = 9)	AR (n = 9)	P	All subjs (n = 24)	P
NDX	210±25	285±29	496±39*	<0.001	330±31	
DX	18±2	21±2	19±1	>0.5	20±2	
Δ	−186±16	−264±21	−477±36*	<0.001	−310±29	<0.001
%Δ	−88	−93	−96		−94	

Note: Values are means ± standard error in nmol/L.
* Significantly different from other groups.
Abbreviations: NDX, absence of dexamethasone; DX, presence of dexamethasone.
(Courtesy of De Souza MJ, Luciano AA, Arce JC, et al: J Appl Physiol 76:1302–1309, 1994.)

tors that increase adrenal responsiveness to ACTH may be implicated. Direct adrenal stimulation with ACTH in the absence of dexamethasone showed reduced adrenal sensitivity to ACTH in amenorrheic athletes. Blunted cortisol responses with both direct and indirect stimulation in the presence of mild hypercortisolism suggest only that the maximal secretory capacity of the adrenal cortex had been attained. No explanation for the hypercortisolism observed in amenorrheic athletes is possible at this time.

▶ There are a number of unanswered questions relating to the changes in reproductive function in amenorrheic athletes. A possible interaction of the hypothalamic-pituitary-adrenal axis with the hypothalamic-pituitary-ovarian axis in other forms of hypothalamic amenorrhea provides the basis for testing the "stress" hypothesis as a cause of menstrual disorders in athletic women. There seems little doubt now that amenorrheic athletes do tend to have elevated levels of cortisol. As yet, there is no explanation for this mild hypercortisolism nor any firm evidence that it adds to the negative impact of the hypoestrogenic state on bone mass in these athletes.—B.L. Drinkwater, Ph.D.

Energy Balance in Endurance-Trained Female Cyclists and Untrained Controls
Horton TJ, Drougas HJ, Sharp TA, Martinez LR, Reed GW, Hill JO (Vanderbilt Univ, Nashville, Tenn)
J Appl Physiol 76:1937–1945, 1994   139-95-7-20

Background.—The report of low caloric intakes among some young female athletes has led to the hypothesis that these athletes are more energy efficient than sedentary women. Differences in energy balance between a group of female cyclists and nontrained women were measured.

Methods.—Five trained female cyclists and 5 noncyclists aged 18–40 years were closely matched in age, body weight, and height. All were healthy nonsmokers. The women completed initial assessments of maximal oxygen uptake, body composition, and determination of menstrual status and then were scheduled for 2 separate measurements of daily energy expenditure in a whole-room indirect calorimeter, once on a cycling day and once on a noncycling day. The normal activity of both groups of women was measured by having them wear a Caltrac accelerometer for 2 separate 7-day periods. All were fed a fixed-composition diet (30% energy from fat, 55% from carbohydrates, 15% from protein) for 5 days before each measurement.

Results.—The cyclists achieved energy balance on the cycling day while consuming 2,900–3,000 kcal (their usual condition), and noncyclists achieved energy balance on noncycling days while consuming 2,100–2,200 kcal (their usual condition). On the cycling day, the daily energy expenditure was significantly higher in the cyclists, compared with the noncycling day, whereas the energy expenditure was not different in the noncyclists on the 2 days. The resting metabolic rate and thermic effect of food and activity (noncycling), the components of daily energy expenditure, were not significantly different between the groups.

Conclusion.—Trained female cyclists demonstrated no evidence of a significant increase in energy efficiency, compared with nontrained women. These results suggest that, in general, energy efficiency in female athletes is not higher than expected.

▶ Numerous reports of a low energy intake but stable body weight in amenorrheic athletes relative to their predicted energy intake has led some investigators to postulate that these athletes were more metabolically efficient than untrained women or eumenorrheic athletes. To date, the results of studies investigating this hypothesis have been inconclusive. The data in this study are unlikely to shed light on that question because these athletes were not amenorrheic and were in energy balance. However, the attention to detail in this protocol lends credence to the authors' conclusion that training does not increase energy efficiency in female cyclists.—B.L. Drinkwater, Ph.D.

The Effect of the Phase of the Menstrual Cycle and the Birth Control Pill on Athletic Performance
Lebrun CM (Univ of British Columbia, Vancouver, Canada)
Clin Sports Med 13:419–440, 1994   139-95-7–21

Introduction.—Very few studies have examined the influence of hormonal cycles on exercise performance. Throughout most of their athletic lives, women are exposed to rhythmic variation in endogenous or, in those taking oral contraceptives, exogenous hormones. Alone or together, estrogens and progestins can affect many metabolic processes; as a result, they may influence athletic performance, especially in elite athletes. Current knowledge of the effects of the menstrual cycle and oral contraceptives on athletic performance was reviewed.

The Menstrual Cycle.—Most early studies of the effects of the menstrual cycle on athletic performance were retrospective and anecdotal. The "phases" of the menstrual cycle were arbitrarily defined and do not correspond well to the follicular, ovulatory, and luteal phases determined by accurate hormonal measurements. Accurate determinations of cycle phase require hormonal measurements, including preexercise estrogen and progesterone levels; even basal body temperature monitoring is not completely accurate. Some studies without hormonal documentation have found little or no difference in athletic performance during various phases, whereas others have found that performance declines in the premenstrual or menstrual phase. Only a few studies using serum progesterone measurements to identify the luteal phase have found any significant changes in performance. In general, these studies suggest that maximal aerobic capacity and submaximal exercise responses are unchanged during the regular ovulatory menstrual cycle. Other studies have examined the effects of the menstrual cycle on metabolic performance, ventilation, cardiovascular response, thermoregulation, and strength.

Oral Contraceptives.—Many elite female athletes use oral contraceptives, but there are no definitive data regarding their potential effects on performance. Most research on this issue has looked at much higher oral contraceptive doses than those in current use. Only 2 prospective studies have been carried out with a low-dose triphasic or monophasic oral contraceptive formulation, the most commonly used types. One found a slight, reversible reduction in functional aerobic capacity after 6 months of a monophasic oral contraceptive; the other reported a similar response to a triphasic oral contraceptive. Other studies have examined the metabolic, respiratory, cardiovascular and hemodynamic, and strength responses to oral contraceptives.

Summary.—There is little agreement regarding the effects of the menstrual cycle phase or oral contraceptive use on athletic performance. Subtle changes have been demonstrated in some variables, but the effect seems to be insignificant for most women. The effects of cycle phase may be clarified by the use of newer techniques to detect ovulation. More studies during the midcycle estradiol surge are needed to separate the relative effect of estrogen and progesterone on performance. Prospective, double-blind, randomized studies of the currently used oral contraceptive formulations are needed.

▶ Although the monthly fluctuations in the gonadal hormones seem to have little effect on athletic performance, the 2 prospective studies of oral contraceptive agents suggesting a slight decrease in aerobic power are a concern. A number of physicians are prescribing oral contraceptives for amenorrheic athletes to guard against premature bone loss rather than as a contraceptive. If an athlete believes that the use of oral contraceptives might detract from her performance, she may elect not to use them, preferring to risk her future health for a better chance of athletic success now. Whether oral contraceptive use actually detracts from performance is not known, but the emphasis on aerobic power in the athletic world will make that a moot point. Perhaps someone will investigate whether the lower dose of estrogen in the medications prescribed for postmenopausal women would be able to protect the bones of young women without affecting their aerobic power.—B.L. Drinkwater, Ph.D.

The Effects of Gymnastics Training on Bone Mineral Density

Nichols DL, Sanborn CF, Bonnick SL, Ben-Ezra V, Gench B, DiMarco NM (Texas Woman's Univ, Denton)
Med Sci Sports Exerc 26:1220–1225, 1994   139-95-7–22

Background.—Recent evidence suggests that the bone loss associated with osteoporosis begins well before the menopause, when symptoms of the disease become apparent. Thus, early prevention techniques, includ-

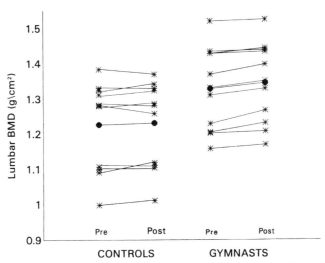

Fig 7–11.—Pregymnastics and postgymnastics training lumbar bone mineral density for controls and gymnasts. (Courtesy of Nichols DL, Sanborn CF, Bonnick SL, et al: *Med Sci Sports Exerc* 26:1220-1225, 1994.)

ing nutritional and exercise factors, are recommended. The effect of a 6-month gymnastics season on bone mineral density (BMD), lean tissue mass, levels of insulin-like growth factor I (IGF-I), and osteocalcin was investigated.

Method.—Eleven eumenorrheic female varsity gymnasts were compared with 11 sedentary, matched controls. During the school year, the gymnasts were involved in 144 days of practice. They trained an average of 4 hr/day, 5 days/wk with weight training, running, stretching, and formal gymnastic training. Bone density measurements were carried out at the beginning of the fall semester and, again, after 27 weeks of training by the gymnasts. The second bone scan was taken at the peak of the gymnasts' competitive season. A nutritional analysis of all participants was also carried out. Finally, hormone levels of IGF-I and osteocalcin were measured before and after 27 weeks of training.

Results.—Age, weight, and percent body fat were the only significantly different variables between the 2 groups. The mean number of years of training for the gymnasts was 9.7. Menarche was similar between the 2 groups (14.4 and 13.3 years for the gymnasts and controls, respectively). The preseasonal BMD values for the lumbar spine and femoral neck of the gymnasts were 1.328 and 1.193 g/cm^2, respectively. Corresponding mean preseasonal BMD values for the controls were 1.225 and 1.079 g/cm^2. After 27 weeks of training, gymnasts experienced a significant increase of 0.017 g/cm^2 in lumbar BMD. However, the increase in the

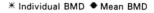

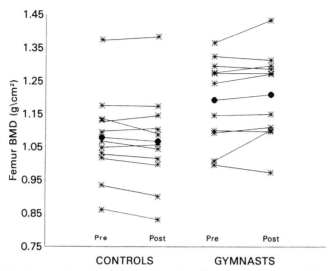

Fig 7–12.—Pregymnastics and postgymnastics training femoral neck bone mineral density (*BMD*) for controls and gymnasts. (Courtesy of Nichols DL, Sanborn CF, Bonnick SL, et al: *Med Sci Sports Exerc* 26:1220–1225, 1994.)

femoral neck density was not significant. Controls had no changes in BMD at either site (Figs 7–11 and 7–12). A significant increase in lean tissue mass was also seen in gymnasts after training. Gymnasts and controls had similar intakes of kilocalories and calcium. As the season progressed, the caloric intakes of the gymnasts tended to decrease slightly. Both groups were below the recommended dietary allowances for calcium. No significant differences in serum levels of IGF-I were seen in the 2 groups; however, osteocalcin levels were significantly higher in gymnasts than controls.

Conclusion.—There were significant increases in lumbar BMD and lean mass tissue in gymnasts after 27 weeks of intense training that incorporated a number of different activities. It would appear, therefore, that gymnastics is an appropriate means of increasing BMD as it places a variety of forces on the bone.

▶ The women in this study were members of an intercollegiate gymnastics team that practiced 4 hours per day, 5 days per week for 6 months. Although it is highly unlikely that large numbers of women will follow this demanding routine to decrease their risk for osteoporosis, the results do suggest that high-impact loading may be more effective in increasing bone mass than many repetitions of a lesser load. An increase of 0.017 g/cm² in lumbar density represents a 1.3% change in bone density, suggesting also that these women may have been at or near their biological potential for peak bone mass. An interesting aspect of these results is the similar finding in young figure skaters (1). Training in both sports begins at a very young age. Is this a factor in the higher bone density of these athletes?—B.L. Drinkwater, Ph.D.

Reference

1. Slemenda CW, Johnston CC: High intensity activities in young women: Site specific bone mass effects among female figure skaters. *Bone Miner* 20:125–132, 1993.

Gymnasts Exhibit Higher Bone Mass Than Runners Despite Similar Prevalence of Amenorrhea and Oligomenorrhea
Robinson TL, Snow-Harter C, Taaffe DR, Gillis D, Shaw J, Marcus R (Oregon State Univ, Corvallis; Palo Alto VA Med Ctr, Calif)
J Bone Miner Res 10:26–35, 1995   139-95-7–23

Background.—Regular weight-bearing exercise is generally thought to have beneficial effects on bone mass. However, athletes with amenorrhea and resultant low circulating estrogen levels appear to have lower than normal bone mineral density (BMD) values. In this study, lumbar spine, proximal femur, and whole body BMD in competitive female athletes who train by techniques that apply different types of skeletal loading and who have oligomenorrhea and amenorrhea were compared with those values for normally menstruating, college-age women.

Methods and Findings.—Twenty-one gymnasts and 20 runners were compared with 19 nonathletic women (Table 1). Values for percentage body fat were similar in runners and gymnasts and were lower than in nonathletes. Lean body mass was comparable among groups. When adjusted for body surface area, however, gymnasts had a greater lean body

TABLE 1.—Group Characteristics for the 3 Groups of Subjects (Mean ± SD)

	Runners (n = 20)	Gymnasts (n = 21)	Controls (n = 19)
Height, cm	167.5 ± 5.6	159.4 ± 4.3*	165.9 ± 7.5
Weight, kg	52.8 ± 4.5	55.0 ± 6.5	60.2 ± 6.5†
% Body fat	14.7 ± 2.2	15.6 ± 2.9	22.3 ± 3.0†
Lean body mass, kg	43.0 ± 3.3	45.0 ± 4.8	44.4 ± 3.0
LBM/Ht², kg/m²	15.3 ± 0.8	17.7 ± 1.2*	16.2 ± 1.6
Age, years	22.0 ± 2.6‡	19.5 ± 1.0	19.2 ± 1.6

* Gymnasts different from runners and controls, $P <0.01$–$P =0.0001$.
† Controls different from runners and gymnasts, $P <0.01$–$P =0.0001$.
‡ Runners different from gymnasts and controls, $P =0.0001$.
(Courtesy of Robinson TL, Snow-Harter C, Taaffe DR, et al: *J Bone Miner Res* 10:26–35, 1995.)

TABLE 2.—Menstrual Cycle Status for the 3 Groups of Subjects (Mean ± SD)

	Runners (n = 20)	Gymnasts (n = 18)	Controls (n = 19)
Age at menarche, years	14.4 ± 1.7[c]	16.2 ± 1.7[a]	13.0 ± 1.2
months	169.5 ± 16.8[c]	193.2 ± 18.8[a]	156.6 ± 14.3
# years since menarche	7.5 ± 2.3[c]	3.4 ± 1.9[a]	6.1 ± 2.1
# cycles since menarche	66.9 ± 37.0	29.7 ± 21.2[a]	70.4 ± 27.3
# cycles/year—current	9.6 ± 4.8	7.2 ± 4.7[a]	12.0 ± 0.4
# cycles/year—since menarche	8.8 ± 3.6	8.0 ± 3.7	11.4 ± 1.1[b]
Prevalence of oligomenorrhea	15%	19%	0%
Prevalence of amenorrhea	15%	28%	0%

[a] Gymnasts different from runners and controls, $P < 0.01$–$P = 0.0001$.
[b] Controls different from runners and gymnasts, $P < 0.01$–$P = 0.0001$.
[c] Runners different from gymnasts and controls, $P = 0.0001$.
(Courtesy of Robinson TL, Snow-Harter C, Taaffe DR, et al: J Bone Miner Res 10:26–35, 1995.)

mass/height² than runners and nonathletes. Gymnasts had significantly greater muscle strength in the quadriceps, biceps, and hip adductor force than runners and nonathletes. The prevalence of oligomenorrhea and amenorrhea was 47% in gymnasts, 30% in runners, and 0% in nonathletes. The gymnasts had a later menarche, fewer cycles per year, and fewer cycles since menarche than runners or controls (Table 2). The groups were comparable in dietary calcium intake. Among the athletes, BMD did not differ at any site according to current menstrual status (Table 3). Compared with those in the other 2 groups, lumbar spine and femoral neck BMD was reduced in runners. Gymnasts had a higher femoral neck BMD than runners and controls and a higher vertebral BMD than runners. After adjustment for estimated bone size, lumbar spine and femoral neck bone mineral apparent density differed among groups, the highest occurring in gymnasts and the lowest in runners.

Conclusion.—Gymnasts had higher femoral neck BMD than runners and nonathletes, as well as an older age at menarche and a slightly increased prevalence of oligomenorrhea and amenorrhea. Compared with gymnasts, runners had lower BMD values, despite similar current and historical menstrual cycle patterns. The mechanical forces generated from high-impact loading and muscular contraction during gymnastics training have powerful osteogenic effects. These effects seem to counteract the increased bone resorption that has been shown to result from oligomenorrhea and amenorrhea.

▶ The specificity of gymnastic training is evident in the bone density and muscle strength of the gymnasts. The bone density data are particularly interesting because 47% of the gymnasts were either oligomenorrheic or amen-

TABLE 3.—Bone Mineral Density (BMD) Values for All Subjects According to Current Menstrual Cycle Status and Past Menstrual History Since Menarche

	FN BMD	LS BMD	WB BMD
Runners			
Category 1 ($n = 3$)	0.781 ± 0.12	0.924 ± 0.12	1.001 ± 0.07
Category 2 ($n = 3$)	0.857 ± 0.06	0.880 ± 0.16	1.014 ± 0.05
Category 3 ($n = 8$)	0.898 ± 0.12	0.982 ± 0.09	1.038 ± 0.07
Category 4 ($n = 6$)	0.939 ± 0.06	1.053 ± 0.09	1.082 ± 0.04
Gymnasts			
Category 1 ($n = 6$)	1.049 ± 0.15	1.146 ± 0.10	1.082 ± 0.06
Category 2 ($n = 4$)	1.044 ± 0.10	1.143 ± 0.08	1.089 ± 0.08
Category 3 ($n = 6$)	1.125 ± 0.14	1.243 ± 0.18	1.170 ± 0.11
Category 4 ($n = 5$)	1.116 ± 0.03	1.140 ± 0.11	1.086 ± 0.04
Controls			
Category 5 ($n = 19$)	0.974 ± 0.10	1.111 ± 0.11	1.092 ± 0.06

*Bone mineral density values are by category as follows: category 1 = amenorrheic athletes with a history of oligomenorrhea and/or amenorrhea; category 2 = oligomenorrheic athletes with a history of oligomenorrhea and/or amenorrhea; category 3 = eumenorrheic athletes with a history of oligomenorrhea and/or amenorrhea; category 4 = eumenorrheic athletes who have always had regular menstrual cycles; category 5 = controls who are currently eumenorrheic and have always had regular menstrual cycles (means ± SD).

† Analysis of variance results:

Femoral neck (FN) BMD: 1 (runners) different from 4 (runners), 1-4 (gymnasts) & 5 controls ($P < 0.05$); 2 & 3 (runners) different from 1-4 (gymnasts); 4 (runners) different from 3 & 4 (gymnasts); 3 & 4 (gymnasts) different from 5 (controls).

Lumbar spine (LS) BMD: 1 & 3 (runners) different from 1-4 (gymnasts) & 5 (controls) ($P < 0.05$); 2 (runners) different from 4 (runners), 1-4 (gymnasts) & 5 (controls); 4 (runners) different from 3 (gymnasts); 3 (gymnasts) different from 5 (controls).

Whole body (WB) BMD: 1-4 (runners), 1 & 4 (gymnasts) & 5 (controls) different from 3 (gymnasts) ($P < 0.05$); 1 (runners) different from 5 (controls).

(Courtesy of Robinson TL, Snow-Harter C, Taaffe DR, et al: *J Bone Miner Res* 10:26–35, 1995.)

orrheic. Yet the bone density was higher than that of the eumenorrheic controls. This may be an example of how bone-loading activities can offset the decrease in estrogen levels if the intensity of the loading stimulus exceeds the threshold for an osteogenic response that has been increased as a result of the decrease in estrogen. However, within each sport group, there is an indication that menstrual history does have an effect on bone density. It will be interesting to see whether the gymnasts retain their advantage once they cease their intensive training.—B.L. Drinkwater, Ph.D.

Long-Term Unilateral Loading and Bone Mineral Density and Content in Female Squash Players

Haapasalo H, Kannus P, Sievänen H, Heinonen A, Oja P, Vuori I (UKK-Inst for Health Promotion Research, Tampere, Finland; Tampere Research Station of Sports Medicine, Finland)
Calcif Tissue Int 54:249–255, 1994   139-95-7–24

Introduction.—The risk of osteoporosis in later life is determined in part by the bone mass acquired during adolescence and early adulthood.

Comparison of Relative Side-To-Side Arm Differences (%) and the Mean BMD and BMC of Right Calcaneus Between Controls and Players (Mean ± SD)

	Difference (%)		
	Controls	Players	P-value
Circumference			
Upper arm	0.5 ± 2.8	3.7 ± 5.7	<0.05
Forearm	0.3 ± 3.1	6.3 ± 6.9	<0.01
Strength measurements			
Elbow extension	3.0 ± 9.9	16.1 ± 24.4	<0.05
Elbow flexion	7.1 ± 11.3	8.8 ± 13.6	ns
Grip strength	15.9 ± 10.3	22.9 ± 22.3	ns
BMD			
Proximal humerus	1.7 ± 2.9	15.6 ± 10.5	<0.001
Humeral shaft	2.5 ± 2.0	15.0 ± 11.2	<0.001
Radial shaft	1.8 ± 3.2	6.5 ± 4.9	<0.01
Ulnar shaft	1.6 ± 2.5	5.6 ± 4.9	<0.01
Distal radius	1.8 ± 3.4	10.0 ± 4.0	<0.001
Distal ulna	3.2 ± 3.5	11.0 ± 3.9	<0.001
BMC			
Proximal humerus	4.1 ± 4.5	17.8 ± 12.9	<0.001
Humeral shaft	3.0 ± 2.4	17.0 ± 13.3	<0.001
Radial shaft	3.2 ± 3.0	8.9 ± 5.7	<0.001
Ulnar shaft	3.5 ± 4.3	7.3 ± 7.2	ns
Distal radius	2.1 ± 4.0	12.4 ± 4.5	<0.001
Distal ulna	3.5 ± 6.1	11.1 ± 6.1	<0.001
Right calcaneus			
BMD ± SD (g/cm^2)	0.676 ± 0.057	0.760 ± 0.081	<0.001
BMC ± SD (g)	9.761 ± 1.240	10.956 ± 1.853	<0.05

Abbreviations: BMD, bone mineral density; BMC, bone mineral content; *ns*, not significant.
(Courtesy of Haapasalo H, Kannus P, Sievänen H, et al: *Calcif Tissue Int* 54:249–255, 1994.)

Acquisition of bone mass is determined by heredity, gender, hormonal status, physical activity, calcium intake, and weight and muscular strength. It is unclear when in life these factors become most important. Studies have established a connection between physical activity and the development of bone mass and density. Female squash players and sedentary controls were examined to determine the association between long-term activity and bone mineral content (BMC) and bone mineral density (BMD), and the effects of age, puberty, and menstrual history on this association.

Methods.—Nineteen national-level female squash players and 19 healthy, sedentary, age-, weight-, and height-matched control women were interviewed to obtain information on the years of squash playing, training intensity, diet, onset of menses, and menstrual status (oral contraceptives, normal cycle, irregular menstrual pattern, or amenorrhea). Height, weight, and upper and lower arm circumferences were measured and the proportion of body fat was determined. Grip strength, elbow extension, and flexion strength were measured in both extremities. The

BMC and BMD were measured with a dual-energy x-ray absorptiometer in the proximal humerus, humeral shaft, radial shaft, ulnar shaft, distal radius, distal ulna, and right calcaneus.

Results.—The players, but not the controls, had significant differences in the arm circumferences between the playing and nonplaying arms (table). There were substantial side-to-side differences in all strength measurements in players, with smaller but significant differences in grip strength and elbow flexion in controls. The players also had significant side-to-side differences in BMD and BMC, with the greatest differences in the proximal humerus and humeral shaft and the least difference in the ulnar shaft. The controls had lesser but significant differences in BMD and BMC. Calcaneal BMD and BMC were higher in the players. Differences in BMD and BMC between the playing and nonplaying arms correlated positively with the number of years of playing, the total time of training, elbow flexion strength; they correlated negatively with the age when training began. Differences were larger for players who began training before or during menarche.

Discussion.—Long-term squash playing produces high BMD and BMC values in the playing arm. The differences between the playing and nonplaying arm are substantial, which gives the playing arm many more years of protection against bone loss in later life. These findings also suggest that physical activity produces its greatest benefits during the rapid bone accumulation phase of puberty, although older individuals may also have significant bone gain with physical activity.

▶ There is a general feeling among those interested in the "exercise and osteoporosis" field that there is a window of opportunity in which to maximize peak bone mass and that that window is in childhood and adolescence. The authors of this study provide strong support for that theory with data showing a larger difference in bone mass and density between the racquet arm and nonracquet arm of women who began training at or before menarche compared with those who began training at an older age, even though the length of training was the same. If this benefit remains after the women cease their activity, it will also provide support for the theory that the effect of activity during childhood is more permanent than that in later life.—B.L. Drinkwater, Ph.D.

Effect of Boron Supplementation on Blood and Urinary Calcium, Magnesium, and Phosphorus, and Urinary Boron in Athletic and Sedentary Women

Meacham SL, Taper LJ, Volpe SL (Winthrop Univ, Rock Hill, SC; Virginia Polytechnic Inst and State Univ, Blacksburg, Va; Univ of Massachusetts, Amherst)

Am J Clin Nutr 61:341–345, 1995   139-95-7-25

Introduction.—Bone hypertrophy and bone mineral density are increased by weight-bearing exercise. However, the exercise-induced menstrual dysfunction that occurs in female athletes can lead to loss of bone mineral, an increased risk of osteoporosis, and increased musculoskeletal injuries. Previous studies have suggested that boron enhances optimal calcium metabolism and, therefore, bone metabolism. The effect of boron supplementation on mineral status in female athletes was assessed, as were some of the effects on serum and urinary mineral concentrations.

Methods.—The study included 28 female college students—17 athletic and 11 sedentary. The women's menstrual statuses were confirmed by monthly calendar recordings of menses and by weekly serum hormone assays during months 0, 6, and 10. The women were randomized in single-blind fashion to receive either boron, 3 mg/day, or placebo. They were allowed to follow their usual diet. Assessments included a Physical Work Capacity 170 Test, skinfold measurements to calculate percentage body fat, and daily food records and a duplicate-plate collection of all food and beverages consumed for 3 days. Blood samples were obtained at 0 and 10 months. Urine samples were collected during the 3-day period in which food collections were made and food records were kept. Urine was also collected at 10 months and again on a day in which food collections and records were made.

Results.—There were no differences between the groups in the daily percentages of energy consumed as protein, fat, and carbohydrate or in intakes of calcium, phosphorus, and magnesium; mineral intakes were low in both groups. At baseline, the dietary boron intake was 0.7 mg/day for the sedentary group vs. 1.5 mg/day for the athletic group. There were no differences in plasma normalized calcium concentrations with time, activity, or supplementation. Athletes who received boron had lower serum magnesium concentrations than their sedentary counterparts; no such difference was seen in women assigned to placebo. For all groups, the amount of calcium excreted in the urine was higher at the end of the study than at the beginning. Urinary phosphorus and magnesium excretion were unaffected by time, activity, or supplementation. Athletes who received boron had a fourfold increase in urinary boron excretion. The sedentary controls had a lesser increase, and the placebo groups had no change.

Conclusion.—Boron supplementation influences serum phosphorus and magnesium concentrations in young women. This effect is modified by exercise. The results suggest that increasing dietary calcium and boron may help balance blood minerals to optimize bone mineralization in young women.

▶ Until markers of bone metabolism are measured at the same time that dietary manipulation is taking place, the effect of specific nutrients on bone metabolism will remain a mystery. Tests for bone-specific alkaline phosphatase and N-telopeptide or pyridinoline and deoxypyridinoline would provide some indication of the rate of bone formation and resorption. The long-term effect on bone will only be determined by actually measuring changes in bone density over an extended period.—B.L. Drinkwater, Ph.D.

Intercondylar Notch Width and the Risk for Anterior Cruciate Ligament Rupture: A Case-Control Study in 46 Female Handball Players

Lund-Hanssen H, Gannon J, Engebretsen L, Holen KJ, Anda S, Vatten L (Trondheim Univ Hosp, Norway; Univ of Trondheim, Norway)
Acta Orthop Scand 65:529–532, 1994   139-95-7–26

Radiographic Measurements

	Injury group		Control group
	Uninjured knee	Reconstructed knee	Average dxt/sin
n	20	20	26
Age	20 (17–28)		21 (16–27)
Weight	64 (53–83)		67 (55–82)
Height	170 (160–180)		173 (163–183)
Anterior outlet mm SD	16.7 2.0*	18.2 2.1	18.5 3.1
Notch width index	0.224 (0.026)†	0.243 (0.028)	0.243 (0.038)
Posterior outlet mm SD	21.8 1.9‡	22.6 2.4	23.1 2.4
Total width mm SD	74.6 2.2§	74.8 2.9	76.2 3.6

*Difference from reconstructed knee, $P = 0.003$, and control group, $P = 0.02$.
†Difference from reconstructed knee, $P = 0.003$, and control group, $P = 0.04$.
‡Compared with control group, $P = 0.05$.
§Compared with control group, $P = 0.07$.
(Courtesy of Lund-Hanssen H, Gannon J, Engebretsen L, et al: *Acta Orthop Scand* 65:529–532, 1994.)

Introduction.—Rupture of the anterior cruciate ligament is a relatively common injury among Norwegian women engaged in high-level handball. A total of 46 female handball players were studied to determine whether a relationship exists between the width of the intercondylar notch of the femur and increased risk of anterior cruciate ligament rupture.

Methods.—Twenty of the handball players had had a previous unilateral anterior cruciate ligament rupture, and 26 had no history of knee ligament injuries. The 2 groups were similar in average age, weight, and height. In the injured group, ruptured ligaments had been reconstructed with a mid-third bone–patellar tendon–bone autograft. The average time from surgery to examination was 15 months. Lachman's test was used in the control group to rule out anterior cruciate ligament deficiency. Intercondylar fossa radiographs were obtained in a posteroanterior axial position, with individuals kneeling on the film with 70 degrees of flexion in the knee and with the tibia parallel to the table.

Results.—In the uninjured group, the notch width of the right and left knees was averaged. Notchplasty had been performed in all reconstructed knees; therefore, the uninjured knee in the injured group was compared with the average control width. The width index (NWI) was calculated as the ratio of the anterior notch width to the total condylar width. The injured group had a narrower anterior opening and NWI than the control group (table). Differences in the posterior opening were of borderline significance. An association was found between decreasing notch opening and an increased risk of anterior cruciate ligament injury. Compared with players with an anterior notch width wider than 17 mm, those with the narrower notch width were 6 times more susceptible to the injury. A similar trend was found using the NWI.

Conclusion.—A narrow anterior opening was associated with an increased risk of anterior cruciate ligament rupture in female handball players. The critical intercondylar notch width was 17 mm. Radiographs obtained using the method described here can be used to screen for rupture risk.

▶ Is anatomy destiny? Not necessarily! As usual, there is considerable overlap between groups whose means differ. Some women in the control group also have an anterior opening 17 mm or less; some injured players have an opening greater than 17 mm. To suggest, as the authors do, that players with an anterior opening less than 17 mm should be "counseled concerning their relatively high risk of ligament injury associated with continued participation in high-level handball" implies that these women should consider dropping the sport. An alternative course of action would be to explore the role of conditioning, skill, shoes, playing surface, etc., in reducing the risk of anterior cruciate ligament injuries for all participants—not just women with a narrow arch.—B.L. Drinkwater, Ph.D.

Gymnast Wrist: An Epidemiologic Survey of Ulnar Variance and Stress Changes of the Radial Physis in Elite Female Gymnasts

De Smet L, Claessens A, Lefevre J, Beunen G (Univ Hosp Pellenberg, Belgium; KU Leuven, Belgium)
Am J Sports Med 22:846–850, 1994   139-95-7-27

Introduction.—Because most female gymnasts begin training at a very young age, the wrist is transformed into a weight-bearing joint and undergoes stress-related changes. A survey of female competitive gymnasts was conducted to determine the occurrence and amount of ulnar overgrowth and its relationship to the weight, height, and chronological age of the athletes.

Methods.—Participants were the 201 female finalists at the World Championships Artistic Gymnastics, held at Rotterdam in 1987. The gymnasts ranged in age from 13.1 to 20.6 years (mean, 15.9 years) and had started formal training at a mean age of 7.1 years. Most were white (119) or Asian (24). Posteroanterior radiographs of the left hand and wrist showed open growth plates in 156 wrists, indicating that the gymnasts tended to have younger bone age than chronological age. For those with open physes, the method of Hafner et al. was used to determine ulnar variance. Palmer's method was used to measure the ulnar variance of the 35 wrists with closed physes. Films in the remaining 10 cases were not suitable for interpretation. Radiographs were also examined for stress-related reaction and other changes, including widened growth plates with irregular margins, ill-defined cystic appearance, and sclerosis.

Results.—When compared with female nonathletes of similar age, the 14- and 15-year-old gymnasts had significantly different ulnar variance characteristics (table). Relationships between measurements A (distance between the most proximal points of the ulnar and radial physes) and B (distance between the most distal points of the ulnar and radial physes) were strong. Ulnar variance showed no relationship to chronological

	Nongymnasts (Hafner et al.)		Gymnasts (Rotterdam 1987)*	
Variable (mm)	14	15	14 (N = 43)	15 (N = 39)
A value	−2.3	−2.3	0.68	0.21
B value	−2.7	−2.8	−0.93	−1.86

Comparison of Ulnar Variance Characteristics in 14- and 15-Year-Old Female Gymnasts and Nongymnasts

*All values significantly different from nongymnasts ($P < 0.02$).
(Courtesy of De Smet L, Claessens A, Lefevre J, et al: *Am J Sports Med* 22:846–850, 1994.)

age, training intensity, or performance score in the competition. Correlations were found between ulnar variance parameters and height and weight. Sixteen wrists showed stress-related changes of the radial physes that appeared as widening of the growth plate with irregular borders and radial side cystic defects. Adult gymnasts in the group also differed significantly from nonathlete adults with a positive ulnar variance.

Conclusion.—Wrist pain and injuries are common in gymnasts. The immature wrists of both male and female gymnasts are exposed to compressive and repetitive impact stress that may lead to premature closure of the distal radial growth plate and relative overgrowth of the ulna.

▶ The long-term consequences of repetitive high-impact loading on immature bone is still a matter of conjecture. Animal models suggest that excessive loading may inhibit growth, whereas low-to-moderate loading has a positive effect. Whether the overgrowth reported in this study will lead to degenerative changes in the future is unknown, but coupled with the other concerns surrounding the intense training schedules of young gymnasts, it is 1 more factor to be considered by the parents and physicians of these girls.

Parents would be well advised to check the credentials of the coach who has control of their child for several hours per day. Does this person have any professional background in the areas of growth and development, exercise physiology, or child psychology? What is the injury rate in this gymnastics program? Are children permitted—or encouraged—to resume training while still recovering from an injury? Physicians treating young gymnasts can educate parents about what to look for in a good program and can emphasize the importance of the parents' role in ensuring the health and safety of their child.—B.L. Drinkwater, Ph.D.

Effects of Chronic Exercise on Blood Volume Expansion and Hematologic Indices During Pregnancy

Pivarnik JM, Mauer MB, Ayres NA, Kirshon B, Dildy GA, Cotton DB (Baylor College of Medicine, Houston)
Obstet Gynecol 83:265–269, 1994   139-95-7–28

Introduction.—Pregnancy and chronic endurance exercise training both increase blood volume significantly. The exercise-induced blood volume changes occurring in endurance-trained gravidas might affect fetal birth weight and pregnancy outcome. To determine whether continuing aerobic exercise during pregnancy further enhances maternal blood volume expansion, blood volumes and hematologic indices were compared between physically active women who continued to exercise throughout pregnancy and healthy sedentary women.

Methods.—Nine aerobically trained, physically active pregnant women and 5 sedentary pregnant women were studied on 3 occasions: 25 and 36 weeks' gestation and 12 weeks post partum. A dye dilution method

Maternal Vascular Volumes and Other Hematologic Indices

	25 wk gestation		36 wk gestation		12 wk postpartum	
	Active	Sedentary	Active	Sedentary	Active	Sedentary
Blood volume						
mL	5777 ± 721	4994 ± 549*	6166 ± 1053	5053 ± 377*	4354 ± 505	3664 ± 414*†
mL/kg	88.5 ± 9.4	75.5 ± 9.8*	88.4 ± 17.3	70.9 ± 7.2*	72.2 ± 8.9	57.6 ± 3.6*†
Plasma volume (mL)	4009 ± 513	3446 ± 331*	4166 ± 785	3342 ± 170*	2800 ± 311	2355 ± 319*†
Red cell volume (mL)	1768 ± 232	1548 ± 236*	2000 ± 350	1711 ± 285*	1554 ± 234	1308 ± 193*†
Hematocrit (%)	34.8 ± 1.7	36.1 ± 1.9	36.6 ± 2.8	37.9 ± 3.4	39.9 ± 2.0	40.6 ± 4.7†
Hemoglobin (g/dL)	11.5 ± 0.5	11.7 ± 0.6	12.1 ± 0.9	12.2 ± 1.0	12.9 ± 0.8	13.1 ± 1.8†
Red blood cells (× 10^6/mm³)	3.64 ± 0.16	3.87 ± 0.18	3.78 ± 0.24	4.10 ± 0.27	4.31 ± 0.23	4.63 ± 0.6†
Plasma protein (g/dL)	6.2 ± 0.2	6.4 ± 0.5	6.4 ± 0.4	6.2 ± 0.4	6.8 ± 0.4	6.7 ± 0.3†

Note: Data are presented as mean ± SD.
*Values of active subjects are significantly ($P < 0.01$) greater than sedentary subjects.
†Values at 12 weeks post partum are significantly ($P < 0.001$) different than at 25 or 36 weeks' gestation.
(Courtesy of Pivarnik JM, Mauer MB, Ayres NA, et al: Obstet Gynecol 83:265–269, 1994.)

was used to estimate plasma volumes. Blood samples—obtained from the antecubital vein with the patients in seated, semirecumbent position—were also assessed for hematocrit ratio, hemoglobin concentration, red blood cell count, and plasma protein concentration. In addition, plasma volume estimates and hematocrit ratios were used to calculate blood and red blood cell volumes.

Results.—The 2 groups were no different in average birth weight and length of gestation. On analysis of variance, the physically active women had significantly greater absolute blood volumes than the sedentary controls at all 3 test intervals. Plasma and red blood cell volumes were also greater in the active women. At 25 weeks' gestation, blood volume relative to body weight was 88.5 mL/kg in the active women vs. 75.5 mL/kg in the controls; corresponding figures were 88.4 vs. 70.9 mL/kg at 36 weeks' gestation and 72.2 vs. 57.6 mL/kg at 12 weeks post partum. Both groups had significant reductions in all vascular volumes at 12 weeks post partum, whereas the hematologic indices—hematocrit ratio, hemoglobin concentration, red blood cell count, and plasma protein concentration—were all increased post partum (table).

Conclusion.—Physically active pregnant women have significantly greater vascular volumes than sedentary gravidas. Physically active women maintain this difference throughout pregnancy as they continue to exercise; however, there is no apparent effect on pregnancy outcome.

▶ As more and more data accumulate relative to exercise and pregnancy, active women can feel more comfortable about continuing to exercise during those 9 months. Whether there are any benefits or liabilities for the fetus or for the woman from this activity is still a matter of disagreement. One benefit on which there is general agreement is that the woman can retain a large portion of her cardiovascular fitness. However, it is incumbent on each woman to discuss her training regimen with her physician to be sure that no contraindications specific to her pregnancy are present. The majority of women, like those in this study, usually choose to moderate their activity by the third trimester.—B.L. Drinkwater, Ph.D.

Effects of Pregnancy and Chronic Exercise on Respiratory Responses to Graded Exercise
Wolfe LA, Walker RMC, Bonen A, McGrath MJ (Queen's Univ, Kingston, Ont, Canada; Univ of Waterloo, Ont, Canada)
J Appl Physiol 76:1928–1936, 1994   139-95-7–29

Introduction.—The endocrine effects of pregnancy lead to changes in many important physiologic functions. There has as yet been no study, however, of the effects of physical conditioning during pregnancy on the onset of blood lactate accumulation (OBLA). Twenty-seven previously sedentary women in their second and third trimesters were examined for

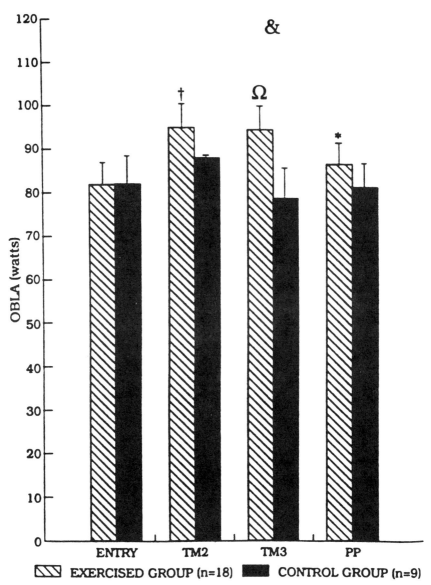

Fig 7–13.—Work rate at onset of blood lactate accumulation (*OBLA*). †Significant difference between group mean changes from entry. ΩSignificant change from entry to TM2 within group. *Significant change from entry to TM3 within group. &Significant change between TM3 and post partum within group. (Courtesy of Wolfe LA, Walker RMC, Bonen A, et al: *J Appl Physiol* 76:1928–1936, 1994.)

changes in respiratory control, gas exchange, and lactate kinetics during graded exercise.

Patients and Methods.—Pregnant women were eligible for the study if they were nonsmokers, were free of metabolic or cardiopulmonary diseases or conditions, had no other contraindications to exercise, and were taking no medications other than prenatal vitamin supplements. Eighteen women took part in a program of cycle ergometer conditioning and 9 served as a nonexercising control group. Both exercise and control groups underwent graded exercise tests at about 17, 27, and 37 weeks of gestation and at 20 weeks post partum. The physical conditioning sessions were conducted 3 days a week by a qualified instructor. Two experienced observers estimated the OBLA—as determined from the plot of respiratory variables vs. work rate—without knowledge of the women's identities, group assignment, or testing times.

Results.—Both exercise and control groups had augmented ventilatory responses to exercise throughout pregnancy. The exercise group demonstrated a 17% increase in oxygen pulse at peak exercise between entry and the third trimester. Their respiratory gas exchange ratio was reduced during standard submaximal exercise, and the work rate at OBLA was increased. The controls had no significant change in work rate at OBLA, either during pregnancy or in the postpartum period (Fig 7–13). For both exercise and control groups, the respiratory exchange ratio at peak exercise was higher in postpartum than in late-gestation tests. Nonexercise controls had significantly lower peak postexercise lactate levels in the second and third trimesters of pregnancy than in the postpartum period. Physical conditioning appeared to prevent this effect in the exercise group.

Conclusion.—In this group of healthy, previously sedentary pregnant women, moderate aerobic conditioning increased aerobic fitness and delayed the OBLA during graded exercise testing. Such conditioning may also lessen pregnancy-induced increases in ventilatory demand at high work rates and the reductions in maximal aerobic power that occur with advancing gestational age.

▶ Doctors are more often asked whether it is wise to continue exercising during pregnancy than whether a training program should be begun at this point in a patient's life. However, as this study shows, there is no reason why moderate training cannot be initiated during the second trimester of pregnancy, and there may be some positive dividends from such action. During the first trimester, it is important to avoid overheating of the body, as this increases the risk of teratoma, and later in pregnancy it is important not to push the exercise to the point of glycogen depletion or to use such a high intensity of effort that the placenta is deprived of blood.

The program adopted here (25 minutes of activity at an average heart rate of 143 beats/min) increased peak oxygen intake by some 17%. However, the study shows that there was a similar gain in the power output at the

OBLA, so this measurement can be used rather than direct maximal testing when assessing the response to training.—R.J. Shephard, M.D. Ph.D., D.P.E.

Fetal Responses to Maternal Exercise: Effect on Fetal Breathing and Body Movement

Winn HN, Hess O, Goldstein I, Wackers F, Hobbins JC (St Louis Univ, Mo; Yale Univ, New Haven, Conn)
Am J Perinatol 11:263–266, 1994   139-95-7-30

Introduction.—There are communities where the proportion of exercising women of reproductive age approaches 90%. A large portion of these women may continue to exercise during pregnancy. The effect of exercise on the health of the fetus is a primary concern of these women. The effects of exercise on 2 common parameters of fetal well-being—fetal breathing and movement—were examined.

Methods.—Entry criteria for the study were an uncomplicated current pregnancy, involvement in an exercise program, a gestational age of 26 to 36 weeks, and no history of abnormal pregnancies. Twelve patients participated in the study. The test exercise was according to a modified Bruce protocol, carried to 75% of the age-adjusted maximal heart rate. With the mother lying in the left lateral position, fetal activities were observed for 20 minutes before and after exercise, using ultrasonography. The fetal heart rate was also monitored during exercise.

Results.—The women averaged 32 years of age, 145 lb, and 30 weeks gestational age. Maternal cardiovascular responses to progressive exercise followed expected trends. The total duration of fetal breathing and body movements was significantly reduced (Tables 1 and 2). Fetal bradycardia was not observed. The average birthweight was 3,378 g, and all but 1 neonate had Apgar scores of at least 7 at 1 and 5 minutes after delivery.

Comment.—The mechanism for the observed reduction in duration of fetal breathing and body movements cannot be determined from these data. Other investigators have suggested that the maternal exercise intensity should not exceed 70% of maximum oxygen consumption, similar to the work rates adopted in this study. Because blood pressure increases during exercise, the hypertensive pregnant patient may be well advised to discontinue training.

▶ The increase in maternal diastolic pressure reported here (from a resting value of 63 mm Hg to a peak value of 73 mm Hg during exercise) is hardly enough to cause concern, but it would seem important to make some observations on women with higher resting blood pressures before concluding too hastily that exercise is either safe or dangerous for the pregnant woman who is showing signs of hypertension.

TABLE 1.—Fetal Activities

	Preexercise (mean ± SD)	Postexercise (mean ± SD)	P Value
Breathing movement			
Frequency of ≥30 sec	2.3 ± 2.4	0.3 ± 0.6	0.02
Total duration (sec)	158.8 ± 108.2	60.9 ± 35.0	0.02
Body movement			
Frequency of ≥30 sec	1.9 ± 1.5	0.8 ± 1.3	0.07
Total duration (sec)	157.2 ± 107.05	96.8 ± 74.9	0.05

(Courtesy of Winn HN, Hess O, Goldstein I, et al: *Am J Perinatol* 11:263–266, 1994.)

The reduction of fetal movements during and after exercise was quite dramatic. Because the decrease in fetal activity continued into the recovery period, it is unlikely to reflect fetal hypoxia; more probably, it is a consequence of a reduction in blood glucose. At least one report (1) has drawn a linkage between fetal breathing movements and plasma glucose levels.—R.J. Shephard, M.D., Ph.D., D.P.E.

TABLE 2.—Total Duration of Fetal Activities

	Preexercise (mean ± SD)	Postexercise (mean ± SD)	P Value
Breathing movement (seconds)	158 ± 108.2	60.9 ± 35.0	0.02
Body movement (seconds)	157.2 ± 107.5	96.6 ± 74.9	0.05

(Courtesy of Winn HN, Hess O, Goldstein I, et al: *Am J Perinatol* 11:263–266, 1994.)

Reference

1. Patrick J, et al: *Am J Obstet Gynecol* 132:507, 1978.

The Initiation of Normal Walking

Elble RJ, Moody C, Leffler K, Sinha R (Southern Illinois Univ, Springfield)
Mov Disord 9:139–146, 1994   139-95-7–31

Objective.—Lower extremity electromyograms, ground reaction forces, and body motion were measured during brisk initiation of forward walking to determine the highly integrated limb movements and postural shifts that underlie gait initiation.

Patients and Findings.—Twelve healthy adults aged 20–82 years participated. Gait was initiated 20 times in response to a visual signal. The center of pressure beneath each foot during quiet stance was 2–9 cm anterior to the ankle for both younger and older participants. Initiation of forward walking started with a posterior movement of the center of pressure beneath each foot (Fig 7–14). During gait initiation, the body rotated about the ankles in a manner similar to a flexible inverted pendulum. The muscles of the lower extremities were activated stereotypically, creating moments of force about the ankles that drove the body toward the stance foot and into forward motion. All participants had similar patterns of gait initiation. The reproducibility of these patterns permitted computer averaging of multiple steps by each individual.

Conclusion.—Gait initiation is a stereotyped sequence of postural shifts that drive the body over the stance leg and into forward motion.

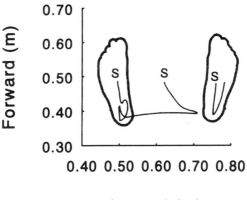

Lateral (m)

Fig 7–14.—Center of pressure beneath each foot and the resultant center of pressure during the initiation of gait. The center of pressure trajectories began at S and are the ensemble averages of 16 trials done by a 23-year-old woman. The woman stepped with her right foot. (Courtesy of Elble RJ, Moody C, Leffler K, et al: *Mov Disord* 9:139–146, 1994.)

Start hesitation and other disturbances of gait initiation may be a result of postural control, movement, or the integration of the two. Because normal gait initiation is sufficiently stereotyped, quantitative studies should provide useful measures of clinical disability and insights into the mechanisms of start hesitation.

▶ Five of the 12 subjects in this study were beyond 70 years of age, with 2 being over 80 years of age. Although they were all classified as being healthy adults, it is interesting that there was little to distinguish these 5 from the other 7 when it came to measuring the variables involved in the initiation of brisk forward walking. It would appear that the image of the shuffling elderly person is not something that is necessarily true among healthy older adults. One must wonder whether the shuffling gait is reversible.—Col. J.L. Anderson, PE.D.

A Comparison of Gait Characteristics in Young and Old Subjects
Ostrosky KM, VanSwearingen JM, Burdett RG, Gee Z (Univ of Pittsburgh, Pa; Leader Nursing and Rehabilitation Ctr, Pittsburgh, Pa)
Phys Ther 74:637–646, 1994   139-95-7–32

Background.—Gait characteristics that have been addressed in many studies comparing young and older subjects include temporal and distance factors with specific joint range-of-motion measurements during gait, or temporal and distance factors alone. The active range of motion during free-speed gait in younger and older individuals was described and compared.

Methods.—There were 60 volunteer participants in good health, 30 between 20 and 40 years of age and 30 between 60 and 80 years of age. Half the individuals in each group were women. Subjects wore 6 reflective markers along their right side as they were videotaped walking down a 6-m walkway. Nine gait characteristics were analyzed, and in both groups, the means and standard deviations were calculated for each characteristic (table).

Results.—Peak knee extension range of motion and stride length were significantly different between groups, and they were significantly less in the older individuals. Differences in speed approached significance; older individuals walked more slowly than younger individuals.

Conclusion.—It may be important to evaluate knee extension in the elderly and develop treatment to normalize knee extension to improve gait pattern or performance. Length of stride and speed could also be measured and addressed during treatment.

▶ Although there is nothing surprising about the data from this study, the question I have is, can anything be done about it? The aging process must account for something, but can we slow the process with conditioning? The

Values for 9 Gait Characteristics by Group

Gait Characteristic	Young People			Older People		
	X̄	SD	Range	X̄	SD	Range
Hip extension (°)	10	9	-4–36	8	6	-1–23
Hip flexion (°)	26	8	15–53	29	8	13–46
Knee extension*(°)	-3	4	-9–8	-7	4	-17–1
Knee flexion (°)	66	4	58–74	69	5	61–81
Ankle dorsiflexion (°)	12	5	4–27	14	3	8–19
Ankle plantar flexion (°)	28	8	12–49	24	6	12–37
Stride length (cm)	152.02	11.94	125.61–177.26	141.80	13.62	115.14–172.89
Stride time (s)	1.12	0.07	0.98–1.28	1.13	0.11	0.95–1.32
Velocity (cm/s)	137.99	13.86	117.20–168.82	127.02	16.02	92.73–170.58

*Positive value represents hyperextension.
(Courtesy of Ostrosky KM, VanSwearingen JM, Burdett RG, et al: *Phys Ther* 74:637–646, 1994.)

lesser knee extension would appear to partially account for the shorter stride length. Is the lesser knee extension caused by the loss of muscle mass that comes from aging?—Col. J.L. Anderson, PE.D.

Muscle Strength and Fiber Adaptations to a Year-Long Resistance Training Program in Elderly Men and Women

Pyka G, Lindenberger E, Charette S, Marcus R (Stanford Univ, Palo Alto, Calif; Dept of Veterans Affairs Med Ctr, Palo Alto, Calif)
J Gerontol 49:M22–M27, 1994   139-95-7–33

Background.—Little is currently known about the long-term adaptive responses to resistance exercise among older men and women. Strength training may provide various health benefits to elderly individuals; however, it is important to determine whether this type of training can lead to persistent improvement, with reasonable long-term compliance, before such strategies are recommended. The effects of resistance training on muscle strength and size were, therefore, investigated in older men and women.

Participants and Methods.—Eight men and 17 women (mean age, 68.2 years) were enrolled in this 1-year exercise trial. Fourteen were randomly assigned to exercise, and 11 were assigned to control groups. Maximum strength was tested in all participants with the 1 repetition maximum (1-RM) method (the maximum weight that can be lifted not more than once with acceptable form), after which the exercise group began a 12-exercise circuit involving all major muscle groups. Three sets of 8 repetitions were done at 75% of 1-RM 3 times per week. Controls were asked to continue their usual activities and not to participate in any exercise program during the 1-year study. In the exercise group, the 1-RM values were determined every 2 weeks during the first 15 weeks and every 3 weeks thereafter. Controls were tested at 15, 20, and 52 weeks. Muscle biopsy specimens were also obtained from 8 exercisers and 3 controls at baseline and at 15 weeks.

Results.—Three of the exercisers withdrew from the study for reasons unrelated to the training program. Muscle strength increased with exercise, with average increases ranging from 30% for hip extensors to 97% for hip flexors. Strength rapidly increased during the first 3 months and then plateaued for the remainder of the study. Strength in the controls did not change. Compared with baseline values, the cross-sectional area of type 1 muscle fibers in the exercise group increased by 29.4% at 15 weeks and 58.5% after 30 weeks. The type 2 fiber area did not change at 15 weeks but increased by 66.6% at 30 weeks of training.

Conclusion.—Prolonged moderate- to high-intensity resistance training may be undertaken by healthy older individuals with reasonable compliance. Such training leads to sustained increases in muscle strength, which are rapidly achieved and accompanied by hypertrophy of type 1 and 2 muscle fibers.

▶ Studies such as this are of significant benefit to the elderly. It should no longer be a question of whether moderate- to high-intensity strength training will be beneficial to the healthy elderly population, but rather we should be asking how we can make such programs available to them. Recent research has suggested that in order to increase bone mineral content in the elderly to help prevent osteoporosis, the skeleton must be subjected to forces greather than the normal forces of everyday living. Lifting weights is one way to introduce those increased forces in a controlled way.—Col. J.L. Anderson, PE.D.

Skeletal Muscle Weakness in Old Age: Underlying Mechanisms
Brooks SV, Faulkner JA (Univ of Michigan, Ann Arbor)
Med Sci Sports Exerc 26:432–439, 1994   139-95-7–34

Objective.—Impairment of skeletal muscle function in old age can lead to physical frailty. Although the causes of frailty are not known, understanding the mechanisms responsible for these changes can shed some light on prevention and treatment. The structural and functional deficits that lead to the frailty associated with aging were reviewed.

Muscle Atrophy.—Muscle mass declines by 25% to 30% by age 70 years, primarily because of the loss of the large type II muscle fibers. This loss could be caused by direct loss of type II fibers or to a conversion of type II fibers to the smaller type I fibers.

Absolute Force.—Between 30 and 80 years of age, muscle strength has declined by 30% to 40% and is related to loss of muscle mass.

Specific Force.—The degree of decline in the force-developing capacity of muscle fiber is related to the number of cross-bridges per unit area in single fibers.

Force-Velocity Relationships.—In old age, muscle strength is much weaker during shortening contractions than in lengthening contractions for reasons that are not clear.

Maximum and Sustained Power Output.—Maximum sustained muscle power and the ability to maintain duty cycles decline significantly with age, possibly because of decreased delivery or use of oxygen by the muscles.

Contraction-Induced Injury.—Muscles in older animals have shown a decreased recovery capacity as the result of reinnervation problems.

Motor Unit Remodeling.—Muscles in humans appear to be susceptible to age-related denervation atrophy.

Conclusion.—Preferential degeneration of faster motor nerves, denervation of faster muscle fibers, type II fiber atrophy, decline in the number of fibers, decrease in muscle mass, increased susceptibility to injury, and decreased ability to heal all contribute to skeletal muscle weakness in old age.

▶ The process of aging is not well understood. We know that certain things happen within muscles as we age, such as muscle atrophy, declining muscle strength and power, more rapid fatigue, and injury. However, we do not understand what the rate of change should be or what we can do about it. For instance, will weight training slow down the rate of change and by how much? Will people who have not been active earlier in their lives benefit from weight training later in their lives and by how much? Do people who have been physically active early in their lives have an advantage in maintaining their muscle through exercise later in life? There are many questions about aging that we must study to arrive at valid answers.—Col. J.L. Anderson, PE.D.

Biomechanics and Muscular Activity During Sit-to-Stand Transfer
Roebroeck ME, Doorenbosch CAM, Harlaar J, Jacobs R, Lankhorst GJ (Free Univ, Amsterdam)
Clin Biomech 9:235–244, 1994   139-95-7–35

Background.—The biomechanics and muscular activity of sit-to-stand (STS) transfer were measured as participants stood up from a chair. Three mechanisms were evaluated in a standardized fashion: the kine-

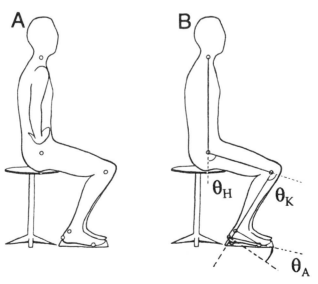

Fig 7–15.—Standardized starting position of the subjects. **A,** positions of the markers applied to the skin of the participants; **B,** definition of joint angles for hip (θ_H), knee (θ_K), and ankle (θ_A). (Courtesy of Roebroeck ME, Doorenbosch CAM, Harlaar J, et al: *Clin Biomech* 9:235-244, 1994.)

matics, kinetics, and muscle activation of STS transfer; the mechanisms applied in STS transfer; and muscle co-contractions in STS transfer.

Method.—Ten healthy persons were studied during 8 trials of STS transfer. Ground reaction forces and electromyograms were recorded on film. Participants began seated, with hands on hips and trunk vertical, and rose naturally to standing. The speed of the rise was standardized with a metronome. Markers were placed on the skin to correspond to the joint angles for the hip, knee, and ankle (Fig 7–15). Kinematics were measured with a high-speed camera. Telemetric electromyography (EMG) measured the activation of 9 leg muscles. Film, force, and EMG data were averaged over 5 trials; the first 3 attempts were practice trials. The standard error of the mean was used to analyze data.

Results.—The total movement time was 2.25 seconds. Typically, the ground reaction force was directed slightly backward and anterior of the hip and ankle and posterior of the knee at seat-off. Three phases of STS transfer were identified: acceleration, transition, and deceleration. Backward rotation of the upper body was noted throughout STS transfer. Electromyography values showed that the activity of all muscles during STS transfer was lower than standard isometric contractions. Joint rotations in hip and knee are most marked during STS transfer. Co-contraction of the hamstrings and rectus femoris occurred in the transition phase.

▶ Although the authors point out that their data are not generalizable to the elderly population, it seems to me that this is the population that can be helped most by this information. Training programs for the elderly are needed to help them to maintain their quality of daily living. Rising from the sitting position is one of the activities that they perform most frequently every day.—Col. J.L. Anderson, PE.D.

Cross-Sectional Areas of Fat and Muscle in Limbs During Growth and Middle Age

Kanehisa H, Ikegawa S, Tsunoda N, Fukunaga T (Toyama Univ, Japan; Univ of Tokyo)

Int J Sports Med 15:420–425, 1994   139-95-7–36

Introduction.—B-mode ultrasonography has been successfully used to determine the cross-sectional area (CSA) of fat and muscle of limbs for children and adults. The relationship between age and CSAs of fat and muscle of limbs during growth and middle age was investigated to provide information for the assessment of development and degeneration in muscle function.

Methods.—Research subjects were 245 Japanese males and 275 Japanese females with an age range of 6-60 years. Children were not involved in any physical training programs outside of school activities.

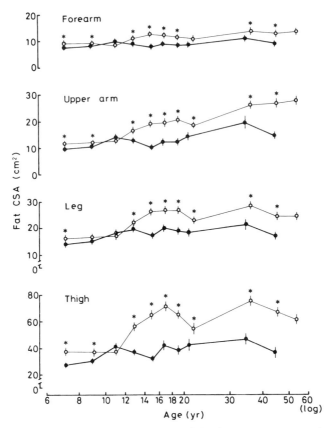

Fig 7–16.—Age changes in fat cross-sectional areas. *Filled and open points* represent the mean values of male and femal subject groups, respectively. The *verticle bars* at each data point indicate the standard errors of the mean. *Asterisks* indicate significant difference between females and males within the same age generation, *P* < 0.05. (Courtesy of Kanehisa H, Ikegawa S, Tsunoda N, et al: *Int J Sports Med* 15:420–425, 1994.)

Adults were mildly active or sedentary. All participants were apparently healthy. Cross-sectional images of the right forearm, upper arm, lower leg, and thigh were measured using B-mode ultrasound. To determine accuracy, male and female cadavers were used for comparison of cross-sectional measurements.

Results.—In males, fat CSAs increased to age 11 years, decreased at age 13–15 years, then increased to middle age, with the exception of a drop in the 40s. In females, fat from early age to 11 years remained about the same, then increased abruptly to age 15 years, dropped in the 20s, then increased again in the 30s (Fig 7–16). Muscle CSAs increased with growth to age 13 similarly in both sexes. From age 13 to 17 years, muscle growth in males increased exponentially; growth was particularly high in the upper extremities, compared with females. Muscle CSA remained almost constant for both sexes through young adulthood and middle age. During and after their 30s, muscle CSA·Ht·BM⁻¹ in females decreased. Fat CSAs and CSA·Ht·BM⁻¹ increased in both sexes during their 30s but decreased during their 40s.

Conclusion.—Results of age changes in fat and muscle CSAs during growth are similar to results of other investigations. However, the lack of fat increase observed after age 40 years varies from other reports. Only Japanese participants were used, so differences may be the result of race.

▶ Although it is true that all of these subjects were Japanese and these data probably cannot be extrapolated to the population of this country, it would be interesting to have similar data regarding the American population. These authors said their subjects were from the Japanese middle class. I wonder what the data from their lower-class population or, for that matter, their upper class would look like. It is my guess that in America we have more obesity within our lower class than we do within our middle class.—Col. J.L. Anderson, PE.D.

Running and the Development of Disability With Age
Fries JF, Singh G, Morfeld D, Hubert HB, Lane NE, Brown BW Jr (Stanford Univ, Calif)
Ann Intern Med 121:502–509, 1994   139-95-7–37

Background.—Although physical activity is known to decrease mortality rates, its effects on morbidity and disability are less clear. An activity such as aerobic running might delay or prevent disability through increased fitness and training; however, it might also accelerate the development of disability because of osteoarthritis or cumulative trauma. An 8-year longitudinal comparison of progression of disability scores between runners and nonrunners was reported.

Methods.—The study included 451 runners selected from the membership of The Fifty-Plus Runners Association and 330 community controls. The average history of running among the runners was 12 years. Persons in both groups were aged 50 to 72 years in 1984 when they responded to a questionnaire on exercise, medical, and dietary history; musculoskeletal injuries; and other variables. They also responded to annual questionnaires during 8 years of follow-up. The main outcome measure was disability, as indicated by responses to the previously validated Health Assessment Questionnaire, which evaluates function in dressing and grooming, arising, eating, walking, hygiene, reach, grip, and activities.

Results.—At baseline, the runners—including controls with a history of running—were leaner, had less frequent joint symptoms, took fewer medications, had fewer medical problems, and had fewer and less severe instances of disability. These differences, which may have reflected either

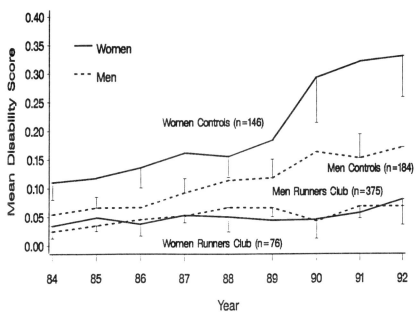

Fig 7–17.—Progression of disability over time by sex. Runners' club compared with community controls. Disability progression is less in the runners' club members. Significant differences were noted for men and women, with the effects more pronounced in women (P < 0.05). *Bars* represent 95% confidence intervals (1992 participants). (Courtesy of Fries JF, Singh G, Morfeld D, et al: *Ann Intern Med* 121:502–509, 1994.)

improved health because of running or self-selection bias, persisted after 8 years. One third of the runners' club members had stopped running; however, the frequency of other vigorous exercise increased in both groups, particularly among runners. During follow-up, disability levels increased steadily from 0.026 to 0.071 for runners and from 0.079 to 0.242 for controls. The difference was significant and consistent between sexes (Fig 7–17). The lower rate of disability among runners' club members persisted after adjustment for age, sex, body mass, baseline disability, smoking history, history of arthritis, and other co-morbid conditions. All age groups had progressive increases in disability; the oldest groups showed an increase in the slope of the disability curve. Mortality was also lower in the runners' club members than in controls (1.5% compared with 7%). The mortality differences remained after adjustment for age, sex, body mass, co-morbid conditions, education level, smoking history, alcohol intake, and mean blood pressure; the conditional risk ratio for controls compared with runners was 4.27.

Conclusion.—Disability develops at a significantly slower rate in older adults who engage in aerobic running and other vigorous exercise. Mortality is lower in runners as well. The benefits of running most likely result from increased aerobic activity, strength, fitness, and organ reserve rather than from postponement of osteoarthritis. The findings have important implications for efforts to increase regular physical exercise throughout the life span. However, it is difficult to remove the influence of self-selection bias—there is no way to tell whether more rigorous exercise could make controls as healthy as runners.

▶ A mere extension of the life span is not a major reason for encouraging regular exercise in an elderly population. The gains in survival among senior citizens are small, as the mortality curves for active and sedentary goups converge to a common value around 80 years of age (1). Indeed, in the oldest age categories, vigorous physical activity may even shorten the lifespan. A much more important reason for advocating regular exercise is to sustain competence in the activities of daily living and, thus, independence.

The average sedentary individual spends a terminal period of perhaps 10 years of partial dependency and 1 year of total dependency, and the quality-adjusted life expectancy is greatly enhanced if this period of disability can be shortened by a program of regular physical activity (2). Given the gains in aerobic power, muscle strength, and flexibility that can be realized by a training program, it is easy to see that, in principle, an exercise training program should increase quality-adjusted life-years by a substantial margin.

This paper points in the direction of a faster deterioration of quality of life in the sedentary group, but, unfortunately, it cannot give conclusive proof of this because the active individuals entered the study with better function than sedentary individuals; their slower rate of deterioration could have arisen in part because of self-selection of exercise by a group with less disability. Nevertheless, it is a sobering thought that a quarter of sedentary people have already lost sufficient strength so that they have difficulty rising from a chair by the age of 66 years. Unless they enter a conditioning program, many of this group are going to be grossly disabled before they die.—R.J. Shephard, M.D., Ph.D., D.P.E.

References

1. Pekkanen J, Marti B, Nissinen A, et al: Reduction of premature mortality by high physical activity: A 20-year follow-up of middle-aged Finnish men. *Lancet* 1:1473–1477, 1987.
2. Shephard RJ. Fitness and aging, in Blais C (ed): *Aging Into the Twenty First Century.* Downsview, Ontario, Captus University Publications, 1991, pp 22–35.

Predictors of Physical Disability After Age 50: Six-Year Longitudinal Study in a Runners Club and a University Population
Hubert HB, Fries JF (Stanford Univ, Calif)
Ann Epidemiol 4:285–294, 1994   139-95-7–38

Introduction.—With the increase in life expectancy, quality of life has become an important issue. Physical and mental health and the ability to remain self-sufficient in managing daily activities have been determined to be 2 important factors in qualify of life. Knowledge of these factors and a determination of the optimal way to preserve them are essential for designing models for successful aging. To identify such factors and their relationship to the development of physical disability, 2 cohorts were evaluated during a 6-year period, with a focus on the effects of running for exercise on disability.

Methods.—Participants aged 50–80 years were recruited from a running club (The Fifty-Plus Runners Association) and a university population (faculty and staff at Stanford University) for a comparison of extremely active and less active individuals. Two cohorts were formed on the basis of response from an initial questionnaire: 539 persons from the running club and 422 persons from the university. Each year from 1984 to 1990, participants were mailed a questionnaire on sociodemographic characteristics relating to health habits, time spent in vigorous exercise, diet, medical and family history, tobacco and alcohol intake, and disability. The Stanford Health Assessment Questionnaire was used to determine physical disability. The relationship between the baseline data collected in 1984 and the disability scores determined in 1990 was evaluated. Data for analysis were selected on the basis of their reported or theorized association with disability, chronic or musculoskeletal disease, and death.

Results.—Questionnaires from 706 persons (407 runners and 299 university participants) were available for analysis. At baseline, those in the runners club had overall better health and less disability than university participants ($P < 0.001$). Runners tended to be leaner and have a lower fat and salt intake than university participants. Runners also reported lower heart rates, systolic blood pressures, less medication use, less arthritis, younger age, and more lifetime physical activities compared with university participants. With the exception of running, there was no difference in vigorous activities between the 2 groups at baseline. Disability scores in 1990 showed university participants to have greater disability in each age group evaluated and a greater increase in disability with age as compared with runners. Older age, higher baseline disability, higher blood pressure, more medications used, family or personal history of arthritis, more cigarette pack-years, single marital status, less physical activity than peers, and more vigorous lifetime work activity were associated with a higher disability rate in 1990 for the university group ($P < 0.05$). For runners, a greater disability was associated with greater baseline disability, lifetime cigarette consumption, greater salt intake and medication use, joint pain and swelling, fewer miles run per week, no current running, and more years running at baseline. Changes in medication use, a decline in alcohol consumption, and the development of joint pain over the 6-year period were associated with greater disability among runners. For university participants, development of joint pain or arthritis, increase in body mass index, and bone fractures were changes associated with greater disability.

Conclusion.—Physical disability appears to be linked to several factors. Less exercise, cigarette smoking, arthritis history, medication use, blood pressure, and single marital status were found to be predictors of disability in the university group. Running status at baseline appeared to be a predictor of disability for running club members. The hypothesis that continuing physical activity into middle and older years will maintain physical ability is supported.

▶ This is an ongoing study of "successful aging." Basically, it follows a group of over-50 runners and a control group of less active people. A companion report adds information (1). At the start of this study, the average age of the subjects was 60 years and the average runner had run about 25 miles per week for 12 years. At the start, runners were healthier than controls; they were leaner and had lower blood pressure, less arthritis, less disability, and fewer doctor visits and took less medication. After 8 years, the "health gap" between runners and controls had widened (1): Male runners were 40% less likely and female runners nearly 90% less likely to have disability (difficulty in performing everyday tasks).

This article explores predictors of such disability in both groups. Predictors in the controls included less exercise, smoking, arthritis history, co-morbidities (reflected by medication use and high blood pressure), and unmarried status. A key predictor in the runners was how much they ran at baseline; those not currently running or running fewer miles per week had more disability later. Self-selection bias cannot be ruled out, but this study suggests that people who stay active in middle age are more apt to "age successfully." In other words, it pays to run for your life.—E.R. Eichner, M.D.

Reference

1. Fries JF, et al: *Ann Intern Med* 121:502, 1994.

The Effects of Nonswimming Water Exercises on Older Adults
Ruoti RG, Troup JT, Berger RA (Warminster, Pa; Temple Univ, Philadelphia)
J Orthop Sports Phys Ther 19:140–145, 1994   139-95-7–39

Background.—Exercise in water may be better for older persons needing rehabilitation because a water medium reduces weight-bearing stresses on joints. The effects of nonswimming water exercises on muscle endurance, body composition, and aerobic work capacity in older adults were investigated.

Methods.—The study started with 44 participants, but, for various reasons, only 12 (mean age, 65 years; 10 women) randomly assigned to the exercise group and 8 (mean age, 56 years; 5 women) to the control group completed the study. During a 1-week period before and again during a 1-week period after 12 weeks of training, each person was evaluated 3 times for resting heart rate (HR), maximum HR, body composition, maximum oxygen consumption (VO_{2max}), and work capacity in water. The exercise group exercised for 60 minutes 3 times weekly; their

HR was monitored periodically to ensure exercise compliance to a target HR of about 80% of maximum.

Results.—Over the 12-week period, the exercise group significantly improved in all evaluated measurements except body composition (percentage of body fat); the control group had no significant improvement in any measurement. In the exercise group, the mean resting HR decreased from 72 to 67 beats/min and the endurance walk HR (at the same workload) decreased from 124 to 98 beats/min. The 15% increase in $\dot{V}O_{2max}$ was similar to the improvement reported for older adults after 8–42 weeks of running exercises.

Conclusion.—Cardiorespiratory function and physical work capacity are improved in older adults by a regular thrice-weekly program of non-swimming exercises. Exercise in water reduces the effects of weight-bearing on skeletal joints and provides exercise loading because of the resistive effect of water on joint movements.

▶ Pool exercises are an attractive social option for seniors. Although it appears to the casual observer that the intensity of activity is quite low, in fact (as this study documents) a substantial training effect can be obtained because of the resistance to movement imposed by the water. If it is necessary to increase the training stimulus, the speed of limb movement can be increased, or the patients can move fins through the water (1). The improvements in flexibility attained by the program of pool exercises in this study are particularly impressive and important from a functional point of view; however, as in many studies of moderate-intensity exercise, the trend to a decrease of body fat content was not statistically significant. One unanswered question is whether such activity provides an adequate stimulus to osteoporotic bone. It is interesting that many of the defections from the study were controls who wished to participate in the pool exercises!—R.J. Shephard, M.D., Ph.D., D.P.E.

Reference

1. Shephard RJ: *Can Assoc Health Phys Educ Rec J* 50:2–5, 20, 1985.

Reanalysis of the 12-Minute Walk in Patients With Chronic Obstructive Pulmonary Disease
Bernstein ML, Despars JA, Singh NP, Avalos K, Stansbury DW, Light RW (VA Med Ctr, Long Beach, Calif; Univ of California, Irvine)
Chest 105:163–167, 1994   139-95-7–40

Introduction.—The 12-minute walking test, developed to estimate exercise tolerance in patients with chronic bronchitis, is often used to determine functional capacity in chronic obstructive pulmonary disease (COPD). Elderly patients with COPD were examined for correlations between the different intervals in the test, which intervals correlated best

Correlation Coefficients Between Volume of Oxygen Use ($\dot{V}O_2$) and Carbon Dioxide Output ($\dot{V}CO_2$) and Various Walking Distances

Walking Distances	$\dot{V}O_2$	$\dot{V}O_2$/kg	$\dot{V}CO_2$	$\dot{V}CO_2$/kg	FEV_1	FEV_1/kg	FVC	FVC/kg
0 to 2 min	0.45	0.55	0.35	0.39	0.08	0.13	−0.04	0.09
2 to 4 min	0.49	0.68	0.36	0.48	0.17	0.26	−0.12	0.12
4 to 6 min	0.46	0.68	0.38	0.52	0.17	0.29	−0.28	0.03
6 to 8 min	0.48	0.71	0.41	0.56	0.13	0.26	−0.18	0.12
8 to 10 min	0.49	0.66	0.41	0.51	0.14	0.23	−0.11	0.13
10 to 12 min	0.49	0.69	0.40	0.58	0.17	0.34	−0.15	0.22
0 to 4 min	0.48	0.62	0.36	0.44	0.12	0.19	−0.08	0.11
0 to 6 min	0.51	0.67	0.40	0.48	0.18	0.24	−0.17	0.05
0 to 12 min	0.49	0.65	0.38	0.53	0.15	0.26	−0.16	0.12

Abbreviations: FEV_1, forced expiratory volume in 1 second; FVC, forced vital capacity.
(Courtesy of Bernstein ML, Despars JA, Singh NP, et al: *Chest* 105:163-167, 1994.)

with maximal oxygen intake and maximal carbon dioxide expelled, whether adding a measure of effort would improve the correlations, and what degree of correlation exists between changes in peak oxygen intake and changes in the walking test or spirometry.

Patients and Methods.—The 9 patients recruited for the study had a mean age of 67 years; all were men with stable COPD of moderate severity. None had known left ventricular disease or other medical problems that would preclude completion of the exercise tests. Patients were seen at baseline and at 3, 6, 8, 11, and 14 weeks, at which time they underwent spirometry, a symptom-limited peak aerobic exercise test, and the 12-minute walk. The modified Borg scale was used to assess breathlessness at the end of each 2 minutes.

Results.—The mean maximal workload achieved in the exercise test was 81 W; the maximal predicted workrate for men older than age 60 years is 180 W. Although walking distances in each 2-minute interval of the walk were similar, a slightly longer distance was attained in the first 2 minutes. Borg scores, however, became progressively higher as walking time increased. The Borg score was 1.64 after 2 minutes vs. 5.7 after 12 minutes. Highly significant correlations were found between the different walking intervals, particularly between 4- and 6-minute, 4- and 12-minute, and 6- and 12-minute walks. There was also a significant correlation between functional capacity as assessed by the symptom-limited peak aerobic exercise test and by the 12-minute walk (table). Changes in oxygen intake per kilogram were more closely correlated with changes in the 12-minute walk than with changes in the 6-, 4-, or 2-minute walks.

Conclusion.—In this group of elderly men with moderate COPD, distances walked in each 2-minute interval of the 12-minute walk were very consistent. Borg scores, in contrast, were progressively higher in succeeding intervals. Changes in the results of the peak aerobic exercise test between testing sessions correlated better with changes in the 12-minute walking distance than with changes in shorter walking distances. Thus, the full 12-minute test is recommended for documenting changes in exercise capacity.

▶ Walking tests are popular for patient evaluation. They have more "realism" than laboratory exercise, no special apparatus is required, and if, by some mischance, an accident is provoked, walking seems less blameworthy than, say, an all-out treadmill test. Nevertheless, if the score is to reflect aerobic power, it is important that patients move as fast as they are able throughout the 12-minute test. This means that time must be allowed for the learning of an appropriate pace (a point appreciated by Bernstein et al.). Moreover, the physical demands on the body may be greater than during a peak-effort treadmill test, in which maximal effort is sustained for no more than 2–3 minutes.

There have been many studies investigating the optimum walking or running distance for the testing of aerobic function in healthy adults; usually, 12–15 minutes of all-out running has been proposed. However, in children (where motivation for prolonged effort is poorer), the optimal time is shorter (corresponding to the completion of a 0.8- to 1.6-km distance (1). Older adults also have problems with sustained effort, and again, some authors have proposed a 6-minute rather than a 12-minute test (2); this might seem to be supported by the data of Bernstein (a correlation of 0.67 against a laboratory "maximal" test for 6 minutes, dropping to 0.65 for 12 minutes). However, in terms of measuring changes in aerobic power, such as might occur with training, the best correlation is seen at 12 minutes ($r = 0.72$, compared with 0.64 for a 6-minute walk). It must finally be recognized that none of these correlations are very strong; they account for less than 50% of the variance in the data, and even this correlation is boosted somewhat because both the peak cycle ergometer test and the 12-minute walk measure not only aerobic power, but also motivation.—R.J. Shephard, M.D., Ph.D., D.P.E.

References

1. Shephard RJ: *Physiology & Biochemistry of Exercise*. New York, Praeger Publications, 1982.
2. Cunningham DA, et al: *Can J Aging* 5:19, 1986.

Effect of Recombinant Human Growth Hormone on the Muscle Strength Response to Resistance Exercise in Elderly Men
Taaffe DR, Pruitt L, Reim J, Hintz RL, Butterfield G, Hoffman AR, Marcus R (Geriatric Research, Education, and Clinical Ctr, Palo Alto, Calif; Veterans Affairs Med Ctr, Palo Alto, Calif; Stanford Univ, Calif)
J Clin Endocrinol Metab 79:1361–1366, 1994   139-95-7–41

Background.—Changes in body composition, muscle strength, and somatotropic function accompany normal aging. Muscle strength reduction contributes to the risk of bone fracture in elderly individuals. Older adults can increase muscle strength through resistance exercise training, but the strength gains quickly level off, with only modest increases accruing during continued training. It is possible that age-related deficits in the somatotropic axis limit the degree to which muscle strength can improve with resistance training in the elderly.

Methods.—Eighteen healthy men aged 65–82 years initially underwent progressive weight training for 14 weeks to invoke a trained state. The men were then randomly assigned to either 0.02 mg/kg of body weight per day of recombinant human growth hormone (rhGH) or placebo subcutaneously while performing another 10 weeks of strength training.

Findings.—Strength increased in both groups for each exercise over the 14 weeks of training, with little improvement thereafter. Muscle strength increases ranged from 24% to 62%, depending on the muscle group. Baseline plasma insulin-like growth factor I (IGF-I) concentrations were comparable in the 2 groups and about half that noted in

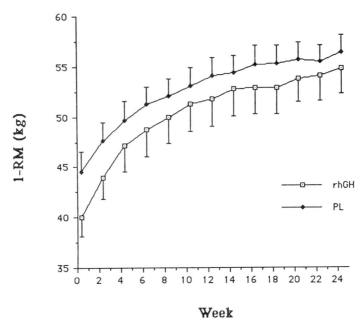

Week

Fig 7–18.—Average muscle strength for the 10 exercises between 0 and 24 weeks. No *difference* exists at any time point between the recombinant human growth hormone (*rhGH*) (*n* = 9) and placebo (*PL*) (*n* = 7) groups. (Courtesy of Taaffe DR, Pruitt L, Reim J, et al: *J Clin Endocrinol Metab* 79:1361–1366, 1994.)

healthy young adults. In the rhGH group, IGF-I levels rose to 255 µg/L by 15 weeks and 218 µg/L at 24 weeks. The IGF-I rose slightly to 119 µg/L by 24 weeks in the placebo group. In addition, IGF-binding protein-3 increased in the rhGH group. The rhGH did not affect muscle strength at any time, and there was no systematic difference in muscle strength between groups during the study (Fig 7–18). Although body weight did not change in either group, lean body mass rose and fat mass dropped in the rhGH group.

Conclusion.—In elderly men, the response to strength training is not augmented by rhGH supplementation. Deficits in GH secretion apparently do not underlie the time-dependent leveling off of muscle strength that occurs with training in the elderly. No support for the popular view of GH as an ergogenic aid was provided.

▶ Now that recombinant growth hormone can be synthesized, there is increasing interest in the possible value of this substance, both as a means of restoring depleted muscle mass in the elderly and as a means of doping in young athletes. The present findings are somewhat paradoxical: Recombinant growth hormone increases muscle mass but does not increase muscle strength relative to control subjects. One possible explanation for this observation is that development of muscle or lean tissue occurs in a body region that is not being evaluated. A second possibility is that the hormone is leading to a retention of water (1) without any synthesis of new tissue.

In this study, all subjects first reached a plateau of strength by exercise alone. This may explain the divergence from other studies, such as that of Cuneo et al. (2); those authors found an increase of strength when rhGH was administered to subjects who had a deficiency of growth hormone.—R.J. Shephard, M.D., Ph.D., D.P.E.

References

1. Yarasheski KE, et al: *Am J Physiol* 262:261, 1992.
2. Cuneo RC, et al: *J Appl Physiol* 70:688, 1991.

β-Adrenergic Effects on Left Ventricular Filling: Influence of Aging and Exercise Training

Stratton JR, Levy WC, Schwartz RS, Abrass IB, Cerqueira MD (Seattle Veterans Affairs Med Ctr; Univ of Washington, Seattle)
J Appl Physiol 77:2522–2529, 1994   139-95-7-42

Objective.—One of the consequences of aging is decreased cardiac response to β-adrenergic stimulation. Although younger and healthier individuals respond well to training, there is no information on the effect of training on the diastolic filling responses to β-adrenergic stimulation in older individuals. The effects of isoproterenol and of intensive endurance exercise training on diastolic filling response in older individuals were determined.

Methods.—Eleven men, aged 24 to 32 years, and 13 men, aged 60 to 82 years, entered the training program. Maximal oxygen consumption and diastolic filling parameters were measured. After baseline data were collected, the men received serial infusions of isoproterenol hydrochloride at 3.5, 7, 14, and 35 ng/kg/min for 14 minutes each.

Results.—Isoproterenol significantly increased all diastolic filling parameters. Age and reduction in peak early filling rates were significantly related at rest and all isoproterenol doses. Endurance training significantly increased maximal oxygen consumption in both groups but did not increase diastolic filling responses to isoproterenol (Fig 7–19). In the older group, diastolic filling responses decreased at rest but not in response to isoproterenol.

Conclusion.—There was no evidence in the older group that isoproterenol decreases diastolic filling responses.

▶ A number of authors have suggested that 1 of the ways an older person adapts to a reduction in peak heart rate is through an increase in end-diastolic volume, and, thus, a larger stroke volume. However, if greater diastolic filling is to be achieved during vigorous exercise, it is desirable that a rapid relaxation of the cardiac muscle occur. β-Adrenergic stimulation is known to

Peak Early and Peak Atrial Filling Rates Pre and Post Training

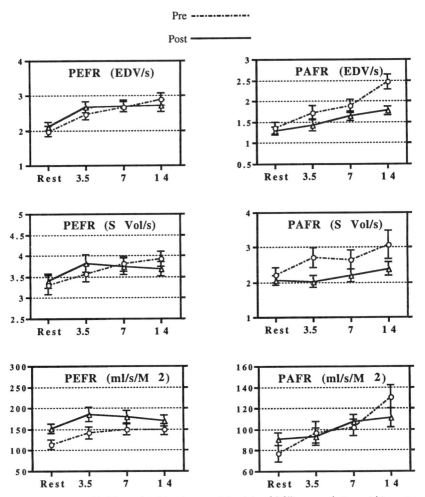

Fig 7–19.—Mean (± SE) pre- (*circle*) and post-training (*triangle*) filling rates during serial isoproterenol doses (rest and 3.5, 7, and 14 ng/kg⁻¹/min⁻¹). (Courtesy of Stratton JR, Levy WC, Schwartz RS, et al: *J Appl Physiol* 77:2522–2529, 1994.)

enhance myocardial relaxation (1, 2), but most of the β-receptors seem to be downregulated in the older person.

The findings of Stratton et al. might suggest that the "widsom of the body" is such that downregulation does not extend to myocardial relaxation, so an increase in end-diastolic volume can occur during vigorous exercise. Nevertheless, it is puzzling that β-adrenergic receptors are affected differentially with respect to their relaxant, inotropic, and chronotropic functions.

Contrary to the view of Stratton et al., Schulman et al. (3) found that β-blockade slowed the ventricular filling rate of young adults but not of older subjects during exercise, suggesting that β-adrenergic function had been suppressed in the younger but not in the older individuals. There are several factors contributing to the discrepant findings of Stratton et al. and Schulman et al., perhaps the most important being that Schulman et al. made their observations during upright exercise, whereas Stratton et al. tested the response to isoproterenol with subjects supine.

All of this may seem rather obscure pharmacology, but there is a practical application in sports medicine. If the body could adjust for the decrease in maximal heart rate by an increase in stroke volume, peak cardiac output would remain unchanged in an elderly person, and there would then be no reason why maximal oxygen intake should decline with age (other than a suboptimal amount of habitual physical activity on the part of the patient). But in my view, peak cardiac output and maximal oxygen intake do decline, regardless of whether the individuals maintain the same training schedule as in their younger years.—R.J. Shephard, M.D., Ph.D., D.P.E.

References

1. Burwash IG, Morgan DE, Koilpillai CJ, et al: Sympathetic stimulation alters left ventricular relaxation and chamber size. *Am J Physiol* 264:1R–7R, 1993.
2. Carmeliet P, Aubert A, Van der Werf F, et al: Evaluation of transmittal pressure gradients at different heart rates: Divergent action of isoprenaline and atropine. *Cardiovasc Res.* 24:560, 1990.
3. Schulman SP, LaKatta EG, Fleg JL, et al: Age-related decline in left ventricular filling at rest and exercise. *Am J Physiol* 263:1932H–1938H, 1992.

Combined Effects of Age and Exercise on Thromboxane B_2 and Platelet Activation

Todd MK, Goldfarb AH, Kauffman RD, Burleson C (West Chester Univ, Pa; Univ of North Carolina, Greensboro)
J Appl Physiol 76:1548–1552, 1994   139-95-7–43

Introduction.—Circulating thromboxane A_2 (TxA_2) is a powerful stimulator of platelet activation, concentrations of which increase with both increasing age and acute exercise. The combined effects of these 2 factors may predispose older adults to platelet activation and perhaps to thrombosis formation. The combined effects of age and acute exercise on circulating TxA_2 and on platelet activation were assessed.

Method.—Two groups of healthy men were studied: 9 young men (mean age, 28 years) and 9 older men (mean age, 55 years). All men performed 30 minutes of treadmill exercise at 70% to 75% of maximal oxygen consumption. Blood samples were obtained for analysis after 15 minutes of rest, immediately after exercise, and at 30 minutes of recovery. These 10-mL specimens were collected in tubes containing 0.5 mL of 4.5 mM of ethylenediamine tetra-acetic acid, 30 mM of acetylsalicylic

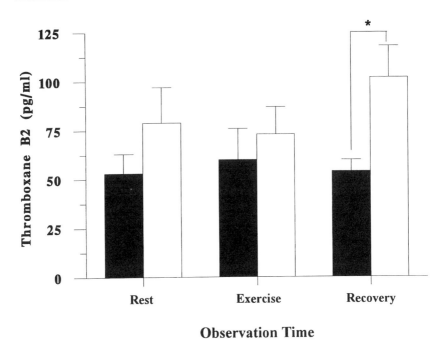

Fig 7–20.—Combined effects of age and exercise on thromboxane B₂ after 15 minutes of rest, 30 minutes of exercise at 70% of maximal O₂ consumption, and 30 minutes of recovery from exercise in young men (*black bars*) and older men (*white bars*). * $P = 0.05$. (Courtesy of Todd MK, Goldfarb AH, Kauffman RD, et al: *J Appl Physiol* 76:1548–1552, 1994.)

acid, and 1 μM of prostaglandin E_1. Radioimmunoassays were performed to measure concentrations of thromboxane B_2 (TxB_2) as a stable metabolite of TxA_2 and of β-thromboglobulin (β-TG) as a marker of platelet activation. Adjustments were made for the hemoconcentration of the samples and for changes in platelet count that were not accounted for by shifts in plasma volume.

Results.—The mean resting plasma TxB_2 concentrations were 53 pg/mL in the young men and 79 pg/mL in the older men. Resting β-TG concentrations were 152 and 114 ng/mL, respectively. Immediately after exercise, there were no significant age group or exercise-induced differences in either marker. At 30 minutes after exercise, the mean TxB_2 concentration was 54 pg/mL in the young men compared with 102 pg/mL in the older men, a significant difference (Fig 7–20). At the same time point, there was no significant difference in β-TG values; which were 170 and 183 ng/mL, respectively.

Conclusion.—Compared with young men, older men may have greater increases in TxB_2 concentrations 30 minutes after moderate exercise. As such, older men may be more predisposed to postexercise platelet activation. In this study, however, the age-group differences in TxB_2

concentrations may have been related to a significantly higher polyunsaturated fat intake in the young men.

▶ This study suggests that in older men compared with younger men, moderately vigorous exercise (running 30 minutes at 70% to 75% of maximum oxygen consumption) may tend to be "thrombotic" because it elevates plasma levels of TxB_2, the stable metabolite of a potent platelet activator. This suggestion is too strong for the data. Plasma levels of TxB_2 tended also to be higher *at rest* in the older men and were not further elevated immediately after the exercise bout, but only 30 minutes later. The pattern here for β-TG, a marker of platelet activation, was inconclusive. Other confounders regarding platelet function were the facts that the older men had higher blood lipids and the younger men ate more polyunsaturated fat.

It seems unlikely that exercise is thrombotic. Probably the opposite is true. In young men and old men (1), regular aerobic exercise expands the plasma volume, lowering the concentration of red blood cells and fibrinogen. Regular exercise can mitigate the hyperreactivity of platelets in overweight men, and exercise triggers the release of tissue plasminogen activator, the "clot-dissolver." All these actions of exercise are "antithrombotic."—E.R. Eichner, M.D.

Reference

1. Carroll JF, et al: *Med Sci Sports Exerc* 27:79, 1995.

8 Hormones, Doping, Immune Function, Metabolism, and Viscera

Gonadal Hormones and Semen Quality in Male Runners: A Volume Threshold Effect of Endurance Training
De Souza MJ, Arce JC, Pescatello LS, Scherzer HS, Luciano AA (Univ of Connecticut, Farmington; New Britain Gen Hosp, Conn)
Int J Sports Med 15:383–391, 1994   139-95-8–1

Background.—Intense endurance training has been associated with a spectrum of menstrual abnormalities in female athletes. In male athletes, endurance training has not been related to a specific "volume threshold" of training. In fact, data showing a distinct, consistent effect of intense endurance training on male reproductive function are very limited.

Methods.—Eleven male high-mileage runners (HRs), 9 moderate-mileage runners (MRs), and 10 sedentary controls (SCs) of similar age were assessed to determine the effects of the volume of endurance training on reproductive function. Levels of reproductive, adrenal, and thyroid hormones were measured during a 1-hour period of serial blood sampling. Urinary excretion of 24-hour luteinizing hormone (uLH) was determined on 2 separate days. Semen examinations and sperm penetration of standard cervical mucus were assessed on 2–5 occasions.

Findings.—Levels of total testosterone and free testosterone were significantly lower in HRs than in MRs and SCs. The 3 groups were comparable in uLH, serum LH, follicle-stimulating hormone, and prolactin. There were no other intergroup hormonal differences. Compared with SCs, in HRs, the total motile sperm count and sperm density were reduced. Compared with MRs and SCs, in HRs, decreased sperm motility and an increased population of immature sperm and round cells were noted. Sperm penetration of bovine cervical mucus was also lower in HRs than in SCs. Training volume was significantly associated with sperm motility, density, and number of round cells. The number of round cells and total testosterone were significantly correlated.

Conclusion.—There appear to be well-defined differences in reproductive function between HRs and MRs. These include reduced gonadal steroids and disturbed semen quality that are seen in HRs but not in those participating in more moderate volumes of training. There seems to be a volume-threshold effect for high volumes of endurance running.

▶ For a number of years, feminists have been anxious to prove that male athletes (like female competitors) have a disturbance of reproductive function if they train too hard. A number of previous investigators have found that heavy training reduces plasma levels of testosterone, but not everyone has observed such an effect. Likewise, the findings from previous examinations of sperm quality have been conflicting. Part of the problem has been that different authors have adopted differing definitions of intense training.

In this study, little difference in reproductive function was seen with a weekly running distance of 40–56 km, and those with disturbed reproductive function had been running a minimum of 104 km/wk for at least 12 months. In some previous reports, the intense exercise has been associated with competitive stress, but in others it has not.

A further important variable is probably the athlete's daily energy intake. De Souza et al. measured this and found no significant intergroup difference between runners and controls. The data had a fairly large variance, but assuming the authors' observation to be correct, it might imply that the distance runners were not consuming enough food to allow for their intensive activity. Even with the very intense exercise that was performed here, the semen quality remained within the low-normal range, so it is doubtful that the changes had much significance for reproductive potency, even on a temporary basis.—R.J. Shepard, M.D., Ph.D., D.P.E.

Weigh Loss Beliefs, Practices and Support Systems for High School Wrestlers
Marquart LF, Sobal J (Cornell Cooperative Extension of Oswego County, Mexico, NY; Cornell Univ, Ithaca, NY)
J Adolesc Health 15:410–415, 1994   139-95-8–2

Background.—Despite numerous warnings from medical, nutrition, and athletic experts, wrestlers continue to use unsafe weight loss practices to achieve a low body weight for competition. Rural high school wrestlers were surveyed regarding their beliefs and practices related to health and weight loss.

Methods.—An investigator-designed questionnaire was distributed before a wrestling practice in the beginning of the season. Wrestlers at all 9 high schools in 1 rural county in New York responded anonymously.

Results.—The questionnaires were returned by 197 wrestlers, 98% of those surveyed. Six percent of these athletes thought they needed to gain weight, 63% thought they needed to lose weight, and 31% wanted to maintain their present weight. "Making weight" was ranked as either very or somewhat important by 93% of the respondents. The most frequent weight loss techniques were running, wrestling practice, eating less, eating nothing, or wearing more to induce sweating. Those for whom wrestling was their major sport were significantly more likely to have abstained from drinking and to have used diet pills, spitting, and rubber suits to induce weight loss. Eleven percent to 75% of the respondents self-identified 1 or more of the weight loss practices they themselves had used as being unhealthy. The vast majority of wrestlers (88%) were receptive to nutrition information and identified coaches and doctors as accurate sources of nutrition information.

Conclusion.—Nutrition counseling extending beyond the provision of information about the risk of rapid weight loss is needed for adolescent wrestlers. Physicians should become more actively involved in motivating wrestlers to adopt healthy weight management strategies.

▶ It seems from this questionnaire study that high school wrestlers still use extreme and bizarre methods—not drinking, sweating, vomiting, laxatives, diet pills, spitting, shivering—to "make weight" and gain an edge. Sadly, 42% of these wrestlers said "nobody" helped them plan a weight loss program. The methods used by wrestlers to lose weight can decrease upper body strength, anaerobic power and capacity, and aerobic performance (1). They can even decrease the testosterone level and sap libido (2). Yet, a recent study finds that neither acute weight gain after the weigh-in nor any weight discrepancy between first-round opponents influences success in a collegiate wrestling tournament (3). This article suggests practical ways to prevent unsafe weight loss by wrestlers in the knowledge that young wrestlers do not take predicted long-term health consequences seriously, but rather only those problems or rules that prevent them from wrestling.—E.R. Eichner, M.D.

References

1. 1991 YEAR BOOK OF SPORTS MEDICINE, pp 143–144.
2. Strauss RH, et al: *Phys Sportsmed* 21:64, 1993.
3. Horswill CA, et al: *Med Sci Sports Exerc* 26:1290, 1994.

Aspirin Does Not Affect Exercise Performance
Roi GS, Garagiola U, Verza P, Spadari G, Radice D, Zecca L, Cerretelli P (Università degli Studi di Milano, Italy; Funzione Medica, Bayer Italia, Milano, Italy; Istituto di Tecnologie Biomediche Avanzate, Milano, Italy)
Int J Sports Med 15:224–227, 1994   139-95-8-3

Background.—Acetylsalicylic acid (ASA) can accelerate glucose utilization and lactate production, thereby decreasing adenosine triphosphate (ATP) production by uncoupling the oxidative phosphorylation in the mitochondria. Clinically, ASA can stimulate respiration rate, with a disproportionate decrease in arterial carbon dioxide pressure. The progressive augmentation of the respiratory quotient suggests a shift toward carbohydrate utilization. Whether these effects can reduce thermodynamic efficiency during exercise, anticipating the onset of the anaerobic threshold, is not clear.

Objective.—The effects of ASA on cardiorespiratory performance during exercise were evaluated in a single-blind, crossover study.

Study Design.—After a single dose of plain aspirin (1,000 mg of ASA), chewable buffered aspirin (1,000 mg of ASA and 600 mg of calcium carbonate), or placebo, 9 athletes and 9 untrained but active individuals completed a progressive maximal exercise test on a cycle ergometer (30-W, 3-minute steps, starting at 60 W) on 3 different occasions. Breath-by-breath ventilation, oxygen consumption, carbon dioxide output, respiratory frequency, and heart rate were monitored continuously at rest and during exercise. Blood lactate levels were measured just before the start of exercise and at the third minute of each step to detect the anaerobic threshold. In 10 participants, the pharmacokinetics of aspirin during exercise were studied.

Findings.—There were no statistically and clinically relevant effects of a single 1,000-mg dose of ASA on oxygen consumption and anaerobic threshold onset during exercise.

Conclusion.—A single dose of ASA at a maximal recommended analgesic dosage has no effect on physical performance during submaximal and maximal exercise. Athletes and active individuals with mild-to-moderate pain before a competition can be treated with aspirin to relieve pain without compromising performance.

▶ This study corroborates an earlier "field" study in trained runners (1) in that a single 1,000-mg dose of plain aspirin taken by young men 30 minutes before exercise did not cause clinically evident hyperventilation, increase oxygen consumption during a maximal effort, or impair submaximal or maximal performance on cycle ergometry. As reviewed before (2), however, anecdotal reports suggest that aspirin or other nonsteroidal anti-inflammatory drugs can predispose to gastrointestinal bleeding in athletes.—E.R. Eichner, M.D.

References

1. Lisse JR, MacDonald K, Thurmond-Anderle M, et al: *J Sports Med Phys Fitness* 31:561–564, 1991.
2. 1992 YEAR BOOK OF SPORTS MEDICINE, pp 246–247.

Sodium Bicarbonate Ingestion Does Not Improve Performance in Women Cyclists
Kozak-Collins K, Burke ER, Schoene RB (Univ of Washington, Seattle; Univ of

Colorado, Colorado Springs; Colorado Altitude Research Inst, Keystone)
Med Sci Sports Exerc 26:1510–1515, 1994   139-95-8-4

Introduction.—The hypothesis that exogenous bicarbonate can enhance buffer capacity in the blood, delay the onset of exhaustion, and improve performance in high-intensity exercise has yet to be proven. Studies evaluating this hypothesis have yielded variable results, but few have controlled for the sodium load ingested with the bicarbonate. The effects of ingesting sodium bicarbonate and sodium chloride before exercise were examined in competitive women cyclists.

Methods.—The study was performed at moderate (2,800 m) altitude. Participants ranged in age from 24 to 32 years and had lived and trained at approximately 2,957 m for a mean of 4.2 years. Each person initially underwent a progressive cycle ergometer test to determine maximal oxygen consumption. Two trials were conducted on separate days and at least 48 hours apart. Four of the 7 cyclists completed the bicarbonate trial as the first experimental trial and 3 completed it as the second trial. Sodium chloride and sodium bicarbonate in gelatin capsules were consumed during a 15-minute period beginning 2 hours before testing. Drinking water was allowed ad libitum. Performance was measured by the number of intervals completed and total time during interval work. An indwelling catheter was placed in a dorsal hand vein to measure arterialized venous blood gases.

Results.—The mean number of intervals completed did not differ significantly between the 2 interventions: 10.0 for sodium bicarbonate and 8.4 for sodium chloride (Fig 8–1). Similarly, there was no difference in maximal heart rate achieved in the 2 trials nor with the preliminary test to exhaustion. There was a tendency for recovery heart rates to be higher and for increases in ventilation and respiratory rate to be lower with bi-

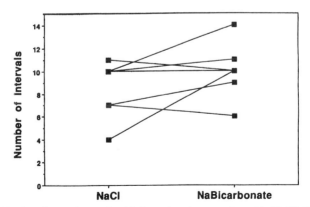

Fig 8–1.—Number of intervals completed before exhaustion on sodium chloride (*NaCl*) and NaBicarbonate. There were no statistical differences between the 2 conditions. (Courtesy of Kozak-Collins K, Burke ER, Schoene RB: *Med Sci Sports Exerc* 26:1510–1515, 1994.)

carbonate, but the differences were not significant. Rates of perceived exertion did not differ under the 2 conditions.

Conclusion.—Bicarbonate rather than sodium chloride ingestion in these women cyclists resulted in a significant alkalemia, but performance was not thereby improved during exhaustive interval tests. This finding brings into question the role of blood acid–base status in exhaustion. The benefit of sodium bicarbonate reported in previous studies may have been secondary to the intravascular volume enhancement from sodium, not from the alteration in pH itself.

▶ Without a third trial of no ingestion of either bicarbonate or sodium chloride, the conclusion that the improved performance reported in previous studies was caused by the expansion of plasma volume is a bit weak. The confounding effect of acclimation to moderate altitude and its accompanying physiologic adjustments emphasize the importance of a nonintervention trial. The variability of results among the subjects seen in Figure 8–1 (an improved performance in 4, a decreased performance in 2, and no change in 1) suggests the need for a larger sample size before concluding that bicarbonate ingestion had no effect on performance. Once again, we have no idea of the power of the test to detect significance.—B.L. Drinkwater, Ph.D.

Anabolic Steroid Use in the Adolescent Athlete
Potteiger JA, Stilger VG (Univ of Kansas, Lawrence; Xavier Univ, Cincinnati, Ohio)
J Athletic Train 29:60–64, 1994   139-95-8-5

Background.—Recent surveys suggest that the use of androgenic-anabolic steroids is prevalent among adolescent athletes, particularly those in high school. The high cost of random laboratory testing for anabolic steroid use is prohibitive. However, if athletic trainers are aware of the clinical signs and symptoms of anabolic steroid use, they can identify athletes' problems and suggest treatment.

Physical signs.—Steroid use combined with a rigorous resistance training program often results in unusually rapid gains in body weight and marked muscular hypertrophy. The trainer should be aware of changes in individuals that are beyond normal development for the adolescent (table). Alterations in body composition, including large increases in lean tissue and reductions in fat, may also be seen. In addition, it is common to notice disproportionate increases in the upper torso, which may cause stretch marks, particularly around the shoulders and chest. An increase in acne, particularly on the upper back and chest regions, is another obvious sign of steroid use. Examination of the large muscles may also reveal evidence of injectable anabolic steroid use. Long-term use may also lead to baldness and breast enlargement. The user may have an increased susceptibility to tendon strains and injuries, particularly involving the biceps and patellar tendons. Bruising, yellowing of the skin, and hyperten-

Physical Signs of Anabolic Steroid Use

1. **Rapid weight gain**
2. **Alterations in body composition with marked muscular hypertrophy**
3. **Disproportionate development of the upper torso**
4. **Severe acne**
5. **Needle marks in large muscle groups**
6. **Development of male pattern baldness**
7. **Gynecomastia (breast enlargement)**
8. **Increased susceptibility to tendon strains and injuries**
9. **More frequent hematoma or bruising**
10. **Jaundice**
11. **Edema**
12. **Elevated blood pressure/epistaxis**
13. **Hirsutism (abnormal development of facial and body hair)**
14. **Atrophied breasts in females**
15. **Deepening of the voice in females**

(Courtesy of Potteiger JA, Stilger VG: *J Athletic Train* 29:60–64, 1994.)

sion may also be apparent. In women, the abnormal development of facial and body hair and breast atrophy are common signs of steroid use. Sometimes there is also a deepening of the voice.

Psychological Signs.—Violent mood swings, increased aggressiveness, and periods of euphoria are some of the signs of anabolic steroid use. Irritability, depression, and anxiety may also be seen. Alterations in the cognitive process and content, along with suicidal or homicidal thought, are also typical of anabolic steroid users. Finally, the trainer should be aware of athletes who become obsessive about spending time in the gym and exhibit extreme body consciousness, such as particularly frequent use of a tape measure and observance of themselves in the mirror.

Counseling the Adolescent Athlete.—It is essential for the trainer to establish trust and to maintain confidentiality with the athlete. One approach is to inquire about the use of legal substances such as alcohol and cigarettes, then about nutritional ergogenic aids, and finally about the use of anabolic steroids. The athlete should be encouraged to discuss the problem with parents. Psychiatric intervention may follow, together with educational intervention, including a problem-oriented approach emphasizing the relationship between steroid use and side effects.

Conclusion.—Athletic trainers are in a position to play a critical role in identifying anabolic steroid use in adolescents. The presence of multiple physical and/or psychological indicators in a high-risk individual should result in the adolescent being entered immediately into an intervention program and referral to the team or family physician for testing.

▶ Steroid use is on the increase in the high school–age population. What can be done to curtail its use? The authors offer a number of solutions. Education of coaches and athletic trainers to recognize the signs of steroid abuse is a key factor. Counseling of the athlete is another factor, and the authors offer various counseling approaches. The authors conclude that "the athletic trainer is often in a position to play a critical role in identifying an athlete's problem and to begin the process of treatment." Trainers must be willing to educate themselves about the signs of steroid abuse and the counseling techniques to use. Each case is individual and should be approached in a different manner.—F.J. George, A.T.C., P.T.

The Effects of Anabolic Steroids on Myocardial Structure and Cardiovascular Fitness

Sachtleben TR, Berg KE, Elias BA, Cheatham JP, Felix GL, Hofschire PJ (Univ of Nebraska, Omaha)
Med Sci Sports Exerc 25:1240–1245, 1993   139-95-8-6

Purpose.—Anabolic steroid use has many well-documented adverse effects. However, there have been few studies of the possible effects on myocardial structure and function. The effects of anabolic steroids on myocardial structure, maximum oxygen consumption ($\dot{V}O_{2max}$), and body composition were assessed in male weight trainers.

Methods.—The individuals were experienced, age-matched male weight trainers (mean age, 26½ years). Eleven of the men used anabolic steroids and 13 did not. For the steroid users, testing was performed while the athletes were off cycle for at least 8 weeks (U-OFF) and again at the peak of their subsequent cycle (U-ON). All individuals underwent

Myocardial Structure and Function			
	Nonusers ($N = 13$)	Users Off ($N = 11$)	Users On ($N = 11$)
LVID (mm)	55.7 ± 4.3	57.5 ± 3.3	59.1 ± 3.5*
IVS (mm)	9.3 ± 1.2	10.3 ± 1.2	11.1 ± 1.2*†
LVPW (mm)	9.5 ± 1.6	10.2 ± 1.0	11.2 ± 1.5*
LV mass (g)	168.5 ± 36.2	182.8 ± 26.9	210.6 ± 42.6*†
Shortening fraction	0.37 ± 0.04	0.37 ± 0.04	0.35 ± 0.06

Note: Values are mean ± SD.
* Significantly different than nonusers ($P < 0.05$).
† Significantly different than users off ($P < 0.05$).
Abbreviations: LVID, left ventricular internal diameter in diastole; IVS, interventricular septal thickness in diastole; LVPW, left ventricular posterior wall thickness in diastole; LV mass, left ventricular mass.
(Courtesy of Sachtleben TR, Berg KE, Elias BA, et al: *Med Sci Sports Exerc* 25:1240–1245, 1993.)

echocardiography to evaluate morphological and physiologic changes in the heart, measurement of $\dot{V}O_{2max}$, and hydrostatic weighing, in addition to various urine and blood tests.

Results.—Left ventricular mass in the steroid users was 183 g in the U-OFF period and 211 g in the U-ON period, compared with 186 g in the nonusers. The intraventricular septum thickness was 10 mm in the U-OFF period and 11 mm in the U-ON period, compared with 9 mm in the nonusers. The differences between the U-OFF and U-ON periods were significant, as were those between the U-ON measurements and the measurements in nonusers. The left ventricular diameter and the left ventricular posterior wall thickness in diastole were also significantly greater in the steroid users in the U-ON period than in the nonusers (table). At both time points, $\dot{V}O_{2max}$ was significantly lower in the steroid users than in the nonusers: U-OFF and U-ON values were 41 mL/kg/min, compared with 50 mL/kg/min in the nonusers. There were no significant differences in shortening fraction or body composition.

Conclusion.—Anabolic steroid use by male weight trainers appears to have significant and sometimes long-term effects on myocardial structure and cardiovascular fitness. There are no acute effects on body composition or $\dot{V}O_{2max}$. Further studies of the adverse myocardial effects of steroids during cycles, as well as of the rate and magnitude of change after steroid cessation, are needed.

▶ Four prior studies are split 50:50 on whether anabolic steroids alter cardiac structure, but this latest study suggests that the myocardium is thickened by as little as 6 weeks of steroid use. "On-cycle" vs. "off-cycle" for 8 weeks was associated with a 15% increase in left ventricular mass and a 1-mm increase in septal thickness. The lack of randomized assignment to user and nonuser groups is a flaw, as is the lack of control of dosages and types of anabolic steroids.

This study raises concern about adverse effects of anabolic steroids on the myocardium, but more and better-controlled studies are needed. The 1992 YEAR BOOK OF SPORTS MEDICINE covered anabolic steroids, muscular strength, and blood lipids (1); the 1994 YEAR BOOK OF SPORTS MEDICINE reviewed abuse of anabolic steroids and other drugs by adolescents, as well as adverse neuropsychiatric effects of anabolic steroids in men (2).—E.R. Eichner, M.D.

References

1. 1992 YEAR BOOK OF SPORTS MEDICINE, pp 120–124.
2. 1994 YEAR BOOK OF SPORTS MEDICINE, pp 345-349.

New Decision Limits and Quality-Control Material for Detecting Human Chorionic Gonadotropin Misuse in Sports

Laidler P, Cowan DA, Hider RC, Kicman AT (King's College London)
Clin Chem 40:1306–1311, 1994   139-95-8–7

Introduction.—The threshold for human chorionic gonadotropin (hCG) in the urine was arbitrarily set at 25 IU/L after the screening of 740 urine samples in 1987. Shortly thereafter, the International Olympic Committee imposed a ban on hCG administration. A statistical evaluation was reported indicating that greater than 5 IU of hCG per liter in the urine of a male athlete is abnormal. The preparation of a freeze-dried urinary quality-control (QC) material for hCG was also reported.

Methods.—Urine samples were collected from 1,400 competing male athletes for measuring hCG concentrations. Reference values were determined from urine specimens from 120 men who were not competing in any national sporting events. The hCG MAIAclone IRMA was used for hCG determination. Freeze-dried urinary QC material was initially separated by size-exclusion chromatography, then passed through a hCGβ (the free β-subunit of hCG) immunoaffinity column to increase its immunoreactive purity. This allowed the removal of hCGβ and hCGβcf (the core fragment of hCGβ) immunoreactivity from the material.

Results.—Statistical evaluation of the results of 1,400 urine samples gave a "far outside" value, defined as $[(3 \times IQR) + Q_3]$, of 5 IU/L. Any value greater than this is extremely rare. The hCG values in the 120 reference urines had a median value of 0.4 IU/L. Values of hCG in concentrated ultrafiltered samples had a median value of 0.7 IU/L, which corresponds to actual hCG concentrations of 0.1 IU/L. The reference preparation of hCG had 3.4 times less hCGβ immunoreactivity than the 3rd International Standard.

Conclusion.—Although the limit for abnormality was set at 5 IU/L, it is proposed that 10 IU/L be used as a decisional limit to eliminate the possibility of false positive results. The value for the QC is equal to the decision limit for positive findings of hCG misuse and should help control drug abuse in sports. The QC is available to interested laboratories upon request.

▶ Dishonest athletes may administer hCG with several objectives: to stimulate the production of endogenous testosterone, to prevent testicular shutdown during administration of anabolic steroids, or to suppress changes in the testosterone-episterone ratio that is currently used to detect exogenous testosterone administration (1).

One study of a large sample of male athletes in the United Kingdom found that 21 of 740 had high levels of hCG in the urine. The current diagnostic threshold of 25 IU/L still allows much abuse to escape attention, given that a typical value for a nonathlete is 0.4 IU/L. The precision of the laboratory test

is now increased by the availability of reference samples of hCG, and a reduction of the threshold to 10 IU/L should go some way to checking
abuse.—R.J. Shephard, M.D., Ph.D., D.P.E.

Reference

1. de Boer D, et al: *Int J Sports Med* 12:46–51, 1991.

On the Origin of Physiologically High Ratios of Urinary Testosterone to Epitestosterone: Consequences for Reliable Detection of Testosterone Administration by Male Athletes

Dehennin L (Fondation de Recherche en Hormonologie, Fresnes, France)
J Endocrinol 142:353–360, 1994   139-95-8–8

Background.—Testosterone administration to male athletes can usually be detected by the urinary excretion ratio of testosterone to epitestosterone glucuronides (TG/EG), which may not exceed 6. There are,
however, some documented cases of physiologically high TG/EG ratios,
and there is a need to discriminate clearly between those who have physiologically high ratios and those whose elevated ratios are pharmacologically high. Individuals with TG/EG ratios greater than 4 and free of any
anabolic steroid supply are characterized by a normal TG/EG plus epitestosterone sulphate (ES) ratio in conjunction with abnormally low EG/
ES ratios.

Methods.—Ninety healthy men and male adolescents aged 15–30
years, free of anabolic steroids and active in sports, were recruited.
Twelve males aged 14–26 years, active in sports and anabolic steroid
free, being followed for TG/EG ratios more than 4 for the previous 3
years, also volunteered. Just before breakfast, a loading test with 1 mg of
deuterium-labeled EG was administered to all the volunteers.

Results.—Compared with the other group, individuals with chronic
TG/EG more than 4 had a decreased output of all 17 α-hydroxyandro-
gen glucuronides, an increased excretion of sulphoconjugates, and similar luteinizing hormone concentrations. All ratios with testosterone as
numerator were higher in the group with TG/EG more than 4, confirming sustained TG production. Between their respective conjugates, significant positive correlations existed for TG and EG. The TG/EG was significantly negatively correlated with EG/ES in both groups. For men
with chronic TG/EG greater than 4, the average EG/ES ratio was 4
times less than in the reference group, denoting preferential sulphocon-
jugate excretion.

Conclusion.—When urinary TG/EG ratios are in the 6–12 range for
the first time in individuals without any previous indication of normal
ratios, some complementary criteria, e.g., excretion of ES and 5-andro-
stene-3β,17α-diol glucuronide, should be taken into account. This will

allow better discrimination between a physiologically high and a pharmacologically high TG/EG ratio.

▶ To find a method of detecting the person who has a naturally high TG/EG ratio, it is logical to begin by asking why the high ratio is occurring. Dehennin suggests one possible explanation: lack of an enzyme that normally splits ES into free EG (usually measured as the glucuronide) and the sulfate radical. This hypothesis implies that the ratio drops to normal limits if the denominator is changed to the sum of EG and ES. In the test population, the ratio dropped from 6.06 to 1.67. However, the practical value of using the more complicated ratio remains in doubt, because in the normal sample the ratio also decreased when EG and ES were summed, from 1.42 to 0.82, a figure still significantly lower than that for the problem group of athletes.—R.J. Shephard, M.D., Ph.D., D.P.E.

Establishing a Ketoconazole Suppression Test for Verifying Testosterone Administration in the Doping Control of Athletes
Oftebro H, Jensen J, Mowinckel P, Norli HR (Aker Hosp, Oslo, Norway; Norwegian Univ of Sport and Physical Education, Oslo, Norway; Medstat Research Ltd, Lillestrom, Norway)
J Clin Endocrinol Metab 78:973–977, 1994   139-95-8–9

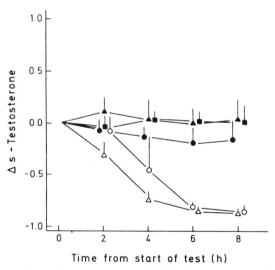

Time from start of test (h)

Fig 8–2.—Relative change in serum testosterone (Δs-T) after ketoconazole administration in T-treated (KETO 3, KETO-10, and HYPO) and untreated (controls and High subjects, compared with basal values at 0 hour. *Filled triangles*, KETO-3; *filled circles*, KETO-10; *filled squares*, HYPO; *open circles*, High; *open triangles*, controls. (Courtesy of Oftebro H, Jensen J, Mowinckel P, et al: *J Clin Endocrinol Metab*: 78:973–977, 1994.)

Background.—To detect testosterone doping, the sports community uses the ratio of urinary testosterone to epitestosterone (T/EpiT). A ratio exceeding 6 is considered an offense. However, the existence of biological outliers is possible. The use of ketoconazole has been proposed to distinguish between such athletes and athletes using testosterone.

Methods.—Ketoconazole was given to 3 groups of men pretreated with testosterone and 2 groups of untreated healthy men. Patients with mild hypogonadism constituted 1 of the pretreated groups. One of the untreated groups included athletes with high urinary levels of T/EpiT after 3 testings. The effects of administering ketoconazole on serum levels of testosterone and the urinary T/EpiT ratio were monitored every 2 hours for 8 hours.

Findings.—The administration of ketoconazole clearly separated testosterone pretreated and untreated individuals into 2 clusters. The T/EpiT ratio rose and the serum levels of testosterone remained unchanged in pretreated men during the ketoconazole test. By contrast, the T/EpiT declined by 60% and the serum level of testosterone declined by nearly 90% in untreated individuals (Fig 8–2). The use of several time points and combining the urinary T/EpiT with the serum level of testosterone data increased the statistical power of the test.

Conclusion.—The suppressive effects of ketoconazole on endogenous androgen production may be used to investigate suspicion of previous administration of testosterone and other androgens. Ketoconazole may be useful as a verification of testosterone doping in athletes.

▶ Although the International Olympics Committee has recommended that a urinary T/EpiT ratio over 6 be considered as proof of the illegal administration of testosterone, there is some evidence that a few athletes who have not engaged in doping can exceed this ceiling. Additional tests are, thus, useful for those individuals with ratios in the range of 6–10. This paper by Oftebro and associates suggests that a very nice separation can be obtained by ketoconazole suppression, even when the sample includes people with high testosterone values who are not doping, and people with relatively low levels who are doping.—R.J. Shephard, M.D., Ph.D., D.P.E.

Lack of Demonstrated Effect of Nandrolone on Serum Lipids
Glazer G, Suchman AL (Highland Hosp, Rochester, NY; Univ of Rochester, NY)
Metabolism 43:204–210, 1994   139-95-8–10

Introduction.—Many previous studies have shown striking adverse lipid profiles, including 50% depression of high-density-lipoprotein cholesterol (HDL-C), in individuals taking 17α-alkylated anabolic steroids (ASs). On the other hand, studies of 17β-esterified ASs have shown mild or no lipid effects. The varying lipid effects of different ASs may therefore be an important clinical consideration. Initial data on the lipid effects of nandrolone, a 17β-esterified AS, were presented.

Methods.—The study sample comprised 21 male and 3 female volunteers. Their lipid profiles were measured before and after administering nandrolone decanoate, 100 mg IM once weekly for 6 weeks. This dose was selected because it is the one most frequently used by athletes who are self-administering nandrolone.

Results.—There were no significant changes after nandrolone administration in lipid profile, including HDL-C, low-density-lipoprotein cholesterol (LDL-C), and total cholesterol; triglycerides; or ratios of total cholesterol to HDL-C or of LDL-C to HDL-C. In men, HDL-C decreased by a mean of only 2 mg/dL, and LDL-C increased by only 5 mg/dL. Power analysis ruled out nandrolone-related HDL-C depressions of 6.3, 7.6, or 8.7 mg/dL with powers of 80%, 95%, and 99%, respectively.

Conclusion.—The 17β-esterified AS nandrolone appears to have only small effects on lipid profile, in contrast to the AS currently available for oral administration. Previous research suggests that steroid-induced HDL-C depression—as well as the greater depression resulting from oral vs. parenteral AS—is primarily mediated by induction of the HDL-C catabolic enzyme hepatic triglyceride lipase. Unless there are contraindications to IM injection or to a particular anabolic agent, parenteral ASs should always be used in preference to oral agents. Patients who are using ASs should be counseled on the particular risks of oral ASs, in addition to the risks of ASs in general.

▶ After reviewing the atherogenic effects of ASs on serum lipid levels and concluding that adverse cholesterol effects were mainly caused by oral (as opposed to parenteral) forms of ASs (1), Glazer and Suchman show here that a parenteral form, nandrolone, used for 6 weeks, has only small adverse effects on the cholesterol profile. Similar results appear in a handful of other studies, notably one that contrasted the major adverse effects of stanozolol with the minor adverse effects of testosterone on serum lipoprotein levels (2).

These studies should not be read as endorsements of the abuse of parenteral ASs. As reviewed in Abstract 139-95-8–6, ASs, often high-dose mixtures of oral and parenteral forms, have adverse effects on the heart and brain and have been implicated in heart attacks in young weight lifters (3) and in peliosis hepatis and/or liver tumors in young bodybuilders (4, 5).—E.R. Eichner, M.D.

References

1. 1992 YEAR BOOK OF SPORTS MEDICINE, pp 121–122.
2. Thompson PD, Cullinane EM, Sady SP, et al: *JAMA* 261:1165–1168, 1989.
3. Huie MJ: *Med Sci Sports Exerc* 26:408, 1994.
4. Cabasso A: *Med Sci Sports Exerc* 26:2, 1994.
5. Klava A, et al: *J R Soc Med* 87:43, 1994.

Bilateral Distal Biceps Tendon Avulsions With Use of Anabolic Steroids

Visuri T, Lindholm H (Central Military Hosp, Helsinki)
Med Sci Sports Exerc 26:941–944, 1994   139-95-8-11

Purpose.—Long-term use of anabolic-androgenic steroids (AASs) is associated with various adverse somatic and psychiatric effects. Experimental data suggest that anabolic steroid use combined with exercise can lead to pathologic conditions of the tendons; however, only 4 cases of AAS-related tendon rupture have been reported. A case of bilateral avulsion of the distal biceps tendon associated with intense, long-term AAS use was reported.

Case.—Man, 23, was admitted with spontaneous rupture of the left distal biceps tendon. He was a long-time bodybuilder who had used AAS in increasing amounts from 17 to 22 years of age. He took 1,500–2,000 mg of various anabolic steroids per week during basic training, increasing his AAS dose to 2,000 mg/day before competitions. The year before the reported admission, the patient reported a sudden snap in his right elbow and biceps pain on lifting a heavy rack of weights. At surgery, the distal head of the biceps was found to be detached from the radial tuberosity. The tendon was reattached by the technique of Body and Anderson. The next year, the patient sustained a similar rupture of the left biceps tendon. It was reattached by the same surgical technique. Both operations produced good results. Other possible adverse effects of steroids in this patient included explosive behavior, painful gynecomastia, and slight hypertrophy of the left and right ventricular walls; at a previous psychiatric admission, an AAS-induced affective syndrome had been diagnosed.

Conclusion.—Use of AAS can lead to biceps tendon avulsion. As in the reported case, many bodybuilders continue using steroids despite knowing about and having experience with their negative effects. Knowing that AAS abuse can cause tendon injuries and, thus, shorten their bodybuilding careers, may temper these athletes' desire to use steroids.

▶ Although anecdotal, accumulating evidence strongly suggests another adverse effect of anabolic steroids: rupture or avulsion of tendons. Bodybuilders who abuse steroids can add this new threat to many other health risks, including myocardial thickening (see Abstract 139-95-8–6), unhealthful blood lipid changes (see Abstract 139-95-8–10), liver tumors, heart attack, psychiatric problems, and HIV infection from sharing needles (1). Sadly, a recent survey of adolescents in Georgia found that 25% of those who abuse anabolic steroids also share needles (2).—E.R. Eichner, M.D.

References

1. Scott MJ, Scott MJ Jr: JAMA 262:207, 1989.
2. 1994 YEAR BOOK OF SPORTS MEDICINE, pp 346–347.

An Acute Myocardial Infarction Occurring in an Anabolic Steroid User

Huie MJ (Univ of California, Berkeley)

Med Sci Sports Exerc 26:408–413, 1994   139-95-8–12

Background.—Anabolic-androgenic steroid abuse may cause abnormalities in lipid profiles. Some cases of acute myocardial infarction (MI) possibly associated with steroid abuse have been reported recently. A young amateur weight trainer without other risk factors sustained an acute MI.

Case Report.—Man, 25, after a heavy weight-training session, experienced severe fatigue followed by a crushing substernal pain. His physical examination was unremarkable except for a blood pressure of 177/75 mm Hg. His ECG showed ST-segment elevations in the anterior and lateral leads, suggesting an evolving MI. The patient had none of the usual cardiac risk factors, except that his grandfather and an uncle both had an MI at around age 40 years. About 16 weeks before his admission, the patient had started taking 100 mg of nandrolone decanoate (Deca-Durabolin) IM once weekly. After 6 weeks, he stopped using the drug for 4 weeks and then started weekly 200-mg injections of a corresponding preparation. The last injection was 2 days before hospitalization.

The patient's initial laboratory findings included a hematocrit of 52.2%, a total unfractionated lactate dehydrogenase value of 1,224 units/L (normal, < 181 units/L), an aspartate aminotransferase value of 272 units/L (< 46 units/L), a cholesterol value of 196 mg/dL (< 231 mg/dL), and a creatine kinase value of 2,831 units/L (< 246 units/L) with a myocardial band fraction of 10.8 ng/mL (< 7.6 ng/mL). He was treated with tissue plasminogen activator, aspirin, metoprolol, nitroglycerin, and heparin. An angiogram showed a large proximal left anterior descending artery thrombus. The coronary blood flow was completely restored after intracoronary urokinase infusion. One day after thrombolytic therapy, his antithrombin III activity was 20% (78% to 177%). At follow-up 8 months after the infarction, his antithrombin III activity and lipid profile values were within normal limits.

Discussion.—The use of nandrolone may have predisposed this patient to platelet hyperaggregation. At least in part, a transient decrease in antithrombin III levels caused by exercise may be responsible for the coronary artery thrombus. Because anabolic-androgenic steroids alter platelet activity, young, otherwise healthy individuals who abuse these drugs are at increased risk for MI, stroke, and pulmonary embolism.

▶ The list of complications from steroid abuse continues to expand. This report supplements 3 others (1–3) that have described incidents of MI in which steroid abuse was probably an etiologic factor. Both changes in lipid profile (3) and alterations in platelet aggregation (4) predispose the steroid abuser to such an outcome.—R.J. Shephard, M.D., Ph.D., D.P.E.

References

1. Bowman SJ, et al: *BMJ* 299:632, 1989.
2. Ferenchick GS, Adelman S: *Am Heart J* 124:507–508, 1992.
3. McNutt RA, et al: *Am J Cardiol* 62:164, 1988.
4. Small M: *Thromb Res* 35:353–358, 1984.

Steroid Abuse in Athletes, Prostatic Enlargement and Bladder Outflow Obstruction: Is There a Relationship?
Wemyss-Holden SA, Hamdy FC, Hastie KJ (Royal Hallamshire Hosp, Sheffield, England; Freeman Hosp, Newcastle upon Tyne, England)
Br J Urol 74:476–478, 1994   139-95-8-13

Introduction.—There are many well-documented side effects of anabolic-androgenic steroid abuse. However, there is little information regarding the effects of steroids on the androgen-sensitive prostate gland, including the possibility of adverse effects on voiding patterns. The effects of steroid abuse on the prostate gland of a bodybuilder were examined.

Methods.—The patient was a 49-year-old male bodybuilder who was routinely using anabolic steroids. He was assessed at regular intervals during a 15-week period of self-administration of steroids. The objective assessments included prostatic volume, as measured by transrectal ultrasound; digital rectal examination; urine flow rate; and serum acid phos-

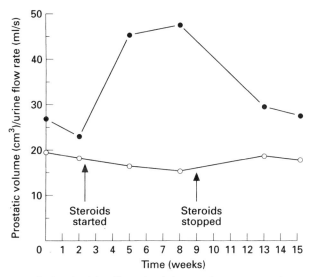

Fig 8–3.—Longitudinal study of the effects of anabolic steroids on prostatic volume and urine flow rate. *Filled circle*, prostatic volume; *open circle*, flow rate. (Courtesy of Wemyss-Holden SA, Hamdy FC, Hastie KJ: *Br J Urol* 74:476–478, 1994.)

phatase and prostate-specific antigen (PSA) values. Subjective assessment included symptom scoring for bladder outflow obstruction and other associated symptoms.

Results.—Prostatic volume increased significantly during the self-administration of steroids and returned to normal thereafter. Urine flow rate decreased during medication and returned to normal after the steroids were stopped (Fig 8–3). There were no significant changes in serum acid phosphatase or PSA values. The patient reported an increase in nocturnal urinary frequency, as well as increased libido and aggression.

Conclusion.—Self-administration of exogenous androgenic-anabolic steroids appears to have profound effects on the human prostate gland. These effects include increased prostatic volume and decreased urine flow rate, as well as subjective alteration in voiding patterns. The effects of steroids on the prostate may prove in the future to be a significant clinical problem and warrant further examination. For young men at risk to come forward for evaluation, the "screening" process will have to be confidential.

▶ The findings of Wemyss-Holden and associates were foreshadowed by a rat study, which also found that testosterone administration caused prostatic enlargement, with a shrinking of the prostate to a more normal size after the drug was withdrawn (1). Freed et al. (2) also noted problems of voiding in 10 athletes who admitted taking Dianabol. Although it would be a difficult study to carry out, there seems to be a need to check whether senile prostatic obstruction develops in former steroid abusers before the "normal" age for such an occurrence.—R.J. Shephard, M.D., Ph.D., D.P.E.

References

1. Kochakian CD, *Anabolic-Androgenic Steroids*. New York, Springer-Verlag, 1976.
2. Freed D, et al: *BMJ* 3:761, 1972.

At What Price, Glory?: Severe Cholestasis and Acute Renal Failure in an Athlete Abusing Stanozolol
Yoshida EM, Karim MA, Shaikh JF, Soos JG, Erb SR (Univ of British Columbia, Vancouver, Canada; Vancouver Gen Hosp, BC, Canada)
Can Med Assoc J 151:791–793, 1994   139-95-8–14

Background.—Equivocal results have been obtained from randomized, controlled studies of the efficacy of anabolic steroids in improving athletic performance. The adverse health effects of these drugs are well documented and extremely serious, but some physicians and athletes believe that the effects of steroid use are potentially dangerous only in the long term. A young athlete in whom acute renal failure and severe liver damage developed after stanozolol use was studied.

Case Report.—Man, 26, who was a power lifter, had generalized malaise, nausea, vomiting, and jaundice during a 4-week period. For 1 month before the onset of symptoms, he had been injecting stanozolol, 125 mg IM, twice weekly. He was taking no other medications, did not drink alcohol or smoke, and had no previous medical history. Physical examination revealed a jaundiced, exceptionally muscled man with a mildly tender liver extending 8 cm below the costal margin. The remaining examination was unremarkable. Laboratory tests revealed that serum creatinine, alkaline phosphatase, total bilirubin, and direct bilirubin levels were all elevated. Treatment was supportive.

In 1 month, he was admitted to the hospital with persistent vomiting, worsening jaundice and renal failure, a weight loss of 8 kg, and jugular venous distention to slightly below the sternal angle. The serum creatinine level was now very markedly elevated, as were urea nitrogen, alkaline phosphatase, total bilirubin, and direct bilirubin levels. Viral hepatitis testing and antinuclear antibody testing were negative, as were chest x-ray films and abdominal ultrasound scan. A percutaneous liver biopsy specimen revealed fibrosis around the portal tracts, marked centrilobular cholestasis, feathery degeneration of hepatocytes, and pericentral fibrosis. Renal biopsy results were consistent with resolving acute tubular necrosis. Supportive treatment was provided, and 2 months after stanozolol use was stopped, serum creatinine, alkaline phosphatase, and biliary enzyme levels began to decline. Five months after discontinuation of stanozolol, biliary enzymes were normal. The patient continued having mild renal impairment, but the serum creatinine level was stable at 142 μmol/L.

Conclusion.—This report should warn athletes and physicians that anabolic steroid use is not only unethical, it can result in severe multiorgan failure.

▶ There seems to be no end to the list of complications that can arise from the administration of massive doses of steroids. A number of investigators have reported cholestasis, with or without obstructive jaundice, in those who are abusing steroids (1–3). However, there have also been growing rumors of outbreaks of HIV and hepatitis epidemics at gymnasiums administering such drugs with improperly sterilized needles, and, although the patient described by Yoshida et al. was supposedly checked for hepatitis, one might wonder whether an acute infectious hepatitis played a role in causing the problem.—R.J. Shephard, M.D., Ph.D., D.P.E.

References

1. Ishak KG, Zimmerman HJ: *Semin Liver Dis* 7:230, 1987.
2. Westaby D, et al: *Lancet* 2:262–263, 1977.
3. Veneri RJ, Gordon SC: *J Clin Gastroenterol* 10:467, 1988.

Leucocytes, Lymphocytes, Activation Parameters and Cell Adhesion Molecules in Middle-Distance Runners Under Different Training Conditions

Baum M, Liesen H, Enneper J (Univ of Paderborn, Germany)
Int J Sports Med 15:S122–S126, 1994   139-95-8–15

Objective.—Immunologic changes occur during chronic recurrent intensive exercise, including an increase in the soluble interleukin-2 receptor. Whether the exercise-induced changes are lasting was determined.

Methods.—Aerobic and anaerobic lactic acid metabolism measurements were made in 20 track-and-field runners and 13 nonathletes. Lymphocyte subpopulations were also measured. Activation and adhesion parameters were determined by measuring the intercellular adhesion molecule (ICAM-1). The oxidation capacity of granulocytes was calculated.

Results.—There was a significant increase in monocytes during training. Expression of ICAM-1 was elevated during the exercise period (table). There was a significant increase in fluorescence intensity. Interleukin-2 increased with increasing levels of exercise. Numbers of B cells and cytotoxic T cells increased. There was a significant decrease in the oxidative capacity of granulocytes.

Conclusion.—There is a connection between susceptibility to infections and overtraining. An increase in the activation and adhesion parameters signals activation of the immune system.

▶ Automated fluorescence staining counting techniques are leading to rapid advances in our understanding of interactions between exercise and immune function, and the implications of such interactions for susceptibility to viral

Activation and Adhesion Parameters			
	First sample	Second sample	Third sample	Control group (4)
ICAM-1 (CD54) on monocytes	54.9 ± 15.3	65.2 ± 12.5	71.2 ± 9.8ˣˣˣ	46.7 ± 7.1
s-ICAM-1 (ng/-1)	371.4 ± 62.6ˣ	328.3 ± 46.1	337.3 ± 42.1	310.6 ± 42.1
IL2-R-pos. helper cells CD4+/CD25+ CD4+	26 % ± 10 %	23 % ± 8 %	34 % ± 7 %○	26 % ± 9 %
s-IL2-R (IU)	624.5 ± 460.0	732.4 ± 522.3	779.0 ± 571.0⊐	364.0 ± 129.5
Neopterin (IU)	10.9 ± 4.8	8.8 ± 1.5	9.4 ± 3.6	10.2 ± 4.0

Note: 3–4 xxx, $P \leq 0.001$; 1–4 x, $P \leq 0.05$; 1–3 circle, $P \leq 0.05$; 3–4 square, $P \leq 0.01$.
(Courtesy of Baum M, Liesen H, Enneper J: *Int J Sports Med* 15:S122–S126, 1994.)

infections. This paper is one of a series in a special issue of the *International Journal of Sports Medicine* that was published to mark the foundation of the International Society for Exercise Immunology.

The observations made show a number of variations relative to other reports in the literature. The resting natural killer (NK) cell count is here not increased by training (although this has been observed in a number of other laboratory studies). Possibly, the interval between fatiguing competition and blood sampling was too short here for full recovery to have occurred. In support of this view, Baum and associates found an increase of CD45 RO–positive T-helper cells, which have been associated with overtraining. The increase of ICAM-1 may be a further pointer in this direction; the adhesion molecule is an indicator of monocyte activation, and it may be that such activation released prostaglandins, which are known to suppress NK cell function (1). An acute bout of exercise can suppress NK cell activity sufficiently to increase the risk of viral infections, but sustained moderate training has a beneficial effect, either through an increase of NK cell count and cytotoxic activity, or through an increase of ICAM-1, which facilitates an interaction between the monocytes and rhinoviruses (2).—R.J. Shephard, M.D., Ph.D., D.P.E.

References

1. Kappel M, Twede N, Galbo H, et al: *J Appl Physiol* 70:2530–2534, 1991.
2. Marlin SD, Staunton DE, Springer TA, et al: *Nature* 344:70–73, 1990.

Effects of Aerobic Exercise Training on Lymphocyte Subpopulations
LaPerriere A, Antoni MH, Ironson G, Perry A, McCabe P, Klimas N, Helder L, Schneiderman N, Fletcher MA (Univ of Miami, Fla)
Int J Sports Med 15:S127–S130, 1994   139-95-8–16

Objective.—Good evidence exists that there is a relationship between exercise and immunologic status. The changes in lymphocyte subpopulations that occur in previously sedentary individuals after an aerobic exercise training program were determined.

Methods.—Fourteen healthy, sedentary men 18–40 years of age were randomly assigned to an assessment-only group or to an aerobic exercise program that met for 45 minutes 3 times per week for 10 weeks. The exercise level was set at 70% to 80% of the age-appropriate maximum heart rate. Aerobic fitness was evaluated, and blood samples were analyzed.

Results.—After exercise, there was a significant decrease in heart rate. Exercise increased the level of lymphocyte subpopulations (table). The increase in the number of CD4 and CD8 cells was probably a manifestation of an increase in immune response because both are necessary for proper immunoregulation. There was also an increase in inducer cells,

Effects of Exercise Training on Lymphocyte Phenotypes
(Mean and SD)

	Exercise (N = 7)		Control (N = 7)	
	before training	after training	before training	after training
CD2+	1 717	2 183†	2 127	1 988
(mm³)	±434	±527	±655	±917
CD2+TA1+	307	681	445	395
(mm³)	±139	±477	±135	±213
CD4+	941	1 280†	1 166	1 043
(mm³)	±226	±383	±433	±483
CD29+CD4+	487	519	559	576
(mm³)	±236	±166	±175	±243
CD45RA+CD4+	312	595†	388	394
(mm³)	±188	±272	±329	±204
CD8+	655	816*	835	777
(mm³)	±180	±293	±238	±489
CD8+12+	101	202	115	118
(mm³)	±79	±240	±57	±119
CD4+/CD8+	1.47	1.49	1.67	1.59
(ratio)	±.25	±.67	±.49	±.97
CD20+	162	244†	260	257
(mm³)	±83	±110	±100	±91
CD56+	319	388	430	403
(mm³)	±148	±82	±92	±291

*Significant increase from before to after training = $P < 0.05$.
†Significant increase from before to after training = $P < 0.01$.
(Courtesy of LaPerriere A, Antoni MH, Ironson G, et al: *Int J Sports Med* 15:S127–S130, 1994.)

lysing cells, and suppressor cells. An increase in CD20 cells indicates a potential for an increased humoral response.

Conclusion.—Aerobic exercise appears to exert beneficial effects by increasing both humoral and cellular immunity. It is unknown whether these effects are lasting; more research is needed to understand how exercise affects these changes.

▶ In this 10-week aerobic training study of healthy young men, modest increases were seen in levels of T-helper lymphocytes and T-suppressor lymphocytes, but not in natural killer (NK) cells. Are these changes clinically important? I doubt it. This study complements 2 training studies of women. In one, a study of middle-aged women, 15 weeks of brisk walking boosted baseline NK cell function and shortened the clinical duration of upper respiratory infections (1). The other training study, of older women, found no enhancement of NK activity but suggested that brisk walkers—and even more so, competitive senior athletes—may have fewer upper respiratory infections than do control women who remain sedentary (2). See also Abstract 139-95-8-17.—E.R. Eichner, M.D.

References

1. Nieman DC, et al: *Int J Sports Med* 11:467, 1990.
2. Nieman DC, et al: *Med Sci Sports Exerc* 25:823, 1993.

Effect of High- Versus Moderate-Intensity Exercise on Lymphocyte Subpopulations and Proliferative Response

Nieman DC, Miller AR, Henson DA, Warren BJ, Gusewitch G, Johnson RL, Davis JM, Butterworth DE, Herring JL, Nehlsen-Cannarella SL (Appalachian State Univ, Boone, NC; Loma Linda Univ, Calif; Univ of South Carolina)
Int J Sports Med 15:199–206, 1994   139-95-8-17

Introduction.—Previous reports indicate that the mitogen-stimulated proliferative response is suppressed after acute bouts of cardiorespiratory exercises as well as after stress/disease events such as spaceflight, myocardial infarction, cancer, severe burns, and psychiatric illness. The mitogen-stimulated lymphocyte proliferative response to high- vs. moderate-intensity exercise was observed in 10 well-conditioned male runners.

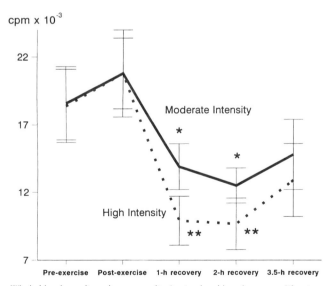

Fig 8–4.—Whole blood, unadjusted concanavalin A–stimulated lymphocyte proliferative response to high- vs. moderate-intensity exercise in 10 well-conditioned young males. The pattern of change was not significantly different between intensity conditions ($P = 0.606$), but a strong time effect ($P < 0.001$) was observed for both conditions. *$P < 0.05$, within condition vs. baseline. **$P < 0.0125$, within condition vs. baseline. (Courtesy of Nieman DC, Miller AR, Henson DA, et al: *Int J Sports Med* 15:199–206, 1994.)

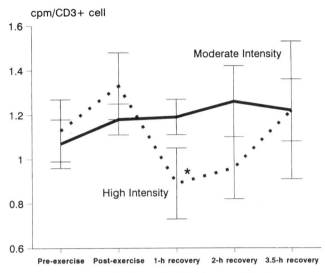

Fig 8–5.—Whole blood, concanavalin A–stimulated lymphocyte proliferative response adjusted per T cell (CD3+) to high- vs. moderate-intensity exercise in 10 well-conditioned young males. The pattern of change was not significantly different between intensity conditions (P = 0.276). $^*P$ < 0.05, within condition vs. baseline. (Courtesy of Nieman DC, Miller AR, Henson DA, et al: *Int J Sports Med* 15:199–206, 1994.)

Methods.—Runners between the ages of 17 and 31 years completed high-intensity and moderate-intensity workouts on separate days, 2 weeks apart. The high-intensity workout took place on a level treadmill for 45 minutes at 80% of maximum oxygen consumption ($\dot{V}O_{2max}$). The moderate-intensity workout consisted of 45 minutes of graded treadmill walking at 50% of $\dot{V}O_{2max}$. Blood samples were assessed for circulating leukocytes, lymphocyte subpopulations, catecholamine and cortisol concentrations, and the mitogen-stimulated lymphocyte proliferative response. The samples were drawn at baseline, immediately after exercise, and at 1, 2, and 3.5 hours during recovery.

Results.—High-intensity exercise, compared with moderate-intensity exercise, was associated with increased neutrophilia and recovery lymphocytopenia; greater lymphocytosis, represented primarily by T and natural killer cells; suppressed concanavalin A (Con A)–stimulated lymphocyte proliferative response at 1 and 2 hours of recovery, adjusted per T cell (CD+3) basis to a 1-hour postexercise decrease (Figs 8–4 and 8–5); and greater increases in both serum cortisol and plasma epinephrine.

Conclusion.—The elevations in both epinephrine and cortisol concentrations after high-intensity exercise may contribute to a temporarily decreased ability of the T lymphocytes to proliferate in response to Con A. Further study is needed to determine whether this has clinical significance.

▶ As noted in Abstract 139-95-8–19, infusion of epinephrine into healthy volunteers mimics many of the immune changes of acute exercise. This careful study of moderate- vs. high-intensity exercise tends to support this "epinephrine thesis" in that the high-intensity exercise here was associated with higher epinephrine (and cortisol) levels, together with greater immediate lymphocytosis (consisting mainly of natural killer cells and T lymphocytes), greater delayed lymphopenia, and greater postexercise depression of lymphocyte mitogenesis. But how important *clinically* are these mild and brief exercise-induced changes in immune markers?—E.R. Eichner, M.D.

Effect of Long-Distance Running on Polymorphonuclear Neutrophil Phagocytic Function of the Upper Airways

Müns G (Kreiskrankenhaus Gummersbach, Germany)
Int J Sports Med 15:96–99, 1994   139-95-8–18

Objective.—Moderate exercise appears to stimulate the immune system. However, intense exercise may cause immune deficiency; several reports have described a high incidence of infections, mainly of the upper and lower respiratory tract, for years after strenuous exercise. The

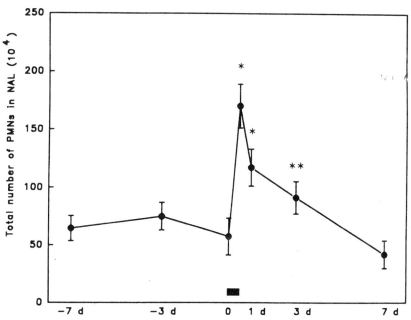

Fig 8–6.—Influence of a long-distance race on the number of polymorphonuclear neutrophils (PMNs) in the upper respiratory tract. Data are expressed as the total number of PMNs recovered by nasal lavage (PMNs/mL × mL of recovered lavage fluid). *Circles* represent the means ± SE; *black box* indicates when the race occurred. *Asterisks* denote significant differences (*P = 0.01; **P = 0.05). (Courtesy of Müns G: *Int J Sports Med* 15:96–99, 1994.)

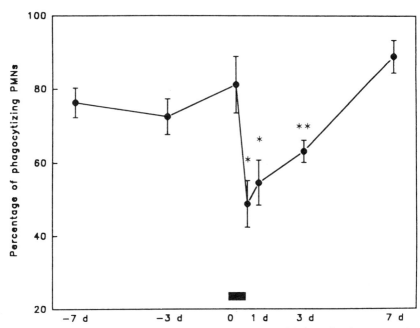

Fig 8–7.—Percentage of phagocytizing polymorphonuclear neutrophils (PMNs) in the upper respiratory tract of amateur runners. Data represent the percentage of phagocytizing PMNs recovered by nasal lavage. *Circles* represent the means ± SE; *black box* indicates when the race occurred. *Asterisks* denote significant differences (*P = 0.01; **P = 0.05). (Courtesy of Müns G: *Int J Sports Med* 15:96–99, 1994.)

primary defense against airborne pathogens is the mucosal surfaces, but there are few data on their function during exercise. The effects of long-distance running on the polymorphonuclear neutrophil (PMN) phagocytic function of the upper respiratory tract were assessed.

Methods.—Twelve male amateur runners (mean age, 34 years) participated in a 20-km race. Each participant underwent nasal lavage for harvesting of PMNs on 7 occasions in the week before and the week after the race, including immediately before and after the competition. The number of PMNs recovered was counted, and the number of phagocytized *Escherichia coli* organisms was measured with a fluorescence-activated cell sorter.

Results.—Immediately after the race, the PMN count was twofold higher than the value before the race. One day after the race, the PMN count was still elevated by 1.6-fold (Fig 8–6). Compared with the immediate postrace value, during training and after the race counts were significantly lower. Before the race, the percentage of phagocytizing PMNs was significantly reduced. However, the most dramatic reductions were seen immediately and 1 day after the race; they were 49% and 55%, respectively (Fig 8–7). Immediately after the race, the number of *E. coli* bacteria ingested by phagocytizing PMNs was 3.2 per PMN, compared with 5.2 per PMN the day after the competition.

Conclusion.—Strenuous exercise may be followed by chronic upper airway inflammation and impaired phagocyte function. These effects may play a role in the high incidence of respiratory tract infections among athletes. Conclusions regarding the mechanisms of exercise-related decreases in mucosal barrier function await further study.

▶ As we have extensively reviewed it (1, 2), exercise can change the levels and functions of white blood cells (especially neutrophils, natural killer cells, and other lymphocytes) and the levels of immunoglobulins, complement, and other immune factors. Generally, however, any exercise-related changes are mild, mixed, and brief, making their clinical import moot. Epidemiologic data, too, are mixed but suggest a slight increased risk of upper respiratory tract and skin infections in athletes in heavy training, a risk that may be enhanced by the psychological stress of competition (3).

This novel study suggests a mechanism for upper respiratory infection in athletes: A distance race doubled the number of PMNs in nasal lavage (suggesting airway inflammation, perhaps) and also decreased the percentage of phagocytizing PMNs and the number of ingested bacteria per PMN. Then again, most upper respiratory infections are viral, defense against which focuses not on PMNs but on salivary immunoglobulins and natural killer cells.—E.R. Eichner, M.D.

References

1. 1993 *Year Book of Sports Medicine*, pp 306–317.
2. 1994 *Year Book of Sports Medicine*, pp 393–395.
3. Brenner IKM, et al: *Sports Med* 17:86, 1994.

Evidence That the Effect of Bicycle Exercise on Blood Mononuclear Cell Proliferative Responses and Subsets Is Mediated by Epinephrine

Tvede N, Kappel M, Klarlund K, Duhn S, Halkjoer-Kristensen J, Kjoer M, Galbo H, Pedersen BK (Univ Hosp, Copenhagen; Bispebjerg Hosp, Copenhagen; Roskilde County Hosp, Copenhagen)

Int J Sports Med 15:100–104, 1994   139-95-8–19

Background.—Physical exercise can induce marked changes in the cellular immune system. Because exercise increases plasma concentrations of several stress hormones, including epinephrine, it was hypothesized that exercise-induced changes in blood mononuclear cell (BMNC) subsets, BMNC proliferative responses, and lymphokine-activated killer (LAK) cell activity are mediated by increased concentrations of epinephrine.

Study Design.—On 2 separate occasions, normal healthy male volunteers exercised on a bicycle ergometer (75% of maximal aerobic power for 1 hour) or they received an IV infusion of epinephrine to obtain plasma concentrations of epinephrine comparable with those seen during exercise. Blood samples were collected before exercise, at the end of exercise, and 2 hours after exercise or epinephrine infusion.

Results.—During both exercise and epinephrine infusion, the percentage of CD3+ T cells and CD4+ T cells decreased, and the percentage of CD 16+ natural killer cells increased more than twofold, whereas the percentage of CD8+ T cells and CD20+ B cells did not change. Two hours after exercise and infusion, the percentage of CD14+ monocytes increased twofold to threefold. When stimulated with phytohemagglutinin, the BMNC proliferative responses declined during both exercise and epinephrine infusion. The LAK cell activity and BMNC proliferative responses after stimulation with interleukin-2 increased, but the changes were more pronounced during exercise. There also were increases in the number of lymphocytes and neutrophils, but the increases were more pronounced during exercise.

Conclusion.—The exercise-induced changes in BMNC subsets can be mimicked by an infusion of epinephrine, resulting in plasma concentrations of epinephrine similar to those obtained during exercise. In response to physical exercise, the rise in plasma concentrations of epinephrine may contribute to the changes in cellular immunity.

▶ As reviewed in Abstract 139-95-8–18, exercise affects various facets of immunity, including lymphocytes, natural killer (NK) cells, and other BMNCs. This article explores mechanisms by which exercise alters immunity. To a great degree, infusion of epinephrine mimics the changes of exercise: leukocytosis, lymphocytosis, increase in the percentage of NK cells, decrease in the percentage of helper T cells, increase in NK activity and decrease in lymphocyte mitogenesis (both caused by changes in relative numbers, not function, of responding cells), and delayed monocytosis. There were minor differences between exercise and epinephrine (with exercise, the lymphocytosis was more pronounced and the neutrophilia more long-lasting), but, in general, the mimicry is striking. Recently, other researchers studying similar facets of immunity in response to high- vs. moderate-intensity exercise also proposed that epinephrine (and perhaps also cortisol) underlies the exercise-induced changes in lymphocyte numbers and function (1). See also Abstract 139-95-8–17.—E.R. Eichner, M.D.

Reference

1. Nieman DC, et al: *Int J Sports Med* 15:199, 1994.

Differential Expression of Interleukin-2 Receptor Alpha and Beta Chains in Relation to Natural Killer Cell Subsets and Aerobic Fitness

Rhind SG, Shek PN, Shinkai S, Shephard RJ (Univ of Toronto; Ehime Univ, Japan)

Int J Sports Med 15:911–918, 1994   139-95-8–20

Background.—Functions of the immune system are modulated by both acute exercise and physical conditioning. Key elements in changes in the immune system are the number and activity of circulating natural killer (NK) cells, interleukin (IL)-2, and the IL-2 receptor (IL-2R). The possible relationship between aerobic fitness and IL-2R expression was evaluated.

Methods.—Thirteen healthy male volunteers, 7 who were endurance trained and 6 who were not, were recruited from the University of Toronto student population. Each volunteer's maximal oxygen intake was determined on a cycle ergometer. A sample of each man's venous blood was collected and analyzed for the expression of alpha (p55)- and beta (p70–p75)-subunits of the IL-2R on various lymphocyte subsets.

Results.—Endurance-trained volunteers had higher percentages and absolute counts of total leukocytes, granulocytes, and NK cells but lower counts for lymphocytes than the nontrained volunteers. The T-cell and B-cell counts and the CD4+/CD8+ ratio did not differ significantly between the groups. The percentage of lymphocytes expressing IL-2Rα was unrelated to training status, whereas the expression of IL-2Rβ was significantly higher in the trained group. There was a strong association between maximal oxygen intake and expression of the IL-2Rβ and a similarly strong association between NK cell subsets and maximal oxygen intake. Compared with the untrained volunteers, endurance-trained men had a significantly higher percentage of CD4+ lymphocytes expressing the IL-2Rα. The IL-2Rβ expression was strongly correlated with aerobic power.

Conclusion.—An association was found between endurance training and circulating counts of peripheral lymphocytes expressing markers for the p70–p75 IL-2Rβ and for NK subsets. Expression of the p55 IL-2Rα is apparently unrelated to aerobic fitness. These findings may have important practical implications with respect to IL-2 treatment of neoplasm and resistance to viral diseases.

▶ This cross-sectional, observational study of selected immune markers suggests that higher levels of physcial fitness are tied to higher levels of natural immunity. The trained men, compared with the untrained men, had twice as many basal NK cells, as well as one third more granulocytes (but lower counts for lymphocytes). Also, maximum oxygen consumption correlated with NK cell subsets and with a receptor for IL-2 on NK cells. A cross-sectional, correlative study like this one cannot, of course, prove cause and effect. However, because NK cells are "minute men" that attack viruses, and because increased sensitivity to IL-2 (which is secreted by helper T cells) suggests a brisk defense, this study offers the promise that we can rev up our natural immunity by becoming fit. A longitudinal training study in women also suggests that becoming more fit via regular, brisk walking can enhance NK cell activity and bolster immunity (1).—E.R. Eichner, M.D.

Reference

1. 1991 *Year Book of Sports Medicine*, pp 134–137.

Immunological Status of Competitive Cyclists Before and After the Training Season

Baj Z, Kantorski J, Majewska E, Zeman K, Pokoca L, Fornalczyk E, Tchórzewski H, Sulowska Z, Lewicki R (Military Med Academy, Łódz, Poland; Polish Academy of Sciences)
Int J Sports Med 15:319–324, 1994   139-95-8–21

Background.—Athletes taking part in long-term, exhausting physical training are prone to recurrent infections, which are thought to be the result of exercise-induced immunosuppression. Although acute exercise is known to produce changes in leukocyte number and function, there are many unanswered questions regarding the changes in specific and nonspecific immunity occurring in response to long-term intensive training. Immunologic parameters were measured in cyclists before and after long-term intensive training and a competitive season.

Methods.—Fifteen male cyclists (mean age, 21 years) and 16 non-trained controls were studied. The cyclists were studied at the beginning of their training season and again after 6 months of intensive training

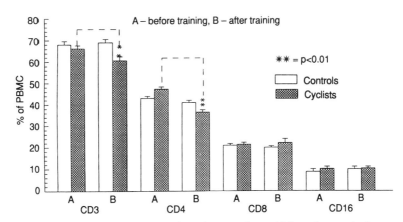

Fig 8–8.—Percentages of T-lymphocyte subpopulations and natural killer cells at rest in the control group and in 15 competitive cyclists. A, values of examined parameters in cyclists during the first test. B, values of the parameters in August after 6 months of intensive training. Each result is mean of *n* individual results ± SEM. *P < 0.05 (Courtesy of Baj Z, Kantorski J, Majewska E, et al: *Int J Sports Med* 15:319–324, 1994.)

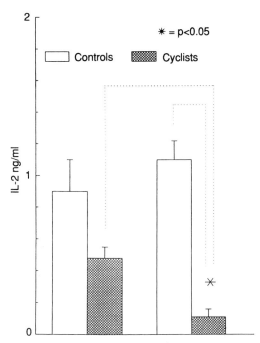

Fig 8–9.—Generation of interleukin-2 (*IL-2*) lymphocytes from controls and cyclists. Concentrations of generated IL-2 were obtained from dose-response curve with recombinant IL-2. (Courtesy of Baj Z, Kantorski J, Majewska E, et al: *Int J Sports Med* 15:319–324, 1994.)

and a racing season. During the training period, the athletes were cycling about 500 km/wk. The immunologic tests included measurement of total number of leukocytes, T-lymphocyte subsets, mitogen-induced lymphocyte proliferation, interleukin-2 (IL-2) generation, adherence capacity, and granulocyte chemiluminescence, as well as a leukergy test.

Results.—The cyclists' baseline values were within the range of the controls' values, with the exception of a significant increase in nonstimulated neutrophil chemiluminescence. At the second test point, the cyclists showed significantly decreased absolute numbers of CD3+ and CD4+ cells, diminished IL-2 generation, and increased neutrophil chemiluminescence stimulated by N-formyl-methionyl-leucyl-phenylalanine and phorbol myristate acetate (Figs 8–8 and 8–9). After the training season, there was a marked increase in phytohemagglutinin antigen-induced lymphocyte proliferation and normalization of nonstimulated neutrophil chemiluminescence.

Conclusion.—Long-term intensive physical training appears to result in significant changes in immunologic parameters, including lymphocyte number and composition and neutrophil oxidative burst capacity. The consequences of these changes for immunity are unknown, however.

Further study is needed to determine whether they represent adaptation or exhaustion of the immune system.

▶ This study differs from Abstract 139-95-8–20 in that, in these athletes (young male cyclists), both at baseline (compared with untrained controls) and after 6 months of heavy training and racing, natural killer cells were not increased in number or activity. Blood lymphocytes did tend to be lower at baseline in the cyclists and fell further after training; this decline was mainly in helper T lymphocytes, which led to the decline in generation of IL-2 after training. In spite of the decline in lymphocyte counts, mitogen-stimulated lymphocyte proliferation increased.

Other changes after training were slight decreases in aggregation of leukocytes (but not in neutrophil adherence) and in chemiluminescence of granulocytes. Lacking data on whether the cyclists got more or fewer infections, we cannot know whether these subtle changes in immune markers are clinically important—or, in the authors' words, whether they reflect "adaptation or exhaustion" of the immune system.—E.R. Eichner, M.D.

Aging and Stress-Induced Changes in Complement Activation and Neutrophil Mobilization

Cannon JG, Fiatarone MA, Fielding RA, Evans WJ (Tufts Univ, Boston; New England Med Ctr, Boston)
J Appl Physiol 76:2616–2620, 1994   139-95-8–22

Purpose.—As a muscle develops tension, repeated forced lengthening results in immediate structural damage to sarcomeres. Afterward, delayed-onset muscle soreness and myocellular enzyme release occur. In quadriceps muscles, this effect can be produced by downhill running or by resisting bicycle pedals that are driven backward by a motor. Various types of exercise are followed by complement activation and neutrophil mobilization. The extent of complement activation and neutrophil mobilization after eccentric exercise was measured, and whether they are age-dependent was studied. The association of these effects with plasma creatine kinase (CK)—a marker of muscle membrane activity—was assessed as well.

Methods.—The study included 21 sedentary individuals with normal weight for their height. Twelve were aged 61–72 years and 9 were aged 20–32 years. All participants performed 1 of the 2 eccentric activities for 45 minutes at an intensity of 78% of maximum heart rate. Plasma des-Arg-C3a concentrations were measured by radioimmunoassay as a marker of complement activation. Hematologic and muscle biopsy studies were performed, and plasma CK and urinary creatinine levels were measured.

Results.—Immediately after exercise, all participants had a median 21% increase in plasma des-Arg-C3a levels. By 4 to 6 hours, the circulat-

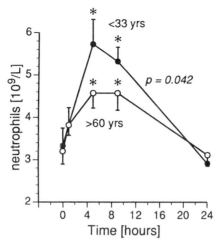

Fig 8–10.—Exercise-induced neutrophilia in younger and older individuals after eccentric exercise. Time points: 0 hours, blood sample taken immediately before exercise; 1 hour, sample taken immediately after exercise; 5 hours, sample taken 4 hours after exercise; and so on. Data from young and old groups overlap at 1-hour time point. Significant age group difference in response over time ($P = 0.042$) was observed. *Significant ($P < 0.0001$) within-group difference compared with time 0. (Courtesy of Cannon JG, Fiatarone MA, Fielding RA, et al: *J Appl Physiol* 76:2616–2620, 1994.)

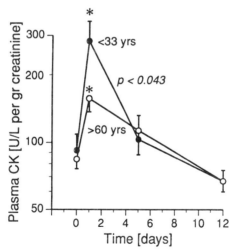

Fig 8–11.—Changes in plasma creatine kinase (CK) activity normalized for muscle mass in response to eccentric exercise in younger and older individuals. Data from young and old groups overlap at 12-day time point. One young individual was omitted from analysis because of CK concentrations that were > 10 SD higher than mean. Significant age group difference in response over time ($P = 0.043$) was observed. *Significant ($P < 0.0001$) within-group difference compared with time 0. (Courtesy of Cannon JG, Fiatarone MA, Fielding RA, et al: *J Appl Physiol* 76:2616–2620, 1994.)

ing neutrophil count increased 66% (Fig 8–10); by 24 hours, the plasma CK increased 135% (Fig 8–11). The peak increases in neutrophils and des-Arg-C3a were significantly correlated, as were the peak increases in CK and the increase in neutrophils. The older participants had significantly smaller increases in neutrophils and plasma CK.

Conclusion.—After muscle injury produced by eccentric exercise, increased concentrations of circulating CK are noted in association with a sequential cascade of inflammatory mediators. In response to this stress, elderly individuals have diminished neutrophil mobilization, but there is no age-related difference in complement activation. Although other mechanism also make important contributions to the CK response, neutrophils may be considered as potential mediators of altered muscle membrane permeability.

▶ This study is part of ongoing research into the "acute-phase response" to muscle-damaging, eccentric exercise (1). Past research suggests that older adults, compared with younger adults, have smaller increases in circulating neutrophils and plasma CK activity after eccentric exercise at the same relative intensity (based on heart rate). This study of older and younger men and women performing eccentric exercise (downhill running or resisting bicycle pedals driven backward by a motor) corroborates the "age difference" in response of neutrophils and CK and suggests this series of events and responses: eccentric exercise, ultrastructural muscle damage, complement activation, neutrophil response, and release of CK. Subjects with the greatest complement activation had the greatest neutrophil response and the highest CK levels.—E.R. Eichner, M.D.

Reference

1. 1992 YEAR BOOK OF SPORTS MEDICINE, pp 183–184.

Lower Limit of Body Fat in Healthy Active Men
Friedl KE, Moore RJ, Martinez-Lopez LE, Vogel JA, Askew EW, Marchitelli LJ, Hoyt RW, Gordon CC (US Army Research Inst of Environmental Medicine, Natick, Mass; US Army Natick Research, Development and Engineering Ctr, Mass; Martin Army Community Hosp, Fort Benning, Ga)
J Appl Physiol 77:933–940, 1994   139-95-8–23

Background.—Quantifying minimum body fat in human beings has been difficult. Anthropometric assessments of body fat, established in comparison with hydrodensitometry, consistently overestimate lean individuals. Dual-energy x-ray absorptiometry (DEXA), a new technology, provides another opportunity to evaluate extremes of body composition.

Methods.—Changes in body composition were assessed in 55 healthy young men during an 8-week Army combat leadership training course. The course involved strenuous exercise and low energy intake, with an

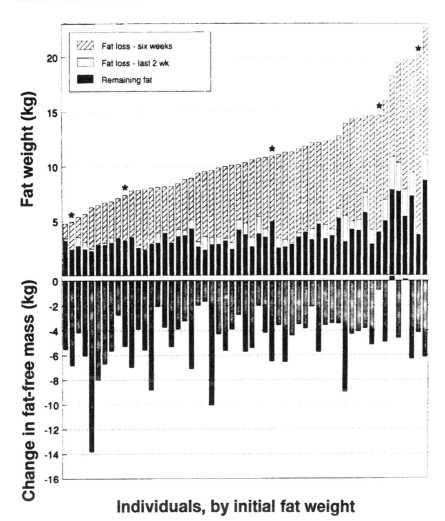

Individuals, by initial fat weight

Fig. 8–12.—Top, individual fat mass at start, 6 weeks, and end of Ranger training. **Bottom,** change in fat-free mass for same idividuals. $n = 55$. *Five men who were not measured at 6 weeks. (Courtesy of Friedl KE, Moore RJ, Martinez-Lopez LE, et al: *J Appl Physiol* 77:933–940, 1994.)

estimated energy deficit of 5 MJ/day and a resulting 15.7% loss of weight.

Findings.—Percentage of body fat, determined by DEXA, averaged 14.3% at the beginning of the course and 5.8% at the end. Men achieving a minimum percentage of body fat—4% to 6%—by week 6 had only small additional total and subcutaneous fat losses in the final 2 weeks, sacrificing increasingly greater proportions of fat-free mass. The percentage of body fat estimated from skinfold thicknesses reflected relative changes in fat mass (Fig 8–12). However, the actual percentage of body fat was overestimated. After fat stores were substantially depleted, abdominal, hip, and thigh girths continued to decrease with body weight loss rather than reaching a plateau.

Conclusion.—A 4% to 6% body fat percentage, or 4 skinfolds under 20 mm, appears to be the minimum achievable in healthy men. In healthy young men with a mean 15% of body fat, the rapid loss of 16% of body weight results in a depletion of fat stores, which is an excessive response.

▶ Despite the growing trend to the use of expensive (and supposedly impressive) methods of measuring body fat content, one important lesson that emerges from this study by Friedl et al. is that even when fat loss is extreme, simple skinfold measurements and use of the equation of Durnin and Womersley (1) provide a reliable guide to the extent of fat loss. All physicians should purchase and become familiar with the use of skinfold calipers! A second point the paper highlights is the fact that body mass index (and other height/weight relationships) is useless as a means of interpreting body fat content in the individual patient. Friedl et al. cite as examples 2 people with body mass index readings of 24.5 kg/m² (a value approaching the threshold for a supposed cardiac risk), yet each has only 6% to 8% body fat!

Finally, it is interesting that the minimum healthy skinfold readings average about 6 mm per fold. This is a level that we observed to be compatible with good health in studies of the Inuit when they were still pursuing the physically active hunter/gatherer lifestyle for which the human race is genetically adapted (2). Unfortunately, the Inuit (like many other indigenous populations) have now become much more obese and are beginning to develop the health consequences of this obesity (such as impaired glucose tolerance and an increasing incidence of cardiovascular diseases).—R.J. Shephard, M.D., Ph.D., D.P.E.

References

1. Durnin JVGA, Womersley JA: *Br J Nutr* 32:77–97, 1974.
2. Rode A, Shephard RJ: *Effects of Modernization on the Health of Circumpolar Peoples.* London, Cambridge University Press, 1996.

Effect of Passive and Active Recovery on the Resynthesis of Muscle Glycogen
Choi D, Cole KJ, Goodpaster BH, Fink WJ, Costill DL (Ball State Univ, Muncie, Ind)
Med Sci Sports Exerc 26:992–996, 1994   139-95-8–24

Introduction.—It is a common practice for athletes to "warm-down" to decrease the accumulation of lactate after intense exercise. However, the effect of active recovery on glycogen resynthesis in muscle after exercise is unclear. The influence of active and passive recovery on the mag-

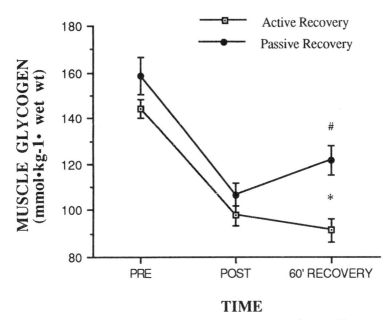

Fig 8–13.—Muscle glycogen response to high-intensity exercise. *Significantly different between trials (P < 0.05). #Significantly different from postvalue (P < 0.05). Values are mean ± SE. (Courtesy of Choi D, Cole KJ, Goodpaster BH, et al: *Med Sci Sports Exerc* 26:992–996, 1994.)

nitude of muscle glycogen resynthesis and lactate removal after high-intensity exercise was examined in 6 untrained college-aged male volunteers.

Methods.—A week before the first exercise trial, research subjects underwent a maximal oxygen consumption ($\dot{V}O_{2max}$) test on a bicycle ergometer to determine trial and active recovery workloads. Research subjects refrained from exercise for 2 days before testing and consumed a 15% carbohydrate solution, in addition to a normal diet, the day before each of 2 trials. The same exercise protocols were used for both trials: three 1-minute exercise bouts at 130% of $\dot{V}O_{2max}$, and a 4-minute rest period between exercise bouts. Research subjects rode at 40% to 50% $\dot{V}O_{2max}$ for 30 minutes, followed by 30 minutes of seated rest for the active recovery trial. In the passive recovery trial, they had 60 minutes of seated rest after the exercise protocol.

Results.—Muscle glycogen significantly increased during the passive recovery phase and significantly decreased during the active recovery phase (Fig 8–13). Muscle lactate and serum glucose concentrations showed a similar pattern of change in each trial. The mean blood lactate levels were significantly higher in the passive compared with the active recovery phase.

Conclusion.—The rate of muscle glycogen resynthesis was significantly greater during passive compared with active recovery. Blood lactate levels decreased more rapidly during active recovery. It is possible that optimal recovery may actually be a combination of both active and passive recovery approaches.

▶ For many athletes, prolonged practices or actual competitions follow in quick succession. The rate of replenishment of glycogen stores is, thus, a key to success; reserves must again be maximized over as little as 1–2 days. Previous generations of physiologists assumed that it was a good idea to speed the elimination of lactate by allowing moderate activity during recovery from a prolonged bout of exercise. However, the downside to this approach is that the lactate is a potential metabolite that could have been used for the resynthesis of glycogen (1); indeed, insistence on active recovery may further deplete glycogen stores.

A prolonged period of active recovery may be important as a means of eliminating lactate in a multibout sport in which further activity is required within 1 hour. However, it is not the optimum tactic when the next bout of sustained activity is 24 hours away.—R.J. Shephard, M.D., Ph.D., D.P.F.

Reference

1. Hermansen L, Vaage O: *Am J Physiol* 233:422E–429E, 1977.

Immediate Post-Training Carbohydrate Supplementation Improves Subsequent Performance in Trained Cyclists
Baker SK, Rusynyk T, Tiidus PM (Wilfrid Laurier Univ, Waterloo, Ont, Canada)
Sports Med Train Rehabil 5:131–135, 1994   139-95-8–25

Introduction.—The daily training intensity required by competitive cyclists can cause continual reduction in muscle glycogen stores if the cyclists are not getting optimal amounts of dietary carbohydrate. This, in turn, may cause a suboptimal training response. The caloric require-

Energy and Macronutrient Content of the Diet of 7 Individuals

		3 Day Self-Selected Diet	24-Hour Post-Training Diet
Daily energy intake	CHO*	34.3 ± 6.3	41.8 ± 9.7
(Kcal·kg⁻¹ body weight)	PLA*	29.3 ± 8.5	34.8 ± 19.2
Daily carbohydrate	CHO	4.2 ± 1.3	6.8 ± 0.9†
(g·kg⁻¹ body weight)	PLA	3.9 ± 1.1	4.7 ± 2.5†
Energy intake as carbohydrate	CHO	51 ± 6	68 ± 6†
(%)	PLA	54 ± 5	55 ± 5

*Carbohydrate (CHO)-supplemented (3 g/kg⁻¹ body weight) and placebo (PLA)-supplemented diets for all 7 individuals in both CHO and PLA conditions.
†Twenty-four-hour post-training diet significantly greater in CHO supplemented condition than in preceding self-selected diet ($P \leq 0.05$).
(Courtesy of Baker SK, Rusynyk T, Tiidus PM: *Sports Med Train Rehabil* 5:131–135, 1994.)

ments for competitive cycling may include carbohydrate supplementation. The effect of carbohydrate supplementation taken immediately after exercise on the next day's performance was studied.

Methods.—Seven healthy, highly trained, experienced competitive road cyclists were studied. The cyclists recorded the quantity and method of preparation of all nutrients in their diet for the 3 days before, the 24 hours between, and the 3 days after testing. Each cyclist rode an ergocycle to exhaustion at 75% of maximal oxygen intake and, immediately after exercise, drank a solution containing either 12% maltodextrin or a noncaloric placebo. The next day, each cyclist rode for 1 hour at 70% of maximal oxygen intake, then to exhaustion at 85% of maximal oxygen uptake. The cyclists repeated the protocol with the alternate solution 2 weeks later.

Results.—The mean carbohydrate intake was significantly increased by the maltodextrin supplement relative to the cyclists' self-selected diets (table). Five of the 7 cyclists had signficantly improved performance the day after ingesting the maltodextrin supplement. The mean ride time with the supplement was 72 minutes, compared with the mean ride time of 64 minutes with placebo.

Discussion.—These data indicate that competitive cyclists choose diets with a suboptimal carbohydrate content. The improved endurance performance 24 hours after the postexercise ingestion of a maltodextrin solution suggests that a postexercise carbohydrate supplement may delay fatigue and maximize muscle glycogen resynthesis, thereby improving daily training performance.

▶ Most athletes are aware that a high-carbohydrate diet can enhance their performance, but surprisingly few choose such a diet in practice. A muscle biopsy study of the Canadian Soccer Team a few years ago demonstrated to our laboratory that when training sessions were closely spaced, the muscle glycogen content was often no more than 50% of the level that could have been attained by conscientious "carbohydrate loading." Much of the glycogen resynthesis occurs in the first few hours after an intensive exercise bout, and it is, thus, a good idea to give any carbohydrate supplements immediately after the activity, as was done in this experiment.—R.J. Shephard, M.D., Ph.D., D.P.E.

Is Exercise Indicated for the Patient Diagnosed as Anorectic?
Michielli DW, Dunbar CC, Kalinski MI (City Univ of New York)
J Psychosoc Nurs Ment Health Serv 32:33–35, 1994   139-95-8–26

Introduction.—Eating disorders associated with a desire to be thin were seen in 18% of athletic and 5% of nonathletic girls, according to a report by Sundgot-Borgan. Many patients with anorexia nervosa exercise daily. Exercise is usually not prescribed for patients with anorexia nervosa. Intense aerobic workouts are prohibited, although short walks are usually recommended. It has been shown that patients with anorexia nervosa have a higher level of motor activity than do healthy females.

Weight Lifting.—Although weight gain is a treatment goal for patients with anorexia nervosa, weight gain in the form of fat may be counterproductive. Resistance training (weight lifting) offers a more modest caloric expenditure, increases lean body mass, gives a more appealing appearance, and may lead to less recidivism compared with putting on fat weight. Other benefits include increased strength, greater self-efficacy, and increased bone density in a population prone to osteoporosis. Although overtraining can be a problem in patients with anorexia nervosa, even vigorous circuit training with free weights burns 18 KJ (4.3 kcal) per minute for a 50-kg woman compared with 52 KJ (12.5 kcal) when jogging at a moderate speed. Additionally, circuit training is likely to tire the patient in a considerably shorter time than jogging.

Conclusion.—Few exercise-related studies in patients with anorexia have been quantified. The need for more research is apparent. Sound exercise guidelines are needed. Examining the effectiveness of a resistance training program on body composition in patients with anorexia would be a starting point.

▶ There is little debate over the concept that contestants in pursuits that are judged, in part, on appearance eat too little and have a negative energy balance. Argument continues as to whether anorexia nervosa is distinct from compulsive exercise, but the patient with a body mass of perhaps 35 kg who is admitted to hospital with an obsessive fear of fatness is clearly in a different category from the rather-thin gymnast, baton-twirler, or ballet dancer.

Our university's Department of Psychiatry shares many of the fears enunciated in this paper. Exercise is allowed only as a reward for the individual who has begun to restore body mass. However, I think the idea of focusing on deliberate weight training is an excellent approach to the treatment of anorexia nervosa from a number of viewpoints. Most such patients have sustained a large loss of muscle mass before hospital admission, and endurance activity will not restore this tissue. Further, resisted exercise can be performed at a small fraction of the energy cost of endurance activity. Finally, if the patient can be shown that the new tissue is muscle rather than fat, her fears of becoming obese may be overcome.—R.J. Shephard, M.D., Ph.D., D.P.E.

The Influence of Endurance Training on Insulin-Like Growth Factor-1 in Older Individuals
Poehlman ET, Rosen CJ, Copeland KC (Univ of Maryland, Baltimore; Univ of Maine, Bangor; Univ of Vermont, Burlington)
Metabolism 43:1401–1405, 1994   139-95-8–27

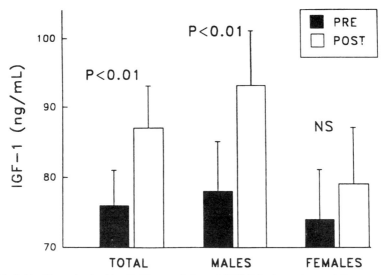

Fig 8–14.—Plasma levels of insulin-like growth factor I (*IGF-1*) in the total group (10 men and 8 women) before (*PRE*) and after (*POST*) training. Significant levels refer to the within-group response of IGF-1 to endurance training. (Courtesy of Poehlman ET, Rosen CJ, Copeland KC: *Metabolism* 43:1401–1405, 1994.)

Background.—Cross-sectional studies have found reduced levels of insulin-like growth factor I (IGF-1) in older adults, partly related to decreased exercise. There are no data regarding whether initiating a long-term exercise program in previously inactive elderly persons results in an increase in IGF-1, or whether this response is any different between the sexes. The effects of short-term endurance training on IGF-1 and on IGF binding proteins (IGFBPs) in elderly men and women were studied.

Methods.—The research subjects were 10 men and 8 women (mean age, 66 years) taking part in an 8-week endurance training program. Levels of IGF-1, IGFBP-1, and IGFBP-3 and maximal aerobic power ($\dot{V}O_{2max}$) were measured before and after training. Changes in body composition, estimated energy intake, and fasting plasma levels of glucose, insulin, and glucagon were assessed as well.

Results.—Both sexes had a significant 14% increase in $\dot{V}O_{2max}$. The men had a significant 19% increase in IGF-1, whereas the women had a nonsignificant 18% increase (Fig 8–14). The changes in $\dot{V}O_{2max}$ and IGF-1 were significantly correlated in men but not in women. There was no mean group change in the IGFBPs; however, individual changes between IGF-1 and IGFBP-3 showed a tendency to be related in men. The men had a decrease in plasma glucose after training, but the women did not. Neither sex had significant changes in fat-free mass, fat mass, or plasma insulin or glucagon.

Conclusion.—In previously inactive older adults, short-term endurance training produces an increase in fasting IGF-1 levels. This change is

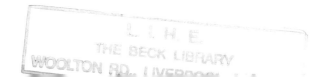

more pronounced in men, in whom it may be growth hormone-mediated. The idea that endurance training can ameliorate some of the hormonal and somatic correlates of aging is supported.

▶ Insulin-like growth factor-I is a peptide that has been attracting increasing attention as the population ages. In addition to its insulin-like properties, it mediates the anabolic effects of growth hormone, and a decline in plasma levels of IGF-I seems to be associated with the accumulation of fat and loss of muscle mass that occur in the elderly patient (1–3).

The authors of this article make the important point that for benefit to be obtained from a training regimen, the exercise sessions should create a positive energy balance; a negative balance can decrease the output of IGF-1 (4). The apparent gender difference in response to training needs exploration in a larger sample. In view of the influence of estrogens on the growth hormone axis, it will be important in such a study to distinguish women who are receiving estrogen supplements after the menopause from those who are not.—R.J. Shephard, M.D., Ph.D., D.P.E.

References

1. Copeland KC, Colletti RB, Devlin JD, et al: *Metabolism* 39:584–587, 1990.
2. Kelly PJ, Eisman JA, Stuart MC, et al: *J Clin Endocrinol Metab* 70:718–723, 1990.
3. Rudman D: *J Am Geriatr Soc* 33:800–807, 1985.
4. Smith AT, Clemmons DR, Underwood LE, et al: *Metabolism* 36:533–537, 1987.

Physical Training Increases Muscle GLUT4 Protein and mRNA in Patients With NIDDM

Dela F, Ploug T, Handberg A, Petersen LN, Larsen JJ, Mikines KJ, Galbo H (Univ of Copenhagen; Rigshospitalet, Copenhagen; Copenhagen Muscle Research Centre)
Diabetes 43:862–865, 1994   139-95-8-28

Introduction.—Increased insulin resistance and decreased glucose transport in skeletal muscle are features of patients with non–insulin dependent diabetes mellitus (NIDDM). Physical training is recommended for patients with NIDDM, even though there are only minor improvements in whole body insulin action. In normal young individuals, training increases glucose uptake, with parallel increases in muscle GLUT4. Similar training responses are seen is aged individuals with impaired glucose uptake. The content of GLUT4 in skeletal muscle is not affected by NIDDM. Muscle GLUT4 messenger RNA (mRNA) content has been reported to be either similar to or increased when compared with healthy controls. The effects of training and aging on muscle GLUT4 and the corresponding mRNA in NIDDM are unknown.

Methods.—Seven men, aged 58 years with a duration of NIDDM of 1.5 to 12 years, and 8 controls, aged 59 years, participated in the study. All performed 1-legged training on a cycle ergometer for 9 weeks, 6 days/wk, 30 min/day at 70% of 1-legged maximal aerobic power. Muscle biopsy specimens were taken from the vastus lateralis before and after training from both legs and analyzed for GLUT4 and GLUT4 mRNA content.

Results.—The aerobic power of all participants was improved by training. The NIDDM patients lost a little weight. Training had no effect on resting plasma glucose and insulin concentrations. Before training, the muscle GLUT4 content was equal across groups; it increased across both groups after training. The mRNA content was 63% and 81% of control values in the untrained and trained legs, respectively. Both the control and NIDDM participants had increases in muscle GLUT4 mRNA content, but the patients with NIDDM had a greater increase (13% vs. 30%). Aging was not a factor in muscle GLUT4 content.

Conclusion.—Muscle GLUT4 and GLUT4 mRNA increase in response to training in both patients with NIDDM and controls. Muscle GLUT4 mRNA content is lower in patients with NIDDM. The GLUT4 content was unaffected by aging.

▶ GLUT4 is the protein associated with glucose transport across the muscle membrane and is important in regulating plasma glucose. The investigation of Dela et al. seems to be the first study to have demonstrated that training can increase not only GLUT4, but also the associated mRNA in patients with NIDDM.—R.J. Shephard, M.D., Ph.D., D.P.E.

Exercise-Training Enhances Fat-Free Mass Preservation During Diet-Induced Weight Loss: A Meta-Analytical Finding
Ballor DL, Poehlman ET (Univ of Vermont, Burlington)
Int J Obes 18:35–40, 1994   139-95-8–29

Background.—Various factors affect the composition of diet-induced weight loss. Meta-analysis was used to determine whether exercise training and gender influence the composition of diet-induced weight loss and whether there are physical characteristics that predict the success of losing body fat and preserving fat-free mass.

Methods and Findings.—Medical reference databases from 1960 to 1991 were searched to locate potential studies. Forty-six papers met the selection criteria. Four groups were examined: men and women on dietary restriction only and men and women on diet-plus-exercise (DPE) programs. The amount of body weight and fat mass lost did not differ among groups. For a given sex, exercise training significantly reduced the amount of body weight lost as fat-free mass compared with dietary restriction alone. The percentage of weight lost as fat-free mass for indi-

Responses of Males and Females to Diet and Exercise Interventions—Post-Test/Pretest Differences

Variable	DO males	DO females	DPE males	DPE females	Main effect ($P < 0.05$)
Body mass (kg)	-12.2 ± 1.5	-10.6 ± 0.9	-8.7 ± 2.3	-9.4 ± 1.1	
Fat mass (kg)	-8.5 ± 1.2	-8.1 ± 0.7	-7.3 ± 1.8	-8.0 ± 0.8	
Percentage fat (%)	-5.0 ± 0.5	-4.6 ± 0.4	-5.8 ± 1.1	-5.7 ± 0.5	
Fat-free mass (kg)	-3.8 ± 0.5[a,b]	-2.5 ± 0.3[a,c]	-1.4 ± 0.8[b]	-1.4 ± 0.4[c]	E
% loss as fat-free mass	28.1 ± 3.7[a]	23.8 ± 2.2[b]	13.4 ± 5.7[a]	11.4 ± 2.7[b]	E

Note: Means ± standard error. Means with the same superscript are significantly different, $P < 0.05$.
Abbreviations: DO, dietary restriction only; DPE, dietary restriction and exercise training; E, a significant main effect for exercise.
(Courtesy of Ballor DL, Poehlman ET: *Int J Obes* 18:35–40, 1994.)

viduals on DPE programs was about half that for persons of the same sex undergoing diet restriction alone. These percentages were 28% for men on dietary restriction alone, 13% for men on DPE, 24% for women on dietary restriction alone, and 11% for women on DPE (table).

Conclusion.—Adding exercise training to dietary restriction is beneficial for both men and women. In both sexes, exercise training decreases the percentage of weight lost as fat-free mass during weight loss regimens.

▶ The likelihood that a combination of exercise and dieting will conserve lean tissue has been a strong argument for the use of exercise programs in the treatment of obesity. Nevertheless, the literature on this question has been conflicting. It is, thus, useful to have it all drawn together in the form of a meta-analysis.

The rigors of meta-analyses vary. Ballor and Poehlman list their criteria for inclusion of a study. They did not go to the lengths that some authors have adopted (searching for unpublished studies and having a panel of experts rate the quality of individual experiments on a double-blind basis). An important criticism of the studies that are included is that their average duration was only 10 weeks. This may suit the convenience of a master of science student, but it is hardly adequate to judge the efficacy of a treatment for obesity.

It is sometimes argued that, because of the needs of lactation, fat is more stable in females than in males (1). No gender difference was observed in the Ballor and Poehlman data set, probably because the initial body fat was far above the minimal requirements for lactation. The loss of body mass averaged about 1 kg/wk, implying a daily energy deficit of about 4 MJ (1,000 calories). Although exercise did help to conserve lean tissue, there was, nevertheless, a decrease in lean mass of about 1.4 kg over the 10 weeks in those who exercised. This emphasizes the point that if exercise is to be effective in preserving lean mass, it is essential that the change of body composition be seen as a long-term project. If a very rapid loss of fat is attempted by creating a large energy deficit, exercise may actually exacerbate the loss of lean tissue. Even when the energy deficit is modest, weighing may overestimate the value of exercise as a means of conserving lean tissue because there is often a substantial training-induced increase in body water content.—R.J. Shephard, M.D., Ph.D., D.P.E.

Reference

1. Murray S, et al: *Eur J Appl Physiol* 55:610, 1986.

Reduced Adipose Tissue Lipoprotein Lipase Responses, Postprandial Lipemia, and Low High-Density Lipoprotein-2 Subspecies Levels in Older Athletes With Silent Myocardial Ischemia

Katzel LI, Busby-Whitehead MJ, Rogus EM, Krauss RM, Goldberg AP (Univ of Maryland, Baltimore; John Hopkins Univ, Baltimore, Md; Univ of California, Berkeley)
Metabolism 43:190–198, 1994   139-95-8–30

Objective.—The enzymes lipoprotein lipase and hepatic lipase play a role in regulating fasting levels of high-density-lipoprotein cholesterol (HDL-C) and postprandial levels of triglyceride-enriched lipoproteins. Individuals who have increased hepatic lipase activity or an abnormal ad-

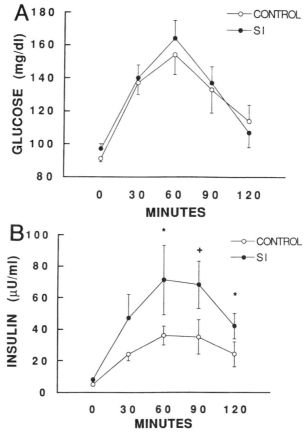

Fig 8–15.—Plasma glucose (**A**) and insulin (**B**) responses during an oral glucose tolerance test in controls and men who had silent myocardial ischemia (*SI*). Plasma insulin levels were higher at 60, 90, and 120 minutes in men who had SI. Data are means ± standard error of the mean, *P < 0.005 (Mann-Whitney U test). (Courtesy of Katzel LI, Busby-Whitehead MJ, Rogus EM, et al: *Metabolism* 43:190–198, 1994.)

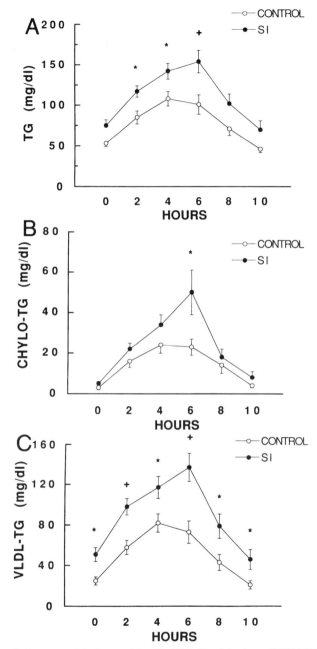

Fig 8–16.—Peak postprandial plasma triglyceride (TG) (**A**), chylomicron (CHYLO)-TG (**B**), and very-low-density lipoprotein (VLDL)-TG (**C**) levels were increased in men who had silent myocardial ischemia (SI). Data are means ± standard error of the mean; °P < 0.05, +P < 0.01 (Mann-Whitney U test). (Courtesy of Katzel LI, Busby-Whitehead MJ, Rogus EM, et al: *Metabolism* 43:190–198, 1994.)

ipose tissue lipoprotein lipase (AT-LPL) response to feeding may demonstrate decreased HDL-C levels, leading to increased postprandial lipemia and, thus, increased risk of atherosclerosis. In a recent study, one third of athletic older men had asymptomatic exercise-induced ST-segment depression, consistent with silent myocardial ischemia (SI). The hypothesis that these men with SI would have decreased LPL activity and increased postprandial levels of triglyceride-enriched lipoproteins was tested.

Methods.—The participants were 13 older male athletes with SI and ST-segment depression on their exercise ECGs. The mean age was 64 years and maximal oxygen consumption was greater than 40 mL/kg/min; all the men were normocholesterolemic and had no history of coronary artery disease. Twelve nonischemic men of similar age, percentage body fat, and maximal oxygen consumption were studied as controls. The 2 groups were compared for their postprandial lipoprotein lipid responses to a standard high-fat meal. The relationship of these responses to LPL activity, measured in both postheparin plasma and AT, was also compared.

Results.—Compared with controls, the men with SI had decreased fasting HDL-C (41 mg/dL vs. 50 mg/dL). They also had decreased %HDL$_{2b}$ subspecies levels, as measured by gradient gel electrophoresis (22 vs. 34). There was no difference in fasting plasma triglyceride or low-density-lipoprotein cholesterol levels. Plasma glucose levels during oral glucose tolerance testing were similar, but total insulin area was greater in those with SI (Fig 8–15).

After the standard high-fat meal, the men who had SI had higher levels of postprandial plasma triglyceride, chylomicron-triglyceride, and very-low-density-lipoprotein triglyceride levels and higher postprandial areas (Fig 8–16). Stepwise multiple regression found that fasting triglyceride levels and log$_{10}$ insulin area were the only independent predictors of postprandial triglyceride areas; these 2 factors accounted for 82% of the variance in triglyceride area. The difference in postprandial triglyceride area was no longer significant after covarying for fasting plasma triglyceride levels and total plasma insulin areas. Postheparin hepatic lipase activity was greater in the SI group, but there was no significant difference in postheparin LPL activity. The men in the SI group had greater fasting abdominal AT-LPL activity, and this value did not change with feeding. In contrast, the controls showed a 57% increase in AT-LPL activity at 4 hours. The percentage changes in AT-LPL activity and postheparin hepatic lipase activity were both positively correlated with postprandial triglyceride area.

Conclusion.—One third of older, normocholesterolemic, nondiabetic, athletic men may have SI. These individuals have increased insulin resistance, increased postheparin hepatic lipase activity, and reduced postprandial response of abdominal AT-LPL activity, with an associated reduction in HDL$_2$ subspecies levels and increased postprandial lipemia. Thus, older athletic men who have SI have abnormalities of HDL and postprandial triglyceride metabolism that may increase their risk for coronary artery disease. There are few treatment options for correcting the dyslipoproteinemia in men who have low HDL levels, particularly those who are already at their ideal body weight and aerobically trained.

▶ What's a man to do? These older, athletic men—most of them runners who jogged an average of 30 miles per week—apparently sustained enough coronary artery disease to have exercise-induced SI, despite maintaining ideal body weight and exemplary aerobic fitness. It seems that they were aerobically fit but not "metabolically fit"; they had signs of insulin resistance, lower HDL-C, and higher postprandial blood triglycerides than did healthy "nonischemic" control men matched for age, body fat, and aerobic capactiy.

This study has limitations: The number of subjects was small and perhaps the matching for body fat was imperfect. The men with ischemia had a slightly greater percentage body fat and waist-hip ratio (neither significantly greater); maybe they had significantly greater visceral fat (not measured). Visceral fat, which is shaped partly by genotype, tends to evoke a cluster of metabolic abnormalities, known as "syndrome X," that some of these men with SI probably had.

What to do? Exercise even more. New evidence in Israeli military recruits shows that 12 weeks of intense physical activity increase HDL-C by 33% (1), and new evidence from the Harvard alumni study suggests that vigorous physical activities more than nonvigorous activities are associated with longevity (2).—E.R. Eichner, M.D.

References

1. Rubinstein A, et al: *Med Sci Sports Exerc* 27:480, 1995.
2. Lee IM, et al: *JAMA* 273:1179, 1995.

Kinetics of Lipids, Apolipoproteins, and Cholesteryl Ester Transfer Protein in Plasma After a Bicycle Marathon
Föger B, Wohlfarter T, Ritsch A, Lechleitner M, Miller CH, Dienstl A, Patsch JR (Univ of Innsbruck, Austria)
Metabolism 43:633–639, 1994   139-95-8–31

Introduction.—The effects of intense aerobic exercise on lipid metabolism were investigated in 8 amateur endurance-trained athletes. Changes in cholesteryl ester transfer protein (CETP) mass and activity were of particular interest regarding its response to strenuous exercise.

Methods.—Body mass index and weight were determined before and after a 230-km bicycle marathon. Serum lipid studies were done 2 days before the race and on days 1, 2, 3, 5, and 8 after the race.

Results.—Cholesterol and low-density lipoproteins (LDLs) were significantly decreased on days 1–3 (Fig 8–17). Triglycerides decreased 63% on day 1, steadily increasing to baseline by day 5. High-density lipopro-

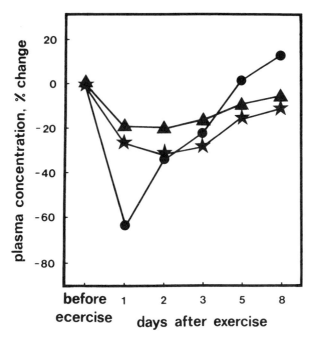

Fig 8–17.—Relative changes in plasma concentrations of cholesterol (*triangles*), triglycerides (*circles*), and low-density-lipoprotein cholesterol (*stars*) after a bicycle marathon compared with preexercise values. (Courtesy of Föger B, Wohlfarter T, Ritsch A, et al: *Metabolism* 43:633–639, 1994.)

teins (HDLs) increased on days 1–5, returning to baseline by day 8, as did HDL_2 and HDL_3 cholesterol (Fig 8–18). The HDL subfraction HDL_2 cholesterol demonstrated the most drastic change, with an increase of almost 100% on day 3. The HDL subfraction HDL_3 decreased below baseline. Significant increases in apolipoproteins (Apo) A-I and A-II were noted on day 8. The mean plasma CETP of the athletes before the race was comparable to that of 8 controls. Post exertion, CETP mass dropped significantly by day 2 and still had not reached baseline by day 8, with similar changes in CETP activity. The CETP mass decrease was directly related to an increase in HDL_2 cholesterol and an increase in the HDL_2 cholesterol to HDL_3 cholesterol ratio. No correlation between CETP mass and HDL_3 cholesterol and HDL Apo was found.

Conclusion.—Major changes in plasma lipids occurred after strenuous exercise, requiring 5 days to return to baseline. The change resulted partly from increases in lipoprotein lipase. Contributing to this was the significant decrease in CETP level and activity, which has not been reported previously. Further study is needed, but a change of this dimension equals or exceeds therapeutic effects of the most potent antilipemic drugs.

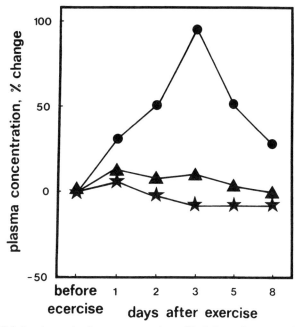

Fig 8–18.—Relative changes in plasma concentrations of high-density-lipoprotein (HDL), cholesterol (*triangles*), HDL₃ cholesterol (*circles*), and HDL₃ cholesterol (*stars*) after a bicycle marathon compared with preexercise values. (Courtesy of Föger B, Wohlfarter T, Ritsch A, et al: *Metabolism* 43:633–639, 1994.)

▶ The authors found favorable lipoprotein changes in the first few days after a single, long episode of heavy exercise: a 12-hour, 230-km bicycle marathon. Even though these trained cyclists had HDL cholesterol values above the 95th percentile for age- and sex-matched controls, their plasma HDL$_2$ cholesterol levels nearly doubled by day 3. Other favorable changes were a decrease in triglycerides and LDL cholesterol and a delayed increase (by day 5 to 8) in apo A-I and apo A-II, the 2 major HDL apoproteins.

Most of these effects can be explained by the well-known exercise-induced increase in activity of lipoprotein lipase, but also playing a role is an exercise-induced decrease in CETP. Others have also reported that exercise training decreases CETP (1, 2). Whatever the mechanisms, it is good to see these exercise-induced lipoprotein changes, all of which are beneficial in terms of preventing cardiovascular disease.—E.R. Eichner, M.D.

References

1. Serrat-Serrat J, et al: *Atherosclerosis* 101:43, 1993.
2. Seip RL, et al: *Arterioscler Thromb* 13:1359, 1993.

Effect of Graded Exercise on Esophageal Motility and Gastroesophageal Reflux in Nontrained Subjects

Soffer EE, Wilson J, Duethman G, Launspach J, Adrian TE (Univ of Iowa, Iowa City; Creighton Univ, Omaha, Neb)
Dig Dis Sci 39:193–198, 1994   139-95-8-32

Purpose.—Previous studies have found that intense exercise can depress esophageal contractility, induce gastroesophageal reflux, and affect intestinal motility in trained athletes. These effects are intensity dependent, and it is unknown whether they occur in nontrained individuals exercising at lower intensities. The effects of differing intensities of exercise on esophageal motor activity and gastroesophageal reflux—and on various regulatory peptides—were evaluated in nontrained individuals.

Methods.—Nine sedentary young adults were studied: 5 women and 4 men. All performed stationary bicycle exercise at 45%, 60%, 75%, and 90% of peak oxygen uptake ($\dot{V}O_{2max}$) with varying durations of exercise sessions and rest periods. The effects of exercise on esophageal motility and gastroesophageal reflux were assessed using a catheter with 3 strain-gauge transducers connected to a solid-state datalogger and an ambulatory intraesophageal pH monitor. The studies were performed in a fasting state; only IV 5% glucose solution was given. Before and after each exercise session and at rest, plasma concentrations of gastrin, motilin, glucagon, pancreatic polypeptide, and vasoactive intestinal peptide were measured.

Results.—As exercise intensity increased, the duration, amplitude, and frequency of esophageal contractions declined (Fig 8-19). The differ-

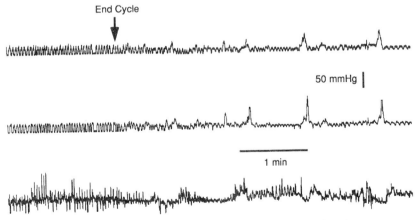

Fig 8–19.—The final phase of exercise at 75% maximal oxygen output. Esophageal contractions are suppressed during exercise and resume soon after it stops. The lower sensor is located at the level of the lower esophageal sphincter (LES), the middle sensor is located 5 cm above the LES, and the proximal sensor is located 10 cm above the LES. The exaggerated baseline represents respiratory oscillations. (Courtesy of Soffer EE, Wilson J, Duethman G, et al: *Dig Dis Sci* 39:193-198, 1994.)

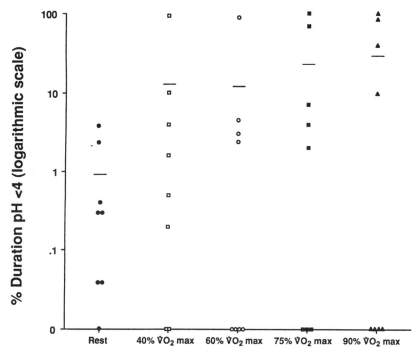

Fig 8–20.—Distribution of percent durations of pH < 4 in each participant in each study period. *Horizontal lines* represent the mean. (Courtesy of Soffer EE, Wilson J, Duethman G, et al: *Dig Dis Sci* 39:193–198, 1994.)

ences for all 3 motility variables were significant at 90% $\dot{V}O_{2max}$. At this exercise intensity, the number of episodes of gastroesophageal reflux and the duration of esophageal acid exposure increased significantly (Fig 8–20). Rest and exercise levels of the regulatory peptides were not significantly different.

Conclusion.—In nontrained as in trained individuals, exercise has profound and intensity-dependent effects on esophageal contractions and gastroesophageal reflux. The various regulatory peptides examined do not mediate these effects. The effects in athletes and nonathletes are similar at similar percentages of $\dot{V}O_{2max}$, even though the absolute levels of exercise performed are different.

▶ This study is a follow-up to 1 reviewed in the 1994 YEAR BOOK OF SPORTS MEDICINE (1). In that study of trained cyclists exercising on a cycle ergometer, the amplitude, duration, and frequency of esophageal contractions steadily decreased, while gastroesophageal reflux increased with increasing exercise intensity. In another study of trained cyclists, intense exercise decreased postprandial small-bowel motility (2). Granted, endurance exercise—especially running—can cause heartburn, belching, and reflux, but most of the studies have been on trained athletes (3). This study finds that in *untrained* subjects, intense cycling (at or above 75% of $\dot{V}O_{2max}$) decreases esophageal motor activity and increases reflux, just as in trained cyclists.—E.R. Eichner, M.D.

References

1. 1994 YEAR BOOK OF SPORTS MEDICINE, pp 319–320.
2. Soffer EE, et al: *Am J Physiol* 260:698G, 1991.
3. Moses FM: *Sports Med* 9:159–172, 1990.

Brief Physical Inactivity Prolongs Colonic Transit Time in Elderly Active Men

Liu F, Kondo T, Toda Y (Nagoya Univ, Japan)
Int J Sports Med 14:465–467, 1993   139-95-8–33

Background.—Cardiovascular events or sports injuries during exercise are common among the elderly. Many must give up exercising after such incidents. Most clinicians are aware of the costive effects of inactivity during hospitalization or bed rest. However, gastroenterologists have been focused on the effect of exercise rather than that of inactivity on gastrointestinal transit. The effect of 2 weeks of reduced activity on gastrointestinal transit time was studied in otherwise active elderly persons.

Methods.—Nine men aged 68–74 years volunteered for the study. All had been exercise-club members for 10 years, exercising for 2 hours a day 3 times a week. All were lactase deficient but asymptomatic. For 2 weeks, the participants' physical exercises were restricted.

Findings.—Mouth-to-cecum transit time was unchanged during physical inactivity. Their average total colonic transit time of 10.9 hours was prolonged significantly to 19.5 hours during physical inactivity. This prolongation resulted from slowed transit through the right and left colonic segments. The transit time of the rectosigmoid segment was unchanged.

Conclusion.—Physical inactivity prolonged colonic transit time in these normally active elderly men. The reason for this is unclear. These findings support the notion that chronic exercise increases colonic transit time. Constipation may occur in active elderly persons shortly after the cessation of physical activity.

▶ As we have stated in previous reviews (1), there is some evidence that regular exercise speeds colonic transit, but this evidence remains mixed. As discussed in this article, of 5 prior studies, 3 find that physical training speeds mouth-to-anus transit, but 2 find no such effect. This report takes the opposite tack, studying the colonic effect not of activity but of inactivity. It finds—at least in these older men who exercised habitually—that 2 weeks of voluntary physical inactivity nearly doubled the colonic transit time, from 11 hours to nearly 20 hours. As we point out frequently in the YEAR BOOK OF SPORTS MEDICINE (2), a good deal of epidemiologic data suggest that regular physical activity helps ward off colon cancer. A recent report from the ongoing, pro-spective-cohort study of male health professionals finds that abdominal adi-posity relates directly, and physical activity relates inversely, to the risk of colon cancer (3). Thus, regular exercise may help prevent colon cancer both by preventing obesity and speeding colonic transit.—E.R. Eichner, M.D.

References

1. 1992 YEAR BOOK OF SPORTS MEDICINE, pp 92–93.
2. 1992 YEAR BOOK OF SPORTS MEDICINE, pp 252–253.
3. Giovannucci E, et al: *Ann Intern Med* 122:327, 1995.

Exercise-Induced Diarrhea: When to Wonder
Swain RA (West Virginia Univ, Charleston)
Med Sci Sports Exerc 26:523–526, 1994   139-95-8–34

Introduction.—Exercise-associated lower gastrointestinal disorders are a fairly common clinical finding. For the colon, difficult physical training sessions may function as a "stress test." A case report of exercise-in-duced diarrhea and proposed methods of management were investi-gated.

Case Report.—Man, 48, had experienced gastrointestinal symptoms for the previous 4 months while running (8 miles per day); he experienced cramping, severe urgency, and diarrhea. The problem rarely occurred at rest and was not accompanied by fever, nausea, vomiting, or abdominal pain between episodes. Abnormalities on initial examination included mild pain on palpation through-out all abdominal quadrants and a guaiac trace positive stool. A complete blood count showed a slightly elevated white blood cell count. Stool cultures were neg-ative, but a stool check for ova and parasites revealed moderate amounts of *En-tamoeba histolytica* in trophozoite and cyst forms. Negative results were ob-tained on an antiamebic antibody test. The patient admitted to drinking out of a stream at some time before the symptoms began. His condition improved after treatment with metronidazole and paromycin and instructions to reduce extra dietary fiber and to eat lightly and use loperamide 30 minutes before exercising.

Discussion.—The symptoms of runners' diarrhea are difficult to quan-titate or qualititate, partly because runners may have subclinical bowel abnormalities such as irritable bowel syndrome or lactose deficiency. This man, although seeming to be a candidate for runners' diarrhea, had an amebic infestation. Previous studies of runners' diarrhea have not been maximally helpful because of small sample size or failure to rule out baseline bowel difficulties. The question remains as to whether hard aerobic work actually stimulates bowel activity or just brings underlying medical disorders to the surface.

Management.—Management of exercise-induced lower-bowel prob-lems should include consideration of age; the most likely differential diagnoses for patients younger than 40 years include infection, malabsorption, inflammatory bowel disease, laxative abuse, and functional conditions; for patients older than 40 years, the list also includes cancer, diverticular disease, and pancreatic disorders. If no specific diagnosis can be made, a primary diagnosis of exercise-induced diarrhea should be considered. Treatment options include suggestions that the patient stay hydrated, avoid caffeine and excess fiber, and evacuate the bowels at the same time each day. A preexercise dose of loperamide may also be considered.

▶ In this patient, running was a "stress test" that provoked diarrhea from the underlying amebiasis, so not all diarrhea in runners is directly and solely caused by the running. But surveys agree that at least 30% of marathoners get abdominal cramps, urgency, and diarrhea, most often during a hard race or training run. A practical approach to exercise-induced gastrointestinal symptoms, using case examples, appeared in 1993 (1); see also the 1993 YEAR BOOK OF SPORTS MEDICINE for more practical tips on overcoming runner's diarrhea (2). Here are my "10 tips to tame the trots": establish a prerun bowel movement ritual; don't eat within 2–3 hours of your run; curb dietary lactose and fructose; cut fiber and, for severe problems, try a liquid prerace meal; cut back on coffee; don't use sorbitol breath mints or gum; avoid large doses of vitamin C; train at a different time of day; remember that conditioning usually helps; and Imodium A-D can help.—E.R. Eichner, M.D.

References

1. Green GA: *Phys Sportsmed* 21:60, 1993.
2. 1993 YEAR BOOK OF SPORTS MEDICINE, pp 376–377.

Physical Activity and Risk of Severe Gastrointestinal Hemorrhage in Older Persons
Pahor M, Guralnik JM, Salive ME, Chrischilles EA, Brown SL, Wallace RB (Catholic Univ, Rome; Natl Inst on Aging, Bethesda, Md; Univ of Iowa, Iowa City)
JAMA 272:595–599, 1994   139-95-8–35

Background.—Although persons older than 64 years of age are 5 times more likely to have a hospital admission for gastrointestinal hemorrhage (GIH) than middle-aged adults, no reports regarding any possible association between personal lifestyle and risk for GIH in the elderly are available. Whether frequent physical activity in older persons is associated with a decreased risk of severe GIH and whether any such association is independent of other risk factors were examined.

Methods.—Included were 8,205 persons older than 67 years of age from 3 communities of the Established Populations for Epidemiologic Studies of the Elderly. The study yielded 22,277 person-years of follow-

Relation of Physical Activities to Severe
Gastrointestinal Hemorrhage

Physical Activity*	RR	95% CI
All Participants		
Walking	0.6	0.4–0.8
Gardening	0.8	0.5–1.1
Vigorous physical activity	0.7	0.4–1.2
Summary variable for physical activity	0.7	0.5–0.9
Mobile Participants		
Walking	0.6	0.4–0.8
Gardening	0.9	0.6–1.3
Vigorous physical activity	0.7	0.4–1.3
Summary variable for physical activity	0.7	0.5–1.0

Note: Separate analyses are presented for all participants (n = 8,205) and for those who were mobile at the time of physical activity evaluation (n = 6,083). Each physical activity variable is entered into a separate multivariate proportional hazards model. Relative risks and 95% confidence intervals are adjusted for age, sex, body mass index, diastolic blood pressure, comorbidity, hospitalization, and intake of coumarin derivatives, corticosteroids, aspirin, and nonsteroidal anti-inflammatory drugs.

* Physical activity was performed frequently 3 years before baseline.

(Courtesy of Pahor M, Guralnik JM, Salive ME, et al: JAMA 272:595–599, 1994.)

up during a 3-year study. Severe GIH was defined as GIH requiring blood transfusion or a death with GIH mentioned on the death certificate. Information about physical activities and risk factors was obtained from in-home interviews completed at a baseline and at the 3- and 6-year follow-ups. After adjusting relative risks (RRs) for many other factors, such as age and medication use, those persons who regularly exercised at least 3 times per week were compared with those who did not.

Results.—The rate of severe GIH was 10.8 per 1,000 person-years (241 individuals). After adjusting for potential confounding variables, the RR for severe GIH associated with walking was .6; it was .8 with gardening and .7 with vigorous physical activity. For the 3 activities together, the RR associated with a summary variable was 0.7 (95% confidence interval, 0.5–0.9). Stratification on health status and disability, or exclusion of those participants who were not very mobile (table), did not change the results.

Conclusion.—Older persons who participate in regular physical activity are at decreased risk for severe GIH. Additional research is needed to discover the mechanisms by which regular physical activity reduces the risk of severe GIH in this age group.

▶ Some papers have suggested that vigorous exercise can increase the risk of both bladder and intestinal hemorrhage. It is, thus, encouraging to have a report that notes a decrease of risk with the levels of habitual activity commonly adopted by the elderly person. Ischemia is the probable cause of exercise-induced hemorrhage (1); whereas very vigorous exercise reduces visceral flow, it may be that moderate activity increases resting cardiac output and, thus, enhances visceral flow in the older person.—R.J. Shephard, M.D., Ph.D., D.P.E.

Reference

1. Reinus JF, Brandt LJ: *Gasteroenterol Clin North Am* 19:293–318, 1990.

Indomethacin Potentiates Exercise-Induced Reduction in Renal Hemodynamics in Athletes

Walker RJ, Fawcett JP, Flannery EM, Gerrard DF (Otago Univ, Dunedin, New Zealand)
Med Sci Sports Exerc 26:1302–1306, 1994   139-95-8-36

Purpose.—Nonsteroidal anti-inflammatory drugs (NSAIDs) are widely used in the management of sports-related musculoskeletal injury. However, there are few data on their potential importance in modifying exercise-induced changes in renal functions. The effects of indomethacin on renal hemodynamics associated with moderate exercise in male athletes were studied.

Methods.—Eight healthy men, 21–42 years of age, who exercised regularly were studied. The study protocol investigated the effects of indomethacin—in a dosage of 50 mg orally every 8 hours for 36 hours—on renal blood flow (RBF) and glomerular filtration rate (GFR). The renal hemodynamic effects were measured before and after 30 minutes of treadmill exercise at 80% of maximum oxygen consumption ($\dot{V}O_{2max}$), as well as during a 120-minute recovery period. The men served as their own controls.

Results.—The control and indomethacin conditions showed no differences in the resting values of RBF, GFR, or renal vascular resistance (RVR). A significant reduction in RBF was noted with indomethacin compared with the control condition on analysis of variance for repeated measures. This change was associated with a significant elevation in RVR. The indomethacin-related changes in GFR paralleled those of RBF, although the differences were not significant. There was significant impairment of free water clearance during the recovery period (Fig 8–21).

Free Water Clearance and Exercise

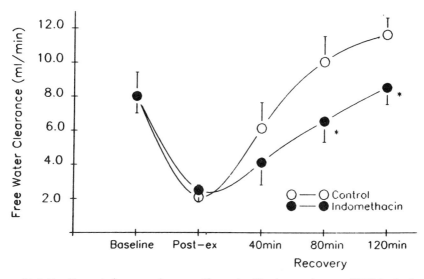

Fig 8–21.—Change in free water clearance with exercise. The data are the mean (SEM) for 8 subjects. Statistical analysis was by analysis of variance for repeated measures comparing control with indomethacin. (Courtesy of Walker RJ, Fawcett JP, Flannery EM, et al: *Med Sci Sports Exerc* 26:1302–1306, 1994.)

Conclusion.—With sustained exercise, the NSAID indomethacin can compromise renal function and potentiate risk of acute renal failure. Athletes should be warned that NSAID use is potentially dangerous when their renal function may be compromised. In addition, they should be cautious about participating in any strenuous or prolonged exercise if they are taking NSAIDS for an injury. Further studies are needed to determine whether other NSAIDs produce similar renal hemodynamic changes.

▶ Athletes are big users of indomethacin, and, thus, this seems to be an important paper. The prostaglandins do not have much effect on renal function at rest, but during stresses such as sodium depletion (1) and hemorrhage (2) (or, in the case of the athlete, dehydration), renal synthesis of the vasodilators PGE_2 and PGI_2 is increased to sustain local blood flow. Indomethacin counters this adaptation (the doses used in this study were sufficient to reduce plasma levels of prostaglandins by at least 50%). Renal failure can be a problem when a person is undertaking prolonged exercise in hot weather, even without administration of indomethacin. Heat plus exercise plus this drug seems to be a very dangerous combination, as has already been observed in a number of marathon events (3).—R.J. Shephard, M.D., Ph.D., D.P.E.

References

1. Donker AJM, et al: *Nephron* 17:288–296, 1976.
2. Bell RD, Sinclair RJ, Parry WL, et al: *Circ Shock* 2:57–63, 1975.
3. Vitting KE, et al: *Ann Intern Med* 105:144, 1986.

PMN Cell Counts and Phagocytic Activity of Highly Trained Athletes Depend on Training Period

Hack V, Strobel G, Weiss M, Weicker H (Med Clinic and Policlinic, Heidelberg, Germany; Univ of Paderborn, Germany)
J Appl Physiol 77:1731–1735, 1994   139-95-8–37

Introduction.—Polymorphonuclear leukocytes (PMNs) are a key part of the "first line of defense" of the human immune system. Previous studies have documented rapid mobilization of PMNs after acute exercise, but they have failed to assess important PMN functions. The available evidence suggests that PMN cell counts and phagocytic activity may be influenced by different training periods. These PMN variables were measured in highly trained athletes during moderate training (MT) and intense training (IT) and compared with the values of untrained controls.

Methods.—Seven competitive male long-distance runners were studied twice in the same training year: during MT, when their weekly training program consisted of endurance running only, and during IT, shortly before their most important competition. Running distances during these

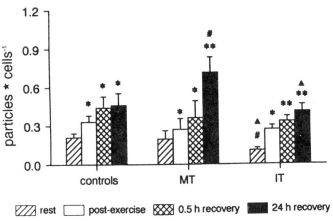

Fig 8–22.—Latex ingestion capacity of polymorphonuclear leukocytes before and immediately after graded exercise to exhaustion on treadmill and after 0.5 or 24 hours of recovery from control subjects and highly trained long-distance runners during moderate training (MT) and intense training (IT). Values are means + SE. Significantly different from rest: *$P \leq 0.05$; **$P \leq 0.01$. Significantly different from MT: ▲$P \leq 0.05$. Significantly different from control: #$P \leq 0.05$. (Courtesy of Hack V, Strobel G, Weiss M, et al: *J Appl Physiol* 77:1731–1735, 1994.)

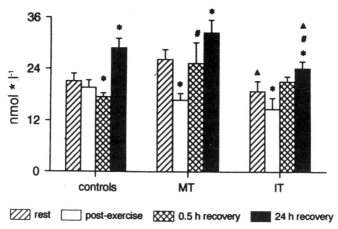

Fig 8–23.—Superoxide anion (O_2) production of polymorphonuclear leukocytes before and immediately after graded exercise to exhaustion on treadmill and after 0.5 or 24 hours of recovery from control subjects and highly trained long-distance runners during moderate training (*MT*) and intense training (*IT*). Values are means + SE. Significantly different ($P \le 0.05$) from: *rest; ▲MT; #control. (Courtesy of Hack V, Strobel G, Weiss M, et al: *J Appl Physiol* 77:1731–1735, 1994.)

periods averaged 89 and 102 km/wk, respectively. Testing consisted of measurement of PMN cell counts and phagocytic activity by latex ingestion and superoxide anion production before and up to 24 hours after a graded exercise test to exhaustion.

Results.—There were no significant differences between the MT and control values for PMN count and phagocytic activity either at rest or after exercise. However, PMN cell counts at rest were significantly decreased during IT compared with MT and control values at 2.55, 3.63. and 3.41 cells/nL, respectively. At-rest and postexercise phagocytic activity was also significantly reduced during IT (Fig 8–22). There was a strong inverse correlation between epinephrine and superoxide anion production (Fig 8–23).

Conclusion.—The phagocytic activity of PMNs appears to be related to the training period. Athletes may have impaired PMN function during IT, which could increase their susceptibility to infection. Careful monitoring of the human immune system as affected by training period, seasonal fluctuation, and hormonal status is needed.

▶ The study presented in Abstract 139-95-8–21 showed slight impairment of the function of PMNs after 6 months of heavy training and racing in cyclists. This study also focuses on PMN function during training in elite male distance runners compared with untrained medical student controls. The absolute number and phagocytic activity of PMNs were unchanged in the runners during MT compared with controls. Lymphocyte counts also were unchanged, and these authors report elsewhere (1) that MT improved the helper/suppressor T-cell ratio. Thus, by these markers, MT did not impair immunity and may have improved it.

In contrast, PMN counts and phagocytic activity were sharply reduced both at rest and after exercise during IT compared with MT and controls, suggesting "exhaustion" of PMNs in the racing season. A possible mechanism: high plasma epinephrine levels, tied here to decreased superoxide anion production by PMNs, a marker of phagocytosis. Epinephrine infusion in healthy volunteers has been reported to decrease chemotactic and phagocytic activities of PMNs. In their other article (1), the authors report a decline in serum immunoglobulin levels during IT, which may further impair phagocytosis. As in Abstract 139-95-8–21, however, we lack clinical data on these runners (did they get more infections, or fewer?), so we do not know the clinical import of these immune changes.—E.R. Eichner, M.D.

Reference

1. Hack V, Weiss M, Weicker H, et al: *Dtsch Z Sportmed* 44:430–436, 1993.

Call Mosby Document Express at **1 (800) 55-MOSBY** to obtain copies of the original source documents of articles featured or referenced in the YEAR BOOK series.

---

9 Cardiovascular and Other Diseases

Exercise and Reduced Health-Care Costs: A Substantial Dividend of Primary Preventive Programs?
Shephard RJ (Univ of Toronto)
J Cardiopulmon Rehabil 14:161–165, 1994   139-95-9-1

Introduction.—It is estimated that at least half the costs of health care could be altered with primary preventive tactics, at least a quarter of which would target personal lifestyle faults, such as inadequate physical activity, alcohol abuse, and cigarette smoking. In calculating the value of mass exercise programs, the personal and fiscal benefits associated with early health improvement and long-term prevention of ill health should be considered.

Early Health Improvement.—Individuals may experience health benefits within a few weeks of beginning an exercise program. Moderate aerobic exercise can enhance immune responses, although this only lasts for 1–2 hours after exercise. Other positive lifestyle changes may also occur, although the association with exercise is not uniformly strong. Physical activity may improve mood to various degrees, reducing medical complaints with a psychological basis. It may also result in a feeling of greater self-efficacy, which is particularly important in the elderly or those with chronic disease.

Long-Term Prevention of Ill Health.—Exercise reduces the risk of cardiovascular disease during the exerciser's working career, which may result in a longer working career. However, the duration of exercise required to provide the various cardiovascular benefits needs further study. In addition, longitudinal experiments are needed that will investigate the potential for reduced medical costs in the geriatric component associated with exercise.

Conclusion.—Current studies have reported early cost savings of $61–$450 per year, because of increased well-being for individuals involved in exercise programs. It is estimated that the long-term reduction of chronic disease and diminished dependency may double those savings. Well-designed research with short- and long-term data documenting both the expenditures involved in providing primary and secondary preventive programs and their fiscal benefits are needed.

▶ This is an interesting article that analyzes discrepancies in the estimates of the presumed reduction of health care cost as a result of the effect of exercise. Presumed fiscal dividends in the United States have been reported to be 4 times those suggested in other countries. It is pointed out that "the main reasons for the discrepancy are higher medical and hospital costs in the United States." It is important to note the primary conclusion of the article, that no conclusive evidence exists on the economic benefits of primary preventive exercise.—J.S. Torg, M.D.

The Public Health Burdens of Sedentary Living Habits: Theoretical But Realistic Estimates
Powell KE, Blair SN (Ctrs for Disease Control and Prevention, Atlanta Ga; Inst for Aerobics Research, Dallas)
Med Sci Sports Exerc 26:851–856, 1994   139-95-9-2

Background.—The public health burden of sedentary living can be estimated by measures of disease and death, the use and cost of medical care, and quality of life factors. Quantitative estimates of mortality attributable to sedentary living were calculated for coronary heart disease (CHD), colon cancer, and diabetes. Physical inactivity has been established as a causal factor for all 3 diseases.

Formulas for Calculating Overall and Stratum-Specific
Population-Attributable Risk

Formula 1.

$$PAR = \frac{Cases_{total} - Cases_{if\ all\ active}}{Cases_{total}} \times 100 \quad \text{Conceptual formula}$$

Formula 2.

$$PAR = \frac{P_{exp} * (RR - 1)}{1 + P_{exp} * (RR - 1)} \times 100 \quad \text{Most commonly used formula, two levels of exposure}$$

Formula 3.

$$PAR = \frac{\sum P_{exp(i)} * (RR_i - 1)}{1 + \sum P_{exp(i)} * (RR_i - 1)} \times 100 \quad \text{Formula for more than one level of exposure}$$

Formula 4.

$$PAR_i = \frac{P_{exp(i)} * (RR_i - 1)}{1 + \sum P_{exp(i)} * (RR_i - 1)} \times 100 \quad \text{Formula for one level exposure if there are several levels}$$

Abbreviations: PAR, population-attributable risk; P_{exp}, prevalance of the exposure; RR, relative risk; $P_{exp\ (i)}$, prevalence of 1 level exposure if there are several (i) levels; RR_i, relative risk for 1 level of exposure if there are several levels.
(Courtesy of Powell KE, Blair SN: *Med Sci Sports Exerc* 26:851-856, 1994.)

Findings.—Quantitative estimates have indicated that sedentary living is responsible for about one third of the deaths caused by CHD, colon cancer, and diabetes, which cost billions of dollars a year. Because not everyone will become physically active and not all active people are equally active, the proportion of the disease burden that would be eliminated by various modifications of the physical activity patterns of the population needs to be estimated. One of the more useful methods of estimating the proportion of a public health burden caused by a particular risk factor is population-attributable risk (table). By assuming modest increases in physical activity practices, mortality from these 3 conditions combined could be decreased by as much as 5% to 6%, or by 30,000–35,000 deaths per year. The overall mortality in the United States might be decreased about 1% to 1.5%. The greatest gains would result from strategies that encourage people who report no leisure-time physical activities to do some and that encourage irregularly active people to participate in 30 minutes or more of light-to-moderate activity for 5 or more days per week.

Conclusions.—Mortality is only 1 component of the public health burden that would be decreased by greater participation in regular physical activity. The authors also claim that the costs of medical care would be reduced and the quality of life would be improved, although the paper does not address these items.

▶ The impact of regular physical activity on such conditions as ischemic heart disease, colon cancer, and diabetes mellitus is sufficiently well established that public health experts are now beginning to assess the beneficial consequences for population health if everyone could be persuaded to undertake more activity. However, the calculations remain somewhat tentative.

Three pieces of information are needed: an accurate dose-response curve for physical activity as a means of preventing each of the diseases under consideration; an accurate assessment of the distribution of current patterns of physical activity among the entire population; and verification of the assumption that if an inactive person becomes active, his or her risk drops to that of an active individual. Patterns of physical activity show so much interindividual variation that dose-response curves have only limited precision. Many national surveys of population activity also quote figures that diverge widely from common observations of how much exercise people actually take. Finally, it is important to recognize that any benefit that is achieved is a change in age-specific mortality rate; premature death is avoided. The authors' summary is unduly optimistic in suggesting that the overall mortality rate will fall from 100%! Thus, another question that may be posed is: If a person does not die of sudden coronary vascular insufficiency at age 65 years, will he or she die a few years later of some less pleasant and more costly disease?—R.J. Shephard, M.D., Ph.D., D.P.E.

Physical Activity Patterns in American High School Students: Results From the 1990 Youth Risk Behavior Survey

Heath GW, Pratt M, Warren CW, Kann L (Ctrs for Disease Control and Prevention, Atlanta, Ga)

Arch Pediatr Adolesc Med 148:1131–1136, 1994   139-95-9–3

Objective.—Physical inactivity during adolescence increases cardiovascular risk factors during adulthood. Accurate and valid data are needed to evaluate the health risks and fitness objectives of adolescents. To determine physical activity patterns, a questionnaire was administered to United States high school students.

Methods.—The Centers for Disease Control and Prevention (CDC) developed the Youth Risk Behavior Survey (YRBS), a self-administered, 75-item questionnaire given to 11,631 high school students in 124 schools.

Results.—A total of 37% of students, 49% of males and 24.7% of females, exercised vigorously 3 times a week. White and Hispanic students were significantly more active than black students, and females in grade 9 were significantly more active than those in grades 11 and 12. Physical activity levels dropped significantly by grade for females and even more significantly for black females. About half of all students were not enrolled in physical education classes. Only one third of students exercised for 20 minutes or more at a time. Approximately 43% of students played on a school sports team, and these represented the majority of vigorously active students. More than 70% of students watched more than 1 hour of television per day, with 35% watching 3 or more hours per day. There was a correlation between television watching and lack of physical activity for females, particularly for black females.

Conclusion.—Low levels of physical activity for women and blacks are apparent by 9th grade. These patterns of inactivity tend to worsen by grade. Attending physical education classes and spending at least 20 minutes per class in vigorous exercise are important.

▶ This survey of physical activity and television watching among American high school students suggests that many of our children are sofa spuds. Less than 40% of high school kids engage in vigorous physical activity at least 3 days per week. Physical activity falls off with increasing grade level, especially among girls. Black women are the least active of all subgroups and also watch the most television. In defense of young black females, they now smoke at only one fifth the rate of white females and are less vulnerable to anorexia nervosa. We have covered the adverse implications of obesity (1). A recent 55-year follow-up of 508 Bostonians found that boys who were chubby adolescents, regardless of whether they later lost weight, were twice as apt as thin cohorts to die prematurely, often of heart disease (2). A typical child in America is blasted with up to 10,000 food commercials per year, none of them for brussels sprouts. The percentage of teens who are now overweight, which held steady at about 15% through the 1970s, rose to 21% by 1991. And the beat goes on.—E.R. Eichner, M.D.

References

1. 1991 YEAR BOOK OF SPORTS MEDICINE, pp xiii–xxv.
2. Must A, et al: N *Engl J Med* 327:1350, 1992.

The Rate of Increase in Blood Pressure in Children 5 Years of Age is Related to Changes in Aerobic Fitness and Body Mass Index

Shea S, Basch CE, Gutin B, Stein AD, Contento IR, Irigoyen M, Zybert P (Columbia Univ, NY; Ctr for Health Promotion, NY; Med College of Georgia, Augusta; et al)
Pediatrics 94:465–470, 1994   139-95-9-4

Background.—One of the most prevalent medical conditions in the United States is hypertension. Many studies have demonstrated a progressive rise of blood pressure with age, beginning in childhood, with the rise greater for systolic than diastolic pressure. Changes in aerobic fitness and body mass index were examined for their association with the rate of blood pressure change in early childhood.

Methods.—Healthy, free-living, preschool children were enrolled in a longitudinal study that measured blood pressure, height, weight, body composition, and aerobic fitness.

Results.—One hundred ninety-six children with an average age of 62 months participated and were followed for a mean of 19.7 months. The children were overwhelmingly Hispanic (91.3%), and there were approximately 50% boys and 50% girls. The mean systolic blood pressure was 95.3 mm HG at baseline, and it increased an average of 4.46 mm HG per year. The mean diastolic blood pressure of 53.9 mm HG did not change significantly with time. Significant increases in aerobic fitness occurred with time. Aerobic fitness was negatively correlated with body mass index at baseline. Aerobic fitness and body mass index were associated with systolic blood pressure, and this relationship remained stable with time. Changes in aerobic fitness and body mass index were significantly, although weakly, related to changes in systolic blood pressure on correlational analysis. A greater increase in fitness and a lesser increase in body mass index were significantly associated with lower rates of increase in systolic blood pressure. An increase in fitness was also significantly associated with lower rates of increase in diastolic blood pressure.

Conclusions.—Lower rates of increase in blood pressure are found in children who increase their aerobic fitness or decrease their body mass index. The implications of these findings for developing interventions for the primary prevention of hypertension are important.

▶ This study shows that young children who increase their aerobic fitness or decrease their body fat reduce the rate of age-related increase in blood pressure. In other words, physical activity and leanness help ward off hypertension. In 1993, we covered the "nondrug" therapy of hypertension in children and adolescents (1). A recent, 6-year study of young Finns shows that regular physical activity promotes less smoking, encourages a healthier diet, and reduces coronary risk factors (2). A study of young Danes shows that higher physical fitness (higher maximal oxygen output) is linked with lower blood pressure (3). Also, a study of former Finnish elite athletes finds that, mainly because of a lifetime of physical activity and other good habits, they have a low prevalence of diabetes, hypertension, and coronary heart disease (4). A recent review of nutrition for young athletes has appeared. (5).—E.R. Eichner, M.D.

References

1. 1993 YEAR BOOK OF SPORTS MEDICINE, pp 252–253.
2. Raitakari OT, et al: *Am J Epidemiol* 140:195, 1994.
3. Andersen LB: *J Intern Med* 236:323, 1994.
4. Kujala UM, et al: *Metabolism* 43:1255, 1994.
5. Steen SN: *Sports Med* 17:152, 1994.

Changes in Physical Activity and Other Lifeway Patterns Influencing Longevity
Paffenbarger RS Jr, Kampert JB, Lee I-M, Hyde RT, Leung RW, Wing AL (Stanford Univ, Calif; Harvard Univ, Boston)
Med Sci Sports Exerc 26:857–865, 1994   139-95-9–5

Background.—Data from a large population of male Harvard alumni were studied to determine whether the adoption or maintenance of physical activity and other optional lifestyle patterns had an influence on the mortality of this group.

Methods.—Men aged 45–84 years in 1977 were surveyed in 1962 or 1966 and in 1977 and were followed up through 1988 or to age 90 years. Of the 14,786 alumni, 2,343 died between 1977 and 1988.

Findings.—The relative risk of death for men who increased their physical activity between questionnaires to 6.3 megajoules (1,500 kcal) or more per week was 0.72, compared with 1.0 for those remaining less active. Physical activity took the form of walking, stair-climbing, and participating in sports and recreational activities. The corresponding relative risk for men taking up moderately vigorous sports was 0.73, compared with 1.0 for those not taking up such activities. For cigarette smokers who quit between questionnaires, the relative risk of death was 0.74

Added Years of Life to Age 90 Years From Adoption or Maintenance of a Favorable Physical Activity Level and Other Lifestyle Patterns Between 1962 or 1966 and 1977

Changed Lifeway Pattern	Age 1977 (yr)						
	35–44 (Extrapolated)	45–54	55–64	65–74	75–84	45–84 (95% CI)	P Value
Physical activity index*increased from <1500 to ≥1500 kcal·wk⁻¹ vs continuing <1500	(1.79)	1.78	1.60	1.28	0.78	1.57 (0.96–2.19)	<0.001
Walking increased from <15 to ≥15 km·wk⁻¹ vs continuing <15	(0.30)	0.30	0.28	0.23	0.14	0.27 (−0.35–0.89)	0.392
Stair climbing increased from <20 to ≥20 stories ·wk⁻¹ vs continuing <20	(1.39)	1.39	1.27	1.02	0.64	1.23 (0.50–1.96)	0.001
Took up moderately vigorous sports play (≥4.5 METs) vs continuing not to play such sports	(1.81)	1.77	1.60	1.25	0.79	1.54 (0.99–2.09)	<0.001
Physical activity index increased by ≥750 kcal·wk⁻¹ vs all other patterns	(1.71)	1.70	1.54	1.23	0.77	1.51 (1.04–1.99)	<0.001
Quit cigarette smoking vs continuing smoking	(2.15)	2.06	1.84	1.45	0.95	1.84 (1.07–2.60)	<0.001
Remained normotensive vs becoming hypertensive	(1.25)	1.21	1.08	0.85	0.54	1.07 (0.48–1.66)	<0.001
Body mass index remained <26 vs increased to ≥26	(0.52)	0.51	0.46	0.37	0.24	0.46 (−0.37–1.28)	0.272
Physical activity index increased from <1500 to ≥1500 kcal·wk⁻¹ and quit cigarette smoking vs opposites	(4.31)	4.17	3.74	2.95	1.90	3.72 (2.70–4.74)	<0.001

Abbreviation: CI, confidence interval; the null value is zero rather than 1.

Notes: As estimated from standardized mortality among 14,786 Harvard alumni from 1977 through 1988. The rates were standardized for differences in age, physical activity, cigarette smoking, hypertension, overweight for height, alcohol consumption, early parental death, and chronic diseases (except for the given lifestyle pattern). Each of the 3 subgroups of physical activity is also standardized for the other 2. A total of 2,343 men died in 165,402 man-years.

*Includes walking, stair-climbing, and sports or recreational activities.

(Courtesy of Paffenbarger RS Jr, Lee I-M, et al: *Med Sci Sports Exerc* 26:857–865, 1994.)

compared with 1.0 for persistent smokers. Men with a recent diagnosis of hypertension had a lower death risk than long-term hypertensive men, as did men with constant normotension. Changes in body-mass index had little effect on mortality during follow-up (table).

Conclusions.—Adopting a physically active lifestyle, quitting smoking, and remaining normotensive independently delay mortality from any cause. Even men who smoked cigarettes and remained inactive until they were aged 65–84 years lived 2 or 3 years longer when they quit smoking and became more active, compared with men who persistently smoked and remained sedentary.

▶ Earlier studies of Harvard alumni measured physical activity at one time point and then examined survival prospects. A repetition of the lifestyle survey after an interval of 11–15 years has now allowed Paffenbarger and his associates to evaluate the consequences of a *change* in lifestyle. The outcome studied continues to be mortality, and a substantial benefit is claimed for vigorous exercise. The required dose of physical activity needed to improve survival prospects is not trivial: an extra energy expenditure of 6.3 megajoules (1,500 kcal) per week, or the equivalent of five 30-minute sessions at around 9 times the resting energy expenditure. Death is a popular end point with epidemiologists because it is unequivocal, although from a practical standpoint, the quality of life (and thus the quality-adjusted life expectancy) probably holds greater importance. Inasmuch as subjects are not randomly assigned to exercise and control conditions, the big question mark is whether due allowance has been made for other factors that go along with a physically active lifestyle. The most important linked variable is cigarette smoking; it is particularly difficult to allow for this because it has 3–4 times as much influence upon survival prospects as does exercise itself. The authors are not very specific about the adjustment they made for smoking habits, but it appears to be, "smoking, any amount." If this was indeed the case, then the study remains vulnerable to the likelihood that more of the "smokers" were occasional smokers in the group that exercised hard than in the group that was sedentary.—R.J. Shephard, M.D., Ph.D., D.P.E.

Heart Rate, Ischaemic Heart Disease, and Sudden Cardiac Death in Middle-Aged British Men
Shaper AG, Wannamethee G, Macfarlane PW, Walker M (Royal Free Hosp School of Medicine, London; Royal Infirmary, Glasgow, Scotland)
Br Heart J 70:49–55, 1993   139-95-9–6

Introduction.—Although a high resting heart rate has been linked to an increased risk of ischemic heart disease, it is not known if the association is dependent on confounding risk factors. The effect of heart rate on the risk of new major ischemic heart disease events and sudden cardiac death was prospectively studied in middle-aged men.

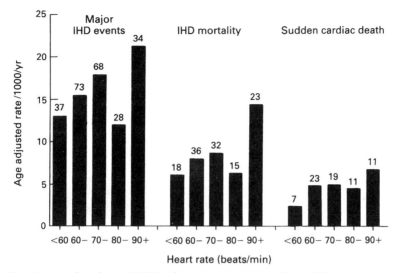

Fig 9–1.—Age-adjusted rates (1,000/yr) for major ischemic heart disease (IHD) events, mortality from IHD, and sudden cardiac death in men with preexisting IHD in the 5 heart rate (beats/min) groups: < 60=341 men, 60–69=605 men, 70–79=482 men, 80–89=287 men, ≥ 90=199 men. Absolute numbers of events are indicated. (Courtesy of Shaper AG, Wannamethee G, Macfarlane PW, et al: *Br Heart J* 70:49-55, 1993.)

Methods.—Study subjects were enrolled in the British Regional Heart Study. A total of 7,735 men aged 40-59 years were randomly selected from general practices in 24 towns. The men completed a standard questionnaire, gave blood samples, and were assessed for body mass, height, forced expiratory volume in 1 second, and heart rate. Also recorded were the men's smoking status, alcohol consumption, and levels of physical activity.

Results.—During 8 years of follow-up, 217 fatal and 271 nonfatal ischemic heart disease events occurred in the study group; 117 of the fatal events were classified as sudden cardiac death. The mean resting heart rate at the time of screening was 70.7 beats per minute in the 7,683 men with available data. Ischemic heart disease was present in 25% of men at the initial examination, and the highest percentage of those men was found in the group with a heart rate of 80 beats per minute or more. In men without preexisting ischemic heart disease, there was a strong, positive association between increasing heart rate and an increasing incidence of fatal and nonfatal ischemic heart disease events, ischemic heart disease mortality, and sudden cardiac death. Those in the highest heart rate group (90 beats per minute or more) were significantly less likely to survive a major ischemic heart disease event. Adjustments for age, systolic blood pressure, blood cholesterol, smoking, social class, heavy drinking, and physical activity did not alter the significance of these associations in men without preexisting heart disease. The heart rate associated risks were also present, although not as strong, in men with preexisting ischemic heart disease at study entry (Fig 9–1).

Conclusion.—Middle-aged men with an elevated heart rate (90 beats per minute or more) and no evidence of preexisting ischemic heart disease were at increased risk of major ischemic heart disease events during the 8-year follow-up. Their risk for sudden cardiac death was particularly high, at 5 times that observed in men with heart rates of less than 60 beats per minute. The effects of a raised heart rate were independent of other established coronary risk factors.

▶ As regular readers of the YEAR BOOK OF SPORTS MEDICINE will know, Shaper and associates have gotten quite a lot of mileage out of their review of 24 family practices. A high resting heart rate is commonly indicative of a sedentary lifestyle, and a number of epidemiologic studies have used resting heart rate in this sense. Unfortunately, the resting heart rate is also increased by a number of other cardiac risk factors, particularly cigarette smoking (1). Shaper and associates were able to counter this criticism (at least partially) by showing that in those who were initially free of known cardiovascular disease, a high heart rate (more than 90 beats per minute) was associated with a doubling of the risk of cardiac mortality and of sudden death in both smokers and "nonsmokers." Unfortunately, the latter category included ex-smokers, who may have stopped smoking because of high cigarette consumption and fears about their hearts.

Perhaps the most puzzling feature of the study is that the adverse effect of a high heart rate supposedly persisted after statistical adjustment of the data for both habitual physical activity and blood lipid levels. A questionnaire initially attempted a 6-level grading of habitual activity, but the statistical adjustment was based on a 2-way classification, with "active" individuals being those who reported activity in the moderate-to-vigorous range. Perhaps it may emerge that the high heart rate is an expression of inactivity, but only if a more detailed and precise grading of physical activity can be obtained. Alternatively, the high heart rate may be serving to identify the sort of individual who becomes anxious in the context of a medical evaluation.—R.J. Shephard, M.D., Ph.D., D.P.E.

Reference

1. Rode A, Ross R, Shephard, RJ: *Arch Environ Health* 24:27, 1972.

Improvement in Exercise Capacity of Candidates Awaiting Heart Transplantation

Stevenson LW, Steimle AE, Fonarow G, Kermani M, Kermani D, Hamilton MA, Moriguchi JD, Walden J, Tillisch JH, Drinkwater DC, Laks H (Brigham and Women's Hosp, Boston; Harvard Univ, Boston; Univ of California, Los

Angeles)
J Am Coll Cardiol 25:163–170, 1995   139-95-9-7

Introduction.—The number of patients currently referred for heart transplantation has increased at a greater rate than the number of donor hearts available, resulting in long waits for surgery. Objective criteria have been established to identify patients for placement on the active candidate list but not for removal from it, even though some patients may show significant clinical improvement with vasodilator and exercise therapy. A strategy for identifying patients who can be safely removed from the active waiting list was investigated.

Methods.—During a 4-year period, 107 ambulatory patients with dilated heart failure were placed on the list for heart transplantation based on achieving a peak oxygen intake less than 14 mL/kg per minute during exercise testing. Patients who survived without transplantation underwent exercise testing again 3–12 months after their initial evaluation. The transplant candidates were followed clinically every 2–4 weeks. Improvements in both clinical and exercise criteria were used to identify patients who should be removed from the list.

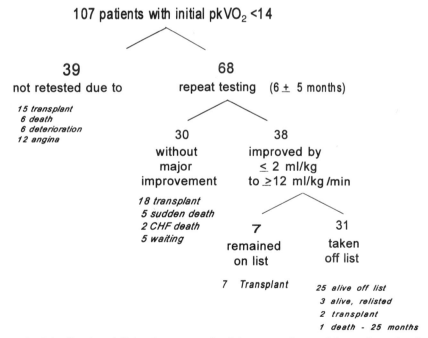

Fig 9–2.—Flowchart depicting the outcome of ambulatory transplant candidates with initial peak oxygen consumption (pkVo$_2$) < 14 mL/kg per minute. The patient who died of respiratory failure at 25 months because of recurrent pneumothoraces is described in the Results section. *Abbreviation:* CHF, congestive heart failure death. (Courtesy of Stevenson LW, Steimle AE, Fonarow G, et al: *J Am Coll Cardiol* 25:163–170, 1995.)

Results.—Of the 107 patients, repeat exercise testing was not performed in 39 patients who either had severe angina, hemodynamic deterioration, intervening transplantation, or death. Of the remaining 68 who underwent repeat exercise testing, 38 had increases in peak oxygen intake of 2 mL/kg per minute or more. These patients also had an improved anaerobic threshold, tolerated a higher work rate, and had an increased exercise heart rate reserve, peak systolic blood pressure, and oxygen pulse. Of the 38 patients with improved exercise values, 31 also met criteria for clinical stability and were removed from the active waiting list. Of these 31 patients, 25 are still alive without transplantation at a mean of 21 months after the repeat test; 5 of the 31 were returned to the active waiting list, and 1 died of respiratory failure caused by pneumothoraces 25 months later (Fig 9–2). Two of the 5 relisted patients underwent transplantation.

Discussion.—Ambulatory patients waiting for heart transplantation often have improved peak oxygen uptake. Those who demonstrate this improvement on repeat exercise testing usually also have significantly improved clinical stability. The tactic of repeat exercise testing identified a group of patients who could be safely removed from the active waiting list. Their short-term survival was similar to that of patients undergoing heart transplantation. This tactic may improve the average overall survival of the transplantation candidates, both by lengthening life before transplantation and by effectively prioritizing donor heart distribution.

▶ A maximal oxygen intake of 14 mL/kg per minute seems a reasonable criterion for deciding which patients require cardiac transplantation. If a patient's peak oxygen intake is less than this, even the simplest tasks of daily living become unpleasantly fatiguing. However, these data suggest that a substantial proportion of patients who are on current surgical waiting lists may move above this threshold because of an improvement in their clinical condition before admission.

It is unclear how much of the improvement is spontaneous and how far it reflects more intensive medical management. The patients studied by Stevenson and associates were not given a specific exercise program, but they were encouraged to exercise at least 4 times per week. Moreover, scores may have improved because of greater confidence during the second laboratory test or a simple "reversion to the mean" of scores in subjects who initially were selected for a low peak oxygen intake. Against this simplistic type of explanation, the average improvement of aerobic power was substantial (5 mL/kg per minute), and there were parallel changes in anaerobic threshold (which is less affected by patient motivation).

It seems important to pursue this research inasmuch as the gain in function from expectant treatment closely matches what is commonly seen in response to surgery. If effective medical management can yield dividends of this order, substantial savings in surgical costs seem possible.—R.J. Shephard, M.D., Ph.D., D.P.E.

Oxygen Uptake Kinetics in Cardiac Transplant Recipients

Paterson DH, Cunningham DA, Pickering JG, Babcock MA, Boughner DR
(Univ of Western Ontario; Univ Hosp, London, Ontario)
J Appl Physiol 77:1935–1940, 1994   139-95-9–8

Introduction.—The heart transplant patient offers a unique look at cardiac control systems because of his or her denervated heart. The cardiac response to exercise is delayed, making cardiac output responsive to Frank-Starling mechanisms, which may not adequately compensate for the slow heart rate. Prior studies have focused on ventilatory responses. However, the kinetics of oxygen consumption at the onset of exercise have not shown consistent results. If oxygen uptake kinetics depend on blood flow, then the kinetics should be slowed. In addition, if the heart rate is slow to recover after exercise, then a second bout of activity should show faster uptake kinetics because the cardiac output is elevated before the second exercise bout.

Methods.—Six men ranging in age from 37 to 57 years had previously undergone orthotopic cardiac transplantation. There was a control group of 8 men aged 37–52 years. Exercise tests were performed an average of 2.3 months after transplantation. All subjects performed a progressive ramp test to volitional exhaustion. A square wave test just below the ventilatory threshold was also performed. This entailed 6 minutes of loadless cycling, 6 minutes at an individually determined work-rate, 6 minutes of loadless cycling, and 6 more minutes of work. This was performed once for the controls and twice, separated by 1 week, for the transplant recipients. Expired gases were monitored using a breath-by-breath system. Onset kinetics were determined for both submaximal work rates by fitting the oxygen uptake to a monoexponential equation that yielded time constants and delay.

Findings.—The onset kinetics (table) time constant was 45 seconds for normal subjects and 77 seconds for the patients. For the second bout of exercise in the transplant patients, the time constant was significantly faster, at 46 seconds.

Conclusion.—The slower-onset time constant reflects a central as well as a peripheral blood flow limitation. Priming the system effectively improves blood flow, allowing the cardiovascular system to deliver the required oxygen in a similar manner to normal subjects. The low fitness of transplant patients may be largely attributable to limitations of the cardiac pump.

▶ The findings of Paterson et al. largely echo what we described to the World Congress of Cardiac Rehabilitation some 3 years ago (1). Because the cardiac transplant operation destroys the sympathetic innervation, the exercising heart lacks the normal inotropic and the chronotropic responses. An increase of end-diastolic volume gives a small increase of heart rate through

Oxygen Kinetics During Initial and Successive Square-Wave Tests in Heart Transplant Recipients

	Initial Square-Wave Test			Second Square-Wave Test	
	Control	Heart transplant	P value	Heart transplant	P value vs. initial square-wave test
Baseline $\dot{V}o_2$, l/min	0.73±0.10	0.78±0.07	NS	0.80±0.19	NS
Amplitude, l/min	0.45±0.15	0.21±0.10	0.004	0.14±0.05	NS
Time constant, s	45±4	77±26	0.027	46±17	0.020
95% confidence interval, s	6.3	13.6		20.4	
Time delay, s	2±5	11±6	0.016	15±15	NS
Goodness of fit, l/min	0.08±0.04	0.04±0.01		0.06±0.04	

Note: Values are mean or mean ± SD. Abbreviation: $\dot{V}o_2$, O_2 uptake. Goodness of fit is SD of sum of squares of differences between data and curve fit.
(Courtesy of Paterson DH, Cunningham DA, Pickering JG, et al: J Appl Physiol 77:1935–1940, 1994.)

the Bainbridge reflex, but the main increase of heart rate and stroke volume does not occur until the arrival of circulating catecholamines from the adrenal glands. The implication is that when assessing exercise performance, the patient should be allowed a longer time to reach a steady state. The sensitivity to catecholamines is increased in the denervated heart, so that tachycardia persists after exercise and the response to the second stage of an exercise test may be faster than the response to the first stage.

At one time, it was argued that denervation was a permanent feature of cardiac transplantation. There is now some evidence that the nerves may regenerate after an interval of 2–3 years; however, this was not an issue with the present group of patients, who were evaluated within a few months of surgery.—R.J. Shephard, M.D., Ph.D., D.P.E.

References

1. Kavanagh T, et al: On the choice of a cycle ergometer exercise test protocol for the heart transplant patient, in: Broustet JP (ed): *Proceedings of the Fifth World Congress on Cardiac Rehabilitation.* Andover, UK, Intercept Ltd, 1993.

Urinary Kallikrein Activity is Increased During the First Few Weeks of Exercise Training in Essential Hypertension
Miura S-I, Tashiro E, Sakai T, Koga M, Kinoshita A, Sasaguri M, Ideishi M, Tanaka H, Shindo M, Arakawa K (Fukuoka Univ, Japan; Univ of Occupational and Environmental Health, Kitakyusyu, Japan)
J Hypertens 12:815–823, 1994   139-95-9–9

Introduction.—Mild-to-moderate hypertension can be effectively treated with exercise training. A reduction of plasma noradrenaline concentration suggests a reduction in sympathetic nerve activity. Plasma volume depletion has also been implicated, as have increases in serum prostaglandin E, serum taurine, and total dopamine excretion. Renal depressor systems include prostaglandins, renal dopamine, and the renal kallikrein-kinin system. The latter system, usually suppressed in patients with essential hypertension, is important in the regulation of body sodium content. The activity of the kallikrein-kinin system early in a training program in patients with mild hypertension was determined.

Methods.—There were 27 nonobese subjects with essential hypertension, ranging in age from 38 to 64 years. They were divided into a training group and a control group. Blood pressure was recorded at weeks 1, 2, 4, and 10. A progressive exercise test to volitional exhaustion was performed to determine the lactate threshold. Subjects trained at the lactate threshold for 60 minutes, 3 times a week for 10 weeks. Parameters evaluated included urinary kallikrein, plasma volume, and plasma concentrations of noradrenaline, albumin, dopamine, aldosterone, prostaglandin E_2, sodium, and renin.

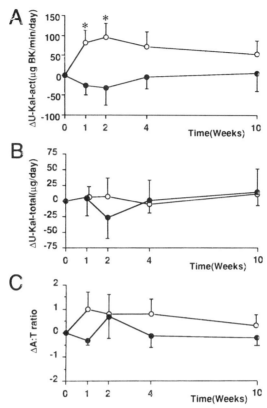

Fig 9–3.—The changes in (**A**) urinary kallikrein activity (ΔU-a-Kal), (**B**) urinary total kallikrein quantity (ΔU-t-Kal) and (**C**) U-a-Kal/U-t-Kal (ΔA:T ratio) between the exercise group (*open circle*) and the nonexercise group (*closed circle*). *Abbreviation:* BK, bradykinin. Values are expressed as mean ± SEM. °$P < 0.05$, vs. nonexercise group. (Courtesy of Miura S-I, Tashiro E, Sakai T, et al: *J Hypertens* 12:815–823, 1994.)

Results.—There were no changes in blood pressure or humoral data in control subjects. In the exercise group, resting blood pressure was significantly reduced after training. The change in systolic blood pressure was inversely related to the change in urinary kallikrein during the first 2 weeks of observation. The change in plasma dopamine was inversely related to the change in diastolic blood pressure, also over the first two weeks. The change in systolic blood pressure during 10 weeks was directly related to the change in plasma noradrenaline. The higher the baseline kallikrein levels, the greater the decline in systolic blood pressure throughout the course of the training (Fig 9–3).

Summary.—During the first weeks of training, changes in the renal kallikrein system may be associated with the reduction in blood pressure. The reduction in activity of the sympathetic nervous system may be involved in maintenance of the lowered blood pressure. These findings add further support to the use of exercise for patients with mild-to-moderate hypertension.

▶ Although it is now widely accepted that regular exercise can yield clinically useful decreases of resting blood pressure in patients with hypertension, the mechanism that is responsible for control of hypertension remains unclear. This study provides good evidence that the kallikrein-kinin and dopamine systems stimulate sodium ion excretion and thus reduce plasma volume. Levels of active urinary kallikrein rise steeply over the first 2 weeks of training. It is interesting that exercise was particularly effective in those who began training with high renal kallikrein-kinin activity and high rates of noradrenaline excretion.—R.J. Shephard, M.D., Ph.D., D.P.E.

Effects of Maximal Exercise and Venous Occlusion on Fibrinolytic Activity in Physically Active and Inactive Men
Szymanski LM, Pate RR, Durstine JL (Univ of South Carolina, Columbia)
J Appl Physiol 77:2305–2310, 1994   139-95-9-10

Objective.—Although habitual exercise is known to play an important role in preventing coronary artery disease, the mechanisms of this protective effect are not entirely clear. There are few data on the effects of exercise—either habitual or single-session—on the components of the fibrinolytic system. Changes in fibrinolytic activity in response to maximal exercise and to 5-minute venous occlusion were assessed. In addition, these responses were compared among men with varying physical activity levels.

Methods.—Forty-five apparently healthy men were studied. Fifteen were classified as inactive, 15 as regularly active, and 15 as highly active. In each subject, tissue plasminogen activator (TPA) and plasminogen activator inhibitor 1 (PAI-1) activity were measured before and after a bout of maximal exercise and before and after a 5-minute venous occlusion test. Three-way analysis of variance with repeated measures was applied to the results.

Results.—The 3 groups had similar baseline TPA activity. However, the postexercise increase in TPA activity was greater among the active men than the inactive men. After venous occlusion, the highly active men also showed a significant increase in TPA activity (Fig 9–4). Baseline PAI-1 activity was significantly different among groups, being highest in the inactive group and lowest in the highly active group. Although PAI-1 activity decreased with exercise, it was unaffected by venous occlusion.

Conclusion.—Physically active men show greater changes in fibrinolytic activity after maximal exercise and venous occlusion than inactive men. Regular physical activity may thus enhance the fibrinolytic effect of an acute bout of exercise, which may be an important mechanism of its cardioprotective effect. Further research on the effects of exercise on

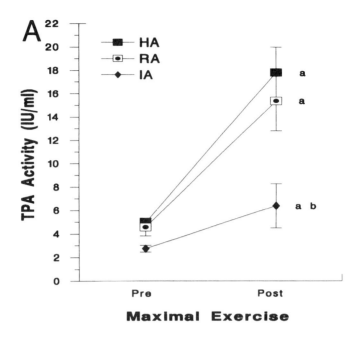

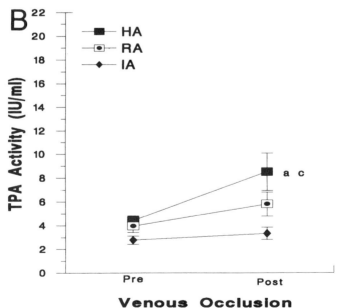

Fig 9–4.—Tissue plasminogen activator (TPA) activity before and after maximal exercise (**A**) and before and after venous occlusion (**B**). *Abbreviations: HA*, highly active; *RA*, regularly active; *IA*, inactive. Values are expressed as means ± SE. Significantly different (P < 0.05) from: [a]preexercise; [b]other groups; [c]IA group. (Courtesy of Szymanski LM, Pate RR, Durstine JL: *J Appl Physiol* 77:2305–2310, 1994.)

fibrinolysis is needed, particularly to evaluate the lower intensity exercise that is currently being recommended and to study fibrinolytic activity in women.

▶ Although there is general agreement that an acute bout of exercise induces an immediate increase in plasma levels of the clot-lysing enzyme plasmin, the overall response is complex, in that vigorous exercise also flushes platelets into the circulation (1), perhaps through an action on β-adrenergic receptors, and there may be changes in adhesion molecules on the surface of the platelets (2).

The data reported by Szymanski et al. were obtained 1 minute after a maximal treadmill test of 11–15 minutes' duration. There is a need not only to examine the response to lower intensity efforts, such as are normally used in preventive programs, but also to follow the dynamics of clotting during and after exercise bouts. The subtle changes associated with platelet release, activation of plasminogen, and possibly, a final depletion of plasminogen activators cannot be studied in a single blood sample!—R.J. Shephard, M.D., Ph.D., D.P.E.

References

1. Pelliccia A: *Medicina dello Sport (Italy)* 30:275-282, 1978.
2. Lee G, et al: Effect of exercise on hemostatic mechanisms, in: *Exercise in Cardiovascular Health and Disease*, Amsterdam EA, et al: (eds): New York, Yorke Medical Books, 1977, pp 122-136.

Adding β-2 Agonism Does Not Improve β-1 Blockade Exercise Responses in Hypertensives

Rueckert PA, Slane PR, Hanson P (Univ of Wisconsin, Madison)
Med Sci Sports Exerc 26:945–950, 1994   139-95-9–11

Background.—The β-1 receptor antagonist celiprolol has the ancillary property of β-2 mediated vasodilation. The hypothesis that celiprolol would allow more blood flow to active muscles and produce less slowing of the heart rate during exercise than the β-1 receptor antagonist atenolol was tested.

Methods.—Eleven untrained men with hypertension (mean age, 40.5 years) were enrolled in this double-blind, crossover study. After a 3-week washout phase, the patients were randomized to receive either celiprolol (200-400 mg daily) or atenolol (50-100 mg daily) for 6 weeks. After an intervening 3-week placebo period, the patients were crossed over to the other drug. At the end of each phase, resting forearm and calf vascular resistance was measured by venous occlusion plethysmography. Also, submaximal and maximal cycle ergometry exercise responses were evaluated.

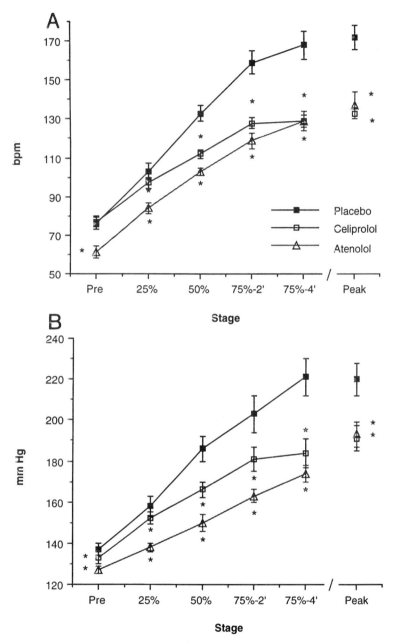

Fig 9–5.—A, preexercise, submaximal (staged protocol), and peak (ramping protocol) heart rates during the treatment and placebo phases. **B**, preexercise, submaximal (staged protocol), and peak (ramping protocol) systolic blood pressures. *Significant difference from placebo. (Courtesy of Rueckert PA, Slane PR, Hanson P: *Med Sci Sports Exerc* 26:945–950, 1994.)

Results.—Resting forearm and calf vascular resistance was significantly decreased by celiprolol but not by atenolol. Atenolol-blunted heart rate increases more than celiprolol during submaximal exercise (Fig 9–5). However, no difference between the 2 drugs in blunting heart rate increases was present at the 75% and peak exercise levels. Although submaximal exercise systolic blood pressure (BP) was lower with atenolol, at 75% and peak exercise the effects of the 2 drugs on systolic BP was similar. Neither drug significantly affected the submaximal exercise oxygen uptake, minute ventilation, rate of perceived exertion, or expiratory gas exchange ratio. Peak oxygen uptake was significantly and similarly decreased by both drugs.

Conclusions.—Resting vascular resistance is decreased by adding β-2 vasodilatory activity to β-1 antagonism; however, this effect is not present while exercising. During exercise, $\beta2$–mediated vasodilation is apparently overridden by factors such as sympathetic vasoconstriction or local metabolic vasodilation.

▶ Beta-1 receptors are concerned primarily with the regulation of cardiac contractility and lipolysis, whereas (at least in resting subjects) β-2 receptors are involved in bronchoregulation, peripheral vasodilatation, and the mobilization of glycogen. Administration of a generalized β-blocker may thus have an adverse impact on a number of aspects of physical performance. Beta-1 blockers avoid some of the undesired responses, although patients still tend to complain of cold extremities, bronchospasm, and generalized fatigue. In theory, an agent such as celiprolol (which combines inhibition of β-1 receptors with stimulation of β-2 receptors) should have many advantages, even over a β-1 selective antagonist such as atenolol.

Under resting conditions, Rueckert and colleagues found that celiprolol did indeed increase peripheral blood flow relative to atenolol, but during exercise both medications produced a similar decrease in performance, including a substantial diminution of maximal oxygen intake. This emphasizes the dominant role of locally accumulating metabolites in regulating muscle blood flow during vigorous exercise.—R.J. Shephard, M.D., Ph.D., D.P.E.

Blood Pressure Responses to a Progressive Step Test in Normotensive Males and Females
Jetté M, Sidney K, Landry F, Quenneville J (University of Ottawa, Ontario; Laurentian Univ, Sudbury, Ontario; Université Laval, Québec)
Can J Appl Physiol 19:421–431, 1994   139-95-9–12

Introduction.—Individuals who experience a hypertensive response to exercise are at increased risk of sustained hypertension. The pathophysiologic changes preceding hypertension may also be associated with an excessive pressor response to exercise. Blood pressure (BP) responses to a progressive step test (a modified version of the Canadian Aerobic Fitness Test [CAFT] using low initial exercise intensities) in an apparently

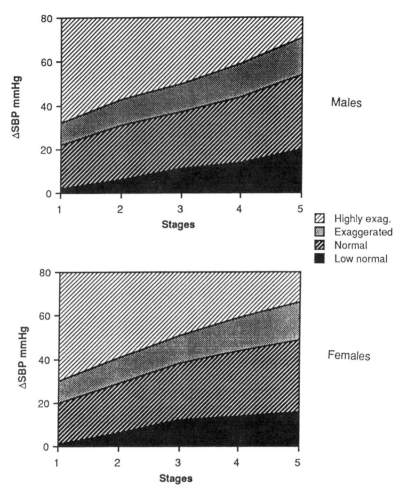

Fig 9–6.—*Abbreviation:* SBP, systolic blood pressure. ΔSBP responses to each stage of the progressive step test. ΔSBP = exercise SBP − resting SBP; *low normal* = < mean ΔSBP − 1 SD; *normal* = mean ΔSBP + 1 SD; *exaggerated* = > mean ΔSBP + 1 SD < mean ΔSBP + 2 SD; *highly exag.* = > mean ΔSBP + 2 SD. (Courtesy of Jetté M, Sidney K, Landry F, et al: *Can J Appl Physiol* 19:421–431, 1994.)

healthy population were documented. The influence of participation in physical activity on blood pressure response to the step test was also evaluated.

Procedure.—Subjects underwent the first five 3-minute stepping stages of the CAFT test in a progressive and discontinuous manner. Of 154 men and 175 women participating, 147 men and 138 women were allowed to complete all 5 stages; individuals were not allowed to complete the test if they experienced exercise heart rates greater than preestablished ceiling heart rates. Exercise heart rate (HR), systolic blood pressure (SBP), diastolic blood pressure (DBP), and ΔSBP (exercise SBP minus preexercise SBP) were measured at each stage.

Results.—Increased exercise intensity was associated with a linear increase in mean HR, SBP, and ΔSBP (Fig 9–6); mean DBP remained stable. Age in men, age and body mass in women, and degree of participation in a physical activity for both sexes were the variables contributing most to ΔSBP. Of individuals who were normotensive at rest, 15% had an exaggerated pressor response (mean ΔSBP + 1 standard deviation [SD] at each exercise stage and 3% had highly exaggerated responses (mean ΔSBP + 2 SD). Individuals with normal resting BP who experienced excessive BP after exercising did so at the lowest levels of stepping intensities.

Discussion.—The cardiovascular responses to graded exercise among this healthy, largely physically active population of subjects were as expected. Because this modified version of the CAFT test begins at a low level of exercise intensity, it represents a range of energy costs observed with daily activity and could elicit fluctuations in BP comparable to those reported during the course of daily activities. Because lower exercise intensities appear sufficient to detect exercise-induced exaggerations in BP, this modification of the CAFT step-test protocol should be useful for assessing the exercise BP response in higher-risk individuals.

▶ There is increasing acceptance of the idea that patients in whom hypertension will later develop can be detected by an unusually large increase in BP during exercise (1). There may thus be value in having fitness testers measure BP during simple field appraisals of physical condition. Those with apparently abnormal values could be referred to their physicians for closer observation. The definition of normal responses to a simple test such as the Canadian Home Fitness Test is a first step in this direction, although a prospective assessment of test sensitivity and specificity will be needed before we can be sure that such an approach has practical value.—R.J. Shephard, M.D., Ph.D., D.P.E.

Reference

1. Wilson MF, Sung BH, Pincomb GA, et al: *Am J Cardiol* 66:731-736, 1990.

Effect of α₁-Adrenoceptor Blockade on Maximal VO₂ and Endurance Capacity in Well-Trained Athletic Hypertensive Men

Tomten SE, Kjeldsen SE, Nilsson S, Westheim AS (Ullevaal Univ Hosp, Oslo, Norway; Norwegian Inst for Sports Medicine Ltd, Oslo)
Am J Hypertens 7:603–608, 1994   139-95-9-13

Background.—The effect of α₁-selective blockage on physical exercise capacity in men with hypertension is not completely known. The effect of an α₁-selective blocker on maximum oxygen consumption ($\dot{V}O_{2max}$)

Effect of α_1-Selective Block on Heart Rate Recorded During the 5,000-m Running Test and Blood Pressure Recorded Immediately After the Finish ($n = 13$)

	Placebo	Doxazosin	Delta	P Value
Mean heart rate (beats/min)	171 ± 3	170 ± 2	−1 ± 2	.85 (NS)
Maximal heart rate (beats/min)	181 ± 2	181 ± 2	0 ± 5	.87 (NS)
Exercise duration (sec)	1377 ± 55	1420 ± 57	43 ± 12	.004
Systolic blood pressure (mm Hg)	181 ± 6	172 ± 8	−9 ± 4	.04
Diastolic blood pressure (mm Hg)	70 ± 7	61 ± 7	−9 ± 6	.13 (NS)

Note: Mean ± SE.
Abbreviation: NS, not significant.
(Courtesy of Tomten SE, Kjeldsen SE, Nilsson S, et al: Am J Hypertens 7:603–608, 1994.)

and the exercise capacity in athletic men with mild hypertension was studied.

Methods.—Sixteen white male marathon runners (mean age, 45 years) with a diastolic blood pressure between 90 and 110 mm Hg (mean, 98) were included in a double-blind, randomized, crossover study. Their physical examination, ECG, and blood hemoglobin were normal. Each morning, the doxazosin group received 1 mg during week 1, 2 mg during week 2, and 4 mg during weeks 3 and 4. Each medication period lasted 4 weeks, and exercise tests were completed at the end of each period. The cycle ergometer tests started at a level of 100 W, and the work-rate was increased by 10 W every minute. The 5,000-m running tests were performed on an indoor track, with 4–5 individuals starting simultaneously. They were extensively monitored during all tests.

Results.—Compared with the study subjects who received a placebo, those who were given doxazosin had a statistically significant reduction of their maximal cycle ergometer power output of 16 ± 3 W and of their $\dot{V}o_{2max}$ by an average of 3 ± 1 mL/(kg/min). In the subjects receiving doxazosin, the 5,000 m running times increased by a mean of 43 seconds (table). No intergroup difference in heart rates during or immediately after the run was found. In the group treated with doxazosin, the systolic blood pressure was reduced by an average of 9 mm Hg immediately after running. While taking doxazosin, 6 individuals complained of headache, fatigue, or leg pain.

Conclusions.—In athletic men with mild hypertension, an α_1-selective blocker (doxazosin) moderately reduces maximal O_2 consumption and endurance for vigorous physical exercise. Immediately after running, the heart rate is unaffected, but the systolic pressure is reduced. Thus, vigorous exercise may be safer when this drug is administered.

▶ α-Blocking drugs are intended to reduce peripheral vascular resistance and maintain blood flow to the capillaries. A previous report suggested that α-blockade had little effect on physical performance (1), and such medication might thus offer a better treatment than a β-blocking agent for the patient with hypertension. In this regard, the present report seems somewhat at variance with earlier studies, although the drug-related impairment of performance was relatively small (5% to 6%); however, the earlier data also showed a nonsignificant trend toward decreased physical performance, as have studies with angiotensin-converting enzyme inhibition and calcium channel blockade. It seems that a small loss of function is the price that must be paid for the control of hypertension. The mechanism for the functional deterioration is unclear; Tomten and associates are inclined to blame hemodilution, although in their study, the decrease in hemoglobin level (from 14.8 to 14.2 g/dL) is quite small.—R.J. Shephard, M.D., Ph.D., D.P.E.

Reference

1. Thompson PD, et al: *Am J Med* 86:104B–109B, 1989.

Role of Myocarditis in Athletes With Minor Arrhythmias and/or Echocardiographic Abnormalities

Zeppilli P, Santini C, Palmieri V, Vannicelli R, Giordano A, Frustaci A (Istituto di Medicina Nucleare, Rome; Istituto di Cardiologia, Rome; Universitá Cattolica del Sacro Cuore, Rome)

Chest 106:373–380, 1994   139-95-9–14

Background.—A variety of endomyocardial abnormalities have been found in biopsies from patients having arrhythmia but no overt heart disease. They include fibrosis, increased interstitial fat, and acute or subacute myocarditis. Myocarditis has been implicated as a possible cause of sports-related deaths, presumably through disposing to ventricular fibrillation.

Series.—The findings were reviewed in 6 young adult sportsmen and sportswomen 17–27 years of age who had minor arrhythmias, echocardiographic abnormalities, or both. The participants underwent endomyocardial biopsy to confirm or rule out myocarditis.

Clinical Findings.—The patients were evaluated by a maximum ECG stress test, 24-hour Holter monitoring, gated blood pool radionuclide ventriculography, and cardiac catheterization with right and left ventriculography. Three patients received a diagnosis of arrhythmogenic right ventricular dysplasia. Two of them had ventricular arrhythmias and left bundle-branch block, whereas 1 had a dilated right ventricle with apical hypokinesia. One patient had a dilated left ventricle and moderately depressed systolic function, ascribed to an athlete's heart.

Biopsy Findings.—Definite myocarditis was found in 4 of the 6 athletes, 2 of whom had changes of fibrosis (Fig 9–7). The appearances of active lymphocytic myocarditis are shown in Figure 9–8. The other 2 patients, whose histories strongly suggested previous acute myocarditis, had findings of nonspecific fibrosis consistent with healed myocarditis.

Implications.—In generally healthy athletes who lack serious ECG abnormalities, minor rhythm disturbances and mild echocardiographic changes may be caused by myocarditis. An early diagnosis of myocarditis will prevent fatal arrhythmia by enforcing the temporary suspension of strenuous physical activity.

▶ This report from Italy reminds us, as reviewed recently (1), that among the causes of sudden cardiac death in athletes is myocarditis. Of these 6 young athletes, 2 had nonspecific fibrosis, but 4 had "definite" myocarditis. The inflammatory infiltrates were mostly lymphomononuclear, suggesting to the authors a viral cause. Past reports (2, 3) of sudden cardiac death in Italian athletes highlight right ventricular dysplasia (RVD), a rare cardiomyopathy of unknown cause, with focal myofibrosis and fatty infiltration. Apparently, RVD can run in some families and is said to be the most common cause of sudden cardiac death in athletes in northern Italy (3).

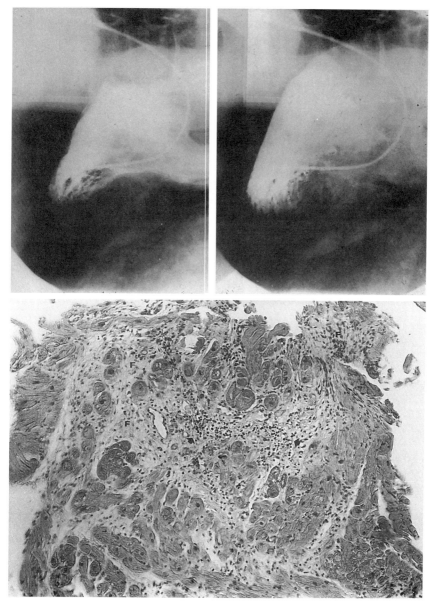

Fig 9–7.—Myocarditis with fibrosis. **Top,** right ventriculogram (*left,* diastolic) (*right,* systolic) showing a moderate enlargement of the right ventricle and a basal-apical hypokinesia. **Bottom,** endomyocardial biopsy specimen showing myocarditis with fibrosis (F) and occasional focus of cellular necrosis (*arrowheads*) (hematoxylin-eosin, original magnification, ×100). (Courtesy of Zeppilli P, Santini C, Palmieri V, et al: *Chest* 106:373–380, 1994.)

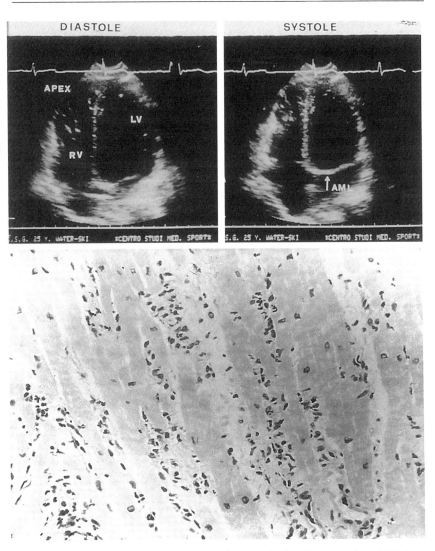

Fig 9–8.—Active lymphocytic myocarditis. **Top,** 2-dimensional echocardiogram in the apical 4-chamber view showing a moderate prolapse of the anterior mitral leaflet (AML), a mild left ventricular enlargement, and a moderate right ventricular dilation with akinesia in the distal two thirds of the diaphragmatic wall and apex. **Bottom,** microphotograph showing active lymphocytic myocarditis. Interstitial lymphocytic infiltrates are present with obvious necrosis of adjacent myocytes (hematoxylin-eosin, original magnification, ×250). (Courtesy of Zeppilli P, Santini C, Palmieri V, et al: *Chest* 106:373–380, 1994.)

These authors seem to think that RVD is overdiagnosed in Italy and that some presumed cases are viral myocarditis. Hypertrophic nonobstructive cardiomyopathy (HNCM) (see Abstract 139-95-6-4) is a rare cause of death in Italian athletes (in contrast to athletes in the United States), perhaps because, as these authors discuss, prescreening in Italy is stringent and any athlete with an abnormal ECG undergoes echocardiography. As a result, HNCM in Italy is detected early and the athlete is precluded from engaging in vigorous sports.—E.R. Eichner, M.D.

References

1. Winget JF, et al: *Sports Med* 18:375, 1994.
2. Thiene G, Nava A, Corrado D, et al: N *Engl J Med* 318:129–133, 1988.
3. Corrado D, Thiene G, Nava A, et al: *Am J Med* 89:588–596, 1990.

Effect of Training on the Blood Pressure Response to Weight Lifting
Sale DG, Moroz DE, McKelvie RS, MacDougall JD, McCartney N (McMaster Univ, Hamilton, Ontario)
Can J Appl Physiol 19:60–74, 1994   139-95-9-15

Background.—Previous studies suggested that weight training would have 2 primary effects. First, the peak pressure response to maximal weight lifting efforts would be expected to increase, probably by increasing motor command to and motor unit activation in the involved muscles. Second, training should cause a decrease in the blood pressure response to lifting a given absolute weight, because a smaller motor command and motor unit activation would suffice in lifting a given absolute weight after training. These expectations were further investigated in a group of untrained young men undergoing weight training using a seated bilateral leg press weight lift exercise.

Participants and Methods.—Six young men (mean age, 22 years), with no previous weight or other form of resistance training, were studied. All men trained on 3 alternate days per week for a total of 19 weeks. Before and after training, the heaviest weight that could be lifted once with isolated concentric action was determined (1-repetition maximum = 1-RM). Each session consisted of 3 warm-up sets of 20 repetitions, followed by 1 set each at 15–20, 10–15, and 7–10 RM (day 1), 3 sets at 15–20 RM (day 2) and 1 set at 15–20 and 2 sets at 10–15 RM (day 3). Arterial and esophageal pressure responses were recorded using a brachial artery catheter and a probe, respectively. Measurements were made before and after training as participants did sets of as many repetitions as possible (up to 20 repetitions), with loads corresponding to 50, 70, 80, 85, and 87.5% of the 1-RM. Right and left knee extensors were also measured with CT.

Results.—Training increased the maximal single leg press lift (1-RM) and knee extensor cross-sectional area by 26% and 12%, respectively. Peak values of systolic pressure obtained during a set (M pre/post, mm Hg) were significantly increased at 85% 1-RM. Significant increases in peak diastolic pressure were observed at 50%, 70%, and 80%. Peak esophageal pressure showed a significant increase at 80% 1-RM (Fig

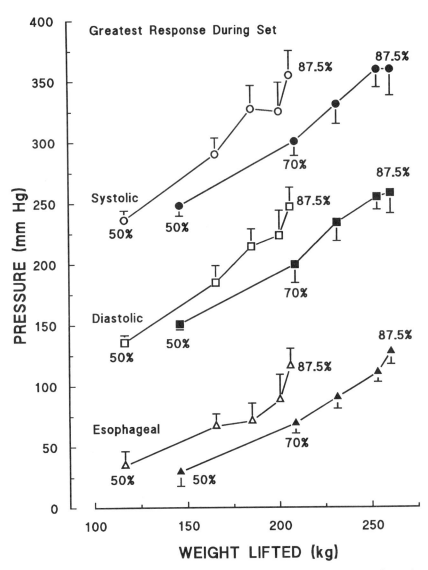

Fig 9–9.—Peak arterial and esophageal pressure (mean and SE) during the repetition producing the greatest response in sets done at 50%, 70%, 80%, 85%, and 87.5% of the 1-RM are plotted in relation to the actual absolute weights lifted at the corresponding percentages of the 1-RM. Pre- (*open symbols*) and post-training (*filled symbols*) values (M and SE) for systolic (*circles*), diastolic (*squares*), and esophageal (*triangles*) pressure are shown. (Courtesy of Sale DG, Moroz DE, McKelvie RS, et al: *Can J Appl Physiol* 19:60–74, 1994.)

9–9). After training, all responses were notably decreased for a given absolute weight lifted.

Conclusions.—Weight training increases the peak arterial and esophageal pressure responses obtained during maximal weight lifting exercise and decreases arterial and esophageal pressure responses to lifting the same absolute weight.

▶ The authors' findings are not unexpected, but they are nevertheless of considerable practical importance. They show clearly that the cardiovascular strain associated with completion of a given lifting task can be appreciably reduced by a weight training program. A 19-week resistance-exercise program was enough to reduce both systolic and diastolic pressures by 20–25 mm Hg, enough to make a substantial difference to the cardiac work-rate, and thus in the likelihood of myocardial ischemia in someone with a marginal coronary vascular circulation.—R.J. Shephard, M.D., Ph.D., D.P.E.

Instituting the Updated CPR Protocol: The Team Physician's Role
Araujo D, Rubin A (Kaiser Permanente Med Ctr, Fontana, Calif; Western Washington Univ, Bellingham)
Physician Sportsmed 22:51–56, 1994   139-95-9-16

Introduction.—In developing an emergency response plan and training personnel, the team physician must know the latest CPR protocol. The new recommendations by the 1992 National Conference on Cardiopulmonary Resuscitation and Emergency Cardiac Care are summarized.

Sequence.—The sequence involves assessment, activation of emergency medical services (EMS), and application of principles of airway, breathing, and circulation (ABCs). Assessment establishes that a patient is not breathing and has no pulse. The new guidelines call for activating the EMS system immediately after assessment for all victims other than infants, whereas previous guidelines recommended beginning the ABCs before calling for help. Defibrillation can increase the chance that a victim will survive cardiac arrest, because more than 80% of victims of sudden, nontraumatic adult cardiac arrest have ventricular fibrillation. A proper airway should be established by using the head tilt–chin lift position. Rescue breathing should be initiated with 2 breaths if victim is not breathing. If the victim has no pulse, external chest compression should be started.

Protocol.—The EMS should be activated after unresponsiveness has been determined. To clear a foreign body, as many as 5 abdominal thrusts should be administered. A finger sweep should be done for an adult. For an infant, as many as 5 back blows and 5 chest thrusts should be administered; the mouth should be checked and visible objects removed; and 2 breaths should be supplied. To prevent communicable diseases, a mask should be used during rescue breathing. The length of an adult rescue breath is $1\frac{1}{2}$–2 seconds per breath. The adult rescue breathing rate is once every 5–6 seconds. The depth of compressions for children is one third to one half total chest depth, or about 1–$1\frac{1}{2}$ inches. For infants, the depth of compressions is one third to one half of the total chest depth, or about $\frac{1}{2}$–1 inch. An unconscious breathing victim should be positioned on her or his side; the torso should not be twisted. The lower arm is placed behind the victim's back, and the upper hand is placed under the chin while the upper leg is flexed.

Planning.—When an emergency action plan is being developed, the role of each person involved should be delineated including ushers, security guards, coaches, administrators, athletic trainers, paramedics, and the team physician. The following should be decided: who recognizes the emergency; who is the first responder; who activates the EMS; how EMS will be activated, whether by cellular telephone, sideline telephone, or radio; and who takes charge when the EMS are present.

▶ Be aware of the changes in CPR protocol. The EMS activation should be done immediately after your assessment. Athletic trainers must always use a mask when performing CPR. Masks are inexpensive and should be available in every athletic training room and every athletic training kit. Your CPR protocol should be practiced frequently so that when an emergency occurs, you will be prepared. Practice placing the victim on his or her side, so that you will be familiar with the proper positioning technique. Develop a plan for spectators as well as injured athletes.—F.J. George, A.T.C, P.T.

Higher Levels of Conditioning Leisure Time Physical Activity are Associated With Reduced Levels of Stored Iron in Finnish Men
Lakka TA, Nyyssönen K, Salonen JT (Univ of Kuopio, Finland)
Am J Epidemiol 140:148–160, 1994   139-95-9–17

Objective.—The coronary protective effect of physical activity cannot be completely explained by the recognized risk factors for coronary heart disease, such as an unfavorable blood lipid profile and increased blood pressure. One possible protective mechanism may be a reduction in body iron stores. Previous studies have found that high serum levels of ferritin are associated with an excess risk of acute myocardial infarction and that endurance athletes have a reduced serum level of ferritin and blood level of hemoglobin. The association between the amount and intensity of conditioning leisure time physical activity and these 2 measures of iron was investigated.

Methods.—The study included 1,743 men aged 42–60 years when first studied from 1984 to 1989. The men were residents of eastern Finland, a population that has a very high incidence of coronary heart disease and mortality. A wide range of variables, including leisure-time physical activity, was measured by questionnaires and laboratory studies.

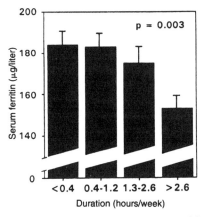 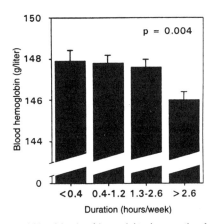

Fig 9–10.—Mean serum concentrations of ferritin and blood levels of hemoglobin by quartile of duration of conditioning leisure-time physical activity, as assessed by the 12-month history questionnaire in 1,743 middle-aged eastern Finnish men. Kuopio Ischemic Heart Disease Risk Factor Study. The *bars* indicate standard error. The data on serum levels of ferritin are adjusted for age; examination year; serum level of γ-glutamyltransferase; body mass index; blood hematocrit; intakes of meat, milk products, alcohol, sugar, coffee, fruits and vegetables, and grain products; regular use of analgesics; and history of liver disease, diabetes, gastritis or peptic ulcer, and colitis or irritable colon. The data on blood levels of hemoglobin were adjusted for age, examination year, body mass index, serum level of γ-glutamyltransferase intakes of meat and coffee, history of colitis or irritable colon, and smoking. (Courtesy of Lakka TA, Nyyssönen K, Salonen JT: *Am J Epidemiol* 140:148–160, 1994.)

Results.—On multivariate regression analyses with adjustment for potential confounders, the duration and frequency of physical activity were inversely associated with both the serum level of ferritin and the blood level of hemoglobin. The serum concentration of ferritin was 17% lower for men in the highest quartile of exercise duration (more than 2.6 hr/wk), compared with those in the lowest quartile (less than 0.4 hr/wk.) Similarly, the serum level of ferritin was 20% lower for men in the highest category of frequency (more than 3 sessions/wk), compared with those in the lowest category (less than 1 session/wk). The differences in blood level of hemoglobin between these groups were 1.3% and 1.0%, respectively (Fig 9–10). Only the blood level of hemoglobin was significantly associated with exercise intensity.

Conclusions.—The serum levels of ferritin are decreased with increasing duration and frequency of exercise. As in previous studies, the results suggest that a reduction in stored levels of iron may be a mechanism by which conditioning leisure-time physical activity decreases the risk of coronary heart disease. A long-term reduction in the serum level of ferritin and blood level of hemoglobin appears to require 2–3 hours per week of regular physical conditioning activity.

▶ These researchers have a knack for offbeat interpretations of their careful epidemiologic work. In 1992, they suggested that high stored iron levels (high ferritin) increase the risk of myocardial infarction in Finnish men (1). This idea, a classic example of "guilt by association," has been debunked (2).

In their study, high ferritin was linked to heart attack only when cholesterol was also high. People who eat a lot of meat end up with high ferritin levels and a high intake of saturated fat. What causes heart attack is the saturated fat, not the ferritin. The ferritin is thus only a *predictor* of heart attack, not a *risk factor.*

Last year, this group reported that a reduction in fibrinogen levels may be one way in which regular physical activity fends off coronary heart disease (3). They were correct—exercise is "nature's anticoagulant." But now they're off-base again. They find that higher levels of physical activity are associated with lower levels of serum ferritin and blood hemoglobin. But instead of the logical interpretation—that both ferritin and hemoglobin are diluted by the expanded plasma volume of the exerciser—they return to their original notion that iron (as a free radical promoter) promotes heart attack. They suggest that physical activity cuts the risk of heart attack by reducing stored iron levels. Wrong! Their iron/heart attack theory is full of holes.—E.R. Eichner, M.D.

References

1. Salonen JT, et al: *Circulation* 86:803, 1992.
2. Sempos CT, et al: N *Engl J Med* 331:1160, 1994.
3. 1994 Year Book of Sports Medicine, pp 396–398.

Effects of Exercise Intensity, Duration, and Time of Day on Fibrinolytic Activity in Physically Active Men
Szymanski LM, Pate RR (Univ of South Carolina, Columbia)
Med Sci Sports Exerc 26:1102–1108, 1994   139-95-9–18

Introduction.—Fibrinolytic activity increases with a single bout of exercise. However, the effects of the primary training variables of frequency, intensity, and duration, as well as initial level of fitness and time of day on fibrinolytic activity, are less well defined.

Methods.—Twelve healthy males (mean age, 34 years) participated. The participants ran 4 treadmill tests, each for 30 minutes duration in the morning and evening, at 50% and 80% of maximal oxygen output ($\dot{V}O_{2max}$), respectively. Energy expenditure was assessed by analysis of expiratory gas. Serial blood samples were drawn for determination of tissue plasminogen activator (TPA) and plasminogen activator inhibitor-1 (PAI-1) activity.

Findings.—Afternoon TPA was significantly higher than that seen in the morning at both intensities of exercise (Fig 9–11). For PAI-1, there was an effect for time of day and time but not for intensity. In 3 of 4 cases, PAI-1 was reduced as a result of exercise.

Conclusion.—Exercise increases TPA activity and decreases PAI-1 activity. Higher intensities and evening exercise produced the greatest changes. The duration of exercise and energy expenditure did not seem to affect the fibrinolytic system.

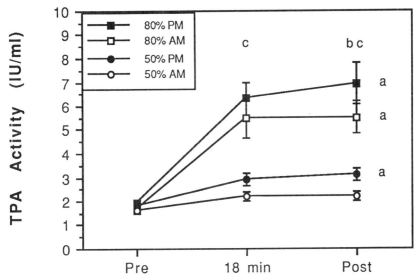

Fig 9–11.—The tissue plasminogen activator (TPA) activity during 4 submaximal exercise sessions. The TPA activity was measured before, during (18 minutes), and after exercise. Values are expressed as mean ± SE. a = 18 minutes, and postexercise values are different from preexercise value (P < 0.05); b = TPA activity in the morning is different from the evening (P = < 0.05); c = TPA activity during the 50% exercise session is different from the 80% session (P < 0.05). (Courtesy of Szymanski LM, Pate RR: *Med Sci Sports Exerc* 26:1102–1108, 1994.)

▶ There is growing evidence that the risk of cardiac events is greatest in the morning, and the diurnal variation of fibrinolytic activity described here may contribute to this phenomenon. Other variables with a circadian rhythm that must be factored into the overall equation include surges in cortisol level (1), increases in circulating catecholamines (2), changes in heart rate and blood pressure (3), and enhanced platelet aggregability (4). It remains difficult to decide what is the optimum time of day for a person to exercise, inasmuch as temperatures and ozone levels are more favorable in the early morning; other factors being equal, the cool of evening may be the best time for the older individual to exercise.

The other issue raised by this paper is the appropriate intensity of exercise for the prevention of cardiac events. Because fibrinolytic activity is more enhanced at 80% than at 50% of maximal oxygen intake, is 50% an adequate intensity of effort? The graphs suggest that although there is some added benefit from exercising at the higher intensity, much of the gain is already realized at 50% of maximum aerobic effort.—R.J. Shephard, M.D., Ph.D., D.P.E.

References

1. Weitzman ED, Fukushima D, Nogeire C, et al: *J Clin Endocrinol Metab* 33:14–22, 1971.
2. Turton MB, Deegan T: *Clin Chim Acta* 55:389–397, 1974.
3. Millar-Craig MW, Bishop CN, Raferty EB: *Lancet* 1:795–797, 1978.

4. Tofler GH, Brezinski DA, Schafer AI, et al: N Engl J Med 316:1514–1518, 1987.

Morning Increase in Ambulatory Ischemia in Patients With Stable Coronary Artery Disease: Importance of Physical Activity and Increased Cardiac Demand

Parker JD, Testa MA, Jimenez AH, Tofler GH, Muller JE, Parker JO, Stone PH (Brigham and Women's Hosp, Boston; Harvard Medical School, Boston; Harvard School of Public Health, Boston; et al)

Circulation 89:604–614, 1994   139-95-9–19

Introduction.—Acute cardiac ischemic events tend to occur in the first hours after awakening in the morning, and reversible episodes of myocardial ischemia exhibit a similar pattern. A better understanding of how ambulatory ischemia develops may help in creating appropriate interventions.

Study Plan.—A double-blind, randomized, placebo-controlled trial was carried out at 2 clinical centers in an attempt to determine whether the concentration of ambulatory ischemia in the morning results from physical activity or whether it reflects a basic endogenous circadian phenomenon such as altered coronary vasomotor tone. Initially, patients received either nadolol, up to a maximum dose of 120 mg daily, or a placebo for 5–7 days. The mean dose was 100 mg daily. The patients then were admitted for ambulatory ECG monitoring during a 2-day period, with 1 day of regular activities and 1 during which the usual morning activities were deferred.

Results.—In the 19 patients evaluated, nadolol reduced the systolic blood pressure and heart rate in the hospital phase. Most ECG manifestations of cardiac ischemia were significantly reduced by nadolol compared with placebo use. In placebo recipients, ischemic episodes were most numerous between 8 AM and noon on the day of regular activity but occurred 3–4 hours later when activity was deferred (Fig 9–12). Nadolol treatment abolished the peak of ischemic episodes at the time activity began in the morning. No circadian variation in ischemic episodes was evident during treatment with nadolol. In patients given nadolol, the increase in heart rate before ischemic episodes occurring in the late afternoon or at night was significantly less than in those occurring at other times.

Implications.—The peak in myocardial ischemia noted in the morning hours is related to physical activity rather than any endogenous phenomenon. β-Blockade is associated with ischemic episodes that do not follow a rise in heart rate, events that may result in part from episodic coronary vasoconstriction. Combined treatment with a β-blocker and either an organic nitrate or a calcium channel antagonist may effectively prevent these episodes.

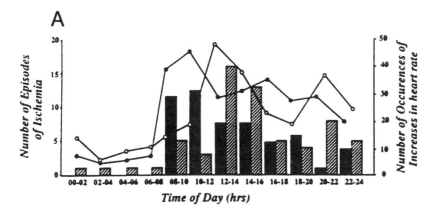

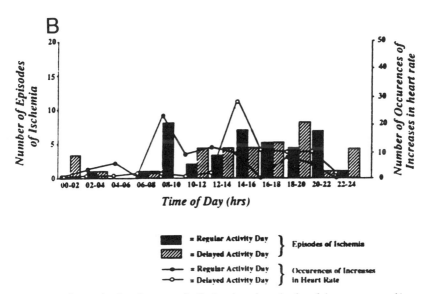

Fig 9–12.—Bar graphs show frequency distribution throughout the day of the occurrences of heart rate increases ≥ 5 beats/min and the number of episodes of ambulatory ischemia. **A,** placebo therapy; **B,** nadolol therapy. (Courtesy of Parker JD, Testa MA, Jimenez AH, et al: *Circulation* 89:604–614, 1994.)

▶ Many middle-aged joggers exercise before work because it arouses them and, in the summer, the weather is cooler. However, recent research show-ing a predominance of ischemic events in the morning has led to the sugges-tion that this practice needs to be changed, particularly in patients in whom there is some suspicion regarding the adequacy of coronary circulation. The authors suggest that the reason for the concentration of ischemic incidents in the morning is an increase in physical activity rather than some intrinsic circadian rhythm. There is about a fivefold increase in the risk of myocardial infarction during physical activity (1, 2), but if this increase in activity is the sole explanation for the morning incidents, it is hard to see why physical activity is greater during the morning than during the afternoon. A more reasonable explanation is that a circadian rhythm of some type leaves the body more vulnerable to the adverse effects of physical activity in the first few hours after waking but that this adverse response can be avoided by resting.

If possible, it seems desirable to move exercise from morning to evening. In most parts of Canada, at least, acceptable temperatures are found in the evening, and problems of sleeplessness can be avoided if the exercise is not done too late in the evening. If morning exercise in unavoidable, this report also suggests that β-blocking agents may offer a useful reduction of danger to the coronary-prone individual.—R.J. Shephard, M.D., Ph.D., D.P.E.

References

1. Shephard RJ: *Br J Sports Med* 8:101–110, 1974.
2. Siscovick DS: Risks of exercising: Sudden cardiac death and injuries, in: Bouchard C, Shephard RJ, Stephens T, et al: (eds): *Exercise, Fitness and Health*, Champaign, Ill: Human Kinetics Publishers, 1990, pp 707–713.

Arrhythmias and ST Segment Deviation During Prolonged Exhaustive Exercise (Ski Marathon) in Healthy Middle-Aged Men
Luurila OJ, Karjalainen J, Viitasalo M, Toivonen L (Lääkäriasema Koe Oy, Helsinki; Central Military Hosp, Helsinki; Helsinki Univ Central Hosp)
Eur Heart J 15:507–513, 1994   139-95-9–20

Background.—Day-long ski marathons have become popular in Europe in recent years. Many participants are middle-aged men who may

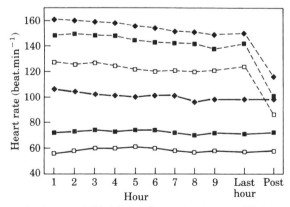

Fig 9–13.—Mean hourly maximal (*filled diamond*), mean hourly average (*filled square*), and minimal (*open square*) heart rate during skiing (*dashed line*) and during regular daily activities (*solid line*) in 37 participants of the skiing marathons. The mean values of the group are indicated by the *arrow*. (Courtesy of Luurila OJ, Karjalainen J, Viitasalo M, et al: *Eur Heart J* 15:507–513, 1994.)

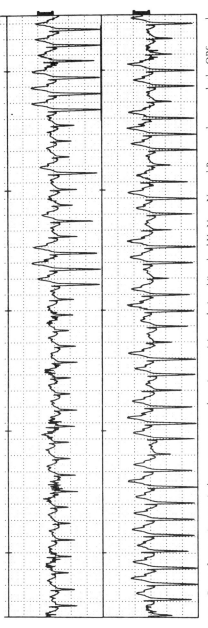

Fig 9–14.—Runs of successive ventricular premature complexes in a participant during skiing, lead V$_1$. Note: Normal P waves also precede the QRS complexes during tachycardia because the sinus and tachycardia frequencies were nearly identical at the beginning of tachycardia. The QRS complexes are fusion beats. (Courtesy of Luurila OJ, Karjalainen J, Viitasalo M, et al: *Eur Heart J* 15:507–513, 1994.)

have unrecognized ischemic heart disease. There is concern that the combination of prolonged strenuous exercise, cold weather, and coronary heart disease could result in an increased risk of sudden death among marathon skiers. Thirty-seven healthy middle-aged men were randomly selected from participants in a ski marathon to evaluate the occurrence of arrhythmias and silent ischemia.

Methods.—Most of the 37 men (aged 40–56 years) had completed at least 4 previous ski marathons. Before skiing, all underwent a chest x-ray examination, 12-lead ECG, and routine laboratory tests. Eighteen men took part in 75-km Finlandia skiing and 19 in 90-km Pirkka skiing; both races began at 7 AM or 8 AM. Ambient air temperatures ranged from −23°C to −5°C Two-channel ambulatory electrocardiographic recorders recorded the ECG during skiing. Immediately after the race, the study participants had another physical examination, underwent blood pressure and axillar temperature measurements, and were interviewed about symptoms.

Results.—The 12-lead ECG was normal in 28 men; 4 had signs of left ventricular hypertrophy. Two men had a history of mitral valve prolapse. All had normal chest radiograph results. The highest and lowest mean hourly heart rates were 150 and 138 beats · min^{-1} during the marathon (Fig 9–13). The mean maximum heart rate, 161 beats · min^{-1}, occurred in most skiers during the first hour of the 7–12 hour races. Thirty-three of 37 men experienced ventricular premature complexes. Complex forms were recorded in 8 men and atrial ectopics in 33 men (Fig 9–14). The frequency of arrhythmias did not increase during the marathon. During the first hour of skiing, 3 men had asymptomatic ST segment depression (0.2–0.3 mV) of 2–10 minutes' duration. One man showed marginal ST segment depression at electrocardiography, but all had normal results at exercise thallium scintigraphy and echocardiography.

Conclusion.—Apparently healthy middle-aged men participating in a day-long ski marathon in extreme weather conditions were found to have a significant increase in cardiac arrhythmias relative to their normal daily activities. The 3 men with short episodes of possible ischemia had no subsequent evidence of coronary artery disease. Although long-distance skiing under these conditions appears to carry few risks of serious cardiac complications, organizers should be aware that the race is potentially more dangerous to participants in the first hour.

▶ In Europe, day-long ski marathons attract more than 30,000 skiers each winter, many of them middle-aged men. Unrecognized coronary heart disease causes an increased risk of sudden death in such men during marathon running and squash playing. This study appraises arrhythmia risk during marathon skiing. Cold activates the sympathetic nervous system and increases vascular resistance and blood pressure, thus increasing myocardial oxygen consumption, especially during the first few minutes of exercise. Ski racing thus seems riskier in the first few minutes; this fits with the finding that all 6 sudden deaths in 10 years of a Swedish ski marathon were during the first hour of the race.

In this study, a significant increase in cardiac arrhythmias was found during an exhaustive day-long ski marathon, but only 8 men (22%) had complex forms of ventricular premature complexes. Three men (8%) had short episodes of possible ischemia, but none had evidence of coronary heart disease on a subsequent exercise thallium scintigram. The frequency of arrhythmias did not increase during the skiing period. The risk of dying during cross-country skiing is estimated to be 1 death in 600,000 hours of skiing. Marathon skiing thus seems safe even in middle-aged men, but a warm-up is key to reducing the risk of arrhythmias during the early phases. Organizers should be alert for possible cardiac arrest, especially during the first hour of a race.—E.R. Eichner, M.D.

Extent of Cardiac Autonomic Denervation in Relation to Angina on Exercise Test in Patients With Recent Acute Myocardial Infarction
Hartikainen J, Mäntysaari M, Kuikka J, Länsimies E, Pyörälä K (Kuopio Univ Hosp, Helsinki; Research Inst of Military Medicine, Helsinki; Central Military Hosp, Helsinki)
Am J Cardiol 74:760–763, 1994   139-95-9–21

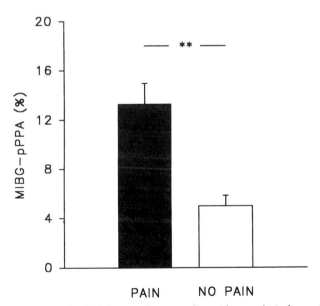

Fig 9–15.—The extent of viable left ventricular myocardium with sympathetic denervation (*MIBG-PPPA*) in patients with (pain, $n = 7$) and without (no pain, $n = 8$) angina pectoris during early exercise testing after myocardial infarction (mean ± SEM). **$P < 0.001$, Mann-Whitney test. (Courtesy of Hartikainen J, Mäntysaari M, Kuikka J, et al: *Am J Cardiol* 74:760-763, 1994.)

Introduction.—The link between ischemia and cardiac pain is still elusive. Documented ischemia is not always accompanied by pain, and more than one third of patients with acute myocardial infarction have no prior symptoms. Anginal pain has been linked to sympathetic nerves within the heart. If so, sympathetic denervation should reduce or remove the anginal pain that comes with myocardial infarction.

Methods.—The 15 men, aged 35–65 years, had survived their first infarction. Before discharge, a symptom-limited cycle ergometer test was performed. Three months after the infarction, single-photon emission tomography with I-123 metaiodobenzylguanidine (MIBG), I-123 paraphenylpentadecanoic acid (pPPA), and Tc-99m sestamibi (MIBI) were used to estimate the extent of denervated myocardium, the extent of the infarction, and myocardial perfusion, respectively.

Results.—There were no significant differences between patients who experienced angina during exercise testing and those who did not. The largest defect was detected with MIBG. This showed a 17% reduction of left ventricular mass. In men in whom angina developed, the area of viable but denervated myocardium was larger than in men who did not have angina develop (Fig 9–15). Defects detected by pPPA and MIBI averaged 8.3% and 8.6%, respectively. Smaller areas of denervated myocardium were found in patients with silent ischemia.

Conclusion.—The extent of viable yet denervated myocardium is associated with increased pain sensitivity in patients with a history of recent infarction. Infarction can result in partial denervation. The remaining myocardium may be supersensitive to increased adrenergic stimulation, or other hormones may increase sensitivity to exercise-induced angina.

▶ Contrary to the predictions of Hartikainen et al., an area of viable but sympathetically denervated myocardium increased the chances of exercise-related angina developing. One limitation of their study is that perfusion measurements were not made during exercise. It may thus be that the patients in whom angina developed had a particularly poor blood flow during exercise. Two possible explanations for the association between denervation and ischemic pain are suggested by Hartikainen and associates: an imbalance between vagal and sympathetic activity may be involved (1, 2); or the sympathetic denervation may not be complete, so that the remaining nerve endings become hypersensitive to humoral stimuli (3).—R.J. Shephard, M.D., Ph.D., D.P.E.

References

1. Foreman RD: Spinothalamic tract and cardial afferents, in: Lown B, Malliani A, Prosdocimi M (eds): *Neural Mechanisms and Cardiovascular Disease.* New York, Springer-Verlag, 1986, pp 169–181.
2. Sheps DS, Maixner W, Hinderliter AL, et al: *Isr J Med Sci* 25:482–487, 1989.
3. Kammerling JM: *Circulation* 76:383–393, 1987.

Composition of Human Pulmonary Surfactant Varies With Exercise and Level of Fitness

Doyle IR, Jones ME, Barr HA, Orgeig S, Crockett AJ, McDonald CF, Nicholas TE (Flinders Med Ctr, Adelaide, Australia)
Am J Respir Crit Care Med 149:1619–1627, 1994   139-95-9–22

Background.—Pulmonary surfactant promotes pulmonary compliance by reducing surface tension at the gas–liquid interface. Variations in surface tension during breathing reflect changes in the mixture of surfactant components of the monomolecular layer at the interface. The changes observed in alveolar surfactant of the rat lung involve the differential handling of disaturated phospholipids (DSP) and cholesterol.

Objective and Methods.—An exercise study was done in 13 men aged 20–46 years to learn whether the amount and composition of alveolar surfactant change in humans as functions of the breathing pattern and the level of fitness. Cycle exercise was done for 30 minutes at 90% of the maximum heart rate. Bronchoalveolar lavage was then repeated, and the samples were analyzed for surfactant protein A (SP-A), DSP, and cholesterol. The work rate–heart rate ratio was taken as a measure of fitness.

Results.—Direct relations were confirmed between the levels of cholesterol and DSP in bronchoalveolar lavage fluid and between both these constituents and SP-A. The change in the cholesterol/DSP ratio correlated negatively with the level of physical fitness, with a correlation coefficient of -0.56. The SP-A/cholesterol and SP-A/DSP ratios correlated directly with fitness, with respective correlation coefficients of 0.75 and 0.62.

Conclusions.—The composition of alveolar surfactant changes rapidly in response to exercise in humans. The findings are consistent with the presence of at least 2 types of surfactant of differing composition in the alveolar compartment.

▶ The surface tension in the pulmonary membrane is so high that in the absence of some agent to reduce tension, the alveoli would quickly collapse. However, the tension also depends on alveolar dimensions, and the body thus needs a substance of variable surfactant properties to stabilize the alveoli during both inspiration and expiration. Alveolar surfactant seemingly accomplishes this remarkable feat by a change in its composition during the breathing cycle. The changes need to be larger during vigorous exercise than during resting ventilation; hence, the rapid alteration in cholesterol/DSP ratio during exercise: There is an associated change in the physical properties of the monomolecular layer, from a liquid crystalline state at high lung volumes to a gel at low lung volumes (1).

Cholesterol is an integral part of the surfactant, and changes in cholesterol/DSP ratios might thus be anticipated during a prolonged training program that reduces body reserves of cholesterol. Cholesterol reduces the viscosity of the DSPs; this allows the layer to spread more easily over the alveolar surface but also facilitates its escape from the air spaces. In the most fit subjects, the cholesterol/DSP ratio decreases during vigorous exercise, presumably optimizing compliance for these conditions. Less fit subjects have a higher cholesterol/DSP ratio during exercise, and this might contribute to the dyspnea that they report.—R.J. Shephard, M.D., Ph.D., D.P.E.

Reference

1. Goerke J, Clements JA: Alveolar surface tension and lung surfactant, in Fishman AP (ed): *Handbook of Physiology: Respiratory System III*, 1985, pp 247–261.

Vertebral-Artery Dissection Following a Judo Session: A Case Report
Lannuzel A, Moulin T, Amsallem D, Galmiche J, Rumbach L (CHU Jean Minjoz, Besançon, France)
Neuropediatrics 25:106–108, 1994   139-95-9–23

Background.—Vertebral artery dissection is well recognized in young adults, in whom it generally occurs after cervical trauma. It is rare in chil-

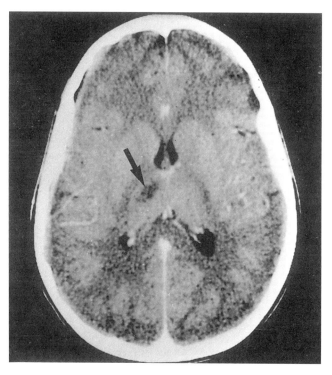

Fig 9–16.—Left thalamic infarct involving the tuberothalamic territory (*arrow*). (Courtesy of Lannuzel A, Moulin T, Amsallem D, et al: *Neuropediatrics* 25:106-108, 1994.)

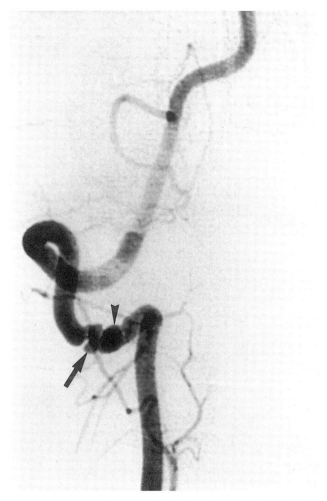

Fig 9–17.—Angiography: type 1 fibromuscular dysplasia ("string-of-beads" lesion) (*arrow*) with arterial dilatations (*arrowhead*) and strictures on the V3 segment of the left vertebral artery. (Courtesy of Lannuzel A, Moulin T, Amsallem D, et al: *Neuropediatrics* 25:106-108, 1994.)

dren, with only a few cases reported. A child with left vertebral artery dissection occurring after a judo session was described.

Case Report.—Boy, 11 years, was admitted a few days after sustaining rotation of the cervical column during a judo session. Signs and symptoms at presentation included dizziness, aphasia, and ataxia with left cervical stiffness. A low-density lesion consistent with an infarct was seen in the left thalamus (Fig 9–16). On selective angiography, the finding of a "string-of-beads" lesion suggested the presence of type 1 fibromuscular dysplasia (FMD) of the left vertebral artery, probably complicated by dissection (Fig 9–17). Treatment consisted of anticoagulation, along with bed rest and cervical support. The child was discharged with-out complaints after 2 weeks. At 3 months' follow-up, when oral anticoagulation was discontinued, the examination was normal.

Discussion.—The diagnosis of vertebral artery dissection should be considered in patients with cervical pain associated with neurologic signs of vertebrobasilar stroke, particularly when occurring after cervical trauma or rotatory motion. The diagnosis is mainly angiographic. The main arteriopathy predisposing to arterial dissection is FMD, the most frequent angiographic sign of which is the so-called string-of-beads sign. If the dissection occurs after unusual activities or minor trauma, it may be best to avoid such precipitating factors in the future.

▶ An excellent clinical depiction and discussion of vertebral artery dissection. The proximate cause seemed to be neck rotation during judo. The root cause was FMD, an uncommon, segmental, nonatheromatous disease of small- to medium-sized arteries, encountered in an estimated 1% of cerebral angiograms. Vertebral artery dissection has also been reported after minor, nonpenetrating neck traumas from ceiling painting, yoga, gymnastics, or chiropractic manipulation. Choking in judo can also cause anoxia, brain damage, and possibly stroke (1).—E.R. Eichner, M.D.

Reference

1. 1993 Year Book of Sports Medicine, pp 235–236.

Length of Postexercise Assessment in the Determination of Exercise-Induced Bronchospasm
Brudno DS, Wagner JM, Rupp NT (Med College of Georgia, Augusta)
Ann Allergy 73:227–231, 1994   139-95-9–24

Background.—Exercise-induced bronchospasm generally is established by a 10% to 20% decline in forced expiratory volume in 1 second (FEV_1). The maximum decrease is observed after 6–8 minutes of continuous exercise, even if exercise continues beyond this time.

Objective.—A group of 397 middle and high school athletes, 12–18 years of age, underwent an exercise challenge to detect exercise-induced bronchospasm.

Methods.—After reproducible baseline spirometric findings were recorded, the participants exercised on a treadmill by warming up and then running for 6 minutes at 6 mph on a 10% grade until 85% of the predicted maximum heart rate was reached, the minimal rate being 170 beats per minute.

Results.—Based on a threshold FEV_1 response of 10% or greater, 187 of the 397 participants had a positive response. One fifth of these responses were noted 20 and 30 minutes after exercise. Sixteen positive

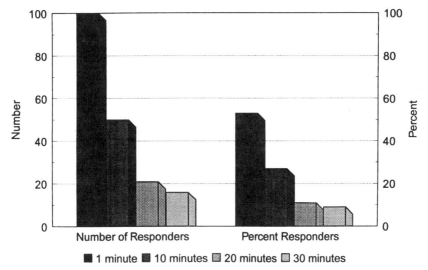

Fig 9–18.—Exercise-induced bronchospasm diagnosed using forced expiratory volume in 1 second (*FEV₁*). Time represents duration after exercise at which testing was performed. The threshold for a positive test is FEV₁ ≥ 10%. (Courtesy of Brudno DS, Wagner JM, Rupp NT: *Ann Allergy* 73:227-231, 1994.)

responders (9%) would have gone unrecognized had the test ended at 20 minutes (Fig 9–18). At a threshold FEV₁ of 15%, 125 subjects had positive test results and 16 would have been missed on a 20-minute test. With a threshold value of 20% and greater, 90 subjects had positive responses, 13 of them only at 30 minutes after exercise.

Implication.—Exercise-induced bronchospasm may be more prevalent than has been suggested by studies that end 20 minutes rather than 30 minutes after an exercise challenge.

▶ Exercise-induced asthma (EIA) goes way back. In the second century A.D., Aretaeus said, "If from running, gymnastic exercise or any other work, the breathing becomes difficult, it is called asthma." Strangely, but perhaps understandably, EIA is on the increase. One reason is clear from this study: diagnosis of EIA depends on how you define it and when you do the test. If you define EIA as a 10% decline in FEV₁, you find twice as many people with asthma than when a 20% decline is your cutoff. Similarly, if you extend testing up to and beyond 30 minutes after exercise, you pick up another 10% of those with asthma. At the elite athlete level, however, probably the main reason EIA is increasing is that athletes believe inhaled bronchodilators are ergogenic.

The general prevalence of EIA is perhaps 15%, yet at the 1994 Winter Olympic Games, nearly 60% of the competitors declared they had EIA. An alarming epidemic! But an epidemic of what? Most, but not all, studies find that the "approved" inhaled bronchodilators (e.g., albuterol, salbutamol) are not ergogenic (1). A recent study finds that the long-acting bronchodilator, salmeterol, is not ergogenic (2). Yet, so far, salmeterol is banned by the United States Olympic Committee. Anyway, the way things are going, soon 100% of Olympic athletes will have "asthma."—E.R. Eichner, M.D.

References

1. 1993 YEAR BOOK OF SPORTS MEDICINE, pp 289–291.
2. Robertson W, et al: *Eur Respir J* 7:1978, 1994.

Effect of Inhaled PGE$_2$ on Exercise-Induced Bronchoconstriction in Asthmatic Subjects

Melillo E, Woolley KL, Manning PJ, Watson RM, O'Byrne PM (McMaster Univ, Hamilton, Ontario)
Am J Respir Crit Care Med 149:1138–1141, 1994   139-95-9–25

Background.—The endogenous release of inhibitory prostanoids appears to restrict the bronchoconstrictor response to repeated exercise. The ability of inhaled prostaglandin (PG)E$_2$ to attenuate exercise-induced bronchoconstriction or methacholine airway responsiveness was studied in patients with asthma.

Methods.—Eight patients with mild, stable asthma and exercise bronchoconstriction were assessed on 4 separate days, 48 hours apart. The patients were given PGE$_2$ or placebo to inhale in a randomized, crossover, double-blind manner 30 minutes before exercise or methacholine challenge.

Findings.—Exercise bronchoconstriction was significantly attenuated by PGE$_2$ inhalation. The mean maximal percentage decrease in forced expiratory volume in 1 second (FEV$_1$) after exercise was 26% after placebo and 9.7% after PEG$_2$. However, methacholine airway responsiveness was not significantly attenuated by PGE$_2$. The geometric mean methacholine provocative level causing a 20% decrease in FEV$_1$ was 0.77 after placebo and 1.41 after PGE$_2$.

Conclusions.—Inhaled PGE$_2$ markedly attenuates exercise bronchoconstriction in individuals with asthma. This effect apparently does not occur through functional antagonism of airway smooth muscle.

▶ The dramatic reduction of exercise-induced bronchospasm by PGE$_2$ is interesting. The authors draw a parallel with the attenuation of allergic responses by PGE$_2$ and suggest that PG may be inhibiting the release of mediators or causing vascular changes that speed the removal of spasmogens. However, the data that are presented seem to be a classic example of an experiment with inadequate statistical power. The observations do not really rule out mediation of the reduction of exercise-induced spasm by an inhibition of bronchial smooth muscle, inasmuch as the dose of methacholine needed to induce a 20% decrease in FEV$_1$ is almost twice the initial amount after PG administration. The authors dismiss this difference as "nonsignificant," but the reason for the nonsignificance is as likely to be the small subject pool and variability of the response as the absence of any effect. Indeed, there is quite a bit of evidence, both in vivo and in vitro, that PGE_2 is a bronchial relaxant (1, 2). —R.J. Shephard, M.D., Ph.D., D.P.E.

References

1. Smith AP, Cuthbert MF, Dunlop MS: *Clin Sci* 48:421–430, 1975.
2. Gardiner PJ: *Prostaglandins* 10:607–616, 1975.

Apple-Dependent Exercise-Induced Anaphylaxis

Añíbarro B, Domínguez C, Díaz JM, Martín MF, García-Ara, MC, Boyano MT, Ojeda JA ("La Paz" Hosp, Madrid)

Allergy 49:481–482, 1994   139-95-9–26

Background.— Exercise-induced anaphylaxis, a form of physical allergy occurring in association with physical exercise, is seen with pruritus, urticaria, and erythema before progressing to upper respiratory obstruction or vascular collapse. A prerequisite for its development in susceptible patients is the ingestion of a specific food. In the case reported here, an apple was the trigger.

Case Report.— Girl, 12 years, who had been playing basketball for 30 minutes was seen at a clinic because of an episode of warmth, intense pruritus of the palms, erythema, facial angioedema, and urticaria, accompanied by dysphonia, difficulty breathing, and weakness. She reported eating an apple immediately before the exercise. Treatment with epinephrine, antihistamines, and corticosteroids relieved cutaneous symptoms, but angioedema persisted for a week. She had a family history of atopy and complained of mild seasonal rhinitis. She had no previous reactions to apples or other fresh fruits and had no similar symptoms when exercising. The physical examination and laboratory assessment were unremarkable when she was asymptomatic. Total IgE level was 60 kIU/L and prick tests were negative except for *Artemisia vulgaris* pollen. The prick-by-prick test with fresh apple was positive, and specific IgE determination revealed class 2 against both apple and *A. vulgaris* pollen. Testing with an open oral challenge with apple was negative. On separate days, indoor exercise challenge tests were given, 1 with the patient fasting and 1 given 1 hour after she had ingested an apple. Both were negative. A free-run outdoor exercise challenge administered 1 hour after eating an apple resulted 10 minutes later in intense pruritus of the palms and fingers and rhinoconjunctivitis. Within another 5 minutes, she had generalized urticaria and facial angioedema develop. Immediate treatment with epinephrine, antihistamines, and corticosteroids was followed, 10 minutes later, with symptoms progressing to cough and difficult breathing. Treatment with inhaled salbutamol and epinephrine resulted in resolution of the episode within 2 hours, although angioedema lasted for several hours. An additional outside exercise challenge after the intake of other foodstuffs was negative.

Conclusion.— Little is known about the physiopathologic mechanisms of exercise-induced anaphylaxis. In this case, it was probably caused by a combined effect of apple allergens, exercise, and environmental factors on mast-cell releasability.

▶ Another case, well studied, of food-dependent, exercise-induced anaphylaxis. This girl had an IgE-mediated allergy to apple, but neither apple alone nor exercise alone evoked anaphylaxis—it took both together. Presumably, the exercise increases the amount of histamine that would be released from just eating the apple. In this case, an apple a day keeps the doctor employed. See past reports of 13 similar cases (1, 2); food triggers include shellfish, peaches, grapes, wheat, fennel, lettuce, tomato, and celery. Proper diagnosis offers prevention by avoiding the culprit food and early self-treatment via an epinephrine kit that the athlete carries.—E.R. Eichner, M.D.

References

1. 1993 YEAR BOOK OF SPORTS MEDICINE, pp 375–376.
2. 1992 YEAR BOOK OF SPORTS MEDICINE, pp 243–245.

Bronchoconstriction Occurring During Exercise in Asthmatic Subjects

Beck KC, Offord KP, Scanlon PD (Mayo Clinic and Found, Rochester, Minn)
Am J Respir Crit Care Med 149:352–357, 1994   139-95-9–27

Objective.—Most studies investigating airway function during exercise in patients with exercise-induced asthma have documented bronchodilation, although many patients with asthma report symptoms that develop during exercise. To investigate further, physiologic changes associated with asthma symptoms were documented using exercise protocols that more closely mimic typical exercise.

Study Design.—Four men and 4 women with exercise-induced asthma were studied during sustained constant-load and interval exercise while breathing dry air at room temperature. In constant-load exercise, the participants pedaled a cycle ergometer at 50% of their maximal power output for 36 minutes. With interval exercise, they pedaled at 60% of maximal power for 6 minutes and then at 40% of maximal power for 6 minutes; the 12-minute cycle was repeated 3 times for a total exercise time of 36 minutes. Maximal expiratory flow vs. volume maneuvers (MEFV) were obtained before, at 6-minute intervals during, and at 5-minute intervals after exercise. Changes in peak expiratory flow (PEF), forced expiratory volume in 1 second (FEV_1), and forced expiratory flow at 50% of preexercise vital capacity (FEF_{50}) were compared with preexercise values.

Results.—Within 15 minutes after a maximal 1-minute incremental exercise protocol, PEF decreased by 22%, FEV_1 fell by 21%, and FEF_{50} decreased by 41% compared with preexercise values. With constant-load exercise, no significant changes in MEFV flows occurred until 18 minutes, when FEV_1 fell by 6% and FEF_{50} decreased by 14%, with minimal changes in PEF. In interval exercise, when exercise intensity was reduced from 60% to 40%, mean PEF fell by 10%, FEV_1 decreased by 10%, and FEF_{50} fell by 24%, but these flows increased toward preexercise values when exercise intensity was increased again to 60% of maximal power.

Discussion.—In patients with exercise-induced asthma, bronchoconstriction can develop during exercise using variable-intensity exercise protocols. Bronchoconstriction occurs when exercise intensity is reduced, although the constriction is reversed by a return to higher exercise intensity. There appears to be no significant refractoriness to the bronchoconstriction at lower intensities during exercise. These findings may explain why some patients with asthma complain of symptoms during exercise. It is hypothesized that airway function during exercise may reflect a dynamic balance between bronchocontriction and bronchodilating influences, and this balance can be altered rapidly by changes in exercise intensity.

▶ Most investigators have reported that patients with asthma show a bronchodilation during exercise, with a larger bronchospasm that develops 5 to 10 minutes after ceasing activity. However, such timing is at variance with what many patients describe. The discrepancy seems caused, in part, by the brief duration of the usual laboratory exercise test. This paper is useful in showing what happens if a patient continues moderate exercise for a longer period. In fact, there then seems to be a tendency to spasm during activity, but this is readily reversed on moving to a higher intensity of exercise. The liberation of catecholamines might be invoked as an explanation of the early bronchodilation, but against this hypothesis the bronchodilation is not prevented by administration of β-blocking drugs (1). It is unclear whether the bronchodilator response is simply a withdrawal of vagal tone or whether vasoactive peptide (2) or relaxing factors (3) are involved.—R.J. Shephard, M.D., Ph.D., D.P.E.

References

1. Larsson K, Martinsson A, Hjemdahl P: *Thorax* 41:552–558, 1986.
2. Hvidsten D, Jenssen TG, Bolle R, et al: *Eur J Respir Dis* 68:326–331, 1986.
3. Tessier GJ, Lackner PA, O'Grady SM, et al: *Respir Physiol* 84:105–114, 1991.

High- vs Low-Intensity Inspiratory Muscle Interval Training in Patients With COPD

Preusser BA, Winningham ML, Clanton TL (Ohio State Univ, Columbus; Ohio State Univ Hosps, Columbus)

Chest 106:110–117, 1994   139-95-9–28

Background.—Respiratory muscle training improves respiratory muscle and exercise performance in patients with chronic obstructive pulmonary disease (COPD), but it is not known whether high-intensity or low-intensity muscle training is most effective. The effect of a high- vs. low-resistive inspiratory muscle interval training protocol was studied in patients with severe COPD.

Methods.—A double-blind, 2-group, repeated-measures design was used in 22 patients with COPD. Of the 20 patients completing the 12-week study, 12 (including 6 women) were randomly assigned to the high-resistance group and 8 (including 7 women) to the low-resistance group. The patients used a threshold trainer (Threshold, Healthscan Products) three times weekly, and the work-to-rest ratio was increased each week. The duration of the training sessions progressed from 5 minutes per session in week 1 to 18 minutes per session in week 12. The high-resistance group trained at 75% of the maximum pressure load achieved during the inspiratory threshold loading test; the low-resistance group trained at 30% of the maximum pressure load. Testing was done at baseline, monthly, and within 3 days of completing the program.

Results.—Compared with their baseline evaluations, both groups improved in incremental inspiratory threshold loading, inspiratory muscle endurance, and the 12-minute distance walking test. Only the high-resistance group showed a significant increase (35%) in the inspiratory muscle strength test. These variables did not differ significantly between the 2 groups, but the patients with the greatest degree of lung hyperinflation appeared to benefit most from high-resistance training. All patients tolerated the interval training well.

Conclusions.—In patients with severe COPD, both high- and low-intensity interval training are effective in conditioning the respiratory muscles. No significant difference in the effectiveness of the 2 methods was found, other than the gain in inspiratory muscle strength in the high-intensity group. The incremental loading test is useful for evaluating these patients.

▶ It is now widely acknowledged that training programs do little to reverse the loss of pulmonary function in COPD (1). Nevertheless, the ventilatory capacity, and thus the effort tolerance, of such patients can be enhanced if they learn a breathing pattern in which inspiration is very rapid and expiration is very slow. To maximize this tactic, it is important to strengthen their inspiratory muscles. Because the sample size was small, only 1 of 4 comparisons of inspiratory muscle function in this study shows a statistically significant advantage to the high-resistance group. Nevertheless, the size of the gains with the high-resistance treatment was larger on all 4 tests. The lesson seems to be that breathing exercises should use the highest resistance the patient can tolerate.—R.J. Shephard, M.D., Ph.D., D.P.E.

Reference

1. Shephard RJ: *Exerc Sports Sci Rev* 4:263–296, 1976.

Strategies for Physical and Ventilatory Training for Patients Before and After Lung Transplantation

Gimenez M, Abril E, Chabot F, Villemot JP, Mattei F, Polu JM (Centre Hospitalier Universitaire de Brabois, Vandoeuvre-lès-Nancy, France)
Médecine du Sport 68:146–156, 1994   139-95-9–29

Introduction.—One reason some institutions are not well suited to doing lung transplantations is the unavailability of a well-equipped exercise physiology laboratory staffed by competent personnel. This institution has a well-equipped, well-staffed facility to train patients with severe chronic obstructive pulmonary disease (COPD) awaiting lung or heart/ lung transplantation and to provide post-transplant cardiopulmonary rehabilitation. Two high-intensity ergospirometric training regimens to improve ventilatory muscle endurance in patients with COPD have been proposed.

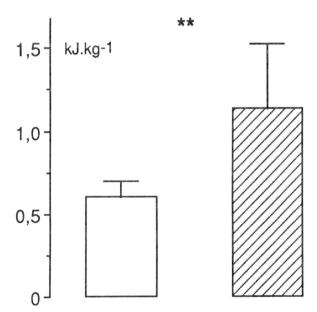

Fig 9–19.—Maximal 45-minute endurance intensity. Average maximal endurance intensity values observed in a group of 8 patients with severe chronic obstructive pulmonary disease who were subjected to a Square Wave Endurance Exercise Test (*SWEET*)-based program. At the end of the program, endurance capacity had nearly doubled. (Courtesy of Gimenez M, Abril E, Chabot F, et al: *Médecine du Sport* 68:146–156, 1994.)

Methods.—Both programs call for 45 minutes of continuous exercise. For patients who cannot exercise continuously for 45 minutes, three 15-minute exercise periods separated by 10-minute rest periods are proposed. Patients with more severe COPD may only be able to exercise for 10 minutes followed by 5-minute rest periods. The original 45-minute Square Wave Endurance Exercise Test (SWEET) was performed to design an individualized exercise program. Patients exercise on a cycle ergometer for 45 minutes while functional and ergometric measurements are obtained. The patient works at a submaximal aerobic exercise intensity for 5 minutes, followed by an intense 1-minute anaerobic peak. This sequence is repeated, and the patient will undertake 9 periods of peak exercise during a 45-minute period. Exercise intensity is increased as endurance increases. This individualized approach enables most patients with COPD to complete a 45-minute program without having to rest.

Patients.—Eight patients with severe COPD were trained, based on data obtained during the SWEET. Patients received oxygen while training, first once daily for 4 weeks, then for 1 week every 1 or 2 months until transplantation. During the SWEET, arterial blood oxygen saturation was monitored continuously for 45 minutes with an oxymeter. Six of the 8 patients improved their physical performance, sometimes dramatically (Fig 9-19). Four patients were able to exercise twice daily during the last 3 weeks of the program.

Conclusions.—The SWEET increases ventilatory and physical muscle power in patients with severe COPD who are awaiting lung transplantation. The SWEET is also suitable for patients who have undergone transplantation.

▶ A preliminary program of physical conditioning can make a major difference in both the ability of many categories of patients to withstand major surgery and also in the rate of recovery after surgery (1). It is interesting that this seems to be true even of the person with COPD. Although considerable symptomatic benefit has resulted from training programs for COPD, it has been harder to demonstrate objective gains in cardiorespiratory function (2). The favorable response seen in this study can be traced to 2 features: the interval training plan and the use of oxygen during training. Although the gains of aerobic performance look very large in the Figure 9–19, it is important to note that this reflects the tolerance of submaximal effort, a variable that is much easier to improve than maximal aerobic power.—R.J. Shephard, M.D., Ph.D., D.P.E.

References

1. Young A: Exercise, fitness and recovery from surgery, disease or infection, in: Bouchard C, Shephard RJ, Stephens T, et al (eds): *Exercise, Fitness and Health,* Champaign, Ill: Human Kinetics Publishers, 1990, pp 589–600.
2. Mertens DJ, Shephard RJ, Kavanagh T: *Respiration* 35:96–107, 1978.

Pre-Participation Physical Evaluations: Development of Uniform Guidelines

Smith DM (Univ of Kansas, Kansas City)
Sports Med 18:293–300, 1994   139-95-9–30

Introduction.—Until recently, no uniform guidelines have existed for the preparticipation evaluation (PPE) of young athletes. Several national medical organizations have now endorsed an educational monograph, *Preparticipation Physical Evaluation*, which was published in 1992 and is scheduled to be updated periodically.

Objectives of PPEs.—The overall goal of the PPE is to ensure the athlete's health and safety. Specifically, the evaluation can detect conditions that might limit participation or predispose athletes to injury; meet legal and insurance requirements and determine general health; counsel on health-related issues; and assess maturity, fitness level, and performance. Objectives considered primary are the detection of preexisting conditions and compliance with legal and insurance requirements. The remaining goals can be fulfilled if time and resources are available.

History and Physical Examination.—Feedback from those who have used the form has been favorable, although the form may have to be modified for different settings. Important additions would be questions designed to identify athletes with pathogenic body weight control behavior or those at risk for substance abuse. Attention to the cardiovascular examination is stressed because of the relation between certain cardiovascular conditions and sudden death in athletes. Areas under debate for inclusion in the PPE are appropriate screening laboratory, radiographic, and cardiovascular tests and HIV and drug testing. At present, HIV testing is neither justified nor recommended.

Frequency of PPEs and Clearance to Play.—Current recommendations are that a complete evaluation be done at least 6 weeks before the season for athletes entering a new program. Thereafter, a limited history and physical examination are conducted annually. Practitioners may not be able to prevent athletes from participating when results of the PPE are unfavorable. In such cases, the athlete or the athlete's parent or guardian may be required to sign an exculpatory waiver, thereby assuming the risk and relieving the physician from liability.

▶ The PPE plays an important role in the athlete's health care. After the original examination, screening physicals must also be done on an annual basis. This may be performed by athletic trainers or by other health care providers with knowledge and experience in this area. The author stresses the importance the PPE plays in detecting preexisting conditions and in meeting legal and insurance requirements. A good history and physical form may easily be adapted to meet the individual needs of your team or institution.—F.J. George, A.T.C., P.T.

Medical Considerations and Planning for Short Distance Road Races

Kleiner DM, Glickman SE (Illinois State Univ, Normal; Tampa Gen Hosp, Fla)
J Athletic Train 29:145–151, 1994   139-95-9–31

Background.—The medical support required to successfully cover long-distance races is well documented. However, little information has been presented on how best to provide for athletes participating in the shorter races that are currently popular in most communities. The types of problems encountered and a protocol for providing optimum care in short race events were documented.

Types of Problems.—In short-distance races, the causes of collapse can be easily defined. It is likely that the runners will be dehydrated and have elevated core temperatures. Short-distance race runners tend to train less and are often unfit. In contrast, runners who are well prepared tend to sprint the short distance and neglect to drink during the race. Combined with high temperatures, this can lead to severe heat illness.

Medical Tent Set-Up.—As an example, the medical tent for a simultaneous 5-km and 15-km race is staffed by 30 volunteers, including a medical director (an emergency room/trauma center staff physician), orthopedic surgeons, podiatrists, and a cardiologist, registered nurses, athletic trainers, and other paramedical staff. An attorney is present to ensure that release forms are signed by each patient before receiving treatment. This is important because of the legal ramifications involved in patient treatment: patients who have heat illness occasionally become incoherent or delirious. The tent is located near the finish line and has 3 areas: critical-medical, noncritical medical, and communications (Fig 9–20).

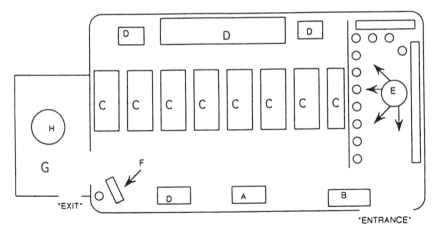

Fig 9–20.—Diagram of the medical tent showing the (A) communications table, (B) registration table, (C) critical-area gurneys, (D) supply table, (E) noncritical area with chairs, (F) checkout table, (G) annex, (H) plastic-covered area. (Courtesy of Kleiner DM, Glickman SE: *J Athletic Train* 29:145–151, 1994.)

Protocol.—Once admitted to the critical area, each patient undergoes triage and is classified. Vital signs are taken along with rectal temperature in those suspected to be hyperthermic/hypervolemic. In patients who have heat illness, intravenous fluid replacement (1,000 mL bag of D5 $1/4$ NS) is started immediately. Oral fluids are administered, and cold towels, mist bottles, and fans are used to cool the patient. Most runners are discharged after receiving 1 L of fluid. Any patient who receives more than 2 L must be reevaluated by the medical director.

Additional Areas of Coverage.—Medical staff are dispersed throughout the race course, at the finish line, and outside the medical tent to deal with overflow and to provide a recovery area for those who have mild symptoms. The finish line and the survey areas are monitored by physical therapists, athletic trainers, and emergency medical technicians who are in constant contact with the medical tent via 2-way radios. Licensed massage therapists are present in the survey areas. Aid stations are positioned along the race at water stations. Two roaming ambulances with advanced cardiac life support patrol the race. Finally, the hospital is placed on alert before the race so that it is ready for patients requiring more advanced care than can be provided by the medical tent.

▶ The authors present a good medical emergency plan for short-distance road races. Anyone who has worked these races will recognize the problems the authors present. Education of these runners can play an important role in preventing injuries. The importance of conditioning must be stressed for those unfit individuals who participate in these races. Proper hydration must be stressed for all runners; both the unfit and the world class runner will often be participating in the same race with as much as a 30- to 60-minute difference in finishing times.—F.J. George, A.T.C., P.T.

Gangrenous Streptococcal Myositis: Case Report
Hird B, Byrne K (Med Univ of South Carolina, Charleston)
J Trauma 36:589–591, 1994   139-95-9–32

Introduction.—Some soft tissue infections continue to have very high mortality. Bacterial infection of skeletal muscle is rarely encountered, and streptococcal infection resulting in gangrenous myonecrosis is rarer still. Occurrence and fulminant course of this infection in previously healthy patients can delay diagnosis and treatment, sometimes with fatal consequences. Gangrenous streptococcal myositis was initially diagnosed as a bruised thigh in 1 patient.

Case Report.—Boy, 17 years, sustained a bruised right thigh in a high school football game. The injury was considered minor, and the patient shortly returned to the game. Pain and swelling increased the next day, and the patient was given a nonsteroidal anti-inflammatory drug. Fever, vomiting and progressive pain and swelling during the next 3 days prompted the patient's referral. At examination,

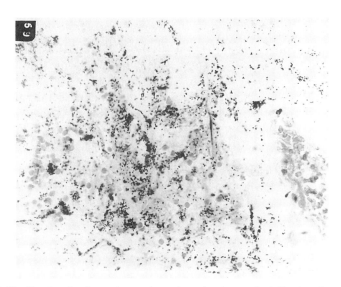

Fig 9–21.—Gram's stain of operative muscle specimen showing massive infiltration of gram-positive organisms. Original magnification, ×800. (Courtesy of Hird B, Byrne K: *J Trauma* 36:589–591, 1994.)

the thigh was swollen from the inguinal ligament to the knee and painful to the touch; the hemoglobin was 15 g/dL, the hematocrit 44%, and the white blood cell count 1.2 k. Magnetic resonance imaging showed no signs of hematoma or abscess; the lateral thigh compartment pressure was 22 mm Hg. Aspiration of the right knee revealed gram-positive bacteria (Fig 9–21).

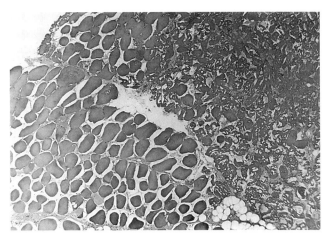

Fig 9–22.—Operative specimen demonstrating areas of normal striated muscle adjacent to areas of muscle necrosis. Hematoxylin-eosin stain; original magnification, ×70. (Courtesy of Hird B, Byrne K: *J Trauma* 36:589–591, 1994.)

The patient died on the thirteenth hospital day, despite high-dose IV penicillin G, exploration of the right thigh, hip disarticulation, and further débridement as the infection spread (Fig 9–22). The cause of death was overwhelming sepsis. All cultures were positive for β-hemolytic group A streptococci.

Discussion.—This case illustrates the consequences of failure to make an early diagnosis of streptococcal myositis. A high index of suspicion for this diagnosis is essential in patients with physical signs and symptoms of unknown cause or out of proportion to the injury. Aggressive antimicrobial and surgical treatment offers the best chance of survival. In this case, the use of a nonsteroidal anti-inflammatory drug may have contributed to the poor outcome.

▶ A tragic, fatal case of streptococcal myositis in a young quarterback who stayed home 3 days with increasing fever, vomiting, and pain and swelling in the right leg after diagnosis of a "thigh bruise" in a game is presented. Bacterial myositis is rare; fewer than 100 cases are cited in the American literature, only about 5% of which are from *Streptococcus*. At least in the early stages, myositis may mimic injury, cellulitis, or thrombophlebitis, and thus be diagnosed late, as happened here. The authors cite reports suggesting that treatment with nonsteroidal anti-inflammatory drugs may accelerate progression of bacterial myositis or necrotizing fasciitis by impeding polymorphonuclear leukocytes. This notion, however, remains anecdotal. Apparently, bacterial myositis may occur in apparently healthy young people with no risk factors and no history of trauma or recent infection. A possible clue in this case, however, is that the patient had been treated with antibiotics within the preceding month for a "soft-tissue infection of his right leg" that was considered "healed." But was it healed?—E.R. Eichner, M.D.

A Swimming-Associated Outbreak of Hemorrhagic Colitis Caused by *Escherichia Coli* O157:H7 and *Shigella Sonnei*
Keene WE, McAnulty JM, Hoesly FC, Williams LP Jr, Hedberg K, Oxman GL, Barrett TJ, Pfaller MA, Fleming DW (Oregon Health Division, Portland; Epidemic Intelligence Service, Ctrs for Disease Control and Prevention, Atlanta; Multnomah County Health Department, Portland, Ore; et al)
N Engl J Med 331:579–584, 1994   139-95-9-33

Background.—A common cause of epidemic and sporadic disease, especially bloody diarrhea and hemolytic-uremic syndrome, is *Escherichia coli* O157:H7. Outbreaks have been traced to contaminated hamburger and other foods, drinking water, and person-to-person transmission. Simultaneous outbreaks of infection with *E. coli* O157:H7 and *Shigella sonnei* in the Portland, Oregon, area were investigated.

Methods.—Cases were identified from routine surveillance reports. The activities of people with park-associated infections with *E. coli* O157:H7 and *S. sonnei* were compared with those of control groups.

Environmental conditions at the park were evaluated and bacterial isolates were subtyped.

Results.—Park-related *E. coli* O157:H7 infections were identified in 21 people, all of them children. *Shigella sonnei* infections were identified in 38 people, most of them children. The infections did not result from food or beverage consumption, sewage leaks, or bathroom facilities. All case patients had been swimming, which was strongly associated with both types of infection. The case patients had spent more time in the lake and were more likely to have swallowed water than were the control patients. Elevated numbers of enterococci, which were indicative of substantial fecal contamination, were detected in the swimming area but not elsewhere in the lake.

Discussion.—The outbreak was caused by ingestion of lake water contaminated by fecal matter. This is supported by the elevated numbers of enterococci in the swimming area of the lake. Many of the bathers were toddlers who were not yet toilet trained. Small children should have alternatives for playing in water at parks.

▶ Who can forget the tragic deaths (resulting from hemolytic-uremic syndrome) of children in the Pacific Northwest who ate undercooked hamburgers at Jack-in-the-Box? The culprit, *E. coli* O157-H7, which can cause bloody diarrhea and hemolytic-uremic syndrome, can be spread via contaminated hamburger, yogurt, apple cider, drinking water, and from person to person. Now add *swimming* as a means of spread—this outbreak was caused by ingesting fecally contaminated lake water. Fortunately, all 21 children in this study who acquired *E. coli* O157-H7 apparently survived. Prevention will depend more on public cooperation than governmental regulation. Infants and toddlers are no longer allowed in this lake; instead, they play in a water-spray area near the beach that drains to the city sewers.—E.R. Eichner, M.D.

HIV/AIDS Policies and Sports: The National Football League
Brown LS Jr, Phillips RY, Brown CL Jr, Knowlan D, Castle L, Moyer J (Columbia Univ, New York; Addiction Research and Treatment Corp, Brooklyn, NY; Tulane Univ, New Orleans, La; et al)
Med Sci Sports Exerc 26:403–407, 1994 139-95-9–34

Introduction.—More than 1 million individuals are estimated to be infected with HIV, with more than 339,250 cases of AIDS reported as of September 1993. Infection with HIV clearly represents an important public health problem in the United States. Because a cure for HIV has yet to be developed, prevention of transmission and education about HIV infection remain the primary way to control the spread of HIV. With the disclosure by well-known sports figures regarding their infection with HIV, the transmissibility of the virus and the participation of HIV-infected athletes in contact sports has become an issue. To address these and related issues, the National Football League (NFL) has developed and implemented a comprehensive HIV/AIDS policy. The policy focuses on 4 areas: HIV/AIDS education; health care procedures; HIV counseling and testing; and participation of HIV-positive players.

HIV/AIDS Education.—As with the rest of society, this portion of the NFL policy focuses on off-the-field activities that may place an athlete at risk for infection with HIV. Until a cure or vaccine is developed, education is the most effective means of controlling the spread of the virus. In conjunction with the Centers for Disease Control and Prevention (CDC), the NFL has provided educational seminars and materials for players. In addition, individual teams are encouraged to provide additional HIV/AIDS education to their players.

Health Care Procedures.—To reduce the risk for transmission of HIV during athletic activities or while medical care is provided or received, the NFL has developed a bloodborne pathogen exposure control plan for use by NFL teams. Universal precautions developed by the CDC are included in the plan. Because of the relatively low incidence of bleeding injuries sustained during NFL games (3.75 bleeding-related injuries per game) compared with other sports, the NFL has not yet adopted a policy of interrupting competition whenever a bleeding injury occurs. Officials have been educated about transmission of bloodborne pathogens and have been directed on how to respond appropriately to severe or significant injuries. Support for the NFL's approach is found in the low risk of HIV transmission from abrasions (the most likely bleeding injury sustained during football competition) and the relation between the volume of blood exposure and risk for infection. Uniforms and protective equipment cover more than 90% of players' bodies, which allows for a limited amount of unprotected skin.

HIV Counseling and Testing.—Mandatory testing of players is not currently a policy of the NFL. Although early diagnosis provides many benefits to infected individuals and may also reduce transmission of the virus, it is not currently considered a guaranteed means of identifying all HIV-infected players. The variations in local and state laws concerning HIV testing and counseling was also a factor in the NFL's determination not to develop a uniform procedure on counseling and testing. The League cautions teams to comply with local laws and regulations regarding HIV testing and counseling.

Participation of Players With HIV Infection.—On the basis of available evidence, transmission of HIV from on-the-field activities in the NFL has been determined to be highly unlikely. This determination is also supported by information on the transmission of hepatitis B virus. Although hepatitis B is a more common and transmissible infection, a survey of the NFL Physicians' Society showed that only 3 cases of hepatitis B have been reported, all associated with the off-the-field activities of players. Moderate athletic training has not been shown to negatively effect the immune system of HIV-infected individuals. The position of the NFL is that the decision for an HIV-infected player to continue to participate in competition is to be made between the player and his physician.

▶ This study concludes that, in the NFL, HIV testing should remain voluntary, and whether an HIV-positive player should continue to play should remain a private decision between player and doctor. A recent study of the NFL concludes that, although there are nearly 4 bleeding injuries per game, the risk of HIV transmission in a game is less than 1 in 1 million (1). There has been no convincing case of HIV transmission through sports. However, in a "sports analogy" (think boxing, wrestling, hockey), there are 2 reports of HIV transmission from bloody fistfights, the second of which is convincing (2). Human immunodeficiency virus testing probably should be mandatory in boxing and wrestling. A practical, legal view of HIV and sports has recently appeared (3).—E.R. Eichner, M.D.

References

1. Brown LS Jr, et al: *Ann Intern Med* 122:271, 1995.
2. Ippolito G, et al: *JAMA* 272:433, 1994.
3. Mitten MJ: *Phys Sportsmed* 22:63, 1994.

Prevention of Hepatitis B Virus in Athletic Training

Buxton BP, Daniell JE, Buxton BH Jr, Okasaki EM, Ho KW (Univ of Hawaii, Manoa; George Washington Univ, Washington, DC; Univ of Tennessee)
J Athletic Train 29:107–112, 1994   139-95-9–35

Background.—Hepatitis B virus (HBV) infection is highly communicable. It is the leading cause of acute and chronic liver disease worldwide. The Occupational Health and Safety Administration has implemented strict regulations and guidelines for the handling of bloodborne pathogens. Athletic trainers must use extensive preventive strategies to reduce exposure to this dangerous infection.

Preventive Procedures.—Adherence to several guidelines can help prevent bloodborne pathogens from spreading in the athletic training room. All athletic training staff and students should be immunized against HBV. The use of protective equipment, such as gloves, eye guards, masks, gowns, and resuscitation devices, will also help prevent spread. Personal hygiene should include hand washing, the availability of towelettes, and avoidance of cosmetics. In addition, all surfaces should be disinfected, and biohazard containers should be available. Staff and students should not be permitted to eat at work stations.

Conclusions.—Information on preventing HBV in the athletic training setting must be disseminated to staff and students through in-service training sessions, symposia, and lectures. The precautions mentioned should be standard practice in all athletic training facilities.

▶ Everyone who works in the training room must have a working knowledge of universal precautions for handling bloodborne pathogens. The HBV presents a real danger (the authors state that 10,000 to 15,000 health care workers are infected annually) to those of us who are exposed to bloodborne pathogens. In his comments on this article, Robert I. Moss makes a strong request for all athletic training educators to include the teaching of disease control in their curricula (1).

The first thing we must do is become immunized and learn how to use universal precautions. The authors have stressed the importance of preventive procedures in this very timely article. Using protective equipment such as gloves must become a habit for all of us. All too often, athletic trainers continue to treat open and bleeding wounds without using universal precautions. The time has come for a change, and this article provides us with guidelines to follow.—F.J. George, A.T.C., P.T.

Reference

1. Moss RI: *Athletic Train: Sports Health Care Perspect* Vol. 1, No. 1, pp 73–74.

Physical Activity and its Relation to Cancer Risk: A Prospective Study of College Alumni
Lee I-M, Paffenbarger RS Jr (Harvard Univ, Boston; Harvard Med School, Boston)
Med Sci Sports Exerc 26:831–837, 1994   139-95-9–36

Background.—Previous studies of the effects of physical activity on cancer risk have typically used a single assessment of physical activity, failing to consider changes with time. However, a single assessment may be imprecise.

Methods.—To overcome such limitations, 17,607 male Harvard alumni aged 30–79 years were followed from 1962 or 1966 to 1988. Physical activity, defined as self-reported stair climbing, walking, and participation in sports or recreational activities, was assessed twice, at baseline and in 1977. During follow-up, 280 men were diagnosed as having colon cancer, 53 had rectal cancer, 454 had prostatic cancer, 262 had lung cancer, and 88 had pancreatic cancer.

Findings.—Among men with a Quetelet's index of 26 units or greater, those who were highly active had 0.19–0.56 times the colon cancer risk of those who were inactive. The risk of colon cancer was unassociated with the level of activity among the men with a Quetelet's index of less than 26 units. Highly active men also had 0.39–0.62 times the lung cancer risks of their inactive colleagues. Physical activity was not significantly related to the risk of rectal, prostatic, or pancreatic cancers (table).

Conclusions.—Increased physical activity may reduce the risk of certain site-specific cancers. Further research is needed to clarify conflicting findings for prostatic and lung cancers, to determine whether Quetelet's

Relative Risks of Selected Cancers Among Harvard
University Alumni

Physical Activity Level* (kcal·wk⁻¹)	No. of Cases/Person-Years of Follow-Up†	Relative Risk‡ (95% Confidence Interval)
Colon cancer		
<1,000	99/116,371	1.00 (referent)
1,000–2,499	100/115,457	1.07 (0.81 - 1.42)
≥2,500	81/93,407	1.08 (0.81 - 1.46)
		P for trend = 0.58
Rectal cancer		
<1,000	16/116,694	1.00 (referent)
1,000–2,499	17/115,807	1.17 (0.59 - 2.32)
≥2,500	20/93,685	1.71 (0.88 - 3.31)
		P for trend = 0.11
Prostatic cancer		
<1,000	166/116,160	1.00 (referent)
1,000–2,499	160/115,290	1.01 (0.81 - 1.26)
≥2,500	128/93,143	1.04 (0.82 - 1.31)
		P for trend = 0.74
<1,000	166/116,160	1.00 (referent)
1,000–3,999	236/169,485	1.04 (0.85 - 1.27)
≥4,000	52/38,948	0.97 (0.71 - 1.32)
		P for trend = 0.98
Lung cancer§		
<1,000	128/105,343	1.00 (referent)
1,000–2,499	80/105,589	0.72 (0.54 - 0.95)
≥2,500	54/85,168	0.62 (0.45 - 0.85)
		P for trend = 0.002
Pancreatic cancer§		
<1,000	35/92,978	1.00 (referent)
1,000–2,499	31/95,313	1.03 (0.63 - 1.68)
≥2,500	22/76,324	0.93 (0.54 - 1.59)
		P for trend = 0.80

Note: According to physical activity level assessed in 1962 and 1966 and updated in 1977.
*Estimated from climbing stairs, walking, and participating in sports or recreational activities.
†Follow-up experience from 1962/1966 to 1977 allocated according to physical activity level assessed in 1962/1966; follow-up experience from 1978 to 1988 allocated according to physical activity level assessed in 1977.
‡Adjusted for age, Quetelet's index, parental history of cancer; for lung and pancreatic cancers, and the number of cigarettes smoked per day as well.
§Analyses include alumni with unknown cigarette habit.
(Courtesy of Lee I-M, Paffenbarger RS Jr: Med Sci Sports Exerc 26:831-837, 1994.)

index and dietary factors modify the physical activity–colon cancer association, and to establish which types and patterns of activity are beneficial.

▶ There is growing evidence that physical activity has a beneficial effect in reducing the likelihood of colon cancers, although the precise mechanism remains unclear. Theories include a reduction of segmentation in the colon, a faster colonic transit time, and a reduction of body fat content. Epidemiologic research unfortunately can only point to associations, although the linkage between physical activity and protection in men with a high Quetelet's index might seem to point in the direction of a mediating role for a decrease in body fat. The prevention of lung cancer through exercise is less commonly observed; one problem here is that although the present data were analyzed "for the number of cigarettes smoked." the classification was crude (1–20 or more than 20), and it could be that the exercisers were much lighter smokers than the sedentary members of the sample were.—R.J. Shephard, M.D., Ph.D., D.P.E.

Physical Exercise and Reduced Risk of Breast Cancer in Young Women
Bernstein L, Henderson BE, Hamisch R, Sullivan-Halley J, Ross RK (Univ of Southern California, Los Angeles; The Salk Inst, La Jolla, Calif)
J Natl Cancer Inst 86:1403–1408, 1994   139-95-9-37

Background.—Findings that ovulatory menstrual cycles, and therefore exposure to ovarian hormones, are a determinant of the risk of breast cancer suggest that any factor that modifies the menstrual cycle pattern might alter the risk that breast cancer will develop. Physical activity may be such a factor, because strenuous exercise markedly alters menstrual activity in adolescence. Even a moderate level of activity at this stage of life may significantly reduce the frequency of ovulatory cycles.

Study Plan.—A large-scale, case-control study was carried out in women 40 years of age and younger with breast cancer to learn whether women who regularly exercise during their reproductive years have a reduced risk of breast cancer. A total of 545 white women with cancer were matched with controls for age and parity.

Findings.—Women who averaged at least 3.8 hours of exercise activity a week had a relative risk of breast cancer of 0.42 compared with inactive women. Among those who participated during the 10 years after menarche, the decrease in breast cancer risk with increasing activity was statistically significant. The risk of cancer in women averaging 5.6 or more hours of physical exercise per week at this time of life was 0.7 relative to inactive women. Similar findings were obtained after adjusting for employment status, age at menarche, and months of oral contraceptive use. Limiting the analysis to women with invasive breast cancer did not alter the findings.

Conclusion.—These results strongly indicate the need to require participation in physical education classes and to encourage lifelong participation in an exercise program.

▶ This solid epidemiologic study adds to the growing evidence that regular physical activity, especially if begun early in life, helps prevent breast cancer, just as it helps prevent colon cancer (see Abstract 139-95-8-33). How exercise may fend off breast cancer is debated. Surely an exercise habit promotes leanness and healthful eating (more fruits and vegetables; less saturated fat; less alcohol), which may help cut the risk of breast cancer. These authors believe that another way that lifelong exercise reduces breast cancer risk is by reducing the cumulative number of ovulatory menstrual cycles and thus the cumulative exposure to the ovarian hormones that shape breast cancer risk.—E.R. Eichner, M.D.

Physical Activity and Risk of Breast Cancer in the Framingham Heart Study

Dorgan JF, Brown C, Barrett M, Splansky GL, Kreger BE, D'Agostino RB, Albanes D, Schatzkin A (Natl Cancer Inst, Bethesda, Md; Information Management Services Inc, Silver Spring, Md; Boston Univ)
Am J Epidemiol 139:662–669, 1994   139-95-9–38

Objective.—It has been suggested that physical activity may protect against breast cancer. Data from the Framingham Heart Study were reviewed to examine the association between the level of physical activity and the risk of breast cancer.

Study Population and Methods.—Physical activity was estimated by a physician-administered questionnaire from 2,321 women at the time of the fourth biennial examination in 1954-1956. Breast cancers were identified by self-reporting, surveillance of hospital admissions, and a review of death records. During 28 years of follow-up, a total of 117 breast cancers developed among 2,307 women for whom data on physical activity and reproductive history were available. The Cox proportional hazards model of analysis was used, with age as the underlying time variable. The models were adjusted for age at the time of activity assessment, age at

Relative Risk of Breast Cancer by Quartile of the Physical Activity Index in the Framingham Heart Study (1954–1984)

Physical activity index by quartile*	Age-adjusted model†			Full model‡		
	Relative risk	95% CI	p value	Relative risk	95% CI	p value
1 (low)	1.0			1.0		
2	1.3	0.7–2.2	0.38	1.2	0.7–2.1	0.52
3	1.3	0.7–2.3	0.37	1.3	0.7–2.4	0.39
4 (high)	1.5	0.8–2.6	0.16	1.6	0.9–2.9	0.13

Abbreviation: CI, confidence interval.
Note: Physical activity index = sleep/rest hours × 1 + sedentary hours × 1.1 + slight activity hours ×1.5 + moderate activity hours × 2.4 + heavy activity hours × 5.
*Quartile cutpoints: 1 = 25–28, 2 = 29–30, 3 = 31–32, 4 = 33–54.
†Relative risks from a proportional hazards model with age as the underlying time variable.
‡Relative risks from a proportional hazards model with age as the underlying time variable, stratifying on age at examination 4, number of pregnancies, and menopausal status and including age at first pregnancy, education, occupation, and alcohol ingestion as covariates.
(Courtesy of Dorgan JF, Brown C, Barrett M, et al: *Am J Epidemiol* 139:662–669, 1994.)

the first pregnancy, parity, menopausal status, education, occupation, and alcohol use.

Findings.—The risk of breast cancer tended to increase with the level of physical activity. Women in the highest quartile of activity had a relative risk of 1.6 compared with those in the lowest quartile (table). Both moderate-to-heavy leisure and occupational activities correlated with an increased risk of breast cancer, but the association was marginally significant only for leisure activity. Each hour spent daily in moderate-to-heavy leisure activities rather than at rest or sleep was associated with a 20% increase in risk.

Conclusions.—These findings fail to confirm a protective effect of physical activity against breast cancer. Instead, they suggest an increased cancer risk for more active women.

▶ The lack of consistency in the results of studies reporting the relationship between breast cancer and physical activity confuses everyone. Surely, someone could examine the literature and determine whether differences in protocols, populations, analytic techniques, confounding factors, etc., account for the different conclusions. The usual explanation for a protective effect is that lifetime exposure to estrogen would be lower in very active women because of the effect of intense activity on the reproductive cycle. Of course, these same women may be at increased risk for premature osteoporosis. Does exercise have a protective effect against breast cancer? We don't know.—B.L. Drinkwater, Ph.D.

Aetiology of Testicular Cancer: Association With Congenital Abnormalities, Age at Puberty, Infertility, and Exercise

Forman D, for the United Kingdom Testicular Cancer Study Group (Radcliffe Infirmary, Oxford, England; Inst of Cancer Research, Sutton, Surrey, England; Royal London Hosp, England; et al)
BMJ 308:1393–1399, 1994   139-95-9–39

Introduction.—The incidence of testicular cancer has been rising among white populations and is now the most common form of cancer in men aged 15–44 years in England and Wales. A case-control study was conducted to determine whether an association exists between the development of testicular cancer and certain urogenital abnormalities, age at puberty, marital status, infertility, and amount of exercise.

Methods.—The study was carried out in 9 health regions of England and Wales. Case subjects were residents, aged 15–49 years, who were given a diagnosis of testicular germ cell tumor between January 1984 and January 1987. Age-matched controls were chosen from the list of each case subject's general practitioner. Nonwhite persons and those with a previous malignancy were excluded. The mean time between case diagnosis and interview was 10 months.

Numbers (Percentages) of Case Subjects and Controls and Odds Ratios (95% Confidence Intervals) by Hours of Exercise per Week and Hours Spent Seated per Day at Age 20 Years and at Reference Age

Variable	No (%) of cases	No (%) of controls	Unadjusted odds ratio	Adjusted odds ratio† (95% confidence interval)
Hours of exercise a week at age 20 (735 matched pairs):				
None	248 (33·6)	217 (29·5)	1·00	1·00
1-2	94 (12·8)	94 (12·8)	0·86	0·91 (0·65 to 1·29)
3-4	101 (13·7)	100 (13·6)	0·87	0·91 (0·64 to 1·29)
5-9	154 (20·9)	157 (21·4)	0·85	0·84 (0·62 to 1·14)
10-14	75 (10·2)	81 (11·0)	0·78	0·79 (0·53 to 1·17)
≥ 15	65 (8·8)	86 (11·7)	0·65	0·62 (0·42 to 0·91)
Not known	0	2		
Younger than age 20	57	57		
Test for trend‡				$\chi^2 = 6·57, P = 0·010$
Hours of exercise a week at reference age (793 matched pairs):				
None	331 (41·7)	309 (39·0)	1·00	1·00
1-2	135 (17·0)	131 (16·5)	0·95	1·00 (0·73 to 1·36)
3-4	115 (14·5)	109 (13·7)	0·94	0·94 (0·69 to 1·29)
5-9	136 (17·1)	144 (18·2)	0·84	0·86 (0·64 to 1·16)
10-14	49 (6·2)	50 (6·3)	0·87	0·85 (0·54 to 1·35)
≥ 15	28 (3·5)	50 (6·3)	0·50	0·54 (0·32 to 0·90)
Not known	0	1		
Test for trend‡				$\chi^2 = 5·63; P = 0·018$
Hours of sitting down a day at age 20 (731 matched pairs):				
0-2	114 (15·6)	104 (14·1)	1·00	1·00
3-4	188 (25·7)	231 (31·4)	0·76	0·77 (0·55 to 1·08)
5-6	166 (22·7)	176 (23·9)	0·89	0·90 (0·63 to 1·30)
7-9	147 (20·1)	134 (18·2)	1·05	1·03 (0·70 to 1·52)
≥ 10	117 (16·0)	91 (12·4)	1·25	1·35 (0·88 to 2·06);
Not known	5	1		
Younger than age 20	57	57		
Test for trend‡				$\chi^2 = 5·11; P = 0·024$
Hours spent sitting down a day at reference age (793 matched pairs):				
0-2	52 (6·6)	62 (7·8)	1·00	1·00
3-4	159 (20·1)	175 (22·0)	1·12	1·20 (0·77 to 1·87)
5-6	192 (24·2)	205 (25·8)	1·18	1·19 (0·76 to 1·86)
7-9	163 (20·6)	168 (21·2)	1·25	1·28 (0·81 to 2·02)
≥ 10	227 (28·6)	184 (23·2)	1·59	1·71 (1·08 to 2·72)
Not known	1	0		
Test for trend‡				$\chi^2 = 7·63; P = 0·006$

* Percentages exclude missing values.
† Adjusted for undescended testis and inguinal hernia diagnosed < 15 years.
‡ Trend test after excluding "not known" and "younger than 20" if appropriate and fitting variables as midpoints of categories presented and median of top group (for exercise 0, 1.5, 3.5, 7, 12, 20; for sitting 1, 3.5, 5.5, 8, 11).
(Courtesy of Forman D, for the United Kingdom Testicular Cancer Study Group: BMJ 308:1393-1399, 1994.)

Results.—Interviews were completed with 794 of 863 eligible case subjects and 609 of 794 matched controls. Most patients had been given a diagnosis between the ages of 20 and 39 years. Both undescended testis and inguinal hernia were found to be significant risk factors for testicular cancer. Bilateral undescended testis was seen in 19 case subjects but in none of the controls; 46 case subjects and 17 controls had unilateral undescended testis. The increased risk did not exist in men successfully operated on to correct the condition before the age of 10 years. The odds ratios were 3.82 for undescended testis and 1.91 for inguinal hernia. There were significant trends of decreased risk of testicular cancer with increasing age at voice breaking, age at the start of shaving, and age at first recalled nocturnal emissions. No associations were found for marital status or having a vasectomy. The risk of testicular cancer increased with a sedentary lifestyle, and exercise offered a moderate protective effect (table).

Conclusion.—This interview-based, case-control study of testicular cancer, the largest to date on the subject, confirms that undescended testis and inguinal hernia are associated with an increased risk of malignancy. Early age at puberty and a lack of exercise may also be risk factors, suggesting hormonal influences in the development of testicular cancer.

▶ This is the first good study to suggest that exercise has a beneficial effect in reducing the risk of testicular cancer. However, there have been previous suggestions linking such cancers to sedentary employment (1–3). The benefit from 15 hours per week of exercise (a halving of risk) is quite impressive, although milder exercise does not seem to offer much protection. Also, as in the earlier studies, there is a graded adverse effect caused by sedentary work.

It is likely that very heavy exercise of the type discussed leads to a suppression of circulating levels of testosterone, which would tie in with some of the other hormonal correlates of cancer risk. However, bearing in mind older hypotheses about testicular temperature and cancer, it is also possible that jogging on a frosty morning reduces the temperature of the germ cells for a substantial part of the day! Given the dedication that is needed to exercise regularly for 15 hours per week, it also remains necessary to check whether other health habits (linked to fanatical exercise) are giving the observed protection.—R.J. Shephard, M.D., Ph.D., D.P.E.

References

1. Coggon D, Pannett B, Osmond C, et al: *Br J Ind Med* 43:381–386, 1986.
2. McDowall, ME, Balarajan R: *J Epidemiol Community Health* 40:26–29, 1986.
3. Swerdlow AJ, Skeet RG: *Br J Ind Med* 45:225–230, 1988.

The Effect of a High Resistance Exercise Program in Slowly Progressive Neuromuscular Disease
Kilmer DD, McCrory MA, Wright NC, Aitkens SG, Bernauer EM (Univ of California, Davis)
Arch Phys Med Rehabil 75:560–563, 1994   139-95-9–40

Introduction.—Studies of the effects of strengthening exercises in patients with slowly progressive neuromuscular diseases (NMD) have yielded varied results. Although overwork weakness has been a concern, one report found that a moderate resistance exercise program did offer benefits to patients with NMD. Ten patients and 6 healthy controls participated in a study of a rigorous, high-resistance protocol.

Methods.—The patients, 8 men and 2 women, all had mild-to-moderate weakness and had not been engaged in a strengthening program in the past year. The controls were untrained volunteers, 3 men and 3 women. Both patients and controls were evaluated at baseline for maximal isometric and isokinetic strength of the elbow flexors and knee extensors. The 12-week, high resistance, home exercise program consisted of sets of 10 repetitions using ankle and wrist cuff weights. The amount of exercise was gradually increased during the course of the exercise protocol by adding to the resistive weights, the number of sets, and the days per week of exercise. One side of the body was randomly chosen for exercise.

Results.—Patients with NMD reported completing 95% of all sessions; control subjects completed 90%. None missed sessions because of excessive soreness or fatigue. There were no significant changes in strength between baseline and 4 weeks. At 12 weeks, the NMD group showed significant improvements in several knee extension isokinetic strength measures. The eccentric strength measures indicated improvement in both the exercised and nonexercised limbs. The upper extremity, however, showed a significant loss of elbow flexion eccentric peak torque and work per degree of rotation. The training responses of individual patients were not dependent on baseline strength. The controls demonstrated significant improvement in all strength measures of knee extension and in elbow isokinetic eccentric work per degree, with overall responses greater than those of the NMD group. Both groups also showed evidence of cross training to the nonexercised limbs.

Conclusion.—These patients with NMD could perform and benefit from a near maximal exercise program, yet a moderate resistance program may prove adequate. The positive benefits of a moderate strengthening program for the elbow flexors were lost in the high-resistance program, suggesting adverse effects to diseased skeletal muscle.

▶ It is necessary to read this study carefully, because both control and experimental subjects participated in the training program! The difference is that the experimental subjects had progressive NMD and the controls did not. Both groups benefited from the knee-strengthening exercises; at the elbow, however, the controls showed small gains of strength, whereas in those with NMD, there was a tendency to a decrease in strength, as much as 10% for some movements. This emphasizes that when dealing with progressive NMD, a standard, vigorous resistance exercise program can be too strenuous, leading to a deterioration rather than an improvement of residual muscle function (1, 2). It is particularly interesting that the deterioration in objectively measured arm performance developed without any reports of pain or muscle soreness.—R.J. Shephard, M.D., Ph.D., D.P.E.

References

1. Johnson EW, Braddom R: *Arch Phys Med Rehabil* 52:333–336, 1971.
2. Peach PE: *Arch Phys Med Rehabil* 71:248–250, 1990.

Autonomic Functions and Orthostatic Responses 24 h After Acute Intense Exercise in Paraplegic Subjects

Engelke KA, Shea JD, Doerr DF, Convertino VA (Univ of Florida, Gainesville; Humana Hosp Lucerne, Orlando, Fla; Kennedy Space Center, Fla; et al)
Am J Physiol 266:R1189–R1196, 1994   139-95-9-41

Background.—In individuals prone to postural hypotension, a single bout of dynamic exercise reportedly increases the sensitivity of cardiovascular reflexes and enhances the maintenance of blood pressure (BP) in the postexercise recovery period. Graded exercise designed to elicit maximal effort may increase the sensitivity of autonomically mediated baroreflexes and increase BP stability in these individuals.

Methods.—Heart rate (HR), BP, forearm vascular resistance (FVR), and vasoactive hormone responses before and during 15 minutes of 70-degree head-up tilt (HUT) in 10 paraplegics were measured on 2 occasions in 10 patients with paraplegia. The first test was 24 hours after maximal arm-crank exercise, and the second was without prior exercise.

Findings.—During HUT, HR rose 30 beats per minute in postexercise and control conditions. However, the reduction in systolic BP was greater during the control condition than that seen after exercise. The

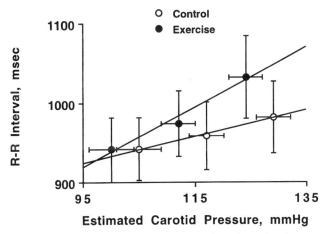

Fig 9–23.—Carotid-cardiac baroreflex stimulus-response relationships, plotted over range of pressures from which maximum slopes were derived, during control (*open circle*) and 24 hours after exercise (*filled circle*). Linear equation for control data is y = 1.7x + 766 (r² = 0.987) and for postexercise data, y = 3.8x + 558 (r² = 0.975). Values are means ± SE. (Courtesy of Engelke KA, Shea JD, Doerr DF, et al: *Am J Physiol* 266:R1189–R1196, 1994.)

postexercise increase in FVR (17–24.8 peripheral resistance units from supine to HUT) was higher than the increase noted in the control condition. The carotid-cardiac baroreflex gain was also increased after exercise (Fig 9–23). Norepinephrine, vasopressin, and plasma renin-angiotensin responses induced by HUT were comparable for control and postexercise conditions. There was no difference in leg vein compliance or plasma volume between conditions. Also, HR and systolic BP responses to phases II and IV of the Valsalva maneuver, indexes of integrated baroreflex sensitivity, were increased after maximal exercise compared with the control condition.

Conclusions.—The elimination of orthostatic hypotension during 70-degree HUT 24 hours after exercise was associated with an increased baroreflex control of HR and FVR but was independent of changes in blood volume and leg compliance compared with the control condition. The improvement in systemic resistance occurred with no changes in circulating norepinephrine, arginine vasopressin, and plasma renin-angiotensin.

▶ Pooling of blood in the paralyzed lower limbs places a major restriction upon the activity of the person with paraplegia, to the extent that some authors have recommended the use of inflatable trousers to return blood from the leg veins to the central circulation. Venous pooling and resulting postural hypotension can also be a problem after space flight. In a healthy individual, it is also well recognized that a period of endurance training can enhance the tone of the leg veins.

The authors have found that even a single bout of exercise can enhance vasoregulation for as long as 24 hours (1). These short-term gains are not associated with any expansion of plasma volume, increase of venous tone, or altered secretion of regulatory hormones. Rather, the explanation seems to be an increased sensitivity of autonomic reflexes. It is encouraging that such a response can be seen in patients who have had paraplegia for many years. This suggests that regular bouts of exercise could conserve postural adjustments for astronauts, even when they are engaged in prolonged space missions.—R.J. Shephard, M.D., Ph.D., D.P.E.

Reference

1. Convertino VA, Adams WC: *Am J Physiol* 260:570R–575R, 1991.

Sports Injury Look-Alikes: When Rheumatologic Disorders Cause Pain or Fatigue
Stiene HA, Hardin GT (Indiana Internal Medicine Consultants, Indianapolis; Specialty Ctrs for Orthopaedic Rehabilitation and Excellence, Indianapolis, Ind)
Physician Sportsmed 22:60–62, 65–70, 1994   139-95-9–42

Background.—Fatigue and the inability to maintain a training regimen may be the only signs of a systemic disorder in active patients with symptoms otherwise consistent with overuse syndromes or chronic injury.

Methods.—Three case studies were presented to illustrate rheumatoid arthritis, systemic lupus erythematosus, and gout.

Case Report.—Man, 33, a white crew member, initially had bilateral shoulder pain. After initial, successful treatment for impingement syndrome, the patient returned 6 months later with complaints of bilateral shoulder, elbow, wrist, hand, knee, and ankle pain for the previous 10 weeks. He described morning stiffness lasting about 2 hours, swelling in his wrists and hands, and progressive swelling of his ankles during the day. During the previous month, his fatigue had increased to the point where he stopped rowing. The diagnosis of rheumatoid arthritis was made after physical examination, joint aspiration, and laboratory tests revealed an elevated erythrocyte sedimentation rate, positive rheumatoid factor, and antinuclear antibody. Treatment led to improvement sufficient to allow him to return to crew.

Systemic Lupus Erythematosus and Gout.—Detailed case studies illustrating systemic lupus erythematosus and gout in athletes were also described. Systemic lupus erythematosus is diagnosed when 4 of the 11 following criteria are present simultaneously or serially: malar rash, discoid rash, photosensitivity, oral ulcer, arthritis, serositis (pleuritis or pericarditis), renal disorder, neurologic disorder, hematologic disorder, immunologic disorder, and positive antinuclear antibody. Gout is associated with obesity and alcohol abuse in middle-aged men. It is a result of an abnormality in purine metabolism leading to deposits of sodium urate crystal in articular cartilage, the synovium, kidneys, and other tissues. Compared with other forms of arthritis, gouty arthritis has an abrupt onset and responds quickly to therapy. Joint aspirate will differentiate gout from other etiologies.

Conclusions.—Although the diagnosis of connective tissue disorders is relatively uncommon in sports medicine, the physician must be aware that not all joint injuries that appear to be recurrent, chronic, or caused by overuse are necessarily the result of athletic activity.

▶ This clinical, practical article reminds us that athletes are not immune to disease, alas, and that acute rheumatologic diseases can, at first glance, resemble sports injuries or overuse syndromes. In this report we see a 33-year-old rower with sore shoulders as the presenting features of acute rheumatoid arthritis; a 21-year-old black female runner with knee pain, "staleness," and fatigue, not from overtraining but from lupus; and a 39-year-old, heavy-set, beer-drinking, recreational basketball player with ankle pain that was not from basketball but from gout. Another recent article covers the case of a 33-year-old runner who precipitated acute gout (in his right knee and ankle) by running in warm weather and quaffing beer afterward (1).—E.R. Eichner, M.D.

Reference

1. Moore GE, Anderson AL: *Med Sci Sports Exerc* 27:626, 1995.

Effects of Strength Training on Neuromuscular Function and Disease Activity in Patients with Recent-Onset Inflammatory Arthritis

Häkkinen A, Häkkinen K, Hannonen P (University of Jyväskylä, Finland)
Scand J Rheumatol 23:237–242, 1994   139-95-9-43

Purpose.—In patients with arthritis, muscular strength can be increased through resistance exercise training, but debate exists over whether exercise may have detrimental effects on disease activity and joint destruction. The effects of prolonged dynamic strength training on maximal strength, explosive force production, the cross-sectional area of the quadriceps femoris muscle, and clinical disease variables were examined in patients with recent-onset inflammatory arthritis.

Design.—Thirty-nine patients with recent-onset arthritis participating in the 6-month trial were randomly divided into 2 study groups: an experimental group that received progressive dynamic strength training and a control group. Antirheumatic medication was administered to all patients throughout the trial. Strength training consisted of twice-weekly exercise of all major muscle groups for 2 months, followed by exercise of greater loading intensity with more repetitions 2–3 times weekly

Clinical Disease Variables (Means ± SD) in the Experimental and the Control Groups Before and After the 6-Month Training Period

	EG	CG
Hemoglobin (g/l)		
before	141.2 ± 15.5	136.4 ± 10.1
after	138.1 ± 13.5	136.5 ± 9.5
Erythrocyte sedimentation rate (mm/1 h)		
before	25.2 ± 24.7	22.0 ± 10.2
after	13.6 ± 19.5*	16.7 ± 11.4
Ritchie's articular index		
before	11.1 ± 5.9	13.4 ± 8.3
after	4.9 ± 4.8†	7.0 ± 7.2*
Number of eroded joints		
before	2.3 ± 4.5	1.7 ± 2.2
after	2.5 ± 4.5	2.2 ± 3.0

Abbreviations: EG, experimental group; CG, control group.
*$P < 0.05$.
†$P < 0.001$.
(Courtesy of Häkkinen A, Häkkinen K, Hannonen P: *Scand J Rheumatol* 23:237–242, 1994.)

thereafter. Other activities such as walking, biking, and swimming were also performed twice weekly.

Findings.—Patients in the exercise group experienced significant improvements in maximal muscle strength, erythrocyte sedimentation rate, Ritchie's articular index (RI), and the Stanford Health Assessment Questionnaire (HAQ) index. The control group experienced a significant decrease in RI. A slight increase in erosive joint changes occurred in both groups but to a lesser extent in the experimental group (table).

Conclusions.—Prolonged dynamic strength training can result in considerable increases in maximal strength of all major muscle groups, including some enlargement in the cross-sectional area of trained thigh muscles, without detrimental effects on disease activity or joint damage in patients with recent-onset arthritis. Hence, the health benefits of dynamic strength training overrule the possible detriments. A dynamic, individually tailored strength training program can safely be included as part of an overall rehabilitation program for patients with recent-onset arthritis to minimize the effects of disease, inactivity, or both on the neuromuscular system.

▶ In the past, physicians have tended to restrict activity during the acute phase of inflammatory arthritis. As with so many medical conditions, rest is not necessarily the best advice. The authors suggest that even in cases of acute inflammatory arthritis, it is better for the patient to maintain a moderate level of physical activity and attempt to strengthen the muscles around the affected joint.—R.J. Shephard, M.D., Ph.D., D.P.E.

Subject Index*

A

A-angle
  in patellar alignment measurement,
    efficacy, 93: 106

Abdomen
  acute, after trauma, 93: 240
  injuries, 94: 27
  muscle training in sport, 94: 252
  trauma, occult injury may be life
    threatening, 94: 47

Absenteeism
  due to illness and injury in
    manufacturing companies, and
    exercise, 94: 367

Abuse
  androgenic anabolic steroids, and
    platelet aggregation in weight
    lifters, 93: 386
  of corticosteroid injections, 95: 33
  of drugs, 94: 319
  of growth hormone during adolescence,
    94: 348
  stanozolol, in athlete, severe cholestasis
    and acute renal failure after
    stanozolol, 95: 390
  steroid, in athletes, prostatic
    enlargement and bladder outflow
    obstruction in, 95: 389

Accelerometer
  measurements of shoe during walking,
    cushioning properties, 93: 28

Accidents
  ski, severity of, alcohol and
    benzodiazepines in, 93: 385

Acetazolamide
  for mountain sickness, acute, 93: 414
  in ventilatory response to high altitude
    hypoxia, 93: 413

Achilles tendnon
  repair, functional postoperative
    treatment, 93: 92

Achilles tendon
  allograft reconstruction of anterior
    cruciate ligament deficient knee,
    94: 134
  injuries in athletes, 95: 193
  overuse injuries, surgery of, long-term
    follow-up, 95: 194
  pain
    peritendinitis causing, 93: 92
    steroids and outcome, 93: 91
  rupture
    acute, immediate free ankle motion
      after surgical repair of, 95: 195

    early controlled motion after surgical
      repair, 93: 93
    operative repair, early mobilization
      after, 94: 168
    operative repair, with polypropylene
      braid augmentation, 95: 197
    operative vs. nonoperative treatment,
      94: 167

Achillis, tendo (see Achilles tendon)

ACOG guidelines
  for exercise during pregnancy, and
    pregnancy outcome, 94: 280

Acromioclavicular
  dislocation, third-degree, strength
    testing after, 93: 38
  joint, arthroscopic resection of, 93: 42

ACSM
  equation for young women, accuracy,
    95: 291

Adhesion molecules
  cell, in middle distance runners under
    different training conditions,
    95: 392

Adipose
  tissue lipoprotein lipase responses, in
    silent myocardial ischemia in older
    athletes, 95: 418

Adolescence
  anabolic steroid use in, 93: 389,
    95: 378
  anterior cruciate ligament tears during,
    93: 135
  athletes, bronchospasm of,
    unrecognized exercise-induced,
    93: 271
  ballet dancers as model of female
    athlete, menstrual cycle and
    exercise, 93: 322
  body image and attitudes toward
    anabolic steroid use during,
    93: 390
  bone mineral density during, diet,
    hormonal and metabolic factors in,
    in amenorrhea and eumenorrhea in
    female runners, 93: 320
  gender difference in aerobic capacity
    after cancer cure in childhood,
    94: 479
  girls during, calcium supplement and
    bone mineral density in, 94: 268
  growth hormone abuse during, 94: 348
  hypertension during, exercising
    non-pharmacologic control,
    93: 252
  multiple drugs with anabolic steroid use
    during, 94: 346

---

* All entries refer to the year and page number(s) for data appearing in this and the
previous edition of the YEAR BOOK.

511

C

Caffeine
  concentration, urinary, and endurance exercise, 93: 392
  doping with, 93: 393
  ingestion
    acute and habitual, and metabolic responses to steady-state exercise, 93: 395
    during exercise to exhaustion in elite distance runners, 93: 394
Calcaneus
  motion in chronic ankle lateral instability, stereophotogrametry of ankle orthosis in, 94: 172
Calcium
  supplement, in girls during adolescence, 94: 268
  urinary, boron supplement effect on, in athletic women, 95: 336
Calf
  muscles, phosphorus-31 nuclear magnetic resonance of, 94: 210
  pain, coagulopathy presenting as, in racquetball player, 94: 465
Cancer
  breast (see Breast cancer)
  endometrial, risk of, and physical activity, 94: 478
  mortality from, heart rate and physical activity in, 94: 474
  ovaries, and occupational physical activity, 94: 476
  risk, and physical activity, in college alumni, 95: 497
  testes, congenital abnormalities, puberty age, infertility and exercise in, 95: 501
  uterus, and occupational physical activity, 94: 476
Canoeist
  world-class, psychologic monitoring and training load modulation of, 95: 255
Capsular
  shift
    inferior, in multidirectional shoulder instability, 93: 56
    procedure, inferior, for anterior-inferior shoulder instability, 95: 53
Capsulolabral
  reconstruction
    anterior, of shoulder in athletes, 93: 58

modified anterior, functional outcomes, 95: 51
Capsulorrhaphy
  of shoulder
    anterior, external rotation loss after, 94: 60
    stable, for anterior instability, 94: 61
Carbohydrate
  oxidation
    exogenous, from maltose and glucose during prolonged exercise, 93: 424
    during prolonged exercise, and gastric emptying and absorption, 93: 420
    during prolonged exercise, carbohydrate type in, 93: 423
  strategies for injury prevention, 95: 13
  supplement, post-training, improving performance in trained cyclists, 95: 410
Cardiac (see Heart)
Cardiography
  impedance, during exercise in coronary heart disease, 94: 435
Cardiomyopathy
  hypertrophic, endurance athletes with, echocardiography of, 95: 241
Cardiopulmonary
  fitness improvement by supervised exercise training in HIV infection, 94: 481
  reserve, and skeletal muscle mass, 93: 264
  resuscitation, updated protocol, instituting by term physician, 95: 465
Cardiorespiratory
  abnormalities, in neurologic decompression illness manifestations, 95: 279
  disease, 93: 209, 94: 419
  fitness, 94: 361
    high, fibrinogen reduction in, 94: 396
    and leisure time physical activity in coronary artery disease, 94: 449
  responses
    to exercise, and maternal aerobic fitness, 94: 282
    in spinal cord injury, and training, 93: 439
  training, 93: 209
Cardiovascular
  aging, and exercise effect, 94: 307
  disease, 95: 435
  fitness, after anabolic steroids, 95: 380
  responses
    to exercise in paraplegia, anti-G suit in, 93: 442
    in paraplegia during exercise, 93: 441

walking and running, interrelationships
with mechanical power and energy
transfers, 94: 234
Ectopic
ventricular activity in physically trained
hypertensive subjects, 93: 238
Edema
dependent, prevented by walking,
plethysmography in, 93: 268
formation with prolonged standing,
93: 268
Education
of sports medicine physician,
understanding, 94: 1
Educational
material readability, in heart disease,
94: 423
Effort
mechanical efficiency of, and thermal
equilibrium in winter sports,
95: xxv
Elastic
soles for running shoes, 93: 174
Elbow
arthroscopy, diagnostic and therapeutic
benefits and hazards, 93: 77
complex, functional anatomy of, 94: 81
epicondylitis, lateral, scientific evidence
lack for treatment, 93: 72
flexion strength curves in untrained men
and women and male bodybuilders,
94: 263
flexor muscles
activation pattern differences during
isometric, concentric and eccentric
contractions, 94: 216
during endurance contractions, and
myo-electric fatigue, 94: 215
instability, medial, in throwing athletes,
93: 75
ligaments, medial, stress radiography of,
95: 68
Little League, treating and preventing,
95: 72
muscle groups, eccentric muscle
performance of, 94: 240
pain and stiffness after trauma,
arthroscopic treatment, 95: 71
problems, common, in athlete, 94: 83
rehabilitation in throwing athlete,
94: 84
tennis (see Tennis elbow)
thrower's, physical examination of,
94: 82
torque production, dual task, surface
EMG amplitude and frequency
measures during, 94: 208

ulnar collateral ligament of (see Ulnar
collateral ligament)
Electrical
capacitive coupling in long bone
nonunion, 95: 203
conductivity, total body, measuring body
composition in ballet dancers,
93: 334
evoked myoelectric signals in back
muscles, side dominance in,
95: 220
stimulation
leg cycle ergometer exercise, 93: 439
motor unit activation during, twitch
analysis of, 95: 266
in paraplegia, cardiovascular
responses during exercise, 93: 441
of quadriceps, torque history of,
94: 242
in triceps surae mechanical and
morphological characteristics,
95: 269
voluntary and neuromuscular,
inducing torque production in
aged, 95: 268
Electrocardiography
in patients admitted for, but without,
confirmed myocardial infarction,
94: 433
vs. seismocardiography of coronary
artery disease diagnosis during
exercise testing, 94: 437
Electrode
position in EMG of upper trapezius
muscle, 94: 214
Electroencephalography
in judo and choking, 93: 235
Electrolyte
alterations after 100-km run, 95: 282
Electromyography
of athletic shoulder, 94: 72
biofeedback for shoulder dislocation,
95: 55
changes
after isometric training, 93: 186
during sustained contraction related
to phosphate accumulation,
94: 210
coefficient method isometric tasks,
muscle forces about wrist joint
during, 94: 211
cross talk, of hamstring muscles,
93: 180
during cycling, lactate manipulation in,
93: 185
of deltoid muscle, arm abduction
activity, 93: 182

G

M

Magnesium
urinary, boron supplement effect on, in
athletic women, 95: 336
Magnetic resonance
nuclear phosphorus-31, of calf muscle,
94: 210
Magnetic resonance arthrography
of labral ligamentous complex of
shoulder, 95: 45
Magnetic resonance imaging
of biceps tendon rupture, distal, 95: 64
in chondromalacia patellae, 93: 119
of cruciate ligament, injuries, anterior,
"bone bruises" in, 94: 123
of cruciate ligament, posterior, tear,
complete vs. partial-thickness,
95: 149
of glenoid labrum in anterior shoulder
instability, 95: 44
gradient-echo, of knee, vs. arthroscopy,
93: 110
of hamstring injury, prognosis, 94: 166
of iliotibial band
friction syndrome, 93: 90
syndrome, 95: 222
for intercondylar notch measurement,
95: 130
of knee
abnormal findings in asymptomatic
subjects, 93: 112
asymptomatic, abnormal findings
prevalence, 95: 98
cost effectiveness of, 93: 112
fracture, occult, 95: 96
replacing diagnostic arthroscopy,
93: 111
tears, recurrent, diagnosis,
intraarticular contrast material in,
94: 114
meniscal tear missed on, relationship to
anterior cruciate ligament tear,
95: 102
of patellar articular cartilage, 93: 120
of patellar tendinitis, 93: 124
for patellar tendon evaluation after use
of central one-third for anterior
cruciate ligament reconstruction,
93: 140
of psoas muscle geometry, 95: 212
of quadriceps tendon rupture, 93: 122
of quadrilateral space syndrome, 94: 68
radial, of meniscus of knee, correlated
with arthroscopy, 93: 113
of suprascapular nerve
entrapment, 93: 51

syndrome, 94: 47
in tibial tendon rupture reconstruction,
93: 95
of ulnar collateral ligament
injury in baseball pitchers, 93: 78
preoperative evaluation in baseball
players, 95: 67
tears, nondisplaced and displaced,
94: 89
ventricular dimensions and mass using,
left, in female endurance athletes,
93: 228
Malignancy (*see* Cancer)
Malleolar
stress fracture, medial, clinical and
imaging features, 93: 97
Maltose
ingestion during prolonged exercise,
93: 424
Maquet procedure
in tibial shingle length in patellofemoral
pressures, 94: 130
Marine
injuries, prevention and treatment,
95: 280
Mask
football helmet face mask removal,
alternative methods, 93: 11
to modify inspired air temperature and
humidity, effect on
exercise-induced asthma, 93: 288
Massage
in delayed onset muscle soreness,
creatine kinase and neutrophil
count, 95: 263
Mast cell
activation not associated with
exercise-induced asthma, 93: 284
McMurray test
evaluation, 94: 104
Meal
standardized, and exercise-induced
myocardial ischemia threshold in
stable angina, 94: 432
Medical
considerations, in short distance road
races, 95: 490
disability, permanent, in intercollegiate
gymnastics of women, 94: 12
insurance practices, athletic, at NCAA
division I institutions, 95: 1
Medicine
environmental, 94: 361
sports (*see* Sports medicine)
Menarche
age at, dietary fat and sports activity as
determinants for, 94: 265
Meniscectomy

Y

Author Index